Essentials of
Ophthalmic Lens
Finishing

Essentials of Ophthalmic Lens Finishing

SECOND EDITION

Clifford W. Brooks, OD
Associate Professor of Optometry
Indiana University School of Optometry
Bloomington, Indiana

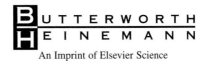

An Imprint of Elsevier Science

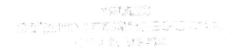

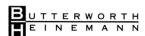

An Imprint of Elsevier Science

11830 Westline Industrial Drive
St. Louis, Missouri 63146

ESSENTIALS OF OPHTHALMIC LENS FINISHING   0-7506-7213-7
Copyright © 2003, Elsevier Science (USA). All rights reserved.

NOTICE

Optometry is an ever-changing field. Standard safety precautions must be followed, but as new research and clinical experience broaden our knowledge, changes in treatment and drug therapy may become necessary or appropriate. Readers are advised to check the most current product information provided by the manufacturer of each drug to be administered to verify the recommended dose, the method and duration of administration, and contraindications. It is the responsibility of the licensed physician, relying on experience and knowledge of the patient, to determine dosages and the best treatment for each individual patient. Neither the publisher nor the author assumes any liability for any injury and/or damage to persons or property arising from this publication.

Previous editions copyrighted 1983.

International Standard Book Number 0-7506-7213-7

Publishing Director: Linda Duncan
Managing Editor: Christie M. Hart
Publishing Services Manager: Linda McKinley
Project Managers: Kristin Hebberd, Julie Eddy
Designer: Julia Dummitt

Printed in the United States of America

Last digit is the print number: 9 8 7 6 5 4 3 2 1

To Him who by wisdom founded the earth;
And by understanding established the heavens.
Proverbs 3:19

Acknowledgments

I would like to thank Ginger Long, Antonio Turner, and Glenn Herringshaw, who have helped considerably in the preparation of the second edition of this book. They also have been a valuable part of both the operation of and education at the optical laboratory at Indiana University.

Ginger Long reviewed the manuscript while it was used in the course on lense finishing. She was helpful in pointing out mistakes and ambiguities in the questions at the back of each chapter. Students were assigned problems and Ginger graded them. (They did not have the answers now found in the back of the book!) Ginger also helped with many of the photos and made suggestions on how to convey certain ideas.

Thanks to Antonio Turner for the help he provided with the photographs in Chapter 13, Drilled, Slotted, and Notched Mountings. He supplied a number of beneficial ideas and his hands are the hands seen in a majority of the photos in that chapter.

I am especially grateful to Glenn Herringshaw, Indiana University's Optical Laboratory Manager, for the valuable help he has given. Glenn carefully reviewed each chapter. When he discovered deficiencies, we worked together to figure out how to overcome them. A number of procedures outlined in the text were a result of his suggestions. Glenn helped in photography and also carefully examined each drawing and pointed out needed improvements. When something did not seem right, Glenn was the first one I would call to discuss the issue. He is optically knowledgeable and equally skilled in the practicalities of optical lens finishing.

Dan Torgersen, OLA (Optical Laboratories Association) Technical Director, was a valuable resource for questions on safety and impact resistance issues. His responses were always thorough and well thought out.

I also appreciate Joe Bruneni's help in answering a spectrum of questions on a number of topics. Joe is a valuable resource for the whole optical industry and much appreciated by all.

And again, as with the first edition, I would like to thank my wife, Vickie, and my children, Debbie, Cliff, Abigail, and Kenneth, for their support and encouragement.

Contents

CHAPTER 1
An Overview of the Fabrication Process, 1

The Optical Laboratory, 1
Finished and Semifinished Lens
    Terminology, 2
Overview of the Lens Finishing Process, 4

CHAPTER 2
Spotting of Lenses, 8

Selecting the Most Appropriate Lens Blank, 9
Using the Lensmeter, 11
Spotting Lenses without Prism, 16
A Lens Prescription that Includes Prism, 18
Spotting Lenses with Prism, 20
Spotting with Autolensmeters, 21
Making the Most of a Blemished Lens, 27
Spotting of Polarizing Lenses, 28
Prescription Verification and Spotting of
    Multifocal Lenses, 29
Progressive Addition Lenses, 32

CHAPTER 3
Lens Shapes, Patterns, and Frame Tracers, 39

The Boxing System of Lens Measurement, 39
Pattern Measurements and Terminology, 44
Positioning the Mechanical Center in the
    Pattern, 50
Pattern Making, 52
Consequences of Using a Noncentered
    Pattern, 57
Pattern Makers that Can Find the Center and
    Decenter, 62
Placing the Pattern on the Edger, 62
Using a Frame Tracer for Patternless Systems
    of Edging, 62

CHAPTER 4
Centration of Single Vision Lenses, 75

Purpose of Centering, 75
Mechanics of Lens Centration, 75
Calculating Horizontal Decentration Using
    the Boxing System, 75

Historical Background, 76
Calculating Vertical Centration of Lenses
    Using the Boxing System, 78
Ensuring Proper Size of the Lens Blank, 83

CHAPTER 5
Centration of Progressive Addition Lenses, 97

Two Major Categories, 97
Progressive Addition Lens, 98
Specialty Progressive Addition Lenses, 105

CHAPTER 6
Centration of Segmented Multifocal Lenses, 112

Segmented Multifocals, 112
Flat-Top Multifocals, 114
Catching Errors before the Lens is Edged, 117
Curve-Top Segment Lenses, 125
Round-Segment Lenses, 126
Blended Bifocals, 129
Franklin-Style Multifocals, 131
Double-Segment Lenses, 131

CHAPTER 7
Blocking of Lenses, 138

Types of Blocking, 138
Pressure Blocking, 138
Blocking with Suction, 139
Metal Alloy Blocking, 139
Precast FreeBlock Blocking, 139
Adhesive Pad Blocking, 140
Lensmeter/Blockers, 146

CHAPTER 8
Edging, 149

Patterned and Patternless Edging, 149
Historical Background, 149
Cutting and Chipping, 150
Automatic Edging with Ceramic Wheels, 151
Edging Process, 152
Variations in Edging Lenses of Different
    Materials, 167
Special Edging Situations, 170

Electronic Shape, 172
Patternless Possibilities, 172

CHAPTER 9
Deblocking, 185

Deblocking Lenses Blocked by Suction, 185
Deblocking Metal Alloy—Blocked Lenses, 185
Deblocking 'Wax'-Blocked Lenses, 186
Deblocking Adhesive Pad–Blocked Lenses, 186

CHAPTER 10
Hand Edging, 190

Rationale for Hand Edging, 190
Types of Hand Edgers, 190
Two Parts to Hand Edging, 192
Edge Smoothing, 192
Basic Rules for Better Results, 194
Pin Beveling, 197
Reducing Lens Size by Hand, 199
Re-edging a Lens for a Different Frame, 202
Changing a Frame's Lens Shape, 203
Correctional Modifications, 205
Edge Polishing, 206
Cleaning Lenses, 208

CHAPTER 11
Lens Tinting, 212

How the Process Works, 212
Ensuring Accuracy of Transmission and
   Color, 217
Styles of Tints, 220
Ultraviolet Dyeing, 225
Effects of Lens Material and Lens Coating on
   the Dyeing Process, 226
Powering Down, Cleaning Up, and Reducing
   Smells, 228
Troubleshooting, 229

CHAPTER 12
Lens Insertion and Standard Alignment, 235

Seeing the Full Picture, 235
Inserting Lenses into Metal Frames, 239
Standard Alignment of Plastic Frames, 239
Standard Alignment of Metal Frames, 243

CHAPTER 13
Drilled, Slotted, and Notched Mountings, 247

Rimless Defined, 247
Types of Lens Drills, 249
Wearer Safety Issues, 249

Edge Thickness for Rimless Lenses, 250
Marking and Drilling the Lens, 251
Notching Lenses, 257
Improvements in Electric Drills, 260
Slotted Lenses, 263
Working with Older-Style, Double-Strap
   Mountings, 266

CHAPTER 14
Nylon Cord and Other Groove Mountings, 276

Wearer Safety Issues, 276
Edge Thickness for Grooving, 277
Grooving Methods, 277
Lens Grooving Method, 278
Grooving in the Edger, 286
Mounting a Grooved Lens, 286

CHAPTER 15
Lens Impact Resistance and Testing, 292

General Eyewear Categories, 292
Requirements for Dress Eyewear, 292
'Duty to Inform,' 296
Safety Eyewear, 298
Impact Requirements for Safety Eyewear, 298
Basic-Impact Requirements for Safety
   Eyewear, 298
High-Impact Requirements for Safety
   Eyewear, 300
Safety Frames, 301
Hardening Glass Lenses, 303
Sports Eyewear, 305

CHAPTER 16
Maintenance and Calibration, 309

Maintenance Schedules, 309
Care of the Lensmeter, 310
Centration Blockers, 311
Calibration of Edgers, 313
Cleaning and Lubricating Edgers, 316
Edger Coolants, 317

CHAPTER 17
Edger Wheels and Cutters, 320

Four Construction Factors, 320
Dressing Diamond Wheels, 322

CHAPTER 18
Safety and Environmental Concerns, 329

Occupational Safety and Health
   Administration, 330

Environmental Protection Agency, 330
Agencies Overseeing OSHA
    Requirements, 330
An Employer's Responsibility under
    OSHA, 330
The Chemical Hazard Communication
    Standard, 331
An Effective Safety Program, 334
Environmental Concerns, 339
Additional Information, 341

APPENDIX 18-1
*What Are My Responsibilities under the
OSHA Act? 344*

APPENDIX 18-2
Sample Hazard Communication Program, 345

Sample Hazard Communication
    Program (B), 345
Our Hazard Communication Program, 345

APPENDIX 18-3
*List of Hazardous Chemicals and Index of
MSDSs, 348*

APPENDIX 18-4
Material Safety Data Sheet, 349

APPENDIX A
Standards of Lens and Frame Measurement, 351

APPENDIX B
*ANSI Z80.1 Prescription Opthalmic
Lenses—Recommendations, 355*

APPENDIX C
FDA Policy, 361

ANSWER KEY FOR PROFICIENCY TEST QUESTIONS, 365

GLOSSARY, 369

CENTRATION SKILLS SERIES, 389

Essentials of
Ophthalmic Lens
Finishing

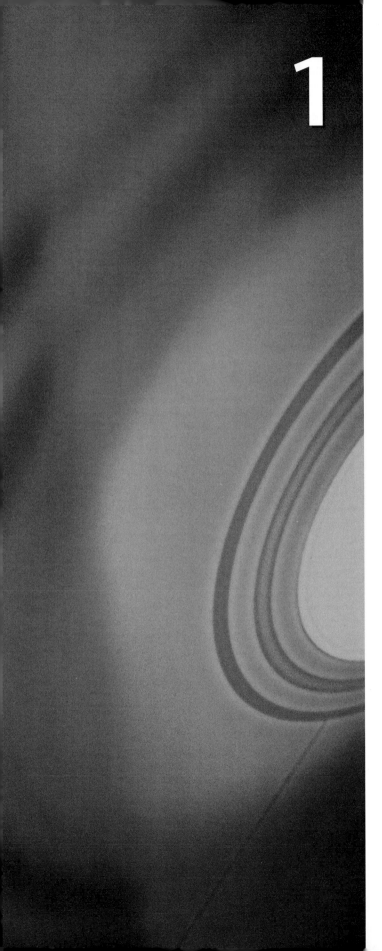

1

An Overview of the Fabrication Process

The Optical Laboratory

When someone needs glasses, the first requirement is an eye examination in the doctor's office to determine the correct lens prescription. The next step takes place in the optical dispensary, where a frame is chosen. The frame should be one that is cosmetically pleasing and appropriate for the type and power of lenses needed. In the dispensary, measurements are taken to ensure the lens will be correctly placed for the location of the eyes, the style of lens chosen, and occupation or avocation of the wearer. Once these are completed, the frame and lens requirements are sent to the optical laboratory.

The optical laboratory may be located in close proximity to the dispensary or halfway across the county. All operations of the optical laboratory may be carried out in one facility, or they may be divided among laboratories. Traditionally the optical laboratory consists of two main areas, a surfacing laboratory and a finishing laboratory.

SURFACING AND FINISHING LABORATORIES

As stated previously, an optical laboratory may consist of two separate areas. One area creates the needed lens power, usually by a process called *lens surfacing*, which is performed at a facility referred to as a *surfacing laboratory*.

The second area takes the correctly powered lens and finishes it. Finishing is accomplished through optical positioning of the lens and grinding of the edges so that the lens fits the shape of the chosen

1

frame. The area where this occurs is known as the *finishing laboratory*. A finishing laboratory is also referred to as an *edging laboratory* because here the lenses are "edged" to the proper shape to fit the spectacle frame.

A great deal more happens in the lens finishing process than just lens edging. This text focuses primarily on the finishing aspect of lens fabrication.

An edging laboratory does not require a surfacing laboratory to function. Most facilities that have a surfacing laboratory also have a finishing laboratory. However, the finishing laboratory has versatility. It may be associated closely with a surfacing laboratory, or it may function independently. Figure 1-1 is an overview of how lenses are processed in the optical laboratory.

Finished and Semifinished Lens Terminology

Ophthalmic lenses may be divided into the following three broad categories:

- Single vision lenses
- Segmented multifocal lenses
- Progressive addition lenses

SINGLE VISION LENSES

Single vision lenses are the most basic type of lens. These lenses have the same power over the entire surface of the lens. Single vision lenses are used when the same optical power is needed for both distance and near vision. They also are used when a person requires no prescription for distance but needs reading glasses. Whenever possible, single vision lenses are edged from lenses kept in stock at the finishing laboratory. Because these lenses are finished optically to the correct power on both the front and back surfaces, they are called *finished lenses*. Finished lenses are also referred to as *uncuts* because they have not yet been "cut" to the correct shape and size (Figure 1-2, *A*). When single vision lenses are in uncut form and do not require surfacing, they are called *stock single vision lenses*.

The finishing laboratory personnel would much prefer to use a stock single vision uncut lens because it is less expensive than a custom surfaced lens. However, if the stock lens is too small for the frame, then a stock single vision lens will not work. Instead the lens must be produced in the surfacing laboratory. The surfacing laboratory starts with a lens having only one surface that is ready to use, or "finished." This is usually the front surface. The laboratory must grind and polish the second surface to the required power. A lens with only one of the two surfaces finished is called a *semifinished lens* because it is only half finished. The prefix *semi-* means half (Figure 1-2, *B*).

Finished uncut and semifinished lenses have not been edged. Before a lens has been edged it is called a *lens blank*.

SEGMENTED MULTIFOCAL LENSES

Segmented multifocal lenses have more than one power. Each power is located in a distinct area of the lens bordered clearly by a visible demarcation line. When two different areas exist, the lens is called a *bifocal* (Figure 1-3, *A*). When three areas exist, the lens is called a *trifocal* (Figure 1-3, *B*).

Multifocal lenses may be made ready for the finishing laboratory in one of several ways:

- **Multifocals may be individually ground and polished to power** by a surfacing laboratory from a semifinished lens blank.
- **Multifocals may be individually cast molded to the prescribed power,** instead of being surfaced from a semifinished lens blank. Cast molding creates the lens from a liquid resin material. It is the same process used to make both plastic semifinished lenses and stock single vision plastic lenses. Cast molding multifocal lenses to power skips the semifinished lens stage. Cast molding to power may be done by a larger wholesale facility or, if equipment is available, in conjunction with a finishing laboratory (Figure 1-4).
- **Multifocals may be made by laminating front and back lens halves together.** In simple terms, the front half of the lens contains the multifocal segment and the back half contains the power. The two are glued together to make one complete lens. This lamination process also skips the semifinished lens stage. It does not require a lot of equipment and, like cast molding, may be carried out at the finishing laboratory (Figure 1-5).
- **Multifocals may be kept as stock, finished bifocals** in the finishing laboratory. This option is possible only if the lens power is spherical. At present, stock, finished bifocals are not often used.[1]

---

[1]Instead of being custom made, stock, finished bifocals may be mass produced with both inside and outside surfaces already ground and polished. Stock, finished bifocals are normally used only when both left and right eyes are spherical in power. Attempting to match one spherocylinder lens from a surfacing laboratory with a prefinished bifocal from another source may create unnecessary problems and mismatches. To prevent optical errors, the exact vertical position of the optical center of the stock, finished bifocal in relationship to the near segment must be known. This position must be duplicated accurately in the custom-surfaced, paired spherocylinder lens.

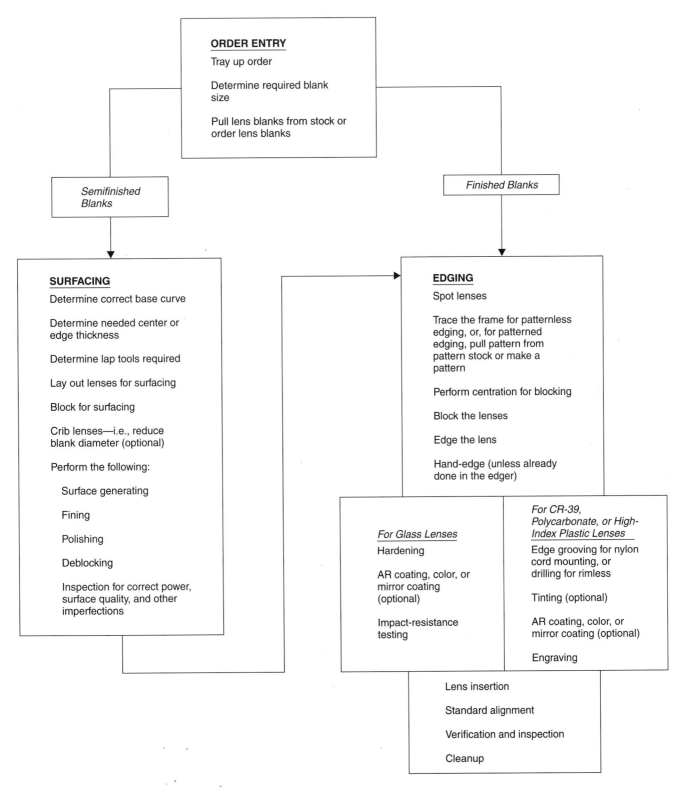

FIGURE **1-1** The processes listed on the right-hand side in the main column sequence may be performed in the finishing laboratory. The processes in the left-hand "loop" are functions of the surfacing laboratory.

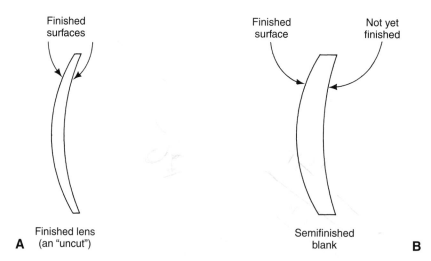

FIGURE **1-2**   **A,** A finished lens is also referred to as an *uncut*. Most single vision lenses are premanufactured to power as finished lenses and are also referred to as *stock single vision lenses*. **B,** Most any type of lens of any material may be made beginning with a semifinished lens. (From Brooks CW: *Understanding lens surfacing,* Boston, 1992, Butterworth-Heinemann, p 17.)

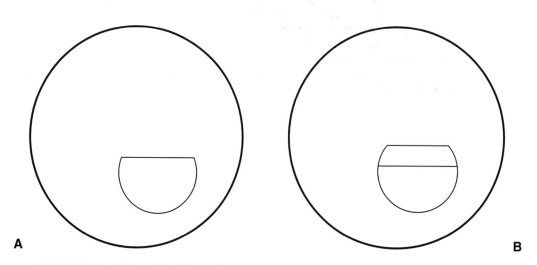

FIGURE **1-3**   When a lens has a different power for near vision than distance vision, the lens area is divided between distance and near powers. **A,** A segment area for near vision is placed within the distance power lens. A lens with two different powers is a bifocal lens. **B,** Two segment areas are included: one for intermediate viewing and one for near viewing. This type of lens is a trifocal lens. Both lenses are flat-top–style multifocals.

PROGRESSIVE ADDITION LENSES

Progressive addition lenses are used as an alternative to a segmented multifocal lens. They have distance power in the upper half of the lens. Lens power gradually increases as the wearer looks down and inward to view near objects.

Progressive addition lenses are prepared for the finishing laboratory in the same way as segmented lenses. These are listed in the previous section.

Overview of the Lens Finishing Process

Edging often is used to denote the entire lens finishing process. In actuality, many steps come before and after the actual edging process. These are outlined in the following section and described in more detail in later chapters.

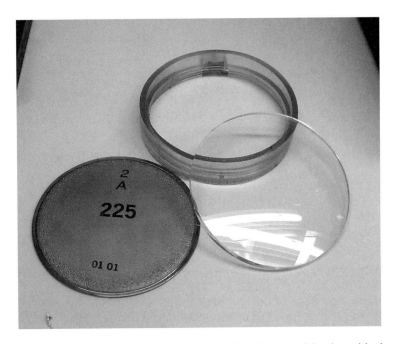

FIGURE **1-4** Cast molding of lenses is done with a front and back mold placed in a gasket to hold the surface molds. The front mold is shown on the left and the back mold on the right. The gasket is at the top. For multifocal lenses, the back mold is rotated so that the prescribed cylinder axis will be correct. Once assembled, liquid resin is poured into the molds to form the lens. The front surface mold may contain a near add power area. This area of different surface curvature turns the lens into a multifocal such as a bifocal or progressive addition lens. The back surface includes cylinder power for astigmatism, when needed.

SELECTION OF THE MOST APPROPRIATE LENS BLANK

Within limitations set by the lens order, a laboratory has the responsibility of choosing a lens blank that gives the best cosmetic and optical results. This is especially important for plus lenses. An inappropriately large plus lens blank creates unneeded lens center and edge thickness. This is explained in more detail in Chapter 2.

SPOTTING THE LENS

A lens-measuring device is needed to determine lens power, optical center location, and other optical characteristics of a lens. It may be referred to as a *lensometer, lensmeter, focimeter, vertometer,* or *lens analyzer,* depending upon the manufacturer. In this text the author uses the more generic term *lensmeter.* The lensmeter precisely determines lens power and exactly locates optical points within the lens. The process of finding these optical points, orienting the lens properly to meet the needs of the prescription, and then placing dots on the lens is referred to as *spotting.* It takes its name from the three horizontally aligned ink "spots"

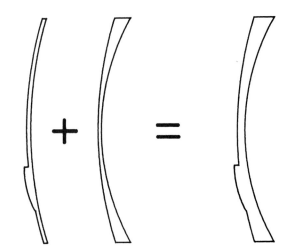

FIGURE **1-5** Another alternative to the lens surfacing process is to create the needed power using a front and a back half. The front half contains the near add power, when needed. The back half completes the distance power and contains any needed cylinder power. The two halves are glued together to create the lens. (From Brooks CW: *Understanding lens surfacing,* Boston, 1992, Butterworth-Heinemann, p 299.)

placed on the lens surface by the lensmeter. See Chapter 2 for a complete discussion of spotting.

CENTRATION AND BLOCKING OF THE LENS

Because the pupil of the eye is seldom found to be directly on line with the middle of the frame's lens opening, the lens must be moved to correspond to the location of the eye. Because the lens is to be centered in front of the eye, this next process is called *centration*. Centration is done by use of the three reference dots that were placed on the lens during spotting. Once the lens has been positioned, a small block is secured to the lens so that it may be edged. Securing the block to the lens is called *blocking*.

Taken together, spotting and centration make up *lens layout*. The instrument used to center and block the lens is called a *layout blocker* or simply a *blocker*.

DETERMINATION OF LENS SHAPE

Before a lens may be cut to the proper shape for the frame, the needed shape must be quantified. Two types of edgers exist—one that uses an actual plastic pattern to guide it in shaping the lens and another that uses an electronic method to supply lens shape. Following are more detailed explanations of both types:

- The first is called a *patterned edger*. A patterned edger operates using a small, flat piece of plastic that matches the lens shape needed for the frame. This pattern itself is either supplied by the frame manufacturer or is made by the laboratory using a *pattern maker*.
- The second type of edger is called a *patternless edger*. It does not use a physical pattern but uses an electronic shape generated from the frame itself by way of a *frame tracer*. The tracer makes an electronic version of the shape needed and downloads it to the edger.

Some edgers operate in both patterned and patternless modes.

EDGING THE LENS

The blocked lens is now placed in the edger and the lens is edged to shape.

DEBLOCKING, TINTING, COATING, ENGRAVING, AND HARDENING

Once the lens is edged to the proper shape and size for the frame, it is taken off the block. The process of block removal is called *deblocking*. Before the lens is placed in the frame, several other possible procedures may be carried out. If the lens is ordered with a specific color and is plastic, it may be *tinted*. Tinting may be performed with hot dyes or by use of a vacuum coating process. Depending on ever-changing fashion, a lens could be decorated with an engraving.

If the lens is glass, it must be treated to increase impact resistance. This hardening process may be done by *heat treating* or *chemical tempering* the lens. Both glass and plastic lenses may be antireflection (AR) coated to reduce surface reflections.

LENS INSERTION OR MOUNTING

The edge of the lens may be angled to a point to allow insertion into a frame with a groove. Lens edges that are angled to a point are called *beveled* lenses. The process of putting beveled lenses in a frame is *lens insertion*.

Alternatively a lens may be held in the frame with a nylon cord, with screws, or by methods closely related to these. If a nylon cord is used, the edge of the lens must be grooved to accept the nylon cord. Some edgers groove the lens during the edging process. If the lens is not grooved in the edger, the edge is made flat. Then a groove is cut into the edge on a separate *lens groover*.

If a lens is to be held in place with screws, the edge is made flat without a bevel. Holes then are drilled in the lens to accept the screws. When lenses are grooved or drilled, the process of placing them in the frame is called *mounting*. (Frames that secure the lenses in place in this manner often are called *mountings* instead of frames.)

STANDARD ALIGNMENT

After the lenses have been placed in the frame, the glasses may not be aligned properly. The process by which the glasses are bent or readjusted to conform to a proper alignment is known as *standard alignment* or *truing*.

VERIFICATION AND CLEANUP

Before a prescription is released to the dispensary, it needs to be verified for accuracy. This is done using the same instrument as was used during lens spotting—the lensmeter. The prescription must optically conform to accepted standards of tolerance. Once judged acceptable, the frames and lenses are cleaned and passed on to the dispensary.

Proficiency Test Questions

1. True or False? Lenses are surfaced in a finishing laboratory.

2. Which of the following lens types has the same power over the entire lens?

   a. A single vision lens
   b. A segmented multifocal lens
   c. A progressive addition lens

3. Which of the following terms is a synonym for a "finished lens"?

   a. Single vision lens
   b. Semifinished lens
   c. Uncut lens
   d. Progressive addition lens
   e. Multifocal lens

4. True or False? It is possible to individually cast mold both segmented multifocal lenses and progressive addition lenses to the prescribed power without surfacing the lens.

5. True or False? Some edgers operate in both patterned and patternless modes.

6. A "frame tracer" is often used in conjunction with which of the following?

   a. Lensmeter
   b. Lens blocker
   c. Lens edger

7. Of the following steps in lens fabrication, which process occurs last?

   a. Blocking
   b. Grooving
   c. Edging
   d. Spotting

8. Arrange the steps in the edging process in their correct order.

   1. blocking
   2. centration
   3. edging
   4. finding lens axis and MRP location

   a. 2, 3, 1, 4
   b. 2, 4, 1, 3
   c. 1, 2, 3, 4
   d. 4, 2, 1, 3
   e. 4, 3, 2, 1

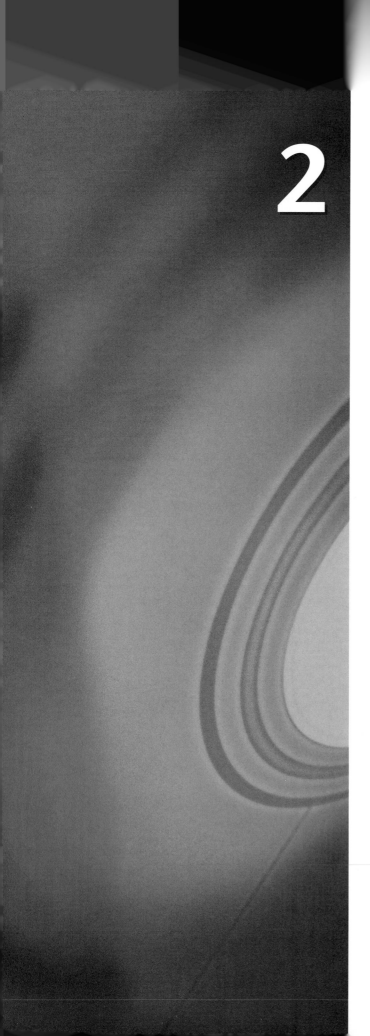

2 Spotting of Lenses

For optical laboratory personnel, the simplest type of lens to work with is the single vision lens. A single vision lens has the same power over the entire lens. Because it is a basic lens, it is usually purchased from a lens manufacturer and kept in stock until needed. Most single vision lenses do not have to be surfaced before edging. As mentioned in Chapter 1, this type of lens may be referred to as a *stock* lens. Stated another way, a stock lens is a ready-made lens with both surfaces already formed.

Once the needed lens is in hand, it must be spotted. To *spot* a lens the practitioner takes a lens and uses a lensmeter to position the lens optically and then places reference dots on the lens for blocking. Following are the steps leading up to and including the actual spotting of the lens:

1. The practitioner decides whether a stock (ready-made) lens is the most appropriate lens.
2. If a stock lens is appropriate, the lens is selected from stock by material (including tint and coating, if applicable), size, and power. If a stock lens is not appropriate, the lens must be obtained from the surfacing laboratory.
3. The lens is inspected visually to be certain it is free from flaws.
4. A lensmeter is used to verify that the lens really is the power needed.
5. The lens is oriented in the lensmeter so that it matches the written prescription.
6. The lens is spotted so that it may be properly blocked for edging.

Selecting the Most Appropriate Lens Blank

A lens either is "pulled" from available stock or must be obtained from a surfacing laboratory. A stock lens is appropriate if it fits the following criteria:

1. Fulfills all the optical requirements of the written prescription
2. Is big enough to cover the frame's lens opening
3. Is appropriately thin for the lens material and frame type[1] and size selected

SELECTING THE MOST APPROPRIATE LENS

In the decision as to whether a stock lens is the most appropriate lens, the first question concerns availability. Is the lens in stock in the finishing laboratory? If not, is it made as a stock lens? It may be appropriate to order a stock lens instead of having one surfaced. However, even if a stock lens is available in the right material and power, it may or may not be used. Stock lenses may or may not work if any of the following are true:

- The prescription requires prescribed prism.
- The lens blank is too small for the frame.
- A plus lens blank is larger than needed, resulting in an unnecessarily thick center and edge.

Size of the Lens

If a lens is too small and gets edged anyway, a gap will exist between the lens and the edge of the frame, making the lens unsuitable (Figure 2-1). Several ways exist to determine whether the lens blank will be large enough.

A blank size determiner may be used in combination with the frame. Another method is to use the following formula:

$$MBS = ED + 2(dec.) + 2$$

where:

MBS = Minimum blank size
ED = Effective diameter of the frame
(dec.) = Decentration per lens

---

[1]For grooved mountings, the lens edge must not end up too thin for grooving. For more information on this, see Chapter 14 on grooved-lens mountings.

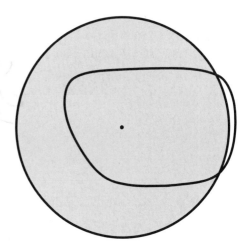

FIGURE **2-1** A lens blank is too small if, when properly decentered, it will not cover the lens opening of the frame.

(The exact use of this formula and the concept of minimum blank size is explained in Chapter 4.)

Minus Lens Center Thickness

Lenses come in both plus and minus powers. Minus lenses are thinnest in the center and get progressively thicker toward the edge. Therefore the final size of a minus lens does not affect center thickness of the lens. Figure 2-2 shows that regardless of whether the lens blank chosen was large or small, edged minus lenses have exactly the same center and edge thickness.

Even though center thickness for minus lenses remains the same if the lens gets larger, edge thickness does increase with increasing lens sizes.

Effect of Blank Size in Plus Lenses

With minus lenses, *edge* thickness increases with lens size. With plus lenses, *center* thickness increases with lens size. The larger the plus lens, the greater the center thickness will be (Figure 2-3).

Unnecessary use of large plus lens blanks results in thick centers, thick edges, glasses that magnify the wearer's eyes, and heavier lenses. Using a smaller lens blank when the frame size is small is much better. Sometimes no stock lens is small enough, and the lens should be ordered from the surfacing laboratory. By knowing the size and shape of the frame and the distance between the centers of the wearer's pupils, the surfacing laboratory personnel are able to grind the lens so that the center and edge thicknesses are minimal.

The worst-looking examples of inappropriately used plus stock lenses are for small children's frames. Using

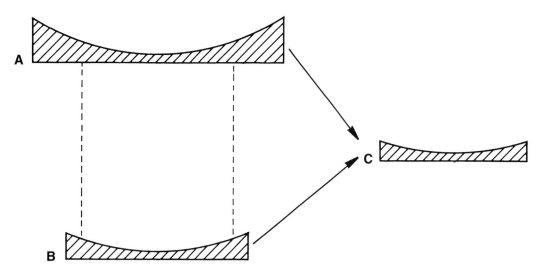

FIGURE **2-2** Whether a large uncut minus lens blank *(A)* or a small uncut lens blank *(B)* is used, the resulting edged lens is exactly the same *(C)*. Dotted lines show the diameter being cut to produce lens C.

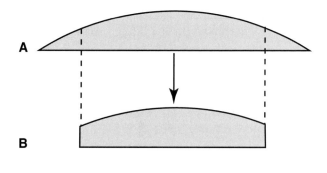

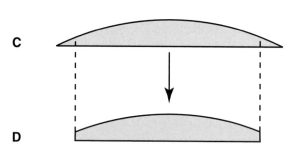

FIGURE **2-3** Lens blank A and lens blank C both have the same plus power. When a larger-than-necessary plus lens blank is used *(A)*, the result is a lens that is too thick in both center and edge *(B)*. When the smallest possible blank is chosen *(C)*, a much better functional and cosmetic result is obtained *(D)*. Dotted lines indicate the diameter being cut from the blank to produce the finished lens.

a large stock lens results in extremely thick edges that are entirely unnecessary. The lenses are much thicker than they need to be, and the size of the child's eyes is magnified. For plus lenses, magnification increases as center thickness increases.

VISUAL INSPECTION OF THE LENS FOR FLAWS

Before edging, the lens should be checked to ensure it is free from flaws. A scratched lens may have the correct power but still be unacceptable. Once a lens has been edged, it is too late to return it to the manufacturer because of a flaw, whether it is a stock or custom surfaced lens. During inspection of an uncut lens for flaws, its front surface quality, back surface quality, and internal lens characteristics are checked.

One method used to inspect surface quality is by use of an unfrosted incandescent bulb. The lens is held as if it were a mirror (Figures 2-4 and 2-5). It is tilted so that all areas of the lens surface are inspected. The image of the light bulb filament must be sharp and clear on all areas of the lens surface. The lens is then turned over and the second surface is inspected in a similar manner.

Internal lens properties may be checked by looking at the lens with a dark background and a light such as a 40-watt, incandescent clear (unfrosted) bulb positioned about 12 inches from the lens, striking it at an angle from behind (Figures 2-6 and 2-7). Any foreign substance in or on the lens scatters the light and causes the area of the foreign substance to be visible.

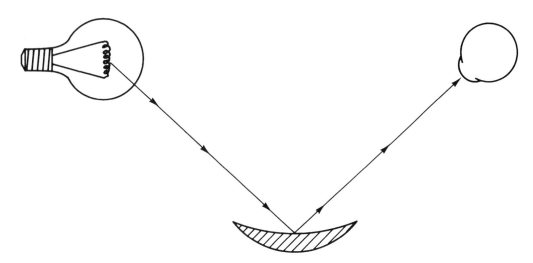

FIGURE **2-4** When the lens is held such that its surface acts as a mirror, surface irregularities cause the reflected unfrosted light bulb's filament image to appear irregularly distorted.

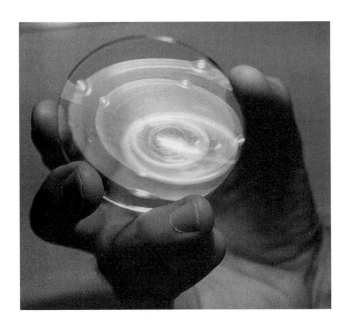

FIGURE **2-5** To inspect the entire surface rapidly, the inspector looks at the bulb filament and tilts the lens slightly.

Assuming that the lens is free of surface deficiencies or internal foreign matter, it may be checked for irregular power variations at this point. This check involves observation of a straight line, such as the edge of a fluorescent tube through the lens. If the straight edge is vertical, the lens is moved left and right along one of its major meridians (Figure 2-8).[2] If the lens has any refractive power, the line observed through the lens

---
[2]The major meridians of a lens are along the cylinder axis and 90 degrees from the axis.

will appear to curve as the lens is moved (Figure 2-9). It should curve evenly. Unevenness in the curve indicates a power variation within the lens. Possible causes of unevenness are a wavy surface or nonuniformity of refractive index within the lens material. A wavy surface usually results from a surfacing problem and is less likely to occur in a quality stock lens.

Using the Lensmeter

The power of a lens may be measured using a lensmeter. A lensmeter also may be called a *lensometer, focimeter, vertometer,* and *vertexometer.* For clarity, the author of this book uses the word *lensmeter* when referring to any of these instrument types. Lensmeters may be manual or automated.

When the power of a lens is measured using a lensmeter, many people refer to the process as *neutralizing* the lens because the instrument is adjusted until the lens system within the lensmeter cancels out, or neutralizes, the power of the lens. For manual lensmeters, this brings the illuminated internal target in focus.

Lenses may be measured for power with the lensmeter before they are edged or after they have been mounted in the frame. The following explanation begins with lenses already edged and mounted in the frame.

FOCUSING THE EYEPIECE

Before attempting to read the power of a lens using a conventional manual lensmeter, the practitioner must first focus the eyepiece. An eyepiece that is not focused for the individual may cause an inaccurate reading.

Dark background

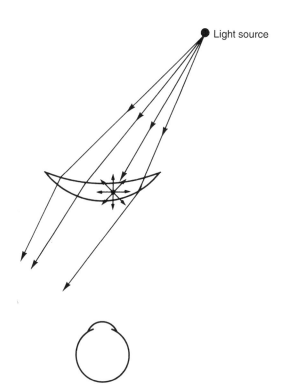

FIGURE **2-6**   A defect within the lens causes a scattering of light. By positioning the light source off to the side and viewing the lens against a matte black background, the main body of a clean, unblemished lens almost will disappear. Any defect becomes easily visible. Inspectors wearing white gloves for factory quality control use this method.

The lensmeter is focused by first turning the eyepiece outward. The practitioner looks into the instrument and rotates the eyepiece slowly inward until the crosshairs and rings within the instrument appear to *first* focus. The eyepiece location should be noted for future reference because it varies from individual to individual (Figure 2-10). When more than one person uses the same lensmeter, it may be helpful to put a colored mark on the eyepiece. Each person has a different color and will be able to quickly turn the eyepiece back to this colored mark each time.

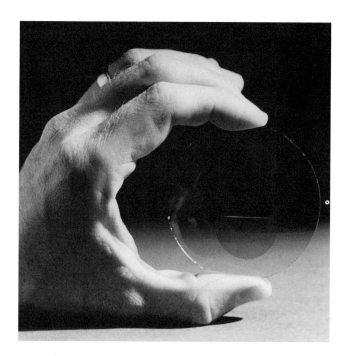

FIGURE **2-7**   A lens is inspected in oblique illumination against a matte black background.

READING A LENS IN MINUS CYLINDER FORM

Lenses with a cylinder component may be written with that cylinder as a plus cylinder or as a minus cylinder. When written with a plus cylinder, the prescription is said to be written in *plus cylinder form*. When written with a minus cylinder, the prescription is in *minus cylinder form*.

To read the power of a lens with a lensmeter such that the prescription may be written directly in minus cylinder form, the lens is placed in the instrument and the power wheel turned to high plus (Figure 2-11). Looking through the eyepiece, the practitioner turns the power wheel slowly in the minus direction until the target within the instrument begins to focus.

The target consists of two sets of lines that run at right angles to each other, forming a cross. One set is a narrowly spaced set of lines (Figure 2-12). (Older instruments have a single line.) This set of lines is known as the *sphere lines*. The set at right angles is a broadly spaced triple set (Figure 2-13). These lines are referred to as the *cylinder lines*.

As the power wheel is being turned in the minus direction, one of the following two things will happen:

1. Both sets of lines will focus simultaneously, indicating that the lens is spherical (Figure 2-14).
2. One set of lines will begin to focus before the other, meaning that a cylinder component is present.

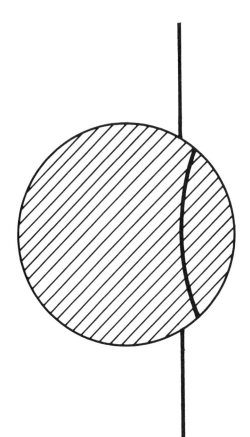

FIGURE **2-8** Lenses free from waviness (caused by either poor surface manufacture or an irregularity in the refractive index of the material) display a uniformly curved image of the straight edge as the lens is moved to either side. This is caused by the refractive characteristics of the lens. Defects discovered in this manner also may be evident through the lensmeter. The lens is moved while the focused target is viewed through the instrument. Defective areas in the lens cause degradation in target clarity.

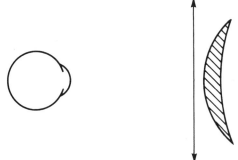

FIGURE **2-9** In this view, the operator checks for waviness by moving the lens left and right and observing a vertical straight edge. The distance between the straight edge and lens must vary depending on lens power.

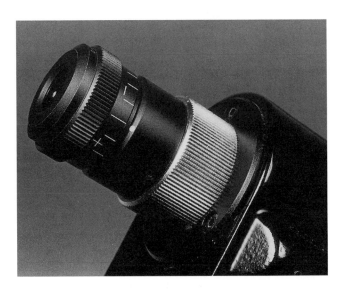

FIGURE **2-10** The lensmeter eyepiece is set for zero. Turning the eyepiece outward adds plus power to the eyepiece; turning inward adds minus power. For practitioners who themselves have only a small spherical eyeglass correction and wish to use the instrument without their glasses, the instrument permits this versatility. The eyepiece should, in any case, be adjusted for the most plus power through which the mires can be seen sharply.

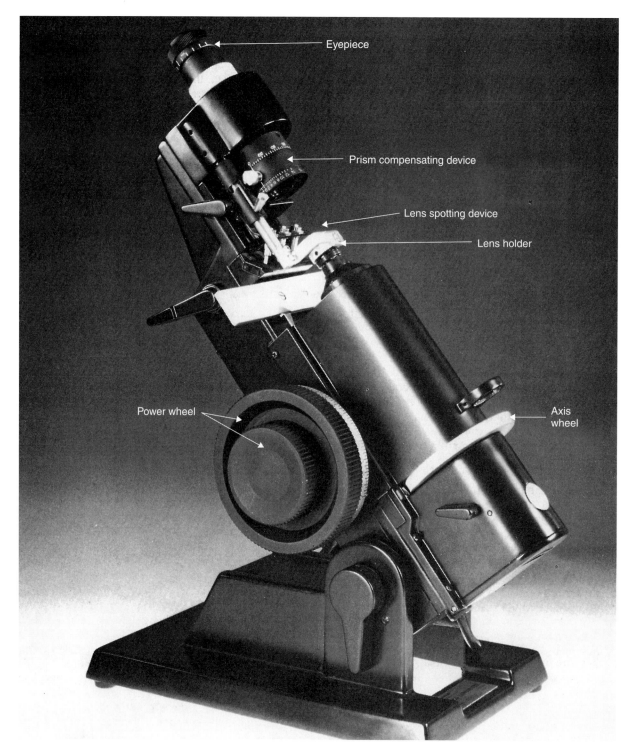

FIGURE **2-11**   Available through a variety of sources, the basic lens measuring instrument is a necessary part of every optically related profession. (Courtesy Marco, Jacksonville, Fla.)

Spherical Lens

In the event that the prescription is spherical, all lines—sphere line and cylinder line sets—come into focus at once. In this case the refractive power is read directly from the power wheel.

Spherocylinder Lens

For a lens with cylinder power the procedure begins the same. The power wheel is turned into the high plus powers and slowly turned back in a minus direction. However, this time the sphere lines may not come

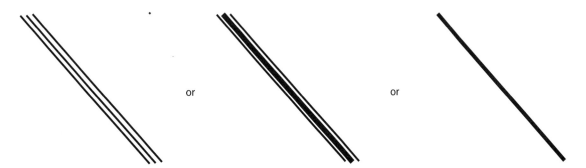

FIGURE **2-12** The exact configuration of the sphere line(s) varies from instrument to instrument. (Some instruments do not use lines at all, but rather a circle of dots that elongate into a circle of short lines when cylinder power is present in the lens.)

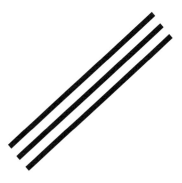

FIGURE **2-13** Cylinder lines appear at right angles to the sphere lines and are usually visible simultaneously, except in the case of extremely high cylinder values. (Instruments using a circle of dots will show elongation of the dots 90 degrees from the original direction of elongation. The original direction of elongation was seen first when the target was viewed for the correct sphere power.)

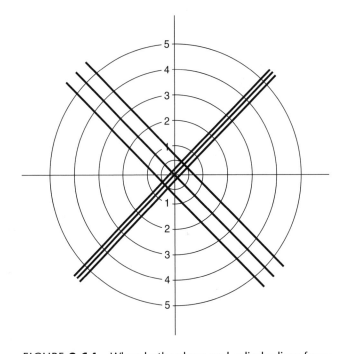

FIGURE **2-14** When both sphere and cylinder lines focus at the same time, the lens has a uniform power in all meridians and is spoken of as being *spherical*. (Instruments using a circle of dots will show no elongation in any direction. The focused target appears to be the same as when no lens is present in the instrument and the power wheel registers zero.) If the sphere and cylinder lines do not intersect at the center of the mires, the lens optical center is not centered in front of the lensmeter aperture and prism is being manifested.

immediately into clear focus. Using the axis wheel of the lensmeter is necessary when a cylinder component is present (see Figure 2-11). As one set of lines begins to clear, rotation of the axis wheel probably will be necessary to increase clarity. As the axis wheel approaches one of two major meridians, one set of lines begins to clear. The sphere lines must be brought into focus first. If the cylinder lines clear up first instead of the sphere lines, the axis wheel is rotated 90 degrees, which brings the sphere lines into focus.

Once the sphere lines are clear, the sphere power and cylinder axis of the prescription are correct. They may be recorded directly from the power and axis wheels.

Next the power wheel is turned slowly once more in the minus direction until the cylinder lines clear. (The axis wheel should not be rotated.) The power wheel reading is noted. The cylinder value is the difference between the first reading (sphere lines) and the second reading (cylinder lines). It is recorded as a minus value (Box 2-1).

Example 2-1

A lens is placed in the lensmeter and the power wheel rotated to a high plus power—+10.00 or +12.00, for example. (The plus power need only be high enough to be certain that it is more plus than the power of the prescription lens.)

While the power wheel is rotated slowly back in the minus direction, the cylinder lines begin to clear. The

---

BOX **2-1**
Finding Spherocylinder Lens Power with a Standard, Crossed-Line-Target Lensmeter

1. The eyepiece is focused.
2. The power wheel is turned into the plus until the illuminated target blurs out.
3. The power wheel is turned slowly in the minus direction until the sphere lines clear.
4. The axis wheel is adjusted for optimum sphere line clarity.
5. Sphere power and cylinder axis are recorded.
6. The power wheel is turned farther in the minus direction until the cylinder lines clear.
7. The difference is taken between the two power wheel readings and recorded as a minus cylinder.

---

axis wheel reads 180. Because the cylinder lines are the wrong lines to start with, the axis wheel is rotated from 180 degrees to 90 degrees. Rotating the axis wheel 90 degrees will blur the cylinder lines and cause the sphere lines to clear. As the power wheel is turned slowly toward minus (away from plus) and the axis wheel slightly adjusted, maximum clarity is obtained. At maximum clarity the power wheel reads +2.50 D and the axis wheel reads 87 degrees. Two parts of the prescription can be recorded as follows:

SPHERE	CYLINDER	AXIS
+2.50		87

Next the power wheel is rotated further in the minus direction. Now the cylinder lines come into focus when the power wheel reaches +1.00 D. The cylinder value is the *difference* between the two major meridians. The difference between +2.50 D and +1.00 D is 1.50 D. This is the correct cylinder value. It is recorded as a minus number. The prescription now reads as follows:

SPHERE	CYLINDER	AXIS
+2.50	−1.50	87

READING A LENS IN PLUS CYLINDER FORM

If a prescription is to be written in plus cylinder form, the lens can be read by the lensmeter in plus cylinder form. This way the power may be written directly from lensmeter values without having to convert or *transpose* the prescription from minus to plus cylinder form.

Direct plus cylinder power readings are carried out as follows:

1. The power wheel is turned into the high *minus* numbers.
2. The power wheel is advanced slowly in the *plus* direction.
3. The axis wheel is rotated to cause the sphere lines to come into focus first. (*Note*: The sphere lines must *always* come into focus first, regardless of whether the lens is being read in plus or minus cylinder form.)
4. When the sphere lines are in focus, the sphere and axis values are recorded.
5. The power wheel is moved a second time in the plus direction, until the cylinder lines come into clear focus.
6. The difference between first and second power readings is the cylinder power. It is recorded as a *plus* value.

The plus cylinder procedure is identical to the minus cylinder procedure, with the exception of the direction of power wheel movement.

Spotting Lenses without Prism

POWER VERIFICATION AND SPOTTING OF SPHERES

When the power of the lens to be verified is of known power, rather than the entire neutralization process being performed, the power simply is checked as the lensmeter is set for the expected sphere value. If the lens is a sphere, the target should be immediately clear, which indicates a lens of the correct power. If the target is unclear, the lens power is incorrect. The actual power may be found through adjustment of the lensmeter power wheel.

Occasionally the lensmeter target will not appear clean and crisp even after being focused correctly. The best focus nevertheless may indicate a correct power reading. If this is the case, the lens is not well polished and should not be used.

When the lens has been determined to be of acceptable quality, it is centered optically in the lensmeter as the lens is moved until the center of the illuminated target crosses the center of the crosshairs in the lensmeter eyepiece or screen (see Figure 2-14). The marking device is then swung into position and the front surface of the lens spotted (Figure 2-15).

POWER VERIFICATION AND SPOTTING OF SPHEROCYLINDERS

When verifying spherocylinder lenses, the practitioner turns the lensmeter power wheel to the expected sphere power. In addition the cylinder axis wheel is turned until the axis indicated for the prescription is correctly

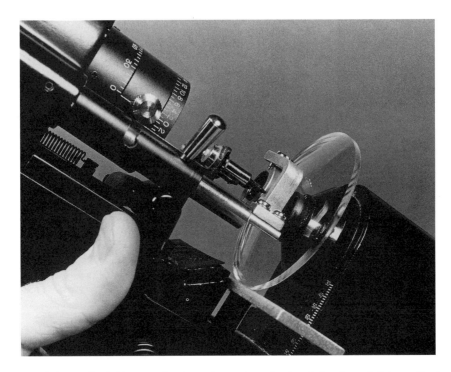

FIGURE **2-15** The inking mechanism places three horizontally aligned dots on the lens. All subsequent steps are based on these dots.

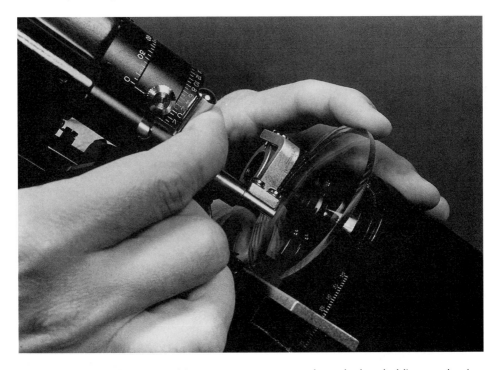

FIGURE **2-16** When a practitioner moves or rotates a lens, the lens holding mechanism is pulled back to prevent possible scratching.

positioned. The lens is placed in the instrument. The lens holding device is not allowed to touch the lens. The lens is rotated (Figure 2-16) until the sphere lines of the lensmeter target are sharp and unbroken. When these lines are clear, the cylinder axis is correct. (The lens also may be moved horizontally and vertically in an effort to begin centering the target lines over the central crosshairs of the eyepiece or screen).

With the lens correctly rotated for axis position, the lensmeter power wheel is turned in the appropriate

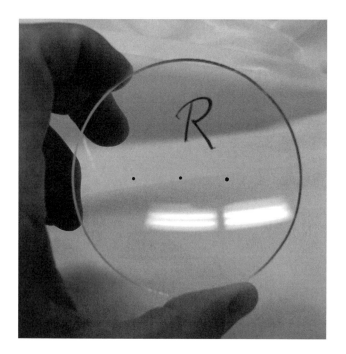

FIGURE **2-17** The lens designation (R or L) is always marked on the upper half of the lens so that the lens will not be blocked upside down. Although not as critical for non-prismatic single vision lenses, an inverted prism lens or multifocal would be useless when inverted. (The lens is pictured from the back side.)

BOX **2-2**
Spotting Single Vision Sphere or Spherocylinder Lenses with a Standard, Crossed-Line-Target Lensmeter

1. The lens sphere power and lens cylinder axis are dialed into the lensmeter.
2. The lens is placed in the lensmeter.
3. The major reference point is located.
4. If the lens is spherical, the lens is spotted.
5. If the lens has a cylinder, the lens is rotated until the sphere lines are clear.
6. If the lens has prescription prism, the illuminated target is moved until it is located at the position at which the prism equals that called for in the prescription.
7. The lens is spotted.

direction to check the cylinder power. (When minus cylinder notation is used, this is always in the minus direction.) The power wheel should read them as the sum of the sphere and cylinder powers. For example, if the lens power is +5.00 −1.00 × 180, the power wheel should read as +4.00 because plus 5.00 minus 1.00 equals +4.00.

Next the lens is moved carefully left, right, upward, or downward until the target is accurately centered. (The lens holding device must be pulled away from the lens surface so that the lens will not get scratched.) If the lens has an especially high cylinder power, it may be necessary to rock the power wheel between sphere and cylinder readings to achieve a correct centration. This is because only one set of target lines may be visible at a time. The lens should not rotate during this process. Rotating the lens causes the axis to be off. When the target is accurately centered, the lens may be spotted (Figure 2-17).

The power verification in a spotting procedure for a spherocylinder lenses is summarized in Box 2-2.

Marking the Lens Right or Left

As soon as the lens is spotted, it should be removed from the lensmeter and marked for the right or left eye.

Lenses are commonly marked on the back surface with a wax pencil. The letter *R* or *L* in uppercase letters is written in the upper half of the lens, above the three spots. Figure 2-17 shows that the letters are written normally (not in mirror image as is commonly done in surfacing procedures).

The lens is then returned to its tray with the back (concave) side down. Placing the lens front side down risks scratching the front lens surface as the lens slides in the tray. Traditionally the right lens always is placed in the right side of the tray and the left lens in the left side (Figure 2-18). In the production process, everyone expects the right lens to be on the right side. If it is not placed correctly in the tray, lenses easily can be marked or edged for the wrong eye.

A Lens Prescription that Includes Prism

OPTICAL CENTER OF A LENS

Up to this point the procedure described has been limited to single vision lenses with no prism power indicated in the prescription. The procedure detailed here includes centering of the illuminated lensmeter target in the middle of the crosshairs. By centering the target in the crosshairs, the optical center (OC) can be found. Locating the OC and spotting it ensures that after the lens is edged, the OC will be positioned before the pupil of the eye. No prism exists at the OC of a lens. When no prescribed prism is in the prescription, the needed point of reference is the OC. The OC becomes

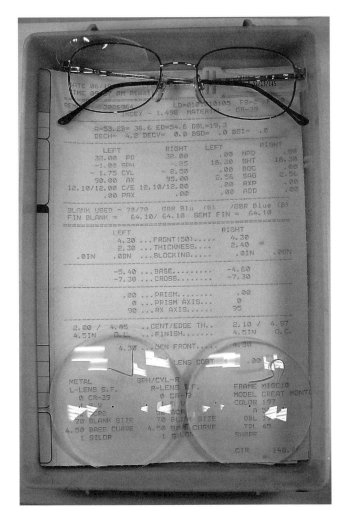

FIGURE 2-18 By convention the right lens is placed on the right-hand side of the tray and is always face up to prevent scratches on the front surface. In spite of this convention the lenses should still be checked before each step in the fabrication process to verify that the correct lens is being used.

the reference point. It is of major importance in aligning the lens. Therefore it is known as the *major reference point,* or *MRP*. So when no prism is in the prescription, the OC *is* the MRP.

OPTICAL CENTERS NOT WITHIN THE LINE OF SIGHT

Whenever the eye looks through a lens at a place other than the OC, the object appears to be displaced from its actual location.[3] This apparent displacement is caused

by the *prismatic effect* of the lens. When the eye looks through the OC of a lens, no apparent displacement exists. However, when the eye looks through an off-center point on the lens, the object does appear displaced.

Most spectacle lens prescriptions have no prescribed prismatic effect. This means that the OC of the lens needs to be in front of the eye. Unwanted prism requires one eye to turn away from the normal direction of gaze to keep from seeing double. This can be very uncomfortable.

Sometimes a prescription includes prescribed prism. The lens must be positioned so that the amount of prism called for will be in front of the wearer's pupil, in the eye's line of sight. When prism is called for in the prescription, the point on the lens with the correct amount of prism becomes the point of reference; it is not the OC. This prismatic point is important in alignment of the lens, and now it becomes the MRP. So when the prescription contains prescribed prism, the OC and MRP are two separate points.

A synonym for the MRP that is perhaps even more descriptive is *prism reference point,* or *PRP.* MRP and PRP are the same.

Prentice's Rule

A relationship exists between prism power and the distance between the OC and the MRP. For a desired prismatic effect the needed distance in centimeters between the OC and the MRP depends upon the power of the lens. It can be calculated using Prentice's rule for decentration. Prentice's Rule states the following

$$\Delta = cF$$

where:

Δ = Prism diopters at the point of reference
c = Distance in centimeters
F = Power of the lens

For spherical lenses the calculation is straightforward.[4]

Example 2-2

How far from each other will the OC and MRP be for a -3.00 D lens when a 1.5Δ prismatic effect is desired?

---

[3]In the case of a plano cylinder, no prismatic effect occurs anywhere along the axis of the cylinder. It might be said that the "optical center" is really an "optical line."

[4]For decentration of plano cylinder lenses along major meridians, the power used is the power of the cylinder in the meridian of decentration. If a cylinder is oriented at an oblique axis and the direction of decentration is horizontal or vertical, prism will be induced with its base oriented obliquely. (For more information on the optical effects of decentration, the reader is encouraged to see Brooks CW, Borish IM: *System for ophthalmic dispensing,* Boston, 1996, Butterworth-Heinemann.)

Solution

In this example,

$$F = -3.00 \text{ D}$$

and

$$\Delta = 1.5\Delta$$

Prentice's Rule states that

$$\Delta = cF$$

This may also be written as

$$c = \frac{\Delta}{F}$$

Therefore

$$c = \frac{1.5}{3} = 0.5 \text{ cm}$$

So the OC is OC = 5 mm from MRP

Spotting Lenses with Prism

SINGLE VISION LENSES

The procedure of spotting single vision lenses with prism is nearly identical to that of nonprism lenses. The only difference is in how the illuminated target is centered. Instead of placing the center of the illuminated target at the center of the crosshairs, the illuminated sphere/cylinder target lines must be positioned to correspond to the location of the desired prismatic effect.

Example 2-3

A right lens calls for 2.0Δ base out prism. How would it be positioned for spotting?

Solution

To correctly position this lens the following steps must be taken:

- The sphere/cylinder target intersection must be on the circular mire marked 2.0.
- Because the prism is horizontal, the illuminated target must be on the 180-degree line.
- Base out for the right eye is to the left. Therefore the center of the illuminated target must be on the 2Δ prism circle where it crosses the 180-degree line to the left.

(*Note:* Before reading prism, the practitioner must be sure that the internal horizontal and vertical lines that are a part of the black lensmeter mires are really horizontally and vertically aligned. If no internal or external degree references are available to use, the cylinder axis is set at zero and the mires are lined parallel to the illuminated target in the lensmeter.)

When the lens is correctly positioned the lensmeter target appears as shown in Figure 2-19.

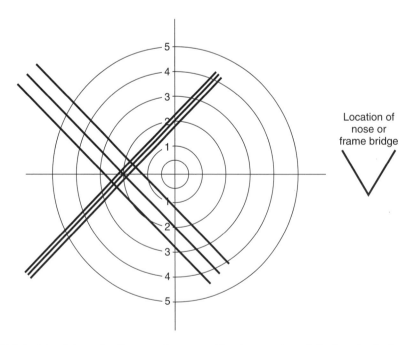

Location of nose or frame bridge

FIGURE **2-19** Prismatic effect can be created by decentering of the lens in the lensmeter until the sphere/cylinder line intersection is positioned for the indicated amount. (Achievement of desired prism by decentration is limited by lens size and refractive power.)

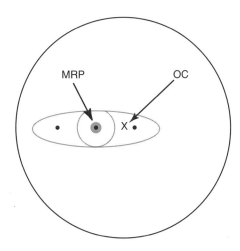

FIGURE **2-20** The major reference point (MRP) of a lens ultimately will be positioned before the wearer's pupil center. If prism is indicated in the prescription, the optical center (OC) is displaced purposely. Therefore the point that will be important in centration and that is consequently spotted is the major reference point—not the optical center.

Once this position is achieved and the cylinder axis is correct, the lens may be spotted. Figure 2-20 shows the lens spotted with the three lensmeter dots. The center lensmeter ink spot is no longer at the center of the uncut lens, but the center dot still indicates the location of the MRP.

PRESCRIBED PRISM WITH BOTH HORIZONTAL AND VERTICAL COMPONENTS

In a case in which both horizontal and vertical prisms are called for simultaneously in the same lens, the target must be moved both laterally and vertically until it reaches the desired position. That position is one where the target center is directly above (or below) the required horizontal prism reading. It is also exactly left or right of the required vertical prism reading.

Example 2-4
A right eye requires 4.0 D base out and 2.0 D base up. How would the lens be positioned for spotting?

Solution
To correctly position the lens, the target must be four full prism diopter units to the left of center *and* two full prism diopter units above center. (The half diopter prism ring should not be counted as a full prism diopter.) This is shown in Figure 2-21.

PRISM RESTRICTIONS WITH ASPHERIC AND ATORIC LENSES

When aspheric or atoric lenses are used, the lens design changes power in a concentric-ring–like manner from the center to the edges of the lens. The center of the "ring" must be in front of the wearer's eye. This means that finished single vision aspheric or atoric lenses cannot be decentered to create prescribed prism. When prescribed prism is present in the prescription, it is necessary to begin with a semifinished lens. The prism must be ground onto the lens precisely at the center of the aspheric "ring." Once a semifinished aspheric or atoric lens has been surfaced for the correct prism amount, it may be spotted in the usual manner as described, with no adverse effects.

Decentering a finished (stock lens) aspheric or atoric places the concentric area in front of the eye. The center of aspheric design will be somewhere else. This destroys the advantage of the aspheric design. It would be optically better not to use an aspheric or atoric design at all. A regular lens gives better optics than an aspheric lens that has the central zone of the lens moved away from where it should be.

Spotting with Autolensmeters

Autolensmeters perform in much the same manner as the manual variety. Their chief advantages are speed of operation when lenses of unknown power are measured and reduced training time for new operators.

Autolensmeters vary in the appearance of the screen and in operation. An example of an autolensmeter is shown in Figure 2-22. This particular instrument includes a measuring mode and a layout mode. In other words, for simple measurement of a lens power, the screen appears as shown in Figure 2-23. In the layout mode the target on the screen is similar to the view into a manual lensmeter (Figure 2-24). It is possible to spot the lens in the measuring mode but is more convenient using the layout mode.

Use of an autolensmeter for spotting lenses requires no presetting of the instrument. Power readings may display in normal quarter-diopter increments or in smaller increments—in some cases down to $\frac{1}{100\text{th}}$ of a diopter.

How the spectacles are physically placed in the autolensmeter varies by manufacturer. For example, if the spectacles are placed in an autolensmeter with an upright design such as the Humphrey autolensmeter, the temples will hang downward and the top of the spectacle frame will be closest to the operator.

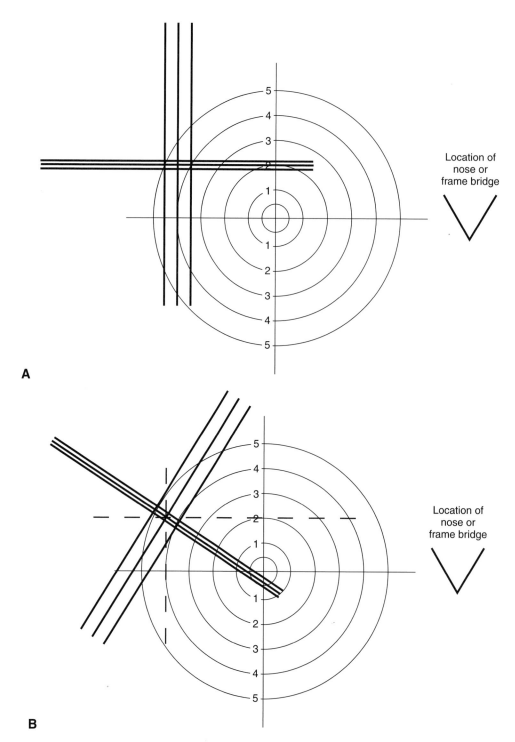

Location of
nose or
frame bridge

A

Location of
nose or
frame bridge

B

FIGURE **2-21** In positioning a prismatic lens, the only important reference is the center of the illuminated target. This is the place where center sphere and cylinder lines cross each other. Where other parts of those lines may cross the circular mires is of no importance. In the example shown, the sphere/cylinder line crossing point must be directly above or below the place where the 4.0 D circle crosses the horizontal line farthest from the "nose." The sphere/cylinder line crossing point must simultaneously also be exactly at the same level as the top of the 2.0 D circle. **A,** This spot is easy to see because the sphere and cylinder lines are aligned horizontally and vertically. However, if cylinder is present at any axis other than 90 or 180, the lines will not look like this. Instead they may appear as shown in **B**. The prismatic effect shown in **B** is exactly the same as in **A**. Both are 4 base out and 2 base up. It may be difficult to tell the exact position of the center of the illuminated target for a spherocylinder lens with an oblique axis. Practitioners who experience difficulty may try this procedure. The cylinder axis is turned temporarily to 90 or 180, causing the illuminated target lines to be exactly horizontal and vertical. Although the lines will be a bit blurred, they will duplicate the situation shown in **A** and make it easier to tell how much vertical and horizontal prism is present.

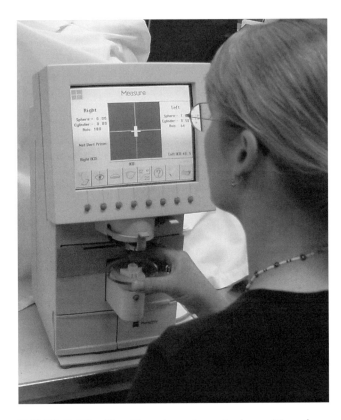

FIGURE **2-22** The Humphrey Lens Analyzer (Humphrey Instruments [division of Carl Zeiss, Inc.], San Leandro, Calif.) is an example of an automated lensmeter.

AUTOLENSMETER SPOTTING WITH NO PRESCRIBED PRISM

To lay out a single vision lens that has no prism in the prescription (Rx), the lens is held over the lens stop (Figure 2-25). When the lens is held in the instrument, the sphere, cylinder, and axis readings on the screen immediately show actual lens power. A gray circle surrounds the cross and represents the lens. The circle and cross move as the lens is moved.

If the lens is a sphere, having no cylinder component, it must now be centered in the lensmeter. The lens is positioned correctly when the gray lens circle surrounds the smallest of the concentric circles on the screen and the cross is exactly in the middle of the simulated lensmeter mires. The screen also reads the amount of horizontal and vertical prism. Both of these readings should be zero. Spherocylinder powers require that the lens be rotated until the correct axis appears.

Example 2-5

A prescription calls for a lens with a power of −5.50 −0.50 × 121. How might this lens be spotted using an autolensmeter?

Solution

The lens is selected from inventory and held in position in the autolensmeter. The axis appears as a number, but the cross on the screen also turns to match the axis of the cylinder. The lens is rotated until the axis shown in the autolensmeter matches the axis called for in the prescription. Next the lens circle is moved on the screen to the central position (Figure 2-26).

The practitioner must verify that the cylinder axis is still correct and check whether the horizontal and vertical prism readings are at zero. If everything checks out correctly, the lens may be spotted with the spotting device (Figure 2-27). The spotting device places three dots on the lens in exactly the same way that the manual lensmeter does.

AUTOLENSMETER SPOTTING WITH PRESCRIBED PRISM

Using the autolensmeter to spot a lens with Rx prism is done much like with a conventional lensmeter. In the layout mode an autolensmeter is likely to have both a simulation of a conventional lensmeter target and a numerical prism reading that tells exactly how much vertical and horizontal prism is showing up in the lens at the measured position. As the lens position changes, the numerical prism readings also are changing.

Example 2-6

A right lens prescription calls for a power of −5.50 −0.50 × 121 with 2.50Δ of base out prism and 0.50Δ base up. How would the lens be positioned and spotted using the example autolensmeter?

Solution

The lensmeter is set for layout mode and for a right lens. The lens is held in the lensmeter and is positioned for the correct 121-degree cylinder axis as in the previous example. Next the lens is moved laterally. The target should move toward the base out and up side of the mires. The circles are used as a general guideline, but the numerical readout is monitored until it shows 2.50Δ of base out horizontal prism and 0.50Δ of base up vertical prism (Figure 2-28). The cylinder axis still must read correctly. The lens may now be spotted.

Story Told by the Numerical Readout

Reading prism with an autolensmeter relies on the numerical readout for prism amount as the final word, not the way the target appears prismatically in the image of the simulated lensmeter target. The simulated position of the target may not exactly replicate the accuracy of the manual lensmeter target, especially for

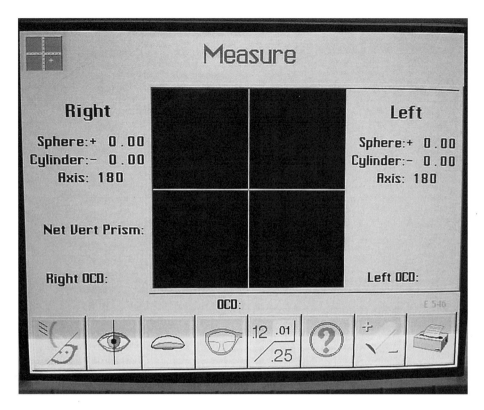

FIGURE **2-23** The Humphrey Lens Analyzer (Humphrey Instruments [division of Carl Zeiss, Inc.], San Leandro, Calif.) has a measuring mode and a layout mode. This is the screen for the measuring mode.

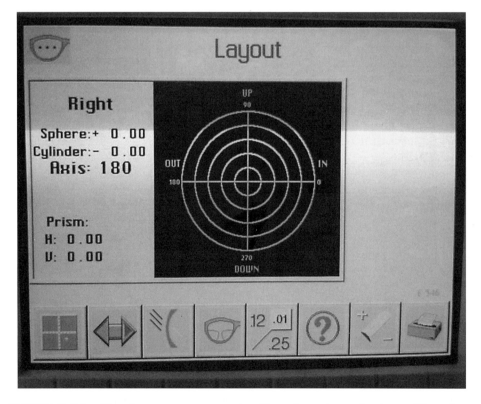

FIGURE **2-24** The layout screen on the Humphrey Lens Analyzer (Humphrey Instruments [division of Carl Zeiss, Inc.], San Leandro, Calif.) looks more like a conventional lensmeter screen.

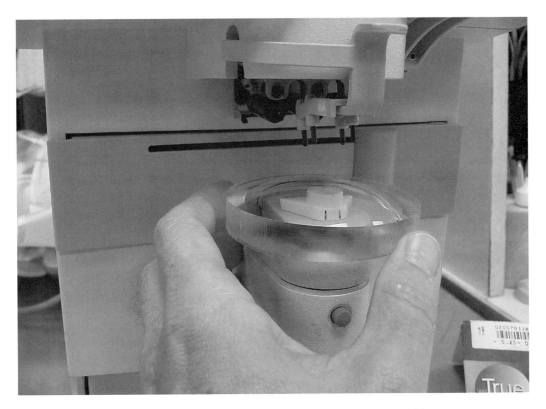

FIGURE **2-25**   Positioning the lens for spotting in an automated lensmeter.

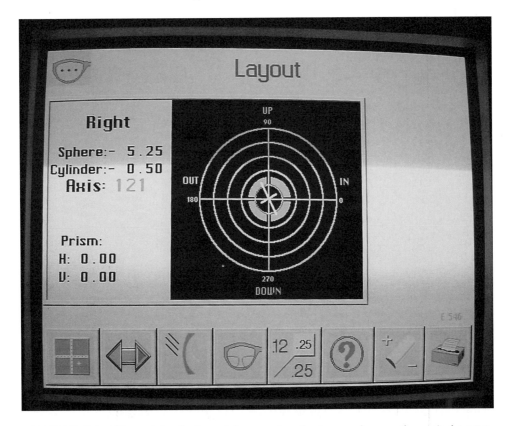

FIGURE **2-26**   When the cylinder axis is correct and prism reads zero, the optical center is correctly positioned.

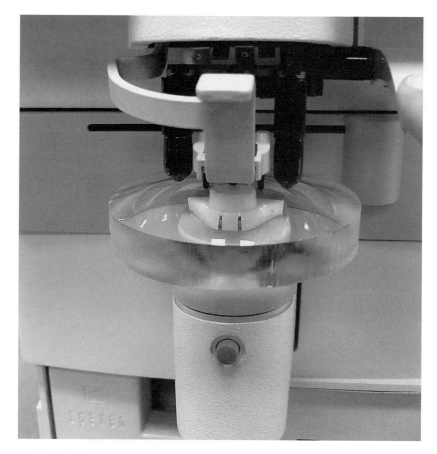

FIGURE **2-27** The spotting mechanism on an autolensmeter is the same as that on the manual lensmeter. (*Note*: This image is for illustration purposes only, as the spotting mechanism is not currently configured to physically spot the lens.)

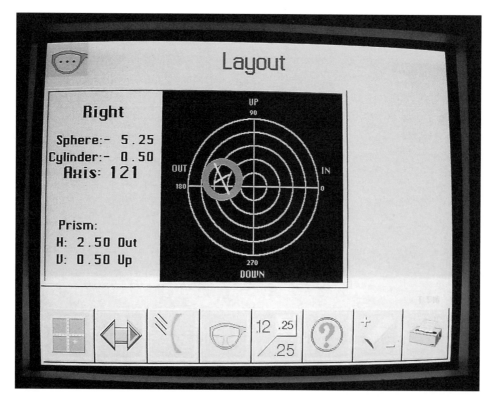

FIGURE **2-28** The mires in the layout mode aide in lens orientation for prism amount, but the numerical readout should be used for exactness.

combined horizontal and vertical prism. However, the numerical readings on the screen are accurate.

Making the Most of a Blemished Lens

Occasionally lenses become chipped or scratched in handling, shipping, or surfacing. Taking full advantage of lens optical properties potentially allows use of the lens without compromise of the quality of the finished product. The crucial factor is the location of the imperfect or damaged portion in relation to the final lens shape and lens power.

A BLEMISHED SPHERE

The most versatile lens type is the spherical lens. Because a sphere is of uniform power in all meridians, it may be rotated around its OC without changing its optical characteristics.[5] Therefore if a large chip were to be broken from its edge as shown in Figure 2-29, *A*, the lens must be turned only so that during the edging process this chipped portion will be edged away (Figure 2-29, *B*).

A BLEMISHED SPHEROCYLINDER

A spherocylinder lens is less adaptable. It has only two possible orientations. The decision on how best to orient a slightly damaged spherocylinder is made after lens spotting but before it is marked at the top with an *L* or *R*.

Example 2-7

A prescription for the right eye has a of power +2.00 -1.00 × 10. The lens is verified and spotted as shown in Figure 2-30, *A*. In recognition that the lens is scratched, the frame shape is checked against the lens. If the scratch appears within the frame shape, the lens is unacceptable (Figure 2-30, *B*). Can this lens be used?

Solution

A cylinder axis goes from one side of the lens to the other. Axis 180 is the same as axis zero. Axis 90 is the same as axis 270. For this reason, cylinder axis is specified only up to 180 degrees. Turning a cylinder lens upside down does not affect the optics. In this example, a 10-degree axis is the same as a 190-degree axis. In the example, turning the lens also repositions it

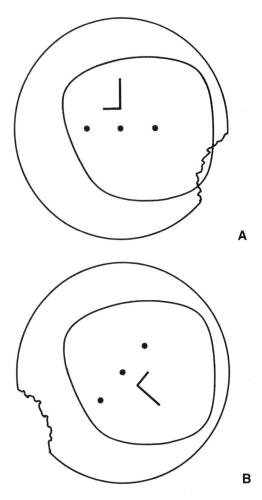

FIGURE **2-29** **A,** The lens will be ruined if edged as marked. By turning this spherical lens, the same optical endpoint is achieved without a sacrifice in quality. **B,** The lens should be remarked so that in marking and blocking the chipped portion will be positioned as shown.

so that the scratch will be ground completely away. This is shown in Figure 2-30, *C*. The lens may now be marked with the appropriate *R* and used.

A BLEMISHED PRISM LENS

When prescribed prism is present, standard lens blanks may be rotated only *before* the MRP is marked for the correct amount of prism. Once the lens is marked for prism, the lens may no longer be rotated.

Lenses that have been specifically surfaced to obtain a prismatic effect that could not be achieved by decentration of a standard lens blank cannot be rotated at all.

---

[5]This does not apply to a polarized lens.

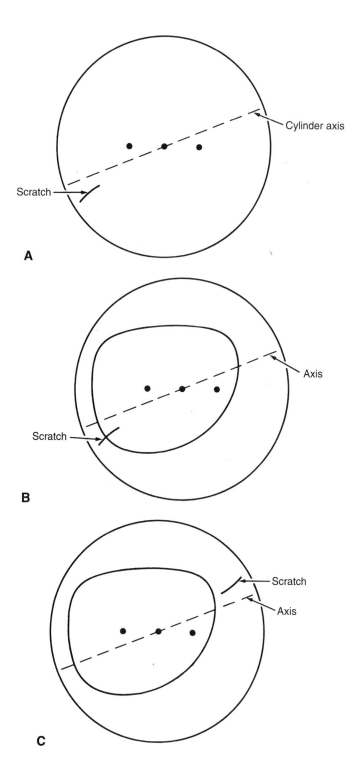

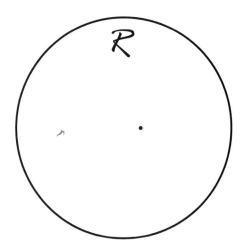

FIGURE **2-31** Occasionally a stock lens will have a misplaced optical center. Before the lens is marked with *R* or *L*, the lens should be turned so that the optical center is toward the nose. If the lens is spherical, the two outer dots are not needed and can be wiped off. They could be confusing if left in place. If the lens is a spherocylinder, the three dots must be left on the lens.

A STOCK LENS WITH AN OFF-CENTER OPTICAL CENTER

Normally the OC of a stock lens is in the middle of the lens. Occasionally this OC is slightly off center. This will not affect the overall quality of the lens. To ensure that the lens will be large enough even with the misplaced center, the lens is turned so that the OC is toward the nasal side of the frame before writing an *R* or *L* on the lens and placing it in the tray (Figure 2-31). Because most lenses are decentered toward the nose for edging, this leaves the larger lens area temporally.

Spotting of Polarizing Lenses

Polarizing lenses block horizontally polarized light that reflects from glare surfaces and allow vertically polarized light to pass through the lens. The lens does this because it has a laminated layer sandwiched within the lens. This laminated layer must be oriented correctly in the frame; otherwise the lens will not work correctly.

To ensure that the lens is oriented correctly, notches are located in the laminated layer on either side of the lens (Figure 2-32). These notches must fall on the 180-degree line.

For sphere lenses, the OC of the lens is located and spotted. Then the outer two lensmeter dots are removed, leaving only the center dot. When the lens is

FIGURE **2-30** A scratch on a lens may not make the lens unusable. Whether it can be used depends on scratch location, frame size, and—in the case of cylinder lenses—axis orientation. **A,** The lens is marked for edging (no prism). If used as oriented, the scratch will appear on the edged lens, as shown in **B.** However, because a spherocylinder without prism can be rotated 180 degrees without any change in optical effect, as **C** demonstrates, this lens is still useful. (Any rotation of the lens must be done after spotting and before the lens is marked.)

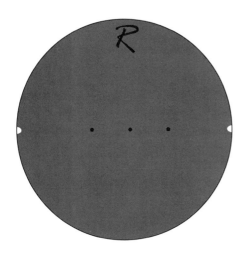

FIGURE **2-32** Polarizing lenses must be spotted so that the two notches in the laminated layer of the lens are oriented on the 180-degree line. If this is not done, the lens will not cut out reflected glare.

ready to be blocked, the central spot indicating the OC and the two notches are used to position the lens. Because it is likely that a polarizing lens will have been custom surfaced from a semifinished lens, it is probable that a number of these lenses will have their OCs displaced nasally. After the lens is spotted, it is turned so that the displaced OC will indeed be nasal before marking an *R* or an *L* on the lens. (This is the same procedure described in the previous section.)

Spherocylinder lenses and most lenses with prescribed prism have to be surfaced so that the cylinder axis is correctly placed in relationship to the lens' direction of polarization.

Prescription Verification and Spotting of Multifocal Lenses

Multifocal lenses are checked for surface defects and internal deficiencies in the same manner as are single vision lenses. They also should be spotted. This marks the MRP and the 180-degree line. This 180-degree line indicates the horizontal plane of the lens. As with single vision lenses, the 180-degree line is not the axis of the cylinder but rather the line from which the axis of the cylinder is measured.

METHOD FOR SPOTTING FLAT-TOP–SEGMENT MULTIFOCALS

For multifocals, the bifocal should be placed in the lensmeter as it will be when mounted in the frame. This

means that for flat-top bifocals, the segment top should be horizontal. The sphere power is dialed into the lensmeter. If the lens has a cylinder component, the axis of the cylinder should be dialed in as well.

Next the MRP of the lens is located. When the lens is spherical, the lens may be spotted. With spherical lenses, if the segment was not placed in the lensmeter exactly straight, the lensmeter-spotted 180-degree line will not be horizontal. It may need to be tilted during the next step of centration so that the segment line will be horizontally straight. This is explained in Chapter 6.

For multifocals with spherocylinder powers, the axis of the cylinder has been custom ground for that particular lens. The lensmeter is set for the axis ordered and the lens rotated to the correct axis. With MRP and cylinder axis correct, the lens is spotted, just like a single vision lens. After the lens has been spotted, the three dots on the 180-degree line should be parallel to the upper edge of a flat-top segment (Figure 2-33, *A*). If they are not parallel to the top of the bifocal segment, the cylinder axis is off and the lens was surfaced improperly. An example of this is shown in Figure 2-33, *B*. When this happens, mounting the lens in the frame with both its segment top straight and cylinder axis correct will be impossible. (Only in the case of an extremely low-powered cylinder may an error like this fall within acceptable quality standards.)

To precheck the lenses as a pair, the lenses are held front-to-front with the segments overlapping (Figure 2-33, *C*). If two different MRP heights or two different segment insets do not exist, the center spots of both lenses should be at the same place. If they are not, a problem with unwanted horizontal or vertical prism is likely after the lenses are edged.

Box 2-3 provides a summary of spotting flat-top multifocals.

HOW TO SPOT ROUND-SEGMENT MULTIFOCALS

For multifocals with round segments and a spherically powered distance portion, the MRP and 180-degree line are marked first by rotation of the lens to the estimated segment position. Segments are rotated inward toward where the nose would be. With a right lens in the lensmeter, the lower part of the lens is rotated inward so that the segment is slightly right of center (Figure 2-34, *A*). The OC is located and the lens spotted (Figure 2-34, *B*). The left lens segment will be rotated likewise somewhat left of center. Even though these left and right inward lens rotations are not likely to be exact, any inaccuracies can and will be corrected later when the lenses are being prepared for blocking.

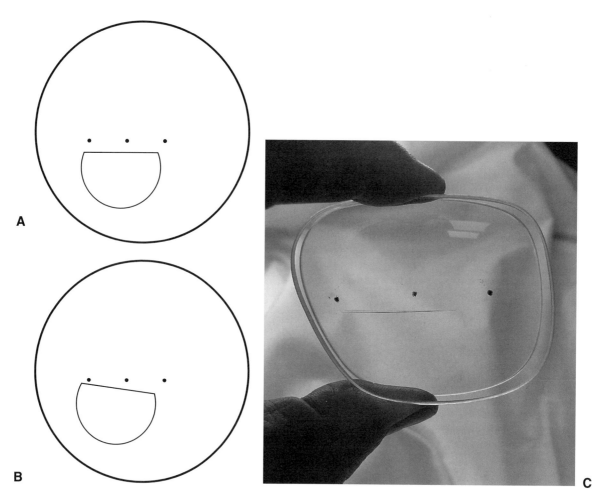

FIGURE **2-33** **A,** For spherocylinder lenses, the three dots should be parallel to the top of the segment. If they are not, the cylinder axis will be wrong. **B,** For spherical lenses that have neither a cylinder nor an axis, an angle between the three dots and the segment top is not a problem, even though it looks off. With a sphere lens, the center dot is the only important point. The lens may rotate around this point at any angle with no change in the optics of the lens. However, if the lens has a cylinder component, the axis of the cylinder will be wrong. **C,** Once flat-top bifocals have been spotted, they may be prechecked before edging. The edged lenses are held front-to-front because the segments and spots are closer to one another and will reduce the amount of parallax. The lenses are not pressed into contact with each other to prevent scratching. The segments must overlap exactly. When both lenses that have equal segment insets and drops, the spots should also overlap as shown. If they do not overlap, a problem may exist with interpupillary distances (PDs) being off or unwanted vertical prism.

For spherocylindrical round-segment multifocals the lens is placed in the lensmeter. The correct sphere power and cylinder axis are dialed into the lensmeter. The OC is found, and the lens is rotated to the correct cylinder axis. Now the lens is spotted. Whether the cylinder axis is within tolerance in reference to the near segment position can be judged only during the centration process that follows.

Invisible segment or "blended bifocal" lenses have round-segment areas with borders that have been smoothed out or "blended" to make them unnoticeable. These blended round-segment lenses are spotted in exactly the same manner as regular round-segment lenses. (Blended bifocals should not be confused with progressive addition lenses. Progressive addition lenses will be considered shortly.) Box 2-4 summarizes the procedure used to spot round-segment lenses and blended bifocals.

To conclude the spotting/verification process, all segments are verified for accuracy of the near addition

> ### BOX 2-3
> ### *Spotting Flat-Top Multifocals*
>
> 1. The lens sphere power and lens cylinder axis are dialed into the lensmeter.
> 2. The lens is placed in the lensmeter.
> 3. The major reference point is located.
> 4. If the lens is spherical, the lens is spotted.
> 5. If the lens has a cylinder, the lens is rotated until the sphere lines are clear.
> 6. If the lens has prescribed prism, the illuminated target is moved until it is located at the position where the prism equals that called for in the prescription.
> 7. The lens is spotted.
> 8. For spherocylinder lenses and lenses with prescribed prism, the practitioner must verify that the segment top and three lensmeter dots are parallel to one another.
> 9. When both lenses have been spotted, the lenses are lined up front-to-front to check for R-L spotting accuracy. The central spots should overlap.

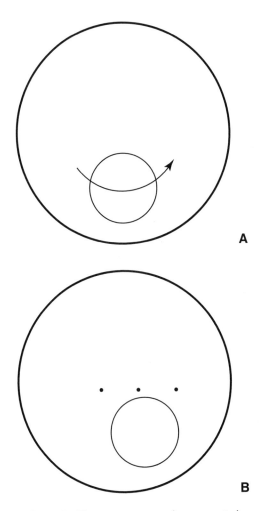

FIGURE 2-34 **A,** To spot a round segment lens for edging, the segment for this right lens is rotated slightly in a direction toward the nose. **B,** The optical center is located, and the lens is spotted. With spheres, this estimated nasalward segment rotation places the lens more as it should be and makes the centration and blocking process easier.

power after the lens is spotted. The lens is removed from the lensmeter and marked with an *L* or *R*.

DISAPPEARANCE OF THE MAJOR REFERENCE POINT INTO THE SEGMENT PORTION

When bifocal and trifocal lenses are surfaced, the distance OC could be ground into the lens so that it will be halfway between the top and bottom of the edged lens shape (Figure 2-35). When the distance OC is placed here, edge thickness will be equal at the top and bottom of the edged lens.

Sometimes bifocal or trifocal lenses are ordered with the bifocal or trifocal segment especially high. In fact, the segment tops occasionally may be higher than the middle of the edged lens. If the distance OC is placed on the 180-degree midline and the segment is higher than the 180-degree midline, the distance OC will be *in* the segment area (Figure 2-36, *A*). With use of the lensmeter, the distance OC becomes "lost" in the segment.

If the distance OC falls within the segment of the lens, distance power measurements cannot be made at the OC. They must be made above the OC and above the segment. For measuring power this is not serious. The process of measuring power above the MRP location is standard for progressive addition lenses.

Unfortunately when the distance OC or MRP cannot be located easily, the lens cannot be spotted and checked for the wearer's interpupillary distance (PD) accurately. Prismatic effects from the segment interfere with distance lens optics and cause the location of the distance OC to appear displaced. For all except round segments, though, lens centration can still be carried out normally. When flat-top lenses are laid out for edging, the segment borders are used for reference instead of the distance OC.

Leaving the OC on the horizontal midline of a multifocal lens, even if the segment is at or above the center of the lens, is not standard procedure for all surfacing laboratories. In cases in which equality of upper and lower lens edge thicknesses is not a factor, the surfacing laboratory commonly places the OC slightly higher than the top of the segment line (Figure 2-36, *B*).

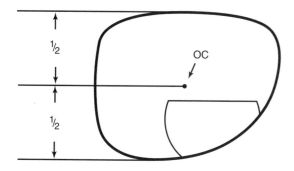

FIGURE **2-35**   A common location for the distance optical center (OC) of a lens is halfway between the top and bottom of the edged lens.

An Alternative Round-Segment Spotting Method

When the distance OC is within the segment area of a round-segment lens, the following process may be used:[6]

1. Distance power is verified at a location just above the segment. This distance should be the same for both left and right lenses.

---

[6]Several factors can prevent this process from being entirely accurate, such as the horizontal prism that may be induced by the presence of a strong oblique cylinder. Yet because the near add can, with higher powers, affect the apparent cylinder axis as well as induce horizontal and vertical prism of its own, the method remains a viable compromise.

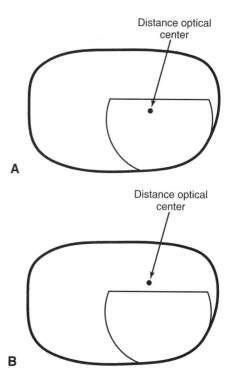

FIGURE **2-36**   **A,** A high bifocal segment combined with conventional vertical placement of distance optical center (OC) "loses" the OC in the segment. It cannot be accurately found with a lensmeter. **B,** Some surfacing laboratories routinely place the distance OC above a highly placed segment top unless it will cause thickness differences between upper and lower lens edges to be cosmetically objectionable.

2. Care should be taken to keep the cylinder axis correct. The lens is moved laterally until no horizontal prism exists. (If prism is prescribed, the lens is adjusted until the correct prism amount appears.)
3. The lens is spotted at this location. As long as the three dots on the lens are kept horizontal, the cylinder axis will be right.

Unless a strong oblique cylinder is present, the OC should be located correctly.

Progressive Addition Lenses

Progressive addition lenses have certain "hidden" markings used in establishment of lens orientation. Lenses coming from the surfacing laboratory also are marked with non–water-soluble ink. If the visible inked marks are applied correctly, the lenses do not need to be spotted. However, they should be verified before edging.

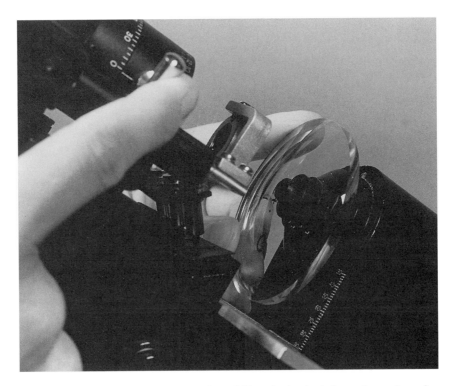

FIGURE **2-37**   The power of a progressive add lens is checked above the major reference point (MRP), at the location of the distance reference point (DRP). The DRP is found within the premarked semicircle. The distance power is not checked at the MRP because the MRP marks the beginning of the progressive zone or corridor leading down into the near portion.

VERIFICATION OF PREMARKED PROGRESSIVES

To check distance lens power, the lens is positioned in the lensmeter to view through the circled area above the MRP (Figure 2-37). (The MRP usually comes marked with a dot.) The center of this circled area used to locate the point for verifying distance power is called the *distance reference point,* or *DRP* (Figure 2-38). Incidentally, some prism will almost always be at the DRP because the DRP of the lens is not the OC of the lens.

To check distance power, the power wheel is set to the sphere power and the cylinder axis wheel to the ordered cylinder axis. The lens is rotated until the target lines are clear and unbroken. The non–water-soluble horizontal reference marks on the lens should be oriented horizontally and not tilted. If they are tilted, the axis of the cylinder is incorrect.[7]

Near lens power is checked through a point well into the near zone so that no intermediate progressive

power is measured. This point usually is marked with a non–water-soluble inked circle and is called the *near reference point,* or *NRP.* The near addition is verified in this specified NRP area.

To check for prism, the lens is centered in the lensmeter at the MRP. A synonym for MRP is *prism reference point (PRP).* However, the lensmeter target may not be altogether clear at the MRP because the progressive zone of the lens starts here. The lens power in the lower half of the measuring area is increasing and may blur the lower half of the target.

Progressive lenses often come with equal amounts of vertical prism in both right and left lenses. This allows the lenses to be made thinner. Equal amounts of "yoked" vertical prism for "prism thinning" purposes are both allowable and usually expected. For example, both right and left lenses may read 1.5Δ base down at the PRP. Because the prism thins the lens and the net binocular prismatic effect is zero, the lenses are considered free of unwanted vertical prism.[8]

---

[7]It is possible that the cylinder axis is correct, but the visible lens marking was applied incorrectly at an angle.

[8]For more information on prism thinning and its workings, consult Brooks CW, Borish IM: *System for ophthalmic dispensing,* ed 2, Boston, 1996, Butterworth-Heinemann (Chapter 11).

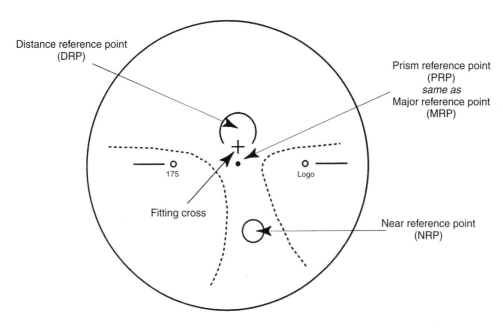

FIGURE **2-38** Points of reference on a progressive addition lens. (From Brooks CW, Borish IM: *System for ophthalmic dispensing,* ed 2, Boston, 1996, Butterworth-Heinemann, p 311.)

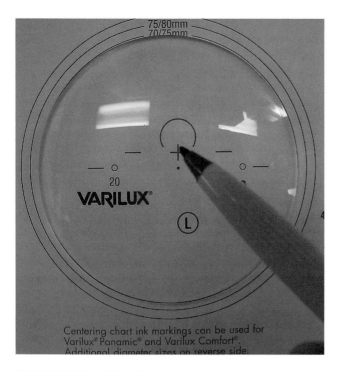

FIGURE **2-39** When the engraved circles on the lens are located and dotted, the guide marks can be reconstructed for use in layout and power verification.

As stated previously, if the lenses are correct and have non–water-soluble progressive lens markings, the lens does not need to be spotted. The existing markings will be used in the blocking process. If the lenses do not come with markings, or if it appears that the markings were applied inaccurately, then the markings must be reapplied.

PROGRESSIVE LENSES THAT ARE NOT PREMARKED

If a progressive addition lens leaves the surfacing laboratory without visible markings, the finishing laboratory should reconstruct the manufacturer's recommended system of identifying marks. This is done as follows:

1. The hidden marks are located on the lens surface. This may be done in several ways.
   - The lens is held under an incandescent bulb. For maximum visibility, the background should be matte black. Two small, etched marks usually are found at about 17 mm from either side of the lens center.

   or

   - The practitioner holds the lens up to a light and looks through the lens.

or

- A commercially available lens mark finder that illuminates and magnifies is used.
2. With a marking pen, a dot is placed on the centers of the small marks on the front surface of the lens.[9]
3. The lens is placed on a verification card and turned so that the dots fall at the indicated "engraved circle" points of the card. The lens manufacturer provides verification cards.
4. The appropriate lines are drawn on the lens from the master markings found on the verification card (Figure 2-39). Some lens manufacturers may provide easily removable decals that may be placed on the lens using the hidden circles for reference (Figure 2-40). This saves drawing the marks on the lens.

Chapter 5 explains more on progressive addition lenses.

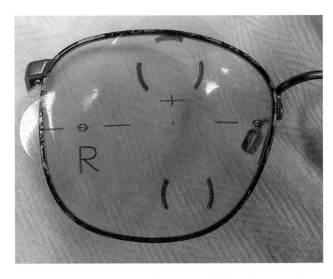

FIGURE **2-40** A decal placed on the lens in accordance with previously located hidden circles is quick and neat.

---

[9]Marking the etchings on the back of the lens when the etchings are actually found on the front can cause a significant amount of error because of parallax.

Proficiency Test Questions

1. True or False? If a stock lens is available, it is normally used instead of a custom surfaced lens.

2. For high plus lens powers, as center thickness increases, which of the following is true?

   a. Magnification of the wearer's eyes increases.
   b. Minification of the wearer's eyes increases.
   c. No relationship exists between lens power, center thickness, and either magnification or minification.

3. Given the generalized formula for minimum blank size, which of the following is the minimum blank size required for a frame having an effective diameter of 53 and a decentration of 3 mm per lens when *no allowance* is made for chipping?

   a. 54 mm
   b. 59 mm
   c. 62 mm
   d. 68 mm
   e. 71 mm

4. Apart from price considerations, in which of the following instances is it critical that the smallest possible lens blank be used?

   a. When the prescription is minus in power
   b. When the prescription is plus in power
   c. Apart from economic considerations, neither plus nor minus prescription power is a consideration.
   d. Using the smallest possible blank size is critical for both plus and minus prescriptions.

5. *Internal* lens deficiencies are inspected for in which of the following ways?

   a. Looking at the filament of an unfrosted light bulb as it reflects from the surface of the lens
   b. Observing a straight line through the lens as the lens is moved back and forth
   c. Looking through the lens at a black background under indirect illumination
   d. All the above
   e. Both *b* and *c*

6. A prescription is –2.00 –1.25 × 30. Which of the following *two* power wheel readings appear when first sphere, then cylinder lines, are brought into focus?

    a. –2.00
    b. –0.75
    c. –3.25
    d. –1.25
    e. +0.75

7. True or False? When the lensmeter is used to neutralize a lens of unknown power and obtain results directly in plus cylinder form, the power wheel is turned into the high minus numbers and slowly moved in the plus direction until the cylinder lines first are brought into sharp focus.

8. The lensmeter power wheel is turned into the high plus power. The power wheel is then turned back slowly, reducing plus power until the sphere lines are clear. (The power wheel now reads +2.00 D; the axis wheel reads 12.) The power wheel is then turned further into the minus until the cylinder lines become clear. (This causes the power wheel to reads –1.00.) Which of the following is the prescription?

    a. +2.00 –1.00 × 12
    b. –1.00 +2.00 × 12
    c. +2.00 –1.00 × 102
    d. +2.00 –3.00 × 12
    e. –1.00 +2.00 × 12

9. The lensmeter power wheel is turned into the high plus power and slowly returned until the *cylinder* lines are clear. (The power wheel reads +4.00 D; the axis wheel reads 180.) The power wheel is turned further into the minus until the *sphere* lines become clear. (The power wheel reads +3.00 D.) Although this is not the correct procedure for lensmeter use, which of the following is the prescription?

    a. +4.00 –1.00 × 90
    b. +4.00 –3.00 × 180
    c. +4.00 –1.00 × 180
    d. +3.00 –1.00 × 90
    e. +3.00 –1.00 × 90

10. When a single vision lens is spotted for edging, in reference to *edged lens orientation*, the lensmeter ink dots will be on which of the following?

    a. The sphere meridian
    b. The cylinder meridian
    c. The 180-degree meridian
    d. The cylinder axis

11. True or False? When a lens is spotted by using plus cylinder notation instead of minus cylinder notation, the lens is turned 90 degrees from where it would otherwise be located.

12. By convention, lenses in the finishing laboratory normally are marked for right *(R)* or left *(L)* on which of the following?

    a. Outside surface, in mirror image, on the upper half
    b. Inside surface, on the lower half
    c. Inside surface, on the upper half
    d. Outside surface, on the lower half
    e. Outside surface, on the upper half

13. True or False? Lenses should never be placed convex-side-down in the job tray.

14. True or False? Lenses are placed convex-side-up in the laboratory tray. The wearer's right lens will be in the lower left half of the tray and the left lens in the lower right half of the tray.

15. For high cylinders in which either the lensmeter sphere or the cylinder lines are visible one group at a time, but not simultaneously, the MRP is found by which of the following?

    a. Centering on the sphere line
    b. Centering on the center cylinder line
    c. Alternately centering on first the sphere line, then on the center cylinder line
    d. Using a lens center locator
    e. Cannot be found by any of the above methods

16. Which of the following points should *always* appear either exactly in front of (or somewhat below) the wearer's pupil?

    a. OC
    b. DBC
    c. Geometric center
    d. MRP
    e. IOP

17. If no prescribed prism is in the prescription, which one of the following points is not the same?

    a. OC
    b. MRP
    c. PRP
    d. NRP

18. For which of the following prescriptions is there a difference in the physical location of the OC and the MRP? (There may be more than one correct response.)

    a. −4.00 D sphere
    b. −4.00 −2.00 × 180
    c. −4.00 D sphere with 0.5Δ base-in prism
    d. −4.00 −2.00 × 180 with 0.5Δ base-up prism
    e. The OC and MRP are synonymous terms and therefore are always at the same point on a lens.

19. True or False? Use of an autolensmeter to spot lenses requires no presetting of the instrument.

20. True or False? With use of most autolensmeters to prepare a lens for edging, the lens is still spotted with three dots, as with a manual lensmeter.

21. A flat-top bifocal is spotted for the MRP. It is immediately evident that the three lensmeter dots are *not* parallel to the segment line. In which prescription is this instance of no consequence?

    a. It is *always* of consequence.
    b. −1.00 −1.00 × 180
    c. pl −1.00 × 70 (*pl* denoting a "plano," or zero power)
    d. −2.25 D sphere

22. True or False? The spotting of blended bifocals is done in the same manner as the spotting of round-segment bifocals.

23. Which of the following is the standard vertical position of the lens MRP?

    a. 3 mm above the horizontal midline of the lens (The horizontal midline is in the middle of the frame B dimension.)
    b. On the horizontal midline of the lens
    c. 3 mm below the horizontal midline of the lens
    d. No standard vertical position exists.

24. True or False? If the MRP "disappears" into the segment, the lensmeter power wheel is refocused so that the target lines come into view through the segment. The MRP, which "vanished," can now be found and spotted.

25. True or False? Spotting a premarked progressive addition lens is done only for verification purposes. The centration process that follows can be accomplished by use of the marks already on the lens.

26. True or False? "Invisible" markings are found on progressive addition lenses. These markings allow the MRP and near portions of the lens to be located exactly.

27. The distance power for a progressive addition lens is verified at which of the following?

    a. OC
    b. MRP
    c. NRP
    d. PRP
    e. DRP

28. Horizontal and vertical prismatic effect for a progressive addition lens is verified at which of the following?

    a. NRP
    b. PRP
    c. DRP

Challenge Questions

29. How far from the MRP must the OC be moved to create the proper prismatic effect by decentration for the following lens?

    +1.50 −1.50 × 90 0.5Δ base out

    a. 3.33 mm
    b. 30 mm
    c. 0 mm
    d. There is no optical "center" for this lens.

30. How far from the MRP must the OC be moved to create the proper prismatic effect by decentration for the following lens?

    $$+1.50 \ +1.50 \times 90 \ 0.5\Delta \text{ base out}$$

    (Notice the plus cylinder form of the prescription.)

    a. 1.67 mm
    b. 3.33 mm
    c. 0 mm
    d. The distance cannot be figured from the measurements provided.

31. The prescription is R: –6.00 D sphere 1.0Δ base out. The lens is in the lensmeter (convex side facing the operator) with the lensmeter target exactly centered. In which of the following directions must the lens be moved before it may be correctly spotted?

    a. It is correct as is and need not be moved.
    b. Operator's left
    c. Operator's right
    d. Up
    e. Down

The following lenses are clear, single vision lenses. Which of the statements apply to each prescription? (*Note:* More than one answer may be appropriate.)

32. –4.25 –1.00 × 035

    a. After this lens has been spotted, it will be *unaffected* by any lens rotation around the center spot.
    b. After spotting, this lens will be *unaffected* if the lens is rotated exactly 180 degrees around the center spot.
    c. After spotting, this lens will be *affected* by any *lens* rotation.

33. –1.00 –2.00 × 018 2Δ base in

    a. After this lens has been spotted, it will be *unaffected* by any lens rotation around the center spot.
    b. After spotting, this lens will be *unaffected* if the lens is rotated exactly 180 degrees around the center spot.
    c. After spotting, this lens will be *affected* by any *lens* rotation.

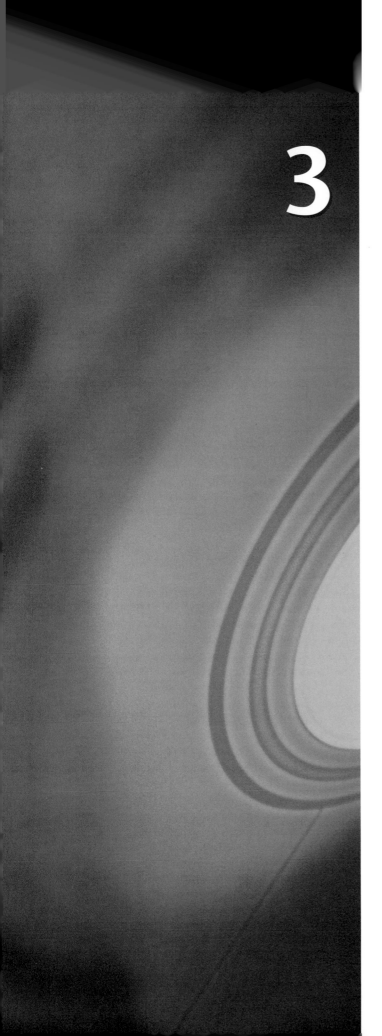

3 Lens Shapes, Patterns, and Frame Tracers

At some point in the lens finishing process, all details about the frame eyesize and shape must be established. A few years ago when the number of available frames was less extensive than it is today, each edging laboratory had a selection of *patterns* that was fairly inclusive of available frame shapes (Figure 3-1). A pattern duplicates the shape of the frame area into which the lens is to be placed.

With the large number of ever-changing frames available, a correct pattern is unavailable more often. To solve the problem the laboratory personnel need to either have a *pattern maker* and make those missing patterns in house or use a frame tracer with a pattern-less edger. A *frame tracer* is like a pattern maker, except that a physical pattern in not produced. The tracer makes a digitized version of the pattern.

A *patterned edger* requires a pattern to edge a lens. A *patternless edger* uses a digitized version of a frame shape to guide the edger. In either case, understanding lens shapes, patterns, and frame tracers relies on knowledge of the basic terminology and standards of frame and lens measurement.

The Boxing System of Lens Measurement

The *boxing system* of lens and frame measurement determines horizontal and vertical lens shape measurements. The smallest possible box is drawn around the lens shape that will enclose the lens completely. The lens shape touches the top, bottom, left, and right sides of the lens or lens shape as shown in Figure 3-2.

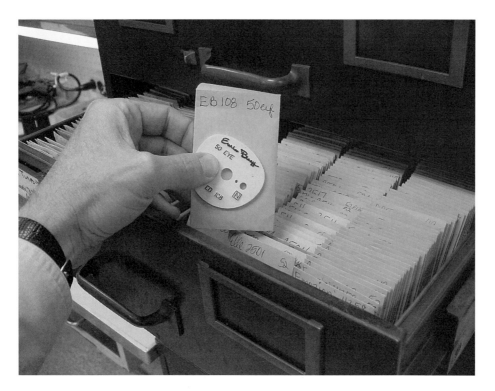

FIGURE **3-1** With new frames coming onto the market at a rapid pace, keeping patterns in stock can be challenging. Maintaining a stock of patterns can be tedious and time-consuming and requires physical space.

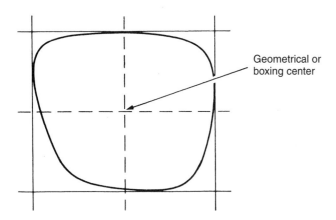

Geometrical or boxing center

FIGURE **3-2** The boxing system bases horizontal and vertical frame shape sizes on the smallest rectangle that completely encloses the shape. The center of that rectangle is the geometrical or boxing center.

HORIZONTAL LENS SIZE

The horizontal size as determined by the box is called the *A dimension* (Figure 3-3) or the *eyesize*. Unfortunately not all frames are marked with an eyesize equal to the A dimension. When calculations are done to determine correct placement of the lens optical center for edging, the A dimension must be known. Using a marked eyesize different from the A dimension results in edging errors.

A common but inaccurate method for measurement of the eyesize of a frame is to measure the width of the frame's lens shape across the center of the lens shape. In certain cases, such as with round or oval frames, this measurement may be equal to the A dimension of the frame. But often this measurement is less than the frame's A dimension. This measurement of lens width at the center of the frame has its own name. It is called the *C dimension*.[1] The C dimension is defined in the boxing system but is not used for lens fabrication purposes.

VERTICAL LENS SIZE

The vertical size as determined by the box is called the *B dimension*. Vertical lens size is needed for correct placement of the optical center for certain types of single vision lenses, bifocal or trifocal height for

---

[1]The C dimension should not be confused with the C size of a lens shape. The C size is the distance around the outside of the lens shape, similar to the circumference of a circle.

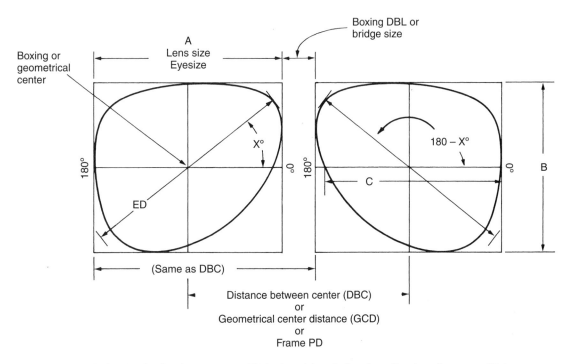

FIGURE 3-3 In the boxing system, *ED* is the abbreviation for effective diameter. ED is twice the longest radius of the shape as measured from the boxing (geometrical) center. The angle from the 0-degree side of the 180-degree line to the effective diameter axis is X for the right lens. The ED is used in accurate calculation of the minimum lens blank size and lens thickness required to fabricate the prescription.

segmented multifocals, and fitting cross height for progressive addition lenses.

HORIZONTAL MIDLINE

The horizontal line passing through the middle of the boxed lens shape halfway between the top and the bottom is known variously as *the 180 line, the datum line,* or *the horizontal midline.*

BOXING CENTER

The center of the boxed lens is called the *boxing center.* It is at the intersection of the horizontal and vertical midlines of the lens. An easier "on paper" way to find the boxing center is to draw corner-to-corner diagonals across the box (Figure 3-4). Another name for the boxing center is the *geometrical center of the edged lens.*

EFFECTIVE DIAMETER

Determining the boxing center of the lens shape makes it possible to find the smallest unedged round lens that could be edged successfully to this shape if the center of that round lens were at the boxing center. This diameter

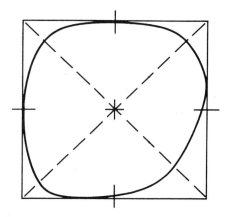

FIGURE 3-4 The geometrical (boxing) center of a pattern or lens is always at the center of the enclosing box, regardless of where pattern holes are drilled or MRPs are placed.

is called the *effective diameter* and is abbreviated *ED.* The ED is found by location of the longest distance from the boxing center to the edge of the lens shape (Figure 3-5, *A*). Next this line is extended an equal amount in the opposite direction (doubled; Figure 3-5, *B*). In other words, the ED is twice the longest radius of the lens shape as measured from the boxing center.

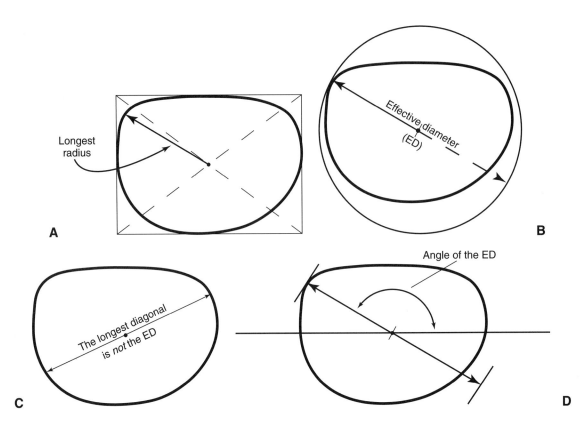

FIGURE **3-5** **A,** To determine the effective diameter (ED) of a lens shape, the practitioner should begin by finding the longest radius from the boxing center to the edge of the lens shape. **B,** Next, that radius is doubled. This is the effective diameter. The ED corresponds to the smallest lens that will completely cover the lens shape before any decentration has occurred. **C,** A common way, but a wrong way, of measuring ED is to measure the longest diagonal of the lens shape. **D,** The angle of the ED is referenced to the right lens and is measured from the horizontal in a counterclockwise manner.

The ED is *not* the longest diagonal of the frame shape (Figure 3-5, *C*). This is the most common *wrong* method of measuring the ED and gives an answer that may be close or at times even equal to the ED but is not really the ED. In some cases it can be considerably different from the true effective diameter. This wrong method is commonly used because no easy way exists to directly measure the ED on a real frame.

ANGLE OF THE EFFECTIVE DIAMETER

As stated previously, when finding the effective diameter for a given lens shape, the practitioner may draw a line from the boxing center to the point on the lens edge farthest from the boxing center. That line is extended equally in the exact opposite direction. The ED line crosses the horizontal midline at an angle. That angle is measured using the right lens. The angle measurement begins from the right side of the horizontal midline of the lens and is called the *angle of the ED* (Figure 3-5, *D*). The angle of the ED is important during the surfacing

process. Knowing the angle of the ED enables the laboratory to grind the lens as thin as possible.[2]

DISTANCE BETWEEN LENSES

Each frame has a measurable distance between lenses (DBL). In the boxing system, the DBL is basically the shortest distance between those lenses. It can be visualized as the distance between the two boxes when those boxes are drawn around each lens in the pair (see Figure 3-3). The DBL also is called the *bridge size*. Like eyesize, the bridge size marked on the frame may not correspond to the bridge size needed in the fabrication of a pair of lenses.

The most common mistake made in measurement of the DBL is to measure the distance between the edges of the lenses along the horizontal midline of the lens (Figure 3-6).

[2]For additional information see Brooks CW: *Understanding lens surfacing,* Boston, 1992, Butterworth-Heinemann.

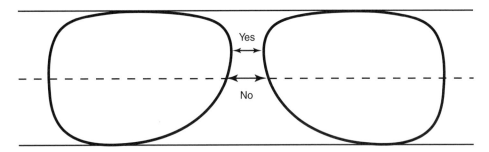

FIGURE **3-6**   The *distance between lenses* is the shortest distance between right and left lenses. It is not the distance between the two lenses along the horizontal midline of the lens.

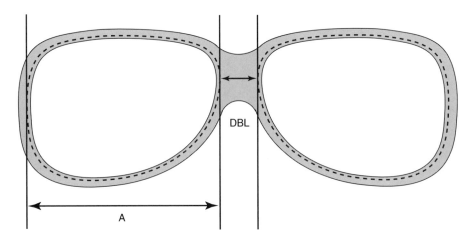

FIGURE **3-7**   When the A dimension and distance between lenses (DBL) are measured on a frame that has a groove for the lens bevel, measurements are taken from the deepest part of the groove.

Measuring the A Dimension and Distance between Lenses on a Grooved Frame

When a practitioner measures the A dimension and DBL of a normal frame with a groove to hold the lenses in place, the starting and ending points are where the beveled lens edges are located. If the groove is a deep groove in a plastic frame, then where does the measurement begin? It does *not* begin at the inside edge of the plastic lens rim. It begins at the deepest part of the groove (Figure 3-7).

GEOMETRICAL CENTER DISTANCE

For a frame or pair of lenses, the distance between the two boxing centers commonly is known as the *geometrical center distance*, or *GCD*. It is called the *geometrical center distance* because the boxing center is also the geometrical center of the edged lens.

The GCD has several other names. One of the most common is *distance between centers*, or *DBC*. A third name is the *frame PD*. *PD* is short for pupil distance or *interpupillary distance*. A PD technically refers only to a person's pupils. Frames do not have pupils and cannot really have PDs. Yet the term *frame PD* is used extensively to mean the GCD. Unfortunately, adding still more to the confusion, this measurement has two other names. These synonyms are the *frame center distance* and *boxing center distance*. So the GCD also can be called the *distance between centers*, the *frame PD*, the *frame center distance*, and the *boxing center distance*.

The distance between centers may be found by adding the A dimension to the DBL (Figure 3-8). It also may be found by directly measuring the frame as shown in Figure 3-9.

MAJOR REFERENCE POINT, FITTING CROSS, AND SEGMENT HEIGHTS

The standard vertical position for the major reference point (MRP) of a spectacle lens is on the horizontal midline of the frame. However, the practitioner may request that the MRP be placed at a different vertical

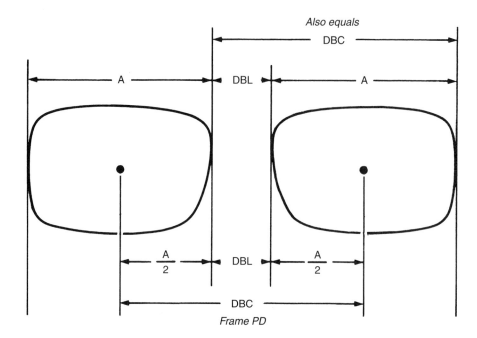

FIGURE 3-8 It can be seen from the figure that the distance between the two centers (DBC) is the same as the A dimension (eyesize) plus the distance between lenses (DBL; bridge size). Because the DBC cannot be directly measured, it may be measured as shown in the upper right-hand corner of the figure.

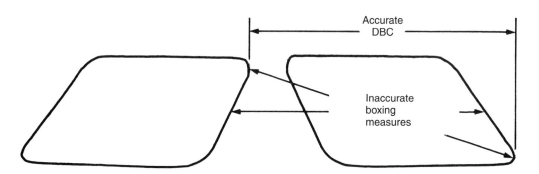

FIGURE 3-9 Measure each of the illustrated dimensions in the figure. Large variations occur between the accurately and inaccurately measured distances.

location. This request is based on the vertical location of the wearer's eyes with reference to the frame. When a practitioner asks for a specific MRP height, that height will be equal to the distance from the lowest point on the lens (the bottom line of the box) up to the desired location of the MRP (Figure 3-10, *A*). MRP height is *not* the distance from the lens edge directly below the MRP to the desired location. This is also shown in Figure 3-10, *A*, and is the most common mistake made when measuring MRP height.

The vertical position of the fitting cross of a progressive addition lens (Figure 3-10, *B*) or the top of a segmented multifocal (Figure 3-10, *C*) is measured in the same way as the MRP is measured. Both are

measured from the level of the lowest point on the lens or the deepest position of the inside bevel of the frame's eyewire.

Pattern Measurements and Terminology

Patterns allow an edger to duplicate the desired lens shape for a specific frame. Their shape and size are critical for the correct duplication of lens shapes. Therefore to maintain accuracy, a standard method of measuring patterns is essential.

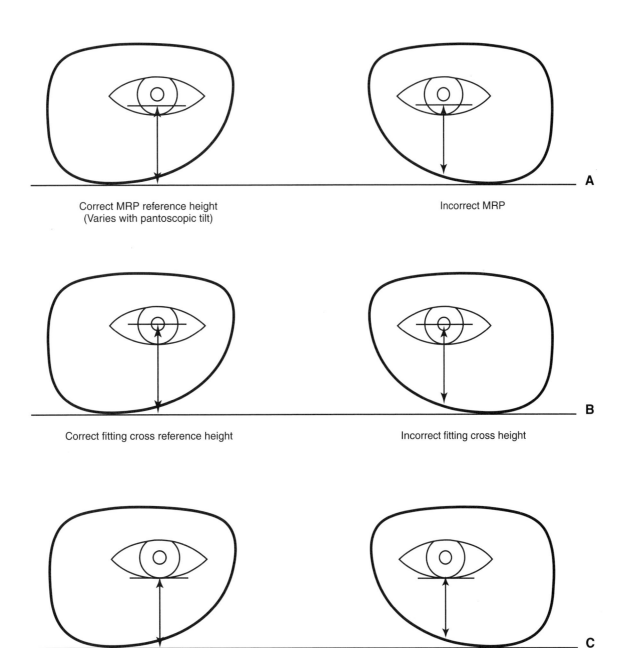

Correct MRP reference height
(Varies with pantoscopic tilt)

Incorrect MRP

A

Correct fitting cross reference height

Incorrect fitting cross height

B

Correct bifocal reference height

Incorrect bifocal height

C

FIGURE **3-10** Reference heights for the major reference point (MRP), progressive addition lens fitting cross, and segmented multifocal height are from the lowest point on the lens. Reference heights are not from the point on the lens directly below the pupil. **A,** The MRP height, when specified, is first measured from the level of the lowest portion of the lens up to the center of the pupil, as shown in **B.** Then 1 mm of height is subtracted for each 2 degrees of pantoscopic tilt, as illustrated in **A** (up to a maximum of 5 mm). (For more information on measuring MRP heights, see Brooks CW, Borish IM: *System for ophthlamic dispensing,* ed 2, Boston, 1996, Butterworth-Heinemann, pp 62–69.) **B,** The fitting cross height for progressives is measured from the level of the lowest portion of the lens up to the center of the pupil. It is not measured from the lower edge of the lens directly below the pupil, as this may not be the lowest point on the lens edge. **C,** Bifocal heights are measured from the level of the lowest portion of the lens up to the lower limbus. The limbus is the place where the cornea ends and the white sclera of the eye begins. It is often at the same location as the lower lid. Again, it is not measured from the lower edge of the lens directly below the pupil.

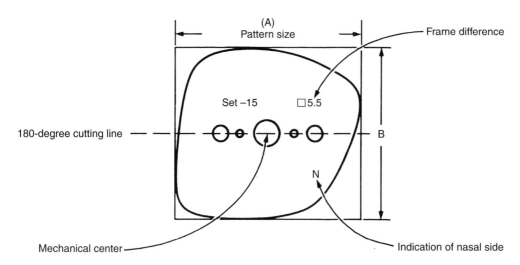

FIGURE **3-11**   The same system of measurement as is used for frames and lenses is also used for patterns. Patterns do not come with A and B dimensions marked. But they do have a pattern set number to help in finding the correct edger setting. The "frame difference" helps in positioning MRP and multifocal heights when the laboratory does not have the frame.

PATTERN SIZE

To determine pattern size, a pattern must be positioned exactly in the same orientation as the frame shape when the frame is held horizontally; in other words, the pattern may not be rotated at an angle. The pattern shape then is enclosed in a box by four tangent lines according to the same boxing system as used for frames and lenses. The perpendicular lines used for boxing in a pattern must be perfectly horizontal and vertical, and each side of the box must touch the pattern, as shown in Figure 3-11. As with frames and lenses, the pattern size for the boxing system is the distance between the two vertical sides of the box. It is *not* the width of the pattern along the center 180 line. Boxing pattern size corresponds to the frame eyesize or A dimension. The vertical dimension of the pattern is measured vertically between the top and bottom of the box and corresponds to the B dimension of the frame. A or B dimensions may not be measured with the ruler held at an angle. Neither may a pattern be measured if it is in a rotated position.

The use of some sort of eyesize gauge may result in pattern measurements (Figure 3-12, *A*) *if* the sides of the measuring portions are high enough to enclose the outermost portions on left and right sides. This same gauge can be used to measure lenses (Figure 3-12, *B*) and other objects. Even with such a handheld gauge, the possibility of a slight rotation of the pattern occurs. Many practitioners choose to use a Box-o-Graph (Kosh Manufacturing Co., Ft. Lauderdale, Fla.) for pattern

and lens size measurements. The Box-o-Graph is shown in Figure 3-13. A Box-o-Graph helps to be certain that no rotation has occurred. It does not give enough accuracy to ensure first-cut sizing when edging but is considerably more accurate than a ruler.

MEASURING FRAME DIFFERENCE

The difference between the horizontal and vertical dimensions of the pattern is the *pattern difference.* Pattern difference has the same numerical value as frame difference. As would be expected, the frame difference is the difference between frame A and B dimensions (Figure 3-14). Therefore the term *frame difference* is used synonymously with *pattern difference.*

Expressed as a simple equation, this takes the following form:

$$A - B = \text{Frame difference}$$

The frame difference number is often printed on the pattern (see Figure 3-11) and does not change, even when the pattern is used to cut out lenses of different sizes.

EFFECT OF EYESIZE CHANGES ON LENS SHAPE

Presumably when eyesize increases or decreases for a given frame style, frame difference should change proportionally. If the lens shape were to stay exactly the same, eyesize changes would result in a proportional change in frame difference.

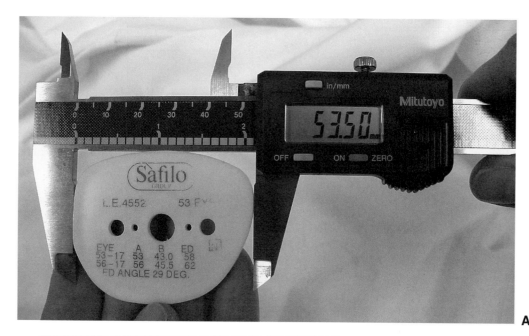

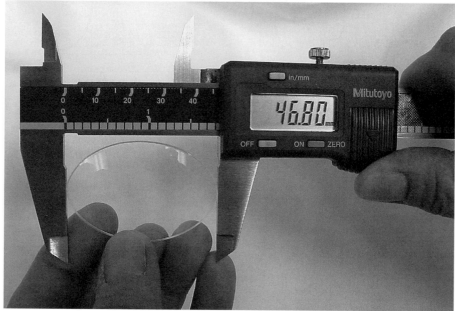

FIGURE **3-12** A pattern or a lens may be measured with a caliper. This particular caliper has a digital readout. To get the correct A dimension, the pattern or lens must have its 180 line parallel to the caliper bar. Turning the lens or pattern will change the measurement obtained. **A,** The caliper is measuring a pattern. The 180-degree line corresponding to the holes is (and should be) parallel to the caliper line. **B,** The A dimension of a lens is being measured with a caliper.

However, because of the way an edger works, each time the lens size is set higher by 1 millimeter, 0.5 millimeter is added to the original pattern shape. This 0.5 mm is added not just left and right in the horizontal direction but in every direction (Figure 3-15).

Example 3-1: The Way the System Works

A particular pattern is rectangular and has an A dimension of 36.5 mm and a B dimension of 26.5 mm. This pattern is put on an edger. If the edger is set to cut a lens having an eyesize of 46.5, what will be the vertical dimension of the edged lens?

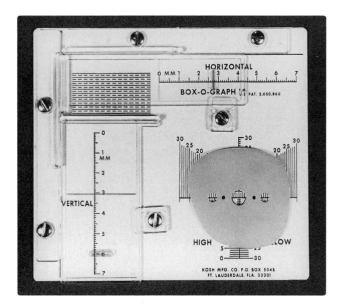

FIGURE **3-13** A pattern may be measured on the Box-o-Graph (Kosh Manufacturing Co., Ft. Lauderdale, Fla.) by placing it over the centrally marked circles to assure horizontal and vertical alignment. The A dimension is the sum of the farthest left and right measures. If only A and B dimensions are needed (and not a check on the accuracy of central hole placement, as shown here), the measurements may be taken in the same manner as with lenses, placing the pattern in the upper left-hand corner of the Box-o-Graph. The pattern holes must nevertheless be perfectly horizontal.

Solution

The newly cut lens will be 10 mm larger in the A dimension than the pattern. Five millimeters have been added to each side of the lens. Because 5 mm also will be added above and 5 mm below the top and bottom edges of the pattern size, the new B_1 lens dimension will be 10 mm larger than the pattern B dimension was. The new B_1 lens dimension will be 36.5 mm. Although this may look more nearly proportional when the two are superimposed as shown in Figure 3-16, the two rectangles are not the same shape.

The phenomenon of nonproportionality occurs with use of a pattern that is not the same size as the lens to be edged. The difference is more obvious the larger the difference between pattern size and actual edged lens size. Therefore use of a pattern that is as close in size to the desired finished lens as possible is advantageous.

For this reason some manufacturers provide different patterns for frames of different eyesize ranges in the same frame design. Others may furnish one size pattern only, but they overcome the problem by manufacturing frames that differ slightly in proportionality from size to size. In this manner any sized lens that is edged with the pattern provided by the manufacturer still fits any eyesize frame.

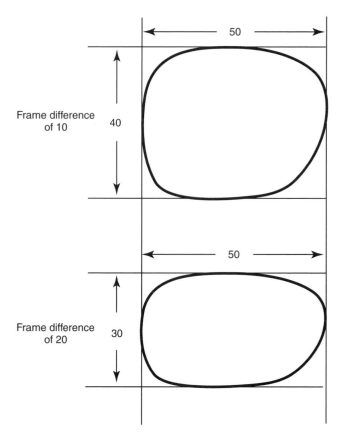

FIGURE **3-14** The difference between the horizontal and vertical measurements of a frame is known as the *frame difference*.

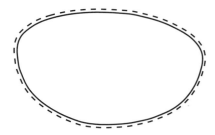

FIGURE **3-15** In the figure, as the horizontal eye (A dimension) increases by 2 mm; the lens increases in size by 1 mm in every direction.

Calculations Based on Frame Difference

Any group of frames capable of having lenses edged from one pattern will, regardless of eyesize, all have the same frame difference. (Frame difference is equal to A − B.) The frame difference number should be marked on the pattern. This marking is for the convenience of the operator during the multifocal lens layout process.

To calculate segment drop or raise, the B dimension of the frame must be known. If the B dimension of the frame to be used is not known, it must be either

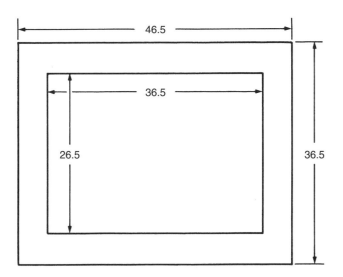

FIGURE **3-16** In this drawing the outer square is created from the inner "pattern." It is not the same shape even though the "frame difference" remains at 10 mm. However, this is the way shapes change when lens sizes increase or decrease using a lens pattern. To be the same shape, both dimensions of the rectangles would have to increase by equal proportions.

measured using the frame itself (if available) or calculated using the pattern as a basis. The B dimension of a lens is found by subtracting the frame difference stamped on the pattern, from the lens eyesize.

Example 3-2

A "lenses only" order must be completed for a frame having an eyesize of 48. The frame is not available at the laboratory. Bifocal height has been specified as 18 mm (Figure 3-17). The frame difference measurement on the pattern is stamped □4.5. (This means that the pattern is made for the boxing system and, according to that system, the difference of A – B is 4.5 mm.) How much segment drop or raise is required?

Solution

Segment drop is the distance from the horizontal midline of the edged lens shape to the top of the bifocal line. To calculate segment drop, the B dimension of the lens must be known. The B dimension is calculated as follows:

$$B = \text{Eyesize} - \text{Frame difference}$$

In this case frame difference will be as follows:

$$B = 48 - 4.5$$
$$= 43.5 \text{ mm}$$

The distance from the horizontal midline of the lens shape to the bifocal line is a downward direction and is technically a negative number. Therefore it is calculated as follows:

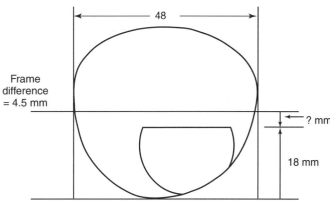

FIGURE **3-17** If segment height, eyesize (A dimension), and frame difference are known, segment drop (or raise) may be found. This is also true in the location of the major reference point or progressive lens fitting cross raise.

$$\text{Segment drop} = \text{Segment height} - \frac{B}{2}$$
$$= 18 - \frac{43.5}{2}$$
$$= -3.75 \text{ mm}$$

So the segment drop will be about 4 mm below the horizontal midline of the lens shape.

(If the frame difference had not been marked on the pattern, it could still have been found by measuring both A and B pattern dimensions with a ruler, a measuring gauge, or a Box-o-Graph.)

MECHANICAL CENTER OF THE PATTERN

No matter how carefully a lens is marked, unless the pattern is accurately made, the optical center of the edged lens will not end up where it should. For the optical center to come out right, the mechanical center of the pattern must be placed correctly. The *mechanical center* of a pattern is the point on the pattern around which the pattern rotates. (Other names for the mechanical center are *rotational center, cutting center,* or *edging center.*) The mechanical center is easy to find because it is found in the middle of the large hole in the pattern (see Figure 3-11). The large hole is used to snap the pattern on the edger.

The horizontal line that passes through the mechanical center of the pattern is sometimes referred to as the *mounting line.*[3] When the mechanical center

---

[3]The mounting line of a pattern is not the same thing as the mounting line of a frame. The mounting line for a rimless frame is the line that passes through the points at which the pad arms are attached. The frame's mounting line serves as a line of reference for horizontal alignment during standard alignment of a frame.

and boxing center of a pattern are at the same location on the pattern, then the pattern's horizontal midline and the pattern's mounting line are also the same.

Positioning the Mechanical Center in the Pattern

The mechanical center is positioned in the pattern in the following two main ways:

1. The pattern is made so that the boxing center and mechanical center are at the same place on the pattern. This is the most common pattern construction. Patterns supplied by the frame manufacturer are made this way.
2. The pattern can be made so that the mechanical center (the large hole in the pattern) is moved intentionally away from the boxing center of the lens shape. This usually happens if the pattern is made for one specific person or one particular edging situation and will never be used for anyone else.

WHEN THE MECHANICAL CENTER IS AT THE BOXING CENTER

When a person wears a pair of glasses, the position of his or her eyes in relationship to the boxing center of the lens shape depends upon the distance between the person's pupils compared with the size of the frame. If the frame is large and the wearer's PD is small, the eyes are nasal to the boxing centers of the lens shape. No matter where the pupils are, the major reference point of the lens should be in front of the pupil.

To be more exact, when the wearer is looking into the distance, the pupil usually is slightly above the major reference point. In other words, the major reference point of the lens should be in the same vertical plane as the wearer's pupil (Figure 3-18). If no prescribed prism is in the prescription, the optical center and MRP are exactly the same.

Centration Process
In the edging process, a lens is first spotted to mark the MRP. The three dots on the lens are reference points to help position the lens in the frame.

The lens must be attached to a block for edging (Figure 3-19, *A*). The block holds the lens in place while it is being edged. If the center dot (MRP) on the dotted lens is placed at the center of the lens block, after the lens is edged the MRP will correspond to the boxing center of the edged lens (Figure 3-19, *B*).

If MRP is at the boxing center of the edged lens, but

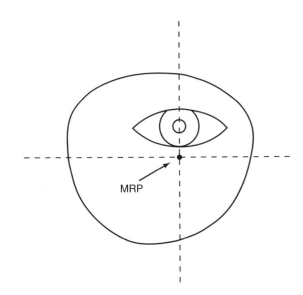

FIGURE **3-18** The standard horizontal major reference point (MRP) location of a single vision lens is on the horizontal midline. It should be in the same vertical plane as the wearer's pupil.

the wearer's eye is not, the position of the lens on the block was not correct. If the wearer's eye is in the nasal half of the frame's lens opening, the prespotted lens has to be moved away from the center of the block and toward the nose so that it will end up in front of the eye (Figure 3-20).

Centration and Decentration
The process of moving a lens so that it will be in front of the eye is called *centration*. To center the lens in front of the eye, the lens must be moved *away* from a given reference point. When a lens is moved away from a given point it is said to be *decentered* from that point. In this case, the lens is moved away from or *decentered* from the location of the mechanical and boxing centers. Taking great care during this process is important because the slightest error results in an inaccurate finished product.

CALCULATION OF HORIZONTAL DECENTRATION WITH THE BOXING SYSTEM

The first part of the centration process involves figuring out exactly where the eye will be in relationship to the boxing center of the edged lens. If the boxing center and the eye are not in the same location, the lens will have to be decentered. The distance and direction of this decentration must be calculated to ensure that the lens optics will be positioned properly before the eye.

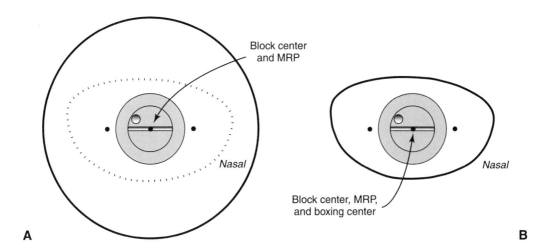

FIGURE **3-19** **A,** A finishing lens block is attached to the lens so that it will be held securely in place during edging. In this case, there is no decentration. The major reference point (MRP) of the lens is right at the center of the lens block. **B,** When edged, the normal position of the block is at the boxing center of the edged lens. In this instance no decentration occurred. The MRP is also at the boxing center. If the A + DBL of the frame equals the wearer's interpupillary distance (PD), the edged lens would be positioned correctly.

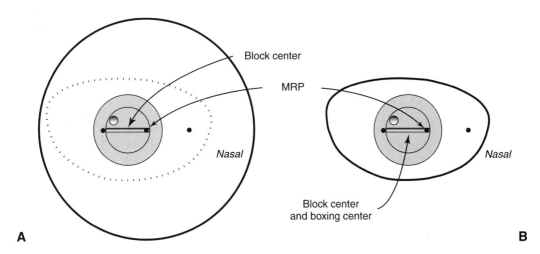

FIGURE **3-20** **A,** Here the lens has been decentered from the location of the block center so that the major reference point (MRP) will be centered in front of the pupil. **B,** Once the lens is edged, the MRP is located in the nasal half of the edged lens and should correspond to the location of the pupil.

Two measurements are required in the calculation of decentration. The first measurement is how far apart the person's pupil centers are from each other. This is called the binocular[4] *interpupillary distance* (PD). The second measurement is the distance between the geometrical (boxing) centers of the frame's two lens openings. This is called the *distance between centers* (DBC), or *frame PD*.

Determinating the Distance between Centers

For frames that conform to the boxing system of measurement, the DBC is equal to the eyesize (abbreviated A) plus the DBL. This is true because the geometrical center is located halfway across each lens opening.

Because the A dimensions of right and left lenses are equal the following equation is used:

---

[4]Decentration may be based on how far the eyes are from one another (the *binocular PD*), or the distance may be figured for each eye separately. The distance of each eye from the center of the bridge measured separately is called the *monocular PD*. Monocular PDs will be covered later.

$$DBC = \frac{\text{Right lens A dimension}}{2} + DBL +$$

$$\frac{\text{Left lens A dimension}}{2}$$

$$= DBC = A + DBL$$

This concept was shown in Figure 3-8.

If the frame is available, the DBC can be measured on the frame. The practitioner starts at the most nasal point on the right lens opening and measures on a straight horizontal to the vertical plane of the most temporal point on the left lens opening. This was shown in Figure 3-9. Because one of these two edge points may be higher or lower than the other, simply measuring in the middle of the frame may not be accurate.

DECENTRATION PER LENS USING BINOCULAR DISTANCE PDS

Most commonly the wearer's PD will be less than the frame PD (DBC). This requires that the lenses be decentered inward (nasally) toward the center of the frame. The amount of decentration per lens can be determined by subtracting the wearer's PD from the DBC (frame PD) and dividing by two.

$$\text{Decentration per lens} = \frac{DBC - \text{Wearer PD}}{2}$$

Decentration (or decentration per lens) refers to the amount one lens is moved. *Total decentration* refers to the sum of both left and right decentrations. Therefore the following equation is used:

$$\text{Total decentration} = DBC - \text{Wearer PD}$$

Example 3-3

The order form indicates that the wearer's PD is 64 mm. The frame size is 53 □ 17. In other words, the eyesize is 53 mm and the DBL 17 mm. The □ symbol indicates that the dimensions are listed according to the boxing system. If the frame is known to conform to boxing measure standards, what is the decentration per lens required?

Solution

To determine initially the difference between the DBC and wearer's PD, the practitioner must know the DBC. By definition, the following is true:

$$DBC = A + DBL$$

Because

$$A = 53 \text{ mm}$$

and

$$DBL = 17 \text{ mm}$$

then

$$DBC = 53 + 17$$
$$= 70 \text{ mm}$$

The following equation is true:

$$\text{Decentration per lens} = \frac{DBC - PD}{2}$$

In this instance the following applies:

$$\frac{70 - 64}{2} = \frac{6}{2} = 3 \text{ mm per lens}$$

(In the unusual case where the wearer's PD was greater than the DBC, a negative decentration would result from the calculations. A negative number indicates that decentration outward is required and the MRP of the lens would be decentered temporally.)

REASONS THE MECHANICAL CENTER OF THE PATTERN AND THE BOXING CENTER MAY DIFFER

As stated previously, pattern boxing and mechanical centers normally coincide so that the pattern hole is in the middle of the pattern. The following list states the four main reasons why the pattern hole (mechanical center) may not be in the center of the pattern:

1. The pattern was intended to be made with the mechanical center at the boxing center, but it was made incorrectly. The hole is simply not where it should be.
2. The pattern is of the old "raised center" type.
3. The pattern was made using some other system besides the boxing system.
4. The pattern is made so decentration does not have to be calculated and is useful for one specific person and one specific frame. (This idea will be discussed later in this chapter.)

Pattern Making

Because of the vast number of available frame styles, having a complete library of patterns so that the correct pattern is available for every frame presented for lens fabrication is impossible. Ordering a pattern for every single frame that passes through the laboratory is impractical. The delays caused would not be acceptable to the wearer, not to mention the volume of paperwork that would be generated. For this reason, when running

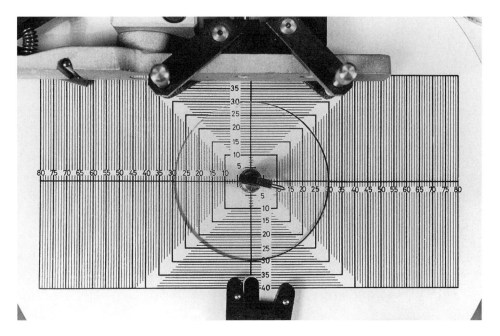

FIGURE **3-21** When a frame is centered on a pattern maker, the grid assists in alignment.

an edger that uses patterns, a system for making patterns is a necessity.

Systems for pattern making vary in methodology and cost, from a system that consists of a marking pen and pair of shears, up to models having automatic tracing systems. In spite of the variety of available products, certain commonalities exist for all systems.

FRAME SETUP FOR PATTERN MAKING

To make a pattern, either the frame must be on hand or, at the minimum, a labeled tracing from that frame. To make a pattern directly from a frame, all pattern makers require that the frame be positioned properly for tracing. The more advanced type of a pattern maker requires only that the frame be horizontally level. After the frame is traced, the pattern maker digitally determines the boxing center and places the mechanical center of the pattern there.

The more traditional pattern maker models require that one eye of the frame shape be centered carefully for tracing according to the boxing center. This is done so that the mechanical center of the pattern will end up corresponding to the boxing center of the lens shape.

The centering grid on a pattern maker may vary in its construction but basically consists of measured distances left, right, up, and down from an origin. This central origin represents the position that the mechanical (rotational) center of the pattern will occupy, as Figure 3-21 shows. The lens opening of the frame must then be centered so that the geometrical center of its

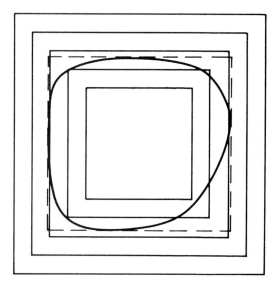

FIGURE **3-22** When a frame's lens opening is centered for pattern making according to the boxing system, the left extremity must be equal to the right; and the upper and lower extremities must also be equal.

shape is precisely at the middle of the grid origin. This is done, as in Figure 3-22, by making sure the outermost points to the left and right fall at the same distance from the origin. The uppermost and lowermost points also must be the same distance from the origin.

To actually carry out this procedure, the frame must be oriented initially with its frame front face down on a centering grid. To ensure that the horizontal midline of

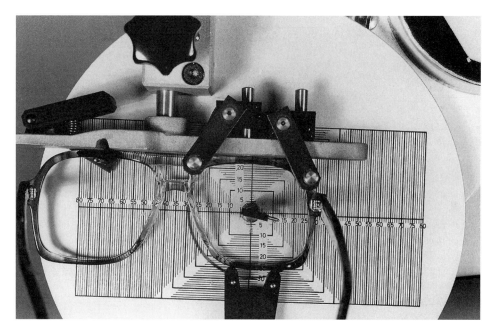

FIGURE **3-23** The horizontal bar on a pattern maker gives stability to the frame during the tracing process while simultaneously keeping it level. If tilted, a correct axis is not possible.

the pattern will correspond to the frame's horizontal midline and not be tilted, the top of the frame is pressed against a horizontal bar (Figure 3-23). This horizontal bar slides up and down but does not tilt. Tilting the frame causes an off-axis pattern, which makes it impossible to cut a cylinder lens for the correct axis. When centering is achieved, the frame is clamped securely into place and is ready for tracing.

Tracing may be accomplished by rotation of the mounted frame on the pattern maker while a stylus rests inside the frame groove. The stylus is linked mechanically to a cutting mechanism that uses a pantographic system to cut the pattern from a pattern blank. The pattern blank is marked with an *N*, indicating the nasal side. This blank should be placed in the pattern maker so that it indeed corresponds to the nasal side of the frame when cut.

Most "homemade" patterns are cut precisely for the size of the frame. This prevents shape distortion caused by large differences in pattern and finished lens sizes, as was described previously. Maintaining a one-to-one eyesize/pattern size ratio understandably may require the use of larger pattern blanks for certain frames. (Pattern blanks are shown in Figure 3-24.) Once the pattern is cut, it may require some smoothing of the edges, depending on the sophistication of the cutting mechanism. When smoothing is necessary, it may be accomplished with a medium-fine file. The practitioner should file only as much as necessary to remove roughness so that the basic shape or size is not changed.

MAKING A PATTERN FROM A LENS TRACING

Occasionally a special order lists no frame name but only a handmade tracing of the lens that is presently being worn in the frame. Such a request is difficult to fill properly. If the tracing is for a metal frame a bad fit is almost certain. With a plastic frame filling the request is possible but difficult. Even for a plastic frame such a request cannot be filled adequately unless certain specifications are given. These are the following:

- The size of the lens (The tracing is the same size as the lens. When a lens is traced, the tracing is naturally larger than the lens, or if the frame eyewire were traced, it is smaller.)
- The distance between lenses (DBL) to allow calculation for decentration
- The 180-degree line (If the lens is traced in an even slightly rotated position, the cylinder axis will be incorrect.)

Using a Similar Pattern
One possibility for filling such a request is to find a pattern that most closely approximates the shape and

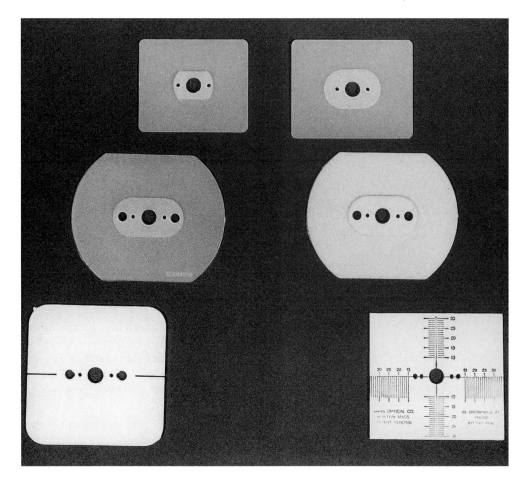

FIGURE **3-24** Pattern blanks come in a variety of shapes and sizes. When cutting patterns on a 1-to-1 ratio, the blank must be large enough to completely cover the frame's lens opening.

will not cut any corners from the required shape. If the pattern is an extra or will be unneeded in the future, it may be reshaped to match the tracing. If not, the lens is edged using the pattern that is close in shape to the drawing, then both edged lenses are reshaped by hand until correct. Each lens is held up to the tracing for comparison.

Making a Pattern to Match

Another method is first to mark carefully the horizontal midline on the tracing. Next a vertical line is drawn through the boxing center. Some pattern blanks already are marked with horizontal and vertical lines as was seen in Figure 3-24.

The tracing is cut out and placed on the pattern blank so that horizontal and vertical markings align, then it is traced with a marking pen. The marked shape is cut from the blank in the manner shown in Figure 3-25 and then smoothed on the edges as shown in Figure 3-26. Such a pattern should be checked for

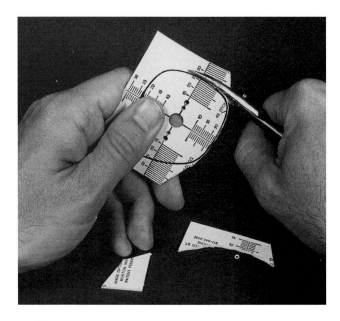

FIGURE **3-25** If a pattern is being cut by hand, curved cutting shears help to cut around corners.

center displacement to ensure accuracy of the PD and segment height. A method of checking for unwanted pattern center displacement is described later in the chapter in the section Checking for Pattern Errors.

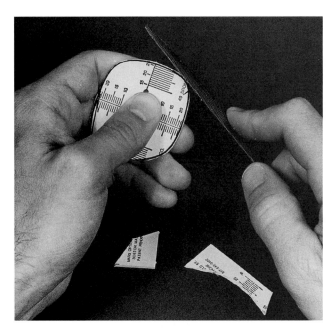

FIGURE **3-26** Smoothing pattern roughness with a file gives better size and shape. This is true not only for hand-cut patterns but also for some patterns made by a pattern cutter.

Recommended Laboratory Requirements for a By-Hand Lens Tracing

If a dispenser sends in a drawing of a wearer's lens traced around the actual lens, then the laboratory has a better chance of success by requesting the following:

- The A and B dimensions of the lens measured on the lens and not on the drawing
- The DBL, also measured using the frame
- A 180-degree line marked on the drawing
- An indication of the type of frame being used. Is the frame metal, plastic, grooved, other?
- An indication of whether the lens is a left or a right lens
- Preferably a circumference measure of the distance around the edged lens

The circumference of a lens is a much more sensitive measure of size than an A dimension. Lens circumference is sometimes called *C-size*. C-size is measured most easily with a circumference gauge (Figure 3-27). If both the dispenser and the laboratory use a circumference gauge, then size errors will be reduced. For those dispensers who send drawings of lenses, using millimeter graph paper will help considerably. A grid, with a form as shown in Figure 3-28, may be helpful to ensure all information is present.

For an electronically equipped laboratory, a much better alternative to lens drawings being sent is to have

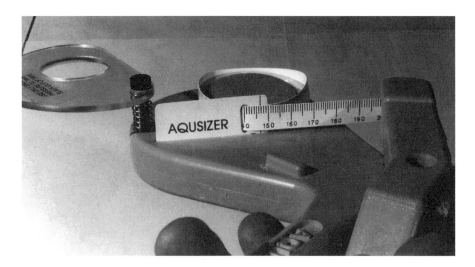

FIGURE **3-27** To measure the circumference of a lens, the lens is placed in the gauge front side up. The tape is closed around the lens and the circumference is read directly from the tape. (From Brooks CW, Borish IM: *System for ophthalmic dispensing*, ed 2, Boston, 1996, Butterworth-Heinemann.)

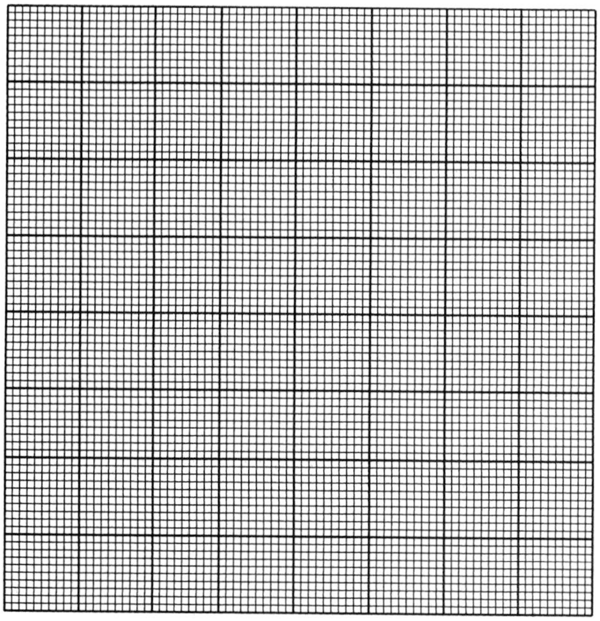

Frame Name _____

Frame Manufacturer _____

Men's/Women's (circle one)

A = _____   Measured DBL _____
                      (or measured frame PD _____)
B = _____

Len circumference = _____

Frame Material (check one)
Plastic _____   Metal _____
Rimless _____   (Grooved? Y/N)
Other _____

Lens traced is a (right/left) lens (circle one)
It is customary to trace the right lens

Right cylinder axis = _____
Left cylinder axis = _____
Right monocular PD = _____
Left monocular PD = _____

Measured pattern A dimension = _____
(Ordered lens size) − (pattern size) = _____
Calculated edger setting size = _____

FIGURE **3-28** An example of one type of form that may be used to trace a lens of unknown shape for a "lenses only" order. (From Brooks CW, Borish IM: *System for ophthalmic dispensing*, ed 2, Boston, 1996, Butterworth-Heinemann.)

the dispenser use a remote site frame tracer. This option prevents many potential problems and saves time. It is explained with the discussion of frame tracers found later in this chapter.

EDGERS THAT MAKE PATTERNS

One type of frame for which traditional pattern makers are usually not capable of making a pattern is a rimless frame. Examples of frames without eyewires include rimless, semirimless, and nylon cord frames. A rimless frame does not have an eyewire that may be traced. However, if a frame tracer is available, then most tracers can be adapted to trace an old lens or the sample lens that comes with the new frame.

If a frame tracer that also can trace lenses is not available, some edgers are capable of making a pattern. To make a pattern with an edger, first the right lens is spotted with the lensmeter while it is still in the frame. This preserves the correct horizontal "180-line" orientation after the lens is out of the frame. Next, the coquille or old lens is centered on a grid to find the boxing center. Using an adapter kit, the lens is clamped and then mounted on the edger as if it were a pattern.

A pattern blank is mounted on a special "lens" block, placed in the grinding chamber of the edger, and edged as if it were a lens.

The head pressure of the edger must be set at its lightest so as not to chip a lens or bend or break a coquille being used as a pattern.

Consequences of Using a Noncentered Pattern

Any calculations for decentering a lens are made on the assumption that the mechanical center of the pattern is at the boxing center of the pattern shape. So if the center of the pattern is off horizontally, the finished PD in the glasses will be off and will not match the wearer's PD. This can cause unwanted prismatic effect and difficulty in comfortably wearing the prescription.

In the same way, when the mechanical center of a pattern is above its geometrical or boxing center, the MRP of the edged lens will be above its boxing center.

If the pattern is off, the difference must either be compensated for, or the pattern should not be used.

USING A NONCENTERED PATTERN

Note: Some readers may wish to skip this section on non-centered patterns and return to it after familiarizing themselves with the centration of lenses presented in Chapters 4 through 6.

Mechanical Center

If the pattern's mechanical center is 3 mm above its boxing center, then the MRP of the edged lens will be 3 mm above the boxing center. Normally both lenses will be edged using the same pattern. Because both MRPs are high by the same amount, for most low-powered prescriptions this will not make much difference. Because both MRPs are elevated to the same level, no unwanted vertical prism will occur. Problems can occur if the MRP is specified, if the lenses are multifocals, or if just one lens is being edged.

Problems Resulting from the Replacement of Just One Lens

Having both lenses edged with a pattern in which the mechanical center is too high may result in future problems. For example, the wearer may return for an eye examination and needs only one lens replaced, or someone comes in with one lens badly scratched and needs a replacement. If the person who replaces the lens does not have the original pattern, a new one will be made according to standard centering methods. Unless a careful check is made, the replacement lens will be made with the MRP at the normal position. Now a difference exists in vertical height between left and right MRPs. This induces an unwanted vertical prismatic effect, which makes the prescription unacceptable.

This is why the MRP height of the nonreplaced lens always should be measured during the replacement process. By always checking vertical MRP height, the practitioner prevents any potential problem. If a difference does exist, the MRP of the new lens may be placed at the appropriate matching height.

If this careful check is not done and only the information given on the order is used, a discrepancy will exist in the vertical heights of the two lenses.

Immediate Multifocal Difficulties

When a pattern with the mechanical center vertically displaced is used to edge multifocals, failure to compensate can be disastrous. For instance, a pattern has a central hole (mechanical center) that is 3 mm higher than the boxing center. For bifocals whose desired height is specified as 18 mm, all calculations for segment drop are made on the assumption that this drop is occurring from the horizontal midline passing through the boxing center. Yet the blocked lens actually is centered 3 mm *above* the horizontal midline. Consequently, instead of having bifocals placed at 18 mm, the top of the bifocal line is at 21 mm.

Compensating for Vertically Displaced Pattern Centers

Compensation for either MRP positioning or multifocal height must be made at the time of lens centration and blocking. Once the lens is blocked, no more compensation is possible.

To compensate, the practitioner needs to know how much higher or lower the pattern's mechanical center is than it should be. In other words, the distance between the pattern boxing and mechanical centers must be known. The following four steps may be used to calculate this distance:

1. The pattern's B dimension is measured and divided by 2.
2. The vertical height of the pattern's mechanical center is measured. This is the distance from the lowest part of the pattern (bottom of the enclosing rectangle) to the mounting line crossing the pattern hole.
3. The result in step 1 is subtracted from the result in step 2. This gives the difference between geometrical and mechanical centers in millimeters.
4. If the mechanical center is high, the MRP or segment height is lowered by the amount found in step 3.

To summarize, if a pattern is made with the central hole too high, the whole lens will be positioned higher in the frame than it should be. To compensate the lens is lowered during layout. If the central hole is too low, the practitioner must raise the lens to compensate.

Example 3-4

During layout the pattern is checked. The central hole is found to be 3 mm above the boxing center. Pertinent prescription data are as follows:

Segment height = 20 mm
Segment style = Flat top 28
Frame B = 42 mm

What is the correct amount of segment raise or drop and how would the correctly positioned lens appear before marking?

Solution

First the practitioner calculates the segment raise or drop in the conventional manner and then compensates for the pattern.

$$\text{Segment raise or drop} = \text{Height} - \frac{B}{2}$$
$$= 20 - \frac{42}{2}$$
$$= 20 - 21$$
$$= -1 \text{ (a minus direction}$$
$$\text{denoting segment drop)}$$

Without compensation the segment would be dropped 1 mm. However, because of the pattern the segment ends up being raised an additional 3 mm. Therefore the segment must be decentered 3 mm lower than it otherwise would be during layout. (A downward direction is minus. So this means an additional −3 mm of vertical segment decentration is required.)

$$\text{Segment drop} = -1 + -3$$
$$= -4$$

Thus the segment is positioned 4 mm below the horizontal reference line and is ready for marking, as shown in Figure 3-29.

Compensating for Horizontally Displaced Pattern Centers

Despite careful setup for cutting patterns, errors can occur that cause a displacement of the pattern's central hole (mechanical center). Unfortunately, the amount of lateral displacement that occurs in the pattern will produce double the amount of error in the resulting PD. This occurs because the two lenses will be displaced in opposite directions. However, if the error is discovered before the lenses are blocked, an appropriate compensation may be made. This compensation is carried out in the same manner as in compensation for a vertically displaced pattern center.

Checking for Pattern Errors

To make any kind of compensation for central pattern hole displacement, the practitioner must first determine if a displacement has occurred. If a displacement has occurred, it is next determined how much that error is.

A simple system can even be made from a piece of centimeter/millimeter graph paper. A cross is drawn on the paper on the centimeter lines. Numbers may be added for ease of reference. Next a pattern is placed on the paper so that the central hole is in the middle of the cross. The other pattern holes should be lined up on the horizontal part of the cross (Figure 3-30). A pen or pencil is used to trace the circles on the paper. These circles must not be displaced and should be checked to ensure that they are absolutely centered.

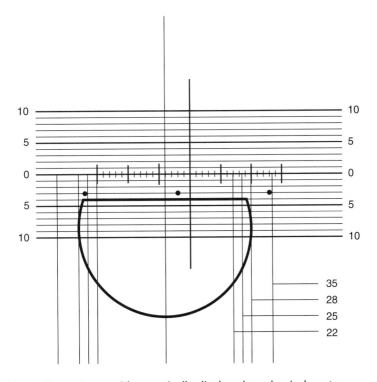

FIGURE **3-29** For patterns with a vertically displaced mechanical center, compensation in centration must occur. In the example shown, a segment drop of −1 mm is calculated, but the pattern's mechanical center is 3 mm above its boxing center. Therefore a −4 mm drop is required to achieve the expected segment height.

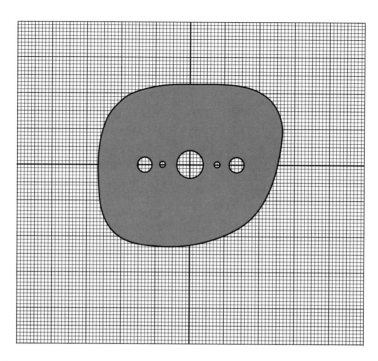

FIGURE **3-30**   A grid to check pattern size and central hole placement can be ordinary millimeter graph paper.

To check a homemade pattern, the pattern is placed on the completed sheet so that the holes in the pattern line up exactly with the drawn circles on the page. The outside edges of the pattern in each direction should be noted. For the pattern to pass as acceptable, top and bottom numbers must be identical. The numbers in the horizontal meridian to the far left and right also must match each other.

As may be remembered from an earlier section in this chapter, a homemade graph paper system is not the only available method for checking of pattern accuracy. A better system that uses identical methods is available on a Box-o-Graph. The Box-o-Graph was seen in Figure 3-13. The figure shows how to check a pattern for accuracy.

Determining Direction and Amount of Error

Once an error has been discovered, the amount of error and its direction must be determined. The easiest way to determine a horizontal error is to center the pattern's central hole on a grid.

In the vertical dimension, the distance above the central hole, plus the distance below the central hole is equal to the B dimension of the pattern. If the pattern is correct, the distances from the central hole to the top and to the bottom will be equal. The distance to the top minus the distance to the bottom should equal zero. If these distances are not equal, the difference between the two measures divided by two is the amount the central hole is off and equals the needed compensation. Expressed as a formula this would be written as follows:

$$\frac{\text{Top} - \text{Bottom}}{2} = \text{Vertical compensation required}$$

If the results are positive the lens must be raised to compensate for the pattern error; if negative, lowered. The same system applies to finding any needed horizontal compensation.

$$\frac{\text{Temporal} - \text{Nasal}}{2} = \text{Horizontal compensation}$$

Suppose the pattern is oriented as if it were a right lens. If the result is a positive number the mechanical center is displaced too far nasalward. This requires that the lens be decentered outward. However, if a negative number results, the mechanical center is too far temporalward. This requires that the lens be decentered inward. Box 3-1 provides a summary of compensation procedures, and Box 3-2 summarizes compensation direction.

Example 3-5

The pattern shown in Figure 3-31 is in error both vertically and horizontally. If this pattern is going to be used, what compensations would be necessary to ensure the accuracy of segment height and PD?

BOX 3-1
Determining the Amount of Compensation for Pattern Center Displacement

Vertical Pattern Dimension

1. The pattern is placed on grid or Box-o-Graph and the pattern's central hole is centered.
2. The grid is used to measure first the distance from the horizontal line to the highest part of the pattern and then the distance from the horizontal line to the lowest part of the pattern.
3. The difference is taken between these two numbers and divided by 2. This is the amount of compensation needed.
4. If the top is the largest measure, the compensating decentration must be upward. If the bottom is the largest measure, the compensation must be downward.

Horizontal Pattern Dimension

1. The pattern is placed on the grid or Box-o-Graph and the pattern's central hole is centered.
2. The grid is used to measure first the distance from the vertical line to the most temporal part of the pattern and then the distance from the vertical line to the most nasal part of the pattern.
3. The difference is taken between these two numbers and divided by 2. This is the amount of compensation needed.
4. If the temporal side is the largest measure, the compensating decentration must be outward or temporally. If the nasal side is the largest measure, the compensation must be inward or nasally.

Solution

Horizontal and vertical components are considered separately. To determine the vertical displacement of the mechanical center, the practitioner must note that it is 21 mm to the top of the pattern and 23 mm to the bottom. The hole is too high in the pattern. To figure how much the MRP or segment height must be lowered, the following equation is used:

$$\frac{\text{Top} - \text{Bottom}}{2} = \text{Vertical compensation required}$$

which in this case is as follows:

$$\frac{21 - 23}{2} = -1$$

This means that the lens MRP or segment height must be lowered 1 mm more than otherwise calculated.

For horizontal compensation, the temporal measurement is 25.5 mm and the nasal 26.5 mm. Therefore to find how far the pattern is off and how much compensation must be made for each lens, the following equation may be used:

$$\frac{25.5 - 26.5}{2} = -0.5 \text{ mm}$$

This means that the MRP must be decentered in by 0.5 mm. This is in addition to the amount of decentration normally required.

BOX 3-2
Pattern Center Displacement Compensation

IF THE LONGEST **VERTICAL** DISTANCE FROM THE CENTRAL PATTERN HOLE TO THE EDGE OF THE PATTERN IS...	THEN THE DIRECTION OF DECENTRATION TO COMPENSATE FOR THE ERROR MUST ALSO BE...	NOTE THAT THE CENTRAL PATTERN HOLE IS DISPLACED...
Downward	Downward (Lower the MRP or segment height.)	Upward
Upward	Upward (Raise the MRP or segment height.)	Downward
IF THE LONGEST **HORIZONTAL** DISTANCE FROM THE CENTRAL PATTERN HOLE TO THE EDGE OF THE PATTERN IS...	THEN THE DIRECTION OF DECENTRATION TO COMPENSATE FOR THE ERROR MUST ALSO BE...	NOTE THAT THE CENTRAL PATTERN HOLE IS DISPLACED...
Nasalward	Nasalward (The lens must be decentered inward more.)	Temporally
Temporalward	Temporalward (The lens must be decentered inward less.)	Nasally

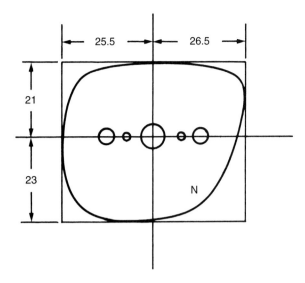

FIGURE **3-31** Were this pattern to be used for a multifocal prescription, the distance and near interpupillary distances (PDs) would both be 1 mm too wide. The segment height would also be a millimeter higher than anticipated.

Pattern Makers that Can Find the Center and Decenter

Pattern makers are similar to the frame tracers used with patternless edgers. (Frame tracers will be discussed shortly.) Much of frame tracing technology is based on principles used in previously existing pattern-making systems. Pattern makers can have some of the same smart features that frame tracers have. In fact, some pattern makers also double as frame tracers. These pattern makers may be hooked to a patternless edger and serve as a tracer or be used by themselves as a pattern maker.

A smart pattern maker can find the boxing center of the lens shape (Figure 3-32, *A*). If a pattern maker is able to determine the boxing center of a lens shape, it can just as easily determine the decentered point on the lens shape where the wearer's eye will be positioned. All that is needed is an A, a DBL, and the wearer's PD (see Figure 3-32, *A*). The A may be determined from the scan. So can the DBL if both lenses are scanned. (If only one lens is scanned, the DBL is entered manually.) The wearer's PD is, of course, entered manually (Figure 3-32, *B*).

In choosing the decentered pattern option, the resulting pattern will be made with the central hole displaced by the needed decentration (Figure 3-33). If the pattern is made this way, the spotted lens does not have to be decentered. The lens block may be placed at the spotted major reference point of the lens without

calculation for decentration.[5] If this type of pattern is used for anyone other than this particular wearer, the lenses will come out incorrectly. (*Note:* If a frame has an especially small eyesize, decentering the pattern may displace the block too far nasally and cause it to strike the edger wheel.)

Pattern makers serving as frame tracers should have the capability of tracing a lens for rimless, semirimless, and nylon cord frames.

Placing the Pattern on the Edger

By convention most people begin the edging process with the right eye. When the pattern is snapped into placed on the edger, it will fit on the edger with either the front or the back of the pattern going on first. Going on one way will edge a right lens shape, whereas the other way will produce a left lens shape.

For most edgers, if the pattern is right-side up and has the nasal edge pointing toward the practitioner, the edger will cut a right lens shape. However, this is not always true. Therefore looking at the way the lens is positioned in the edger first is important, and the pattern is placed accordingly. For example, if the convex side of the upright lens faces left, then a right lens will require that the nasal side of the upright pattern be nearest the operator (Figure 3-34). If the convex side faces right, however, the pattern must be positioned in the opposite direction.

The pattern orientation for the left lens is exactly opposite from what it was for the right.

Using a Frame Tracer for Patternless Systems of Edging

Patternless edgers that do not use a physical pattern still need a shape to go by. This shape is given to the edger in digital form. Still, in order to get a digital version of the shape, that shape must sooner or later be physically traced and transferred to the edger digitally.

The most common method for generating a pattern shape is by using a frame tracer. A *frame tracer* is an apparatus that traces the shape of the frame's lens area and converts it into digital form.

---

[5]Incidentally, this also allows high plus aspheric lenticular lenses to be blocked on the optical center, where the block has better adherence, instead of on the side of the aperture portion of the lens. It also holds the lens at a better angle in the edger when the lens is edged so that the bevel will not "drop off" the side of the lens.

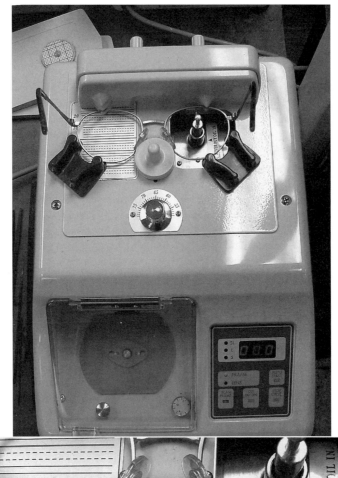

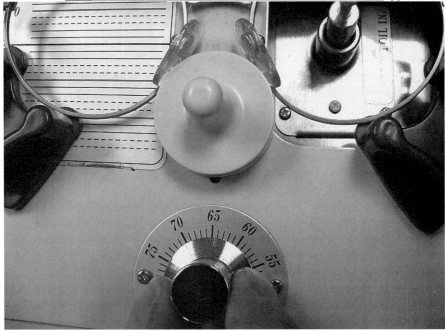

FIGURE **3-32** **A,** When the pattern maker can determine the boxing center of the lens, it is no longer necessary to tediously search for the boxing center as was shown in Figures 3-22 and 3-23. The frame must simply be straight. If it is tilted, the lens shape will be tilted and the cylinder axis will be incorrect. **B,** The wearer's interpupillary distance (PD) is being set for the pattern maker. When the PD is used instead of A + DBL the pattern will be decentered. If this is done, no decentration is required during layout. (This type of decentered pattern works well with lenticular lenses. The pad adheres better when in the center of the highly curved lenticular portion of the lens.) *DBL,* Distance between lenses.

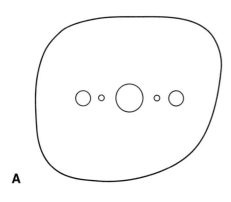

A

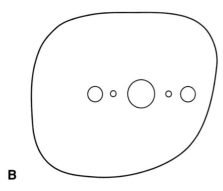

B

FIGURE **3-33** If a pattern is made in the standard way, the mechanical center is at the boxing center as shown in **A**. If the pattern is custom made to avoid decentering the lens, it may appear more as shown in **B**.

ADVANTAGES OR DISADVANTAGES OF A FRAME TRACER

At first it would appear that a frame tracer is really no different from a pattern maker. It does everything that a pattern maker does, except for making a physical pattern. However, frame tracers are more than just digital pattern makers. Although not all frame tracers can do all of these extra functions, following are some of the things that frame tracers may be capable of doing:

- Trace both right and left lenses to determine size and shape consistency
- Trace the frame shape in three, instead of two, dimensions
- Work together with an edger to demonstrate what the placement of the bevel will look like ahead of time at any given point on the lens edge
- Trace a shape from an old lens or a coquille
- Transfer data to a surfacing laboratory to help determine how thin a lens may be surfaced

In spite of the many things frame tracers can do well, certain pitfalls with frame tracers exist. These pitfalls

are also present with pattern makers. However, with a pattern maker, the physical pattern shape is immediately visible and it is easier to detect a potential problem ahead of time. Following are some of the potential pitfalls:

- Frame tracers tell it like they trace it. A plastic frame may not retain the same shape it had with the demonstration lenses in place. If it flexes to a different shape, the tracer will trace the shape the frame has at that moment, not the shape it may have been designed with originally.
- Frame tracers may change the shape of the eyewire as they trace. If a frame has an especially thin plastic or metal eyewire, the tracer pin may exert enough outward force on the frame groove to cause the eyewire to give slightly. The tracer records this distortion as part of the intended lens shape.
- When a frame is traced from a remote site on one lens only, the new lens may not exactly match the old lens.
- Some frames have such narrow B dimensions that certain frame tracers are not able to trace the frame at all.

Tracing Both Eyes

Frame tracers usually trace both right and left sides of a frame. Some trace it with a single stylus doing first the right, then the left eye. (The *stylus* is the small pin that rides in the groove of the frame.) Other tracers, to increase speed, trace both eyes simultaneously.

The following list includes several reasons that both eyes are traced:

- The two sides of the frame may have slightly different sizes. Usually the lens is made for the larger eye so that the lens is not inadvertently small.
- If the tracer picks up a difference in shape between the two eyes, the differences may be averaged for consistency.
- By tracing both lenses the tracer is determining the size and shape of the lens and measuring the distance between lenses. Thus the tracer is capable of determining A, B, ED, angle of the ED, and DBL.
- In knowing all of the lens and bridge size measurements, with only the addition of the wearer's PD, the tracer has furnished all the data to automatically calculate lens decentration. This can be used to simplify further lens layout.

Tracing the Frame Shape in Three Dimensions

The type of pattern used in the optical laboratory is a flat piece of plastic. It tells exactly what the shape of the frame's eyewire looks like in two dimensions: up and down (the y axis) and left and right (the x axis), as it

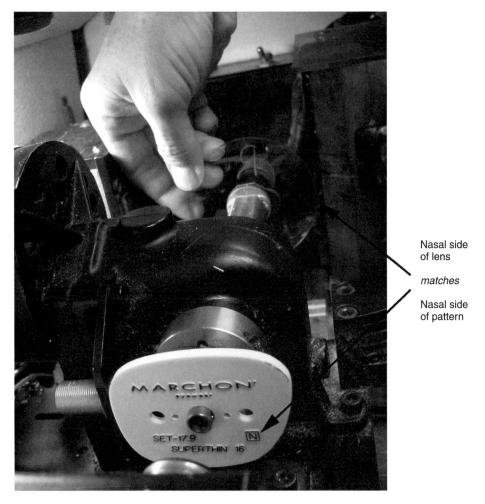

Nasal side
of lens

matches

Nasal side
of pattern

FIGURE **3-34** A pattern should be placed on the edger so that the nasal side of the pattern matches the nasal side of the lens to be edged.

would appear drawn on a piece of paper. A lens is not flat. It is arched as the result of a front surface that is usually convex and a concave back surface. Frame manufacturers make their frames to fit the average lens. This adds the third "in and out," or z-axis, dimension. The frame front is not just flat. The eyewires are curved to accept the curve of the lens.

Unfortunately, because lenses come in a wide variety of lens powers, not all lenses are curved the same (Figure 3-35). When the curve of the lens does not match the curve of the frame, either the frame has to be reshaped or the bevel on the lens must be custom cut (Figure 3-36).

When a tracer traces the frame, the stylus does not move in a flat plane as it travels around the groove. If the frame is arched, the stylus moves up and down to keep from slipping out of the groove. Some tracers do not record up-and-down movement but instead report

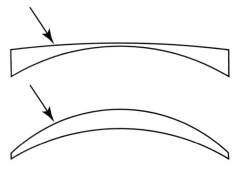

FIGURE **3-35** Because not all lenses are curved the same, a lens bevel that follows the front surface of a minus lens will not fit into a frame in the same way that the bevel on a plus lens will.

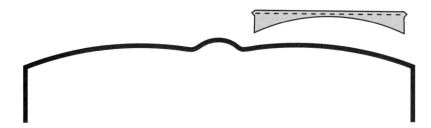

FIGURE **3-36** When the curve of the lens does not match the curve of the frame, either the frame has to be reshaped or the bevel on the lens must be custom cut.

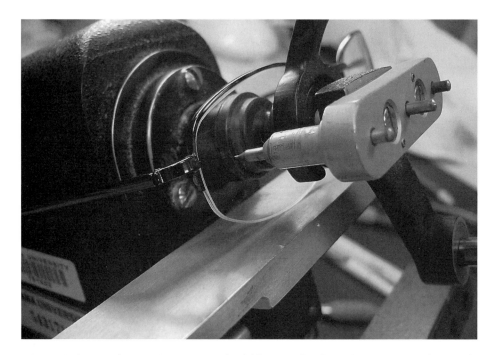

FIGURE **3-37** Before tracing a wearer's old lens or the demo lens in a new frame, the 180-degree line must be spotted on the lens. Otherwise, after the lens is out of the frame, the practitioner will have no way of knowing whether it is tilted improperly. An improperly tilted lens results in cylinder off axis once the prescription lens is made and mounted in the frame.

the flat shape of the eyewire. These are called *2-axis frame tracers*. Others record and use the third axis movement. These are called *3-axis frame tracers*. If the edger is unable to use the third (z) axis information, the 3-axis tracer loses its advantage.

Recording the third dimension permits the following two things:

1. If the tracer or edger has a screen, it allows the operator to view what the bevel will look like in the frame. Some edgers even make suggestions as to how the bevel should be positioned as it tracks around the shape to make the glasses look the best.
2. It decreases the possibility of making a shape error on frames with a lot of face form. Measuring

in three dimensions helps get a tighter, more consistent lens fit and prevents possible gaps at outside corners.

Tracing a Shape from a Pattern, an Old Lens, or a Coquille

When a frame is rimless or of nylon cord, no rim exists to guide the stylus. A frame tracer may be adapted so that the stylus will trace the outer shape of an old lens or coquille.

To trace a lens from the old prescription, or to trace a dummy lens from a new frame, the frame is placed in a lensmeter. The lens is spotted with three dots along the 180-degree line (Figure 3-37). These three dots are necessary to be certain that the shape of the lens will

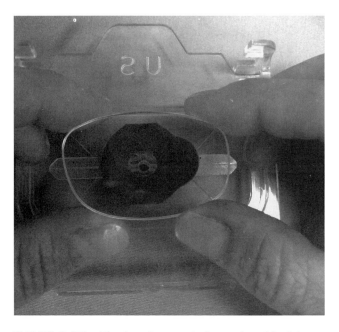

FIGURE **3-38** The lens is mounted on a lens block in an adapter. The tracer needs to know if the lens being traced is a right or a left lens.

not be rotated off axis, causing the cylinder axis to be wrong. Once the lens is spotted, it is blocked on an adhesive padded block that has been placed in an adapter in preparation for tracing (Figure 3-38). The lens and adapter is placed in the tracer (Figure 3-39) and traced.

Most patternless edgers cannot directly use a pattern. Therefore being able to trace an existing pattern becomes an important frame tracer feature. The same mechanism used to trace lens shape from an existing lens is also used to trace a lens pattern (Figure 3-40).

Transferring Data to a Surfacing Laboratory

For the surfacing laboratory to grind a lens to the optimum thickness, the laboratory needs accurate data. This is especially true for plus lenses. The size and shape the lens will have when edged are essential for calculating plus lens thickness. The more exact the data, the more precisely the thickness may be controlled. If the lens is traced, those tracing values may be sent to more places than just the edger. Values can be sent to a surfacing program that calculates lens curves and thickness then controls the lens generator.

USING A FRAME TRACER IN A VARIETY OF LOCATIONS

A frame tracer can be used in a variety of locations and situations. Each has certain advantages and disadvantages.

Adjacent to the Edger

When a tracer is situated right next to the edger, the person doing the edging has the frame in front of them (Figure 3-41). The advantage to this set up is ease in visualizing what bevel placement will look best. This works best if the tracer is interactive with the edger. If the tracer is not interactive, it simply feeds the shape into the edger. Any further adjustments are dependent upon the edger's stand-alone capabilities. Feeding information to more than one edger from the same tracer still may be possible.

Part of the Edger

A tracer that is part of the edger has the advantage of requiring less working space (Figure 3-42). When laboratory space is limited, this may be very helpful. The amount of interactivity and capabilities of the combination of tracer and edger depends solely upon the number of functions built into the system. It can be very basic or quite advanced. The disadvantage is that such a tracing system is possible to use only with that one edger.

In the Order Entry Area of a Laboratory

When the tracer is placed in the order entry area of the laboratory, information is entered only once. The laboratory that has a tracer at "order entry" will be wired with a central laboratory computer. That computer tracks the job and is capable of downloading needed information into any piece of surfacing or edging equipment that is hooked into the system when the tray number of the job is keyed in. The information on shape and eye and bridge sizes are used to calculate lens thickness for surfacing and decentration for edging.

Placing a Tracer in a Remote-Site Dispensary

One of the biggest headaches for dispensers is the situation in which a wearer wants to keep his or her old frame but cannot or will not give it up long enough to send it to the laboratory. This is especially troublesome if the frame is a metal frame and/or a frame that cannot be identified. If a frame tracer is on site, the dispenser can remove one or both lenses, trace the shape, reinsert the lens or lenses, and give the spectacles back to the wearer (Figure 3-43).

The information is then sent to the laboratory electronically. It enters the computer system just as if it had been entered in the laboratory order entry area.

Once the lenses are completed, just the lenses are sent to the dispensary. There, with the wearer present, the dispenser removes the old lenses from the wearer's frame and replaces them with the new ones.

Such a system is capable of speeding up the process for all prescriptions. Because most dispensaries acquire

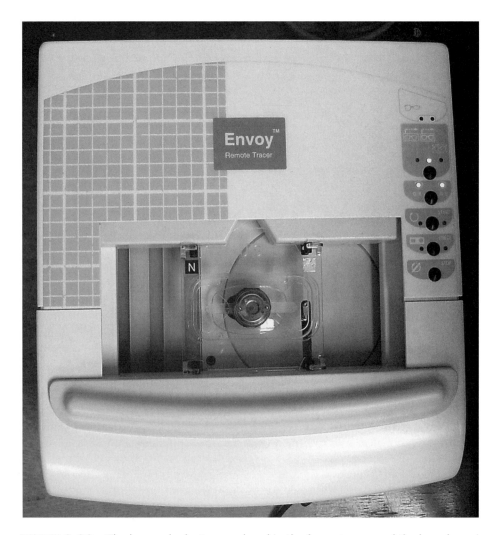

FIGURE **3-39**   The lens and adapter are placed in the frame tracer, and the lens shape is traced.

frames directly from frame manufacturers and distributors, they will be using the frame selected from the display board. In a dispensary without an in-house optical laboratory, the frame must be sent to the laboratory, fabricated, and sent back. In cases in which the shape of the frame is unknown, the laboratory will be reluctant to start the job until all information is present. When the dispensary uses a frame tracer to send that information, the laboratory can get a head

start on the prescription before the new frame arrives. To save time, dispensary personnel may choose to not send the new frame but insert the lenses themselves.

The disadvantages of a frame tracer are also present in a remote setting. The frame may be distorted before tracing, or flex during tracing and not retain the same shape it had with the old lens or demonstration lens in place. This can be a problem when ordering either one or both lenses.

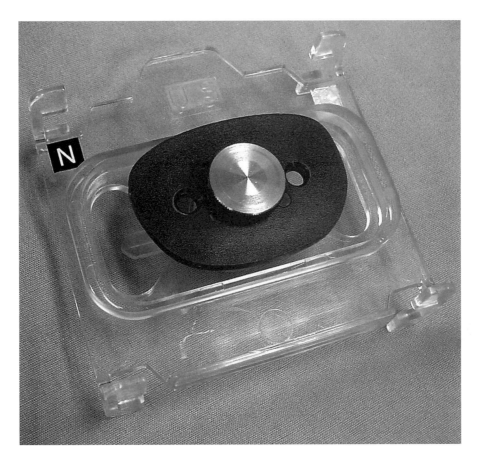

FIGURE **3-40** Most patternless edgers cannot use patterns. When a frame is not available, but a pattern is, the pattern can be mounted on an adapter. It is the placed in the frame tracer and traced for shape.

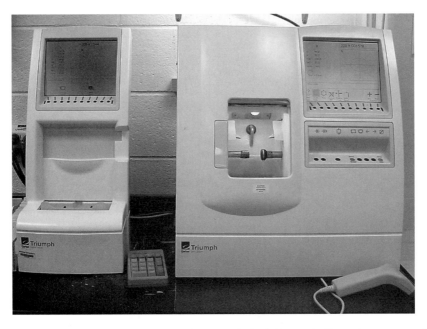

FIGURE **3-41** A tracer is next to the edger. It is linked electronically to the edger and has a screen to allow the traced shape to be viewed before edging.

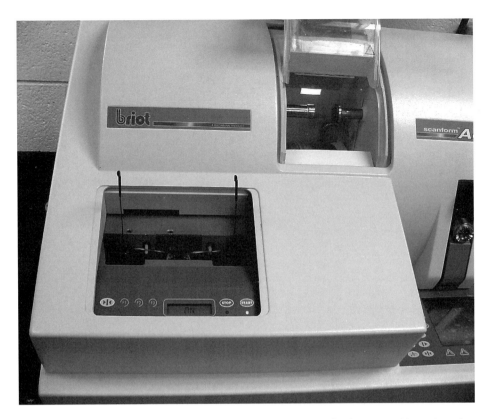

FIGURE **3-42**   Both a frame tracer and a layout blocker can be integrated into the edger and save space in the laboratory.

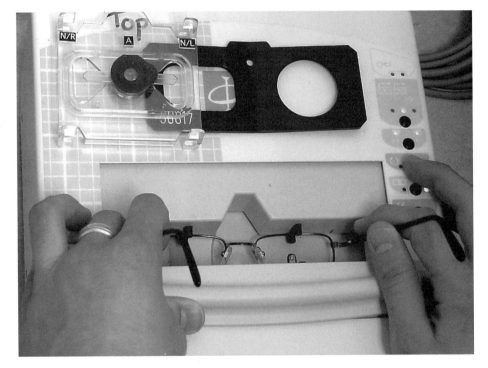

FIGURE **3-43**   A frame tracer may be used at a remote, off-site location. This ensures that the frame dimensions as read at the dispensary are exactly what will be input into the edger.

Proficiency Test Questions

1. According to the boxing system, which of the following is the measurement for the horizontal size of the edged lens?

   a. ED
   b. GCD
   c. A dimension
   d. B dimension
   e. C dimension

2. Which of the following describes the effective diameter of a lens shape?

   a. The longest horizontal dimension of a lens shape that passes through the boxing center
   b. The longest vertical dimension of a lens shape that passes through the boxing center
   c. The longest diagonal of the lens shape that passes through the boxing center
   d. Twice the longest radius of a lens shape as measured from the boxing center
   e. The smallest lens size that will be possible to use after allowing for lens decentration

3. The angle of the effective diameter is measured as which of the following?

   a. The angle from the 90-degree line to the effective diameter line, measured clockwise for the right eye
   b. The angle from the 90-degree line to the effective diameter line, measured counterclockwise for the left eye
   c. The angle from the 180-degree line to the effective diameter line, measured clockwise for the right eye
   d. The angle from the 180-degree line to the effective diameter line, measured counterclockwise for the right eye
   e. The angle from the 180-degree line to the effective diameter line, measured counterclockwise for the left eye

4. To measure the DBL on a metal or plastic grooved frame made to hold beveled lenses in place, measurements are made in which of the following ways?

   a. From the deepest part of the groove on one nasal eyewire to the deepest part of the other nasal eyewire on the horizontal midline of the frame
   b. From the two nasal-most edges of the eyewire rims along the horizontal midline of the frame
   c. From the deepest part of the groove on one nasal eyewire to the deepest part of the other nasal eyewire at the location where the distance between those lenses is smallest
   d. From the two nasalmost edges of the eyewire rims at the place where the distance between those lenses is smallest

5. Which of the following is not a synonym for geometrical center distance?

   a. Distance between centers
   b. Frame PD
   c. Frame center distance
   d. Boxing center distance
   e. All the above are synonyms.

6. When using a metal or plastic frame, the practitioner makes the correct measures for MRP height, segment height, and fitting cross height beginning at which of the following?

   a. The point on the inside of the eyewire groove directly below the center of the pupil
   b. The level of the lowest point on the inside of the eyewire groove. This will not necessarily be at the same level as the point on the eyewire groove directly below the pupil

7. True or False? Horizontal pattern size is measured horizontally through the central hole in the pattern.

8. If a pattern is made for use with the boxing system, at which of the following will it have its central hole?

   a. Boxing center
   b. Datum center
   c. Optical center
   d. Major reference point

9. Which of the following is the point on a pattern around which it *always* rotates?

    a. Boxing center
    b. Datum center
    c. Mechanical center
    d. Optical center

10. Which of the following terms does not mean the same thing as the other three terms?

    a. Cutting center
    b. Mechanical center
    c. Boxing center
    d. Edging center

11. Frame difference is calculated by which of the following equations?

    a. A + DBL
    b. A – DBL
    c. A – C
    d. B – C
    e. A – B

12. True or False? Using the same pattern for frames having two different sizes means that the frame size and the frame's lens shape may be altered somewhat.

13. True or False? One frame style is available in several different eyesizes. All those eyesizes are able to have lenses edged from the same pattern. Therefore all of these frames, regardless of eyesize, will have the same "frame difference."

14. A pattern has a frame difference of 10. A 50-mm eyesize frame of the same shape has a B dimension of 40. Which of the following B dimensions does an identically shaped frame with a 55-mm eyesize have?

    a. 44 mm
    b. 45 mm
    c. 46 mm
    d. 40 mm
    e. None of the above

15. A pattern has an A dimension of 46 and a pattern difference of 5. If the A dimension of the lens to be cut is 50, which of the following will be the B dimension of the lens?

    a. 45
    b. 55
    c. 46
    d. 54
    e. 41

16. A frame has a B dimension of 40 mm. If the segment height of the lens is 17 mm, what is the segment drop? (Segment drop will be listed as a negative number because it is below the midline of the lens.)

    a. –2
    b. –3
    c. –4
    d. –17
    e. –23

17. A pattern is marked with a frame difference of 7 mm. If the lens eyesize is 50 mm and the segment height is to be 19 mm, which of the following indicates the segment drop?

    a. –2.5 mm
    b. –6 mm
    c. –9.5 mm
    d. –1 mm
    e. None of the above

18. A pattern has a pattern difference of 7. Which of the following indicates the amount of segment drop for a frame with an A dimension of 52 and a segment height of 17 mm?

    a. –12.5 mm
    b. –9 mm
    c. –7.5 mm
    d. –5.5 mm
    e. None of the above

19. A lens is to be edged for a frame with an A dimension equal to 48 mm and a DBL of 18 mm. If the wearer has a PD of 60 mm, which of the following indicates the decentration per lens?

    a. 6 mm
    b. 5 mm
    c. 4 mm
    d. 3 mm
    e. 2 mm

20. A lens is to be edged for a frame with an A dimension of 47 mm and a DBL of 19 mm. If the wearer has a PD of 60 mm, which of the following is the *total* decentration?

    a. 6 mm
    b. 5 mm
    c. 4 mm
    d. 3 mm
    e. 2 mm

21. A pattern is made with the hole intentionally displaced nasally in order to avoid having to decenter the lens. If the pattern is made for a frame having an eyesize of 46 mm and a DBL of 18 mm—and the wearer's PD is 60 mm—which of the following distances from the boxing center of the pattern would you expect the hole to be placed?

    a. 4 mm nasally
    b. 3 mm nasally
    c. 2 mm nasally
    d. 0 mm (because the pattern should never be made this way)

22. A pattern with its mechanical center 3 mm above the geometrical center of the pattern is used. To make sure that the optical center of the lens ends up as ordered, how much horizontal and vertical decentration per lens is needed?

    +4.75D sphere
    +4.50D sphere
    Height of OCs = 25 mm
    A = 49
    B = 47
    ED = 54
    DBL = 18
    PD = 63

23. If a lens is to be made from a tracing that was done from an old lens, which of the following need not be measured?

    a. Eyesize
    b. 180-degree line
    c. DBL
    d. C-size
    e. ED

24. If a pattern center is displaced too far nasally, in which of the following directions must the lens be decentered to compensate for the error?

    a. Nasally
    b. Temporally
    c. Decentration dependent on lens power

25. A homemade pattern is placed on a Box-o-Graph to check it for accuracy. From the mechanical center, the outermost tangents in each direction are as follows:

    Top: 23 mm
    Bottom: 23 mm
    Nasal: 26 mm
    Temporal: 24 mm

    Which of the following choices indicates how far the mechanical center of the pattern is located from the boxing center of the pattern? (Remember, the mechanical center is where the hole is located.)

    a. The mechanical center is displaced 1 mm nasally from the location of the boxing center of the pattern.
    b. The mechanical center is displaced 1 mm temporally from the location of the boxing center of the pattern.
    c. The mechanical center is displaced 2 mm nasally from the location of the boxing center of the pattern.
    d. The mechanical center is displaced 2 mm temporally from the location of the boxing center of the pattern.

26. For the pattern described in the question above, which of the following decentration compensations must be made during layout so that the PD comes out correctly?

    a. Decenter each lens in an additional 1 mm.
    b. Decenter each lens 1 mm *less* in than would be otherwise indicated.
    c. Decenter each lens in an additional 2 mm.
    d. Decenter each lens 2 mm *less* in than would otherwise be indicated.

27. A frame has the following dimensions:

    A = 46
    B = 42
    DBL = 18

    The pattern to be used has its mechanical center 2.5 mm above the boxing center. The ordered MRP height for the prescription is 25 mm. Which of the following choices indicates how much the MRP should be raised to be sure it ends up in the frame where it belongs?

    a. 5.5 mm
    b. 3.0 mm
    c. 2.5 mm
    d. 1.5 mm
    e. None of the above

28. A pattern made on a pattern maker has the central hole displaced 1 mm too high and 1 mm too far nasally. For a single vision lens, which of the following choices indicates how much vertical and horizontal decentration is required to obtain a properly centered lens when the lens with the following dimensions is placed in a frame?

    A = 46
    B = 43
    C = 45
    ED = 48
    DBL = 18
    Wearer's PD = 60

    a. 2 in, 1 up
    b. 3 in, 1 up
    c. 3 in, 1 down
    d. 1 in, 1 down
    e. None of the above

29. True or False? Although pattern makers sometimes make a pattern with the center displaced too far nasally or temporally through human error, pattern makers cannot and should not make a pattern with the center hole laterally displaced on purpose.

30. Which of the following is not a valid function for a frame tracer?

    a. To gather shape data to transfer to a patternless edger directly wired to that edger
    b. To gather shape data to transfer to a patternless edger to a remote location using phone lines
    c. To allow the collection of three-dimensional frame information to better locate the bevel on the edge of the lens
    d. To determine the DBL of the frame
    e. All the above are possible functions.

31. True or False? Frame tracers are capable of tracing a shape from a pattern, an old lens, or a frame's demonstration lens.

Challenge Question

32. Which choice indicates how far away from the boxing center of the edged lens the optical center would be for the following lens? (Because the prismatic effect was achieved by surfacing the lenses, rather than by decentering a standard, uncut lens blank, the distance between these two points may not be directly measurable.)

    −0.50 D sphere 3.5Δ base out
    A = 48
    B = 43
    ED = 53
    DBL = 18
    PD = 62

    a. 1.75 mm
    b. 17.5 mm
    c. 14.3 mm
    d. 72 mm
    e. None of the above

4

Centration of Single Vision Lenses

Purpose of Centering

During the edging process the lens rotates around a central point while being ground to a specific shape to fit the frame. This central point of rotation corresponds to a hole in the pattern. This hole always should be in the middle of the pattern used on the edger to generate the shape. This middle point, the *geometrical* or *boxing center* of the lens, is defined as being the center of the smallest rectangle that encloses the lens shape using horizontal and vertical lines.

For the major reference point (MRP) of the lens to be centered before the wearer's pupil, the lens must be moved, or decentered, from the boxing center of the lens.

Mechanics of Lens Centration

The first part of the centration process involves the calculation of exactly where the major reference point of the lens will be in relationship to the boxing center of the edged lens. If these two points are not coincident, the lens is *decentered*. The distance and direction of this decentration must be calculated to ensure that the lens optics will be positioned properly before the eye.

Calculating Horizontal Decentration Using the Boxing System

Two measurements are required in the calculation of decentration. One depends on the wearer, the second on the frame being worn. The first measurement is how far apart the person's pupil centers are from each other. This is known as the *interpupillary distance* (PD). The second measurement is the distance between the geometrical (boxing) centers of the frame's two lens openings. This is known as the *distance between centers* (DBC).

DETERMINATION OF DISTANCE BETWEEN CENTERS

For frames that conform to the boxing system of measurement, the DBC is equal to the eyesize (abbreviated *A*) plus the *distance between lenses* (DBL).

$$DBC = A + DBL$$

DECENTRATION PER LENS

Most commonly the wearer's PD will be less than the distance between centers. This will require that the lenses be decentered inward (nasally) toward the center of the frame. The amount of decentration per lens can be determined by subtracting the wearer's PD from the DBC (frame PD) and dividing by 2.

$$\frac{DBC - Wearer\ PD}{2} = Decentration\ per\ lens$$

Example 4-1

A wearer's PD is 62 mm. The frame size has an A dimension of 48 mm and a DBL of 20 mm. What is the decentration per lens required?

Solution

The following formula is used to find decentration per lens:

$$Decentration\ per\ lens = \frac{DBC - PD}{2}$$

and because

$$DBC = A + DBL$$

$$Decentration\ per\ lens = \frac{(A + DBL) - PD}{2}$$

then

$$Decentration\ per\ lens = \frac{(48 + 20) - 62}{2}$$
$$= \frac{68 - 62}{2}$$
$$= \frac{6}{2}$$
$$= 3\ mm$$

So for the example, the decentration needed per lens is 3 mm inward.

DETERMINING DECENTRATION FROM MONOCULAR INTERPUPILLARY DISTANCES

When a prescription specifies the wearer's PD in reference to each eye individually, PDs were taken one eye at a time. This measurement is referred to as the *monocular PD*. For a monocular PD the reference is basically from the center of the bridge of the nose to the center of the pupil. A more conventionally measured *binocular PD* of 64, for example, may result in a right monocular PD of 31 and a left monocular PD of 33. This difference between left and right PDs is not unusual considering the asymmetry of facial features of many healthy individuals.

For a monocular PD, decentration is determined *first* by dividing the DBC of the frame by 2, *then* subtracting the monocular PD; thus the following equation is true:

$$Decentration = \frac{DBC}{2} - Monocular\ PD$$

or

$$Decentration = \frac{A + DBL}{2} - Monocular\ PD$$

DECENTRATION FOR READING GLASSES

Laboratory personnel may not know whether the prescription is being fabricated is for distance vision or near vision. A single number given for PD could be either the distance PD or the "near PD." Near PD designates a smaller separation of the MRPs of the finished lenses to allow for convergence. *Convergence* is the inward turning of people's eyes that occurs when they do close work.

Occasionally an order for single vision lenses is received that lists distance and near PDs. This would be written as *65/62*, for example. Unless otherwise noted, it must be assumed that the distance PD (65) is desired, even if the prescription is for low plus lenses. When the order form also contains the instructions "for reading glasses," the smaller measure is chosen (62). This is the near PD.

When in doubt as to which measurement to use, the practitioner should check with whomever ordered the glasses.

Historical Background

Most lens centration is done using an instrument specially designed for this purpose. However, in the past the centration of lenses was carried out with only

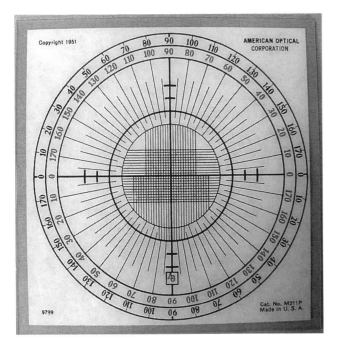

Copyright 1951   AMERICAN OPTICAL CORPORATION

9799   Cat. No. M211P Made in U. S. A.

FIGURE 4-1 A lens protractor may be used in lens layout for edging but has been used more traditionally in the lens layout for surfacing process. The inner degree scale is used when the lens is placed convex side up (as when glasses are being worn). The outer scale is appropriate when the convex side is facing down.

a minimal amount of equipment. Centration may be done accurately this way, but it requires a steady hand. Historically this was done by hand with a *lens protractor.* A lens protractor is shown in Figure 4-1. Centration really could be done with only a sheet of millimeter-ruled graph paper.

THE LENS PROTRACTOR

A few lens protractors have three raised pegs that hold the surface of the lens without allowing it to come directly in contact with the face of the protractor. These pegs hold the lens steady, which keeps it from rocking, and prevent the ink spots on the lens from smearing or rubbing off.

The degree scales on a lens protractor are used mainly for marking the lens axis for surfacing and are not used in the edging process.[1]

---

[1]A lens protractor has two or three degree scales. The lens degree scale that increases in value in a counterclockwise direction is the scale of reference when the front surface of the lens faces up. The clockwise numbered axis scale is the reference scale when the front surface of the lens faces down. A third scale, normally 90 degrees away from the other two, would be used if the lens were turned sideways.

The intersection of the cross in the center of the protractor corresponds to the boxing center of the edged lens.

LENS CENTRATION USING A LENS PROTRACTOR

Step 1
The lens is spotted in the manner that is described in Chapter 2 for correct MRP orientation and correct cylinder orientation.

Step 2
The amount of decentration per lens required is calculated using the following formula:

$$\text{Decentration per lens} = \frac{(A + DBL) - PD}{2}$$

The practitioner then determines if the lens must be decentered to the right or to the left. If the lens is a right lens and is facing down, decentration "in" is to the left (Figure 4-2, *A*). A left lens facing down would be decentered to the right.

Note: If the right lens were facing up, the lens would be decentered to the right (Figure 4-2, *B*). A left lens would be decentered left (Box 4-1).

Step 3
The right lens is placed face down (front surface down) on the protractor.[2] The three spots on the lens are aligned with the main horizontal line on the protractor. The central dot is placed at the intersection of the cross (Figure 4-3). Horizontally the lens is decentered the number of millimeters calculated.

In the example previously given, the required decentration was 3 mm per eye nasally—that is, 3 mm in. If this right lens is to be decentered *in,* it must be moved to the left 3 mm. The three dots remain on the horizontal line and the central MRP dot is 3 mm to the left of center (Figure 4-4).

---

[2]By placing the lens face down, the spot on the front surface of the lens is closer to the protractor grid surface. This helps to prevent parallax error. *Parallax* is the phenomenon that occurs when someone attempts to align visually an object with a scale when the object is not directly in contact with the scale. If the viewer's eye is not on a line directly perpendicular to the correct reading on the scale above or below the object, an error results. The most common example of a parallax error occurs when the front seat passenger attempts to read the speedometer of a car. Parallax error also can be prevented by using a centration device. A centration device such as a marker/blocker allows the lens to be positioned face up and then blocked while still in the instrument.

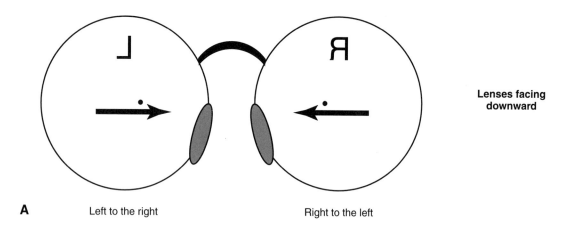

A   Left to the right   Right to the left

Lenses facing downward

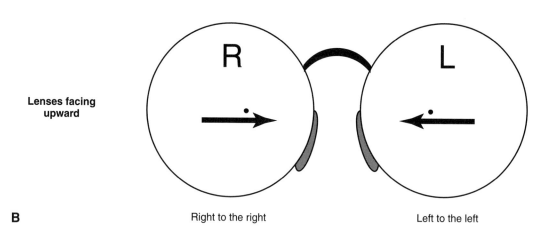

B   Right to the right   Left to the left

Lenses facing upward

FIGURE **4-2**   **A,** If the lenses are facing down for lens layout, the direction of inward decentration is opposite to the named lens; that is, left decentration for a right lens and right decentration for a left lens. If the lens is facing up, inward decentration is the same direction as the named lens, as shown in **B;** that is, right decentration for a right lens and left decentration for a left lens.

Step 4

The lens is decentered vertically if an MRP height is ordered. Exactly how this decentering is done is explained later in this chapter. In the example given here, no vertical decentration is required.

Step 5

Using the horizontal protractor line as a guide, a long horizontal line is hand drawn through the central part of the lens. (Alternatively a flexible ruler may be used to help in drawing a line if the lens has been reference dotted ahead of time as seen in Figure 4-4. Figure 4-5 shows a lens being marked with a ruler.)

A shorter, vertical line is drawn at the center of the protractor. Figure 4-6 shows the vertical line. This line

should only be about 10 mm long. The difference in length between the two lines gives an immediate visual cue as to the orientation of the lens. The intersection of the two crossed lines shows exactly where the lens will be blocked. The center of the marked cross indicates the future boxing center of the edged lens. These steps are summarized in Box 4-2.

Calculating Vertical Centration of Lenses Using the Boxing System

When no preference is expressed on the order form about MRP height, the height is presumed to be in the standard position. In most cases this standard height will be at the level of the boxing center of the edged lens. This means that the three dots on the lens remain on the 180-degree line of the lens centration device throughout centration.

<table>
<tr><td colspan="2" style="background:black;color:white">BOX **4-1**
Lens Decentration Direction</td></tr>
<tr><td>WHEN DECENTERING A FACE-DOWN LENS INWARD</td><td>WHEN DECENTERING A FACE-UP LENS INWARD</td></tr>
<tr><td>For a right lens, decenter the lens to the left.
Right/Left
For a left lens, decenter the lens to the right.
Left/Right</td><td>For a right lens, decenter the lens to the right.
Right/Right
For a left lens, decenter the lens to the left.
Left/Left</td></tr>
<tr><td colspan="2">The direction of decentration depends on whether the lenses are facing up or down. With a centration device, most of the time the lens will be facing up. It is facing up so that it can be blocked in the centration device. So if the lens is a right lens, inward decentration is to the right: "right/right." The left lens decentration direction will be "left/left." By-hand decentration with the lens face down is just the opposite.</td></tr>
</table>

SPECIFICATION OF VERTICAL PLACEMENT

For edging a lens, the MRP location must be given in terms of how far it is above or below the horizontal midline of the lens. However, when the order arrives from the dispensary, MRP height is not specified this way. Instead MRP height is the distance from the lower line of the box enclosing the shape of the lens up to the MRP location. The laboratory must convert from MRP height to MRP raise (or drop).

To make this conversion from MRP height to MRP raise (or drop), the vertical dimension of the frame must be known. Then half the vertical dimension of the frame (the B dimension) is subtracted from MRP height to find MRP raise or drop. (*Note*: MRP height almost always results in "raise." An MRP drop may indicate a mismeasurement.)

Example 4-2
An order specifies an MRP height of 25 mm. The frame has a vertical dimension (B) of 46 mm. What will the MRP raise be?

Solution
Vertical decentration is calculated as follows:

$$\text{Vertical decentration} = \text{MRP height} - \frac{B}{2}$$

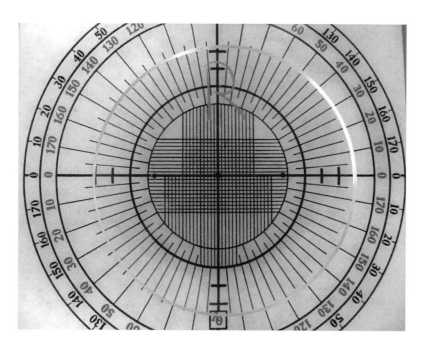

FIGURE **4-3** The lens is seen positioned on a lens protractor before any decentration occurs. All three dots are on the 180-degree line with the center dot at the center of the grid.

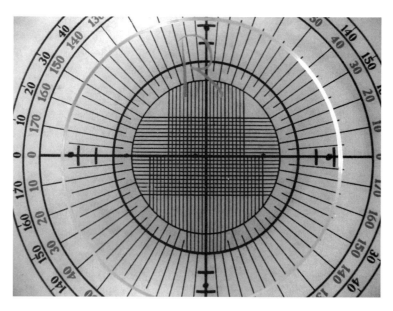

FIGURE **4-4**   For a right lens with its concave side (back surface) up, the direction of decentration is inward (left) toward the nose. The place where the boxing center of the lens will be once the lens has been edged must be marked. (The boxing center is the point around which the lens rotates during edging.) In preparation for hand-marking a lens (the old-fashioned way), the lens is dotted near the edges on the x,y coordinates of the grid. (See the four dots at the top, bottom, and sides of the lens.)

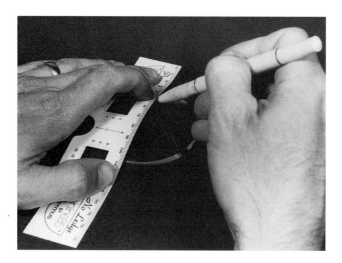

FIGURE **4-5**   Before centration instruments were used, lenses were centered on a lens protractor, then marked by hand, sometimes using a ruler, sometimes freehand.

In the example, because MRP height is 25 mm and the frame B is 46 mm, then the following is true:

$$\text{Vertical decentration} = 25 - \frac{46}{2}$$
$$= 25 - 23$$
$$= 2 \text{ mm}$$

Because the MRP height is greater than half the B dimension, the vertical decentration is positive and the lens is moved up by 2 mm. The height above (or below) the horizontal midline of the lens may be visualized from Figure 4-7.

VERTICAL COMPENSATION FOR PATTERN ERRORS

As discussed in the previous chapter, some patterns may not have the center of rotation of the pattern at the boxing center. This may happen because the pattern is old and uses a different standard or because it is a homemade pattern and was made incorrectly.

When the rotational center of patterns are above the boxing center, the difference between these two locations must be compensated for. If the rotational center is *above* the boxing center, the distance between these two centers must be subtracted from the calculated MRP raise. (If the rotational center is *below* the boxing center, the difference is *added* to the MRP raise.)

Example 4-3

In this example, vertical decentration is 2 mm above the boxing center. A pattern has its mechanical center (center of rotation) 3 mm above the boxing center. How will the MRP raise have to be compensated?

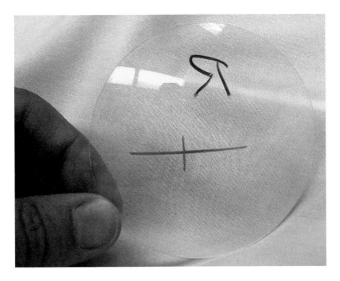

FIGURE **4-6** A marked cross on a lens has a short vertical and long horizontal component. This provides an immediate visual cue on where the 180-degree midline is located and where the boxing center of the edged lens will be. However, it is at the future location of the boxing center of the lens once the lens has been edged. Because of decentration, the cross is no longer at the geometrical center of the uncut lens blank. Is the lens concave side up or convex side up?*

———

*Answer. The lens is convex side up.

Solution

A pattern with its center of rotation 3 mm above its boxing center will cause the MRP to be 3 mm above the boxing center of the edged lens. Therefore 3 mm are subtracted from the normally calculated vertical decentration.

$$+2 \text{ mm} - 3 \text{ mm} = -1 \text{ mm}$$

In other words, when this particular pattern is used, the MRP must be positioned 1 mm below the horizontal

180-degree reference line to make the lens center properly.

LENS CENTRATION INSTRUMENTS

A centration instrument has many advantages over a lens protractor, even though the process is basically the same. These advantages are as follows:

1. The optical system of the instrument eliminates most parallax problems.
2. Internal illumination makes viewing of marks on the lens and lens segments easier.
3. The instrument contains a movable vertical reference line. This reference line may be moved left or right and makes horizontal alignment for decentration easier.
4. If the instrument just marks the lens, the system contains a lens-marking stamp that always strikes at the location of the boxing center. It gives a consistent, straight set of marks. This type of centration device is called a *lens marker.*

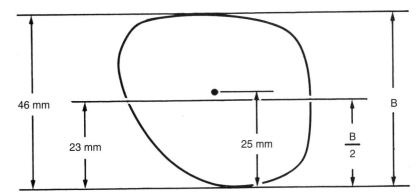

FIGURE **4-7** If the position of the major reference point (MRP) is given in terms of height from the lowermost portion of the shape, drop or raise can be calculated by subtracting one half of the B dimension from MRP height.

Instruments that only mark a lens are now rare. Most lens centration devices also include a lens-blocking mechanism. Instead of stamping the lens and having to carry out an additional step of blocking the lens at the location of the stamp, the lens is blocked directly. This type of device is called a *marker/blocker.*

LENS CENTRATION WITH A CENTRATION INSTRUMENT

The following are the steps for use of a centration instrument for single vision lenses.

Step 1

The lens is spotted (as described in Chapter 2).

Step 2

If the instrument has blocking capabilities, a double-sided adhesive blocking pad is stuck on a lens block and the block is mounted on the instrument. Then the paper is peeled off the pad to expose the adhesive.

Step 3

The amount of horizontal decentration per lens required is calculated using the following formula:

$$\text{Decentration per lens} = \frac{(A + DBL) - PD}{2}$$

Step 4

The practitioner must determine whether the lens must be decentered to the right or to the left. In most centering devices the lens is face up. If the lens is a right lens and is facing up, decentration "in" is to the right. (see Figure 4-2, *B*). A left lens facing up would be decentered to the left (see Box 4-1).

Step 5

The position of the movable vertical reference line[3] in the instrument is adjusted to the right or left by the amount of decentration calculated.

Step 6

The right lens is placed face up (front surface up) on the screen. The three spots on the lens are aligned with the horizontal line on the instrument screen.

Step 7

The center lens dot is placed on the movable vertical reference line. (The position of this line corresponds to horizontal decentration.)

Step 8

When the MRP height is specified, the lens is decentered up (or in rare instances, down). The amount of decentration is according to the correct number of millimeters of MRP raise (or drop).

Step 9

The handle is grasped and swung into place, or the button or footswitch is pressed. This blocks (or marks) the lens[4] (Figure 4-8).

Example 4-4

A frame has an eyesize (A) of 54 mm and a DBL of 20 mm. The wearer's PD is 66 mm. The lenses are already spotted. How must the instrument be set, and how must the lens placed in order to properly block the lens? The reader should assume that the lens is a *left* lens.

Solution

Lens decentration is calculated as follows:

$$\begin{aligned}
\text{Decentration per lens} &= \frac{(A + DBL) - PD}{2} \\
&= \frac{(54 + 20) - 66}{2} \\
&= \frac{8}{2} \\
&= 4 \text{ mm}
\end{aligned}$$

To preset the movable vertical line in the instrument for the left lens, the practitioner should first recall in which direction the MRP should be moved. Because the wearer's PD is smaller than the frame's geometrical center distance or "frame PD,"[5] the lenses will decenter nasally or inward. The lens is placed convex side up. Therefore the left lens is moved to the left. As Figure 4-9 shows, the movable vertical line is positioned 4 mm to the left of the central reference line.

Now the lens is placed face up in the instrument. It is aligned so that the central dot is at the intersection of the horizontal line and the movable vertical line. Figure 4-10 indicates that the other two dots must fall directly on the horizontal reference line.

The lens is blocked. The lens block is positioned at what will become the boxing center of the edged lens (Figure 4-11).

---

[3]For single vision lenses, the movable vertical line is basically used as a place marker. When laying out single vision lenses, some people prefer not to use the movable vertical line at all. Instead they move the dot on the lens directly to the desired amount of decentration.

[4]To check for calibration, the practitioner views a marked or blocked lens through the instrument *before* it leaves the grid. This shows whether the mark or block is really at the origin of the instrument grid and is straight.
[5]"Frame PD" is equal to A + DBL.

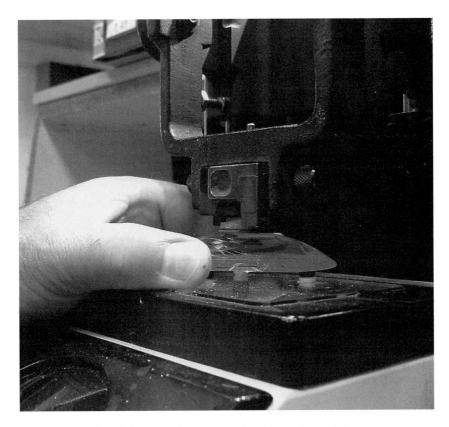

FIGURE **4-8** The lens is being blocked for edging.

INCREASING ACCURACY

The dots that are applied by the lensmeter can be small, as they should be. However, sometimes these dots tend to "disappear" into the black horizontal line of the centration device. One "cure" is to make the center dot larger than it might otherwise be by remarking with a marking pen.

Instead of increasing the size of the dots, an easy way to eliminate the problem of disappearing dots while simultaneously increasing accuracy is to position the dots 0.5 mm above the 180 line until all decentration positioning is completed. As a last step, when everything is completed, lower the lens back down 0.5 mm so that the dots disappear into the line.[6]

Ensuring Proper Size of the Lens Blank

Nobody wants to intentionally waste a lens. To help avoid edging a lens that is not quite large enough, some centering devices use a system that visually compares the blank to the required size. Two main systems exist.

CENTRATION UNITS THAT USE EFFECTIVE DIAMETER CIRCLES

The first system is a series of circles of known diameter that appear on the screen of the instrument (Figure 4-12). These show possible *effective diameters* (ED). The effective diameter of a frame is on the frame package or package insert, is listed in a frame reference catalog, or can be measured. (See Chapter 3 for how to measure the ED.)

When properly positioned, the decentered lens blank must enclose completely the circle of the same diameter as the effective diameter of the frame (Figure 4-13).

CENTRATION UNITS THAT USE SUPERIMPOSED PATTERNS

A second system used in centration devices to ensure that a lens is large enough superimposes the shadow of the pattern on the screen of the centering device. The scale used in decentration, the lens blank, and the shadow of the pattern are seen at the same time.

---

[6]Thanks to Glenn Herringshaw of Bloomington, Ind., for contributing this hint.

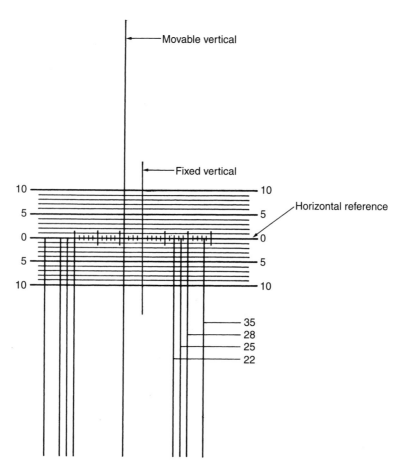

FIGURE **4-9**   In the case of single vision lenses, the movable line indicates the positioning of the major reference point and the fixed vertical line the position of the geometrical center of the lens after edging. In this illustration, the movable line is set for 4 mm of decentration. The vertical position of the major reference point is not always specified by the practitioner. When it is, the procedure is carried out through a simple raising or lowering of the central lensmeter dot, exercising care to maintain parallelism between the three dots and the x axis of the grid.

This system works best when the pattern is exactly the same size as the frame. If the pattern size is the same size as the frame, the shadow of the pattern must be enclosed completely by the decentered lens blank. If it is not, any part of the pattern found outside of the lens blank will end up as "air space" (Figure 4-14). (This is the system used on many patternless edgers. The edged lens shape is drawn over the unedged lens on the screen.)

This pattern shadow system still can be used with patterns somewhat larger or smaller than the finished lens, but compensation must be made. To compensate, the size of the pattern must be known. This can be measured directly.[7]

_____
[7]Pattern size can be calculated by adding the absolute value of the "set number" printed on the pattern to 36.5 mm.

Example 4-5
The eyesize of a particular frame is 50 mm and the pattern size is 46 mm. How much larger in every direction will the edged lens be?

Solution
The eyesize minus the pattern size is 50 minus 47, or 3 mm. This means that the lens will be larger by half that amount in every direction. The lens will be three halves or 1.5 mm larger than the pattern in every direction.

Knowing this, the practitioner can make a visual estimate with the use of the pattern shadow system, even if the pattern is smaller than the frame's eyesize. For the lens to be large enough, the edge of the lens blank must clear the pattern shadow by half the difference between pattern size and eyesize—in this

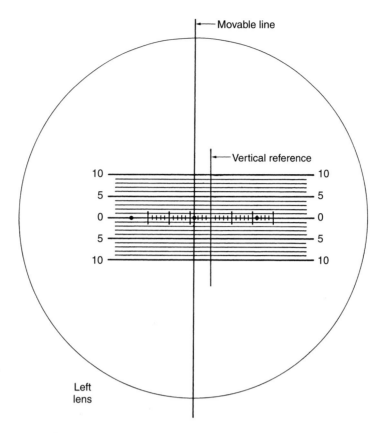

FIGURE **4-10** The movable line is preset to the correct decentration. The movable line helps to prevent the dot on the lens from getting "lost" on the grid. With the movable line pointing out the desired major reference point (MRP) location, the lens is positioned as shown.

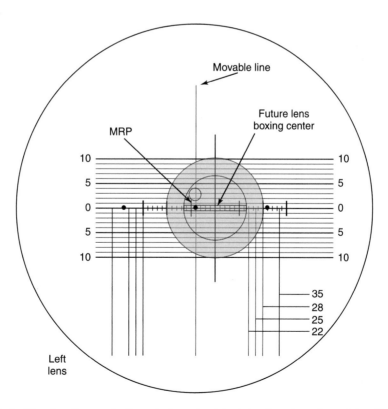

FIGURE **4-11** On the centration device, the block is placed at the origin. The block center corresponds to the *future* geometrical or boxing center of the *edged* lens. *MRP,* Major reference point.

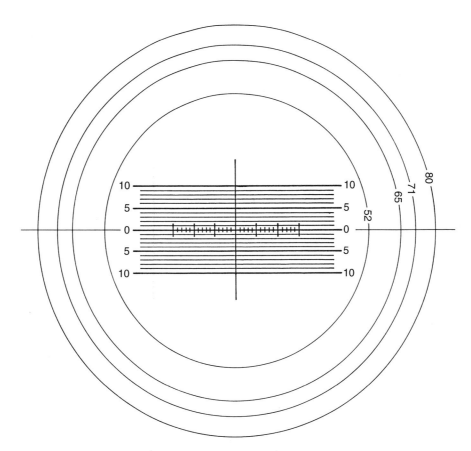

FIGURE **4-12** When a centration device contains a series of concentric circles, the correctly centered uncut lens must enclose completely the circle equal to the *effective diameter (ED)* of the frame. (It cannot be assumed that because the circle equal to the frame *eyesize* is enclosed, the uncut lens will be large enough.)

case, 1.5 mm. If this amount of clearance is not present, the lens will not cut out.

Example 4-6

A lens has an eyesize of 58 mm. The pattern is measured and found to be 52 mm. The wearer's PD is 68 and the frame DBL is 18, giving a 4 mm decentration per lens. When the lens is prepared for edging and viewed through the instrument, it appears as shown in Figure 4-15. Will the lens be large enough to cut out?

Solution

Answering the question requires finding the minimum distance from the edge of the pattern to the edge of the lens. To do this, the pattern size is subtracted from the eyesize and divided by 2:

$$\frac{\text{Eyesize} - \text{Pattern size}}{2}$$

or

$$\frac{58 - 52}{2} = 3 \text{ mm}$$

The practitioner must add 3 to the superimposed pattern shadow in every direction to simulate edged lens size. Applying this to Figure 4-15, it is evident that less than 3 mm is between the pattern edge and lens edge. This means that the lens will not cut out.

MINIMUM BLANK SIZE

The smallest lens blank that can be used for a given prescription lens and frame combination is called the *minimum blank size* (MBS). The MBS depends on the following:

- The effective diameter of the frame
- The amount of decentration of the optical center away from the boxing center

If no decentration occurred and the lens optical center was positioned exactly at the boxing center, the minimum blank size would be equal to the effective diameter (Figure 4-16).

Minimum blank size also must allow for extra size required because of lens decentration. When 1 mm of

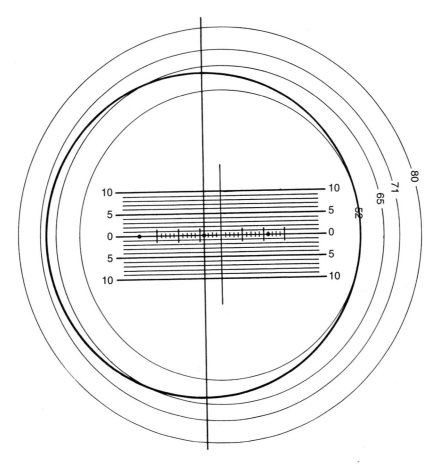

FIGURE **4-13** If the frame to be used has an effective diameter greater than 52 mm, the 63 mm lens blank shown in this illustration will not be large enough when decentered for the wearer's interpupillary distance (PD), as it has been in this drawing.

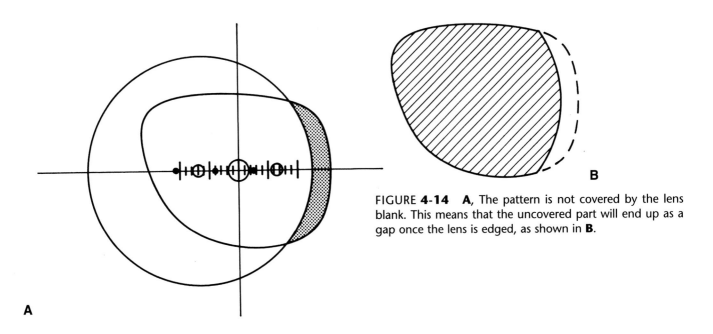

A

B

FIGURE **4-14** **A**, The pattern is not covered by the lens blank. This means that the uncovered part will end up as a gap once the lens is edged, as shown in **B**.

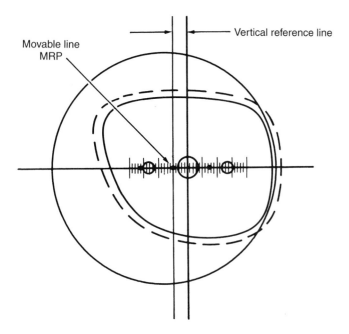

FIGURE **4-15** Centration devices using a shadow projection of the pattern work best when the pattern size equals the frame eyesize. When a pattern is smaller than the frame's eyesize, compensation must be made by visualizing whether the lens will cut out. In this figure, the dotted line represents the "visualized" increase in pattern size that must be estimated to determine whether the lens blank size is sufficient. As shown, the lens blank will be too small. *MRP,* Major reference point.

decentration inward occurs, the minimum-sized lens must be 1 mm larger temporally. However, because uncut lens blanks are made round—with the optical center in the middle of the blank—they must increase equally in all directions. Therefore for every millimeter of decentration, the MBS also must increase 2 mm (Figure 4-17).

In addition, allowing an extra 2 mm is advisable for the possibility of lens chipping or other error. The extra 2 mm is only 1 mm on each side, so really only 1 mm of leeway exists.

Written mathematically and not including the extra 2 mm, the MBS is the following:

$$MBS = ED + 2(decentration)$$

Written to include the extra 2 millimeters, the formula is as follows:

$$MBS = ED + 2(decentration) + 2$$

Blank size charts and devices are available that allow the frame to be used in the determination of lens blank size. One such chart, and the explanation of how to use it, is shown in Figure 4-18.

LENSES OF INSUFFICIENT SIZE

Sometimes a lens blank is only slightly too small. A temptation exists to use the lens blank anyway by moving it

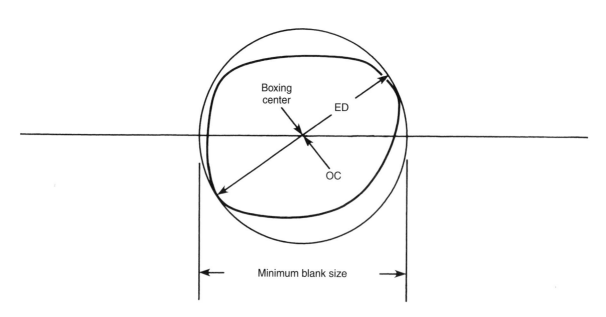

FIGURE **4-16** When there is no decentration, minimum blank size equals effective diameter (ED). (No allowance for lens chippage is shown.) *OC,* Optical center.

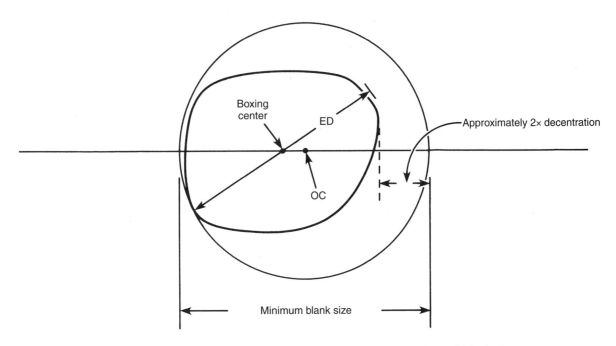

FIGURE **4-17**   For each millimeter of decentration, 2 mm of additional blank size must be added to the effective diameter (ED) to determine the minimum blank size. (No allowance for lens chippage is shown.) *OC,* Optical center.

outward slightly. This causes the distance between optical centers to be larger than ordered and is called "pushing" the PD. By pushing the PD, the small lens blank may be used. But because the lens optical center will be decentered from its intended position before the eye, unwanted prism may result.

The amount of prism that will be induced by altering the ordered PD varies considerably with the power of the lens being used. The amount of prism that results is predictable using Prentice's Rule.

INCORRECT INTERPUPILLARY DISTANCE

As mentioned in Chapter 2, Prentice's Rule states the amount of prism (Δ) induced by decentration of a lens. Prism amount is equal to the number of centimeters (c) the lens is moved times the power of the lens (F). In equation form this appears as follows:

$$\Delta = cF$$

The stronger the power of the spectacle lens *(F),* the more unwanted prism will be induced for the same amount of lens decentration *(c).* Once this relationship is understood, it is relatively easy to estimate the amount of prism induced by a given amount of lens decentration.

Example 4-7
A −5.00 D lens blank is not large enough to cut out. If the PD is "pushed" 2 mm out for this lens, how much unwanted prism is induced?

Solution
The amount of unwanted prism can be calculated with the following equation:

$$\Delta = cF$$

The absolute value for *F* is used, so 5.00 is substituted for *F* in the equation. The decentration amount per lens is 2 mm. Because *c* is measured in centimeters and 2 mm = 0.2 cm, the equation becomes the following:

$$\Delta = (0.2)\ (5.00)$$
$$= 1.00$$

A prism has both an amount and a base direction. For this eye the base direction will be base in. This is evident when the lens is seen in cross-section. This cross-section is shown schematically in Figure 4-19.

Base-in prism forces the eyes of the wearer to turn outward to keep from seeing double. For example, a pair of glasses with great amounts of unwanted prism is dispensed. If this happened, it would be better if the lenses were uncomfortable and rejected. The worst

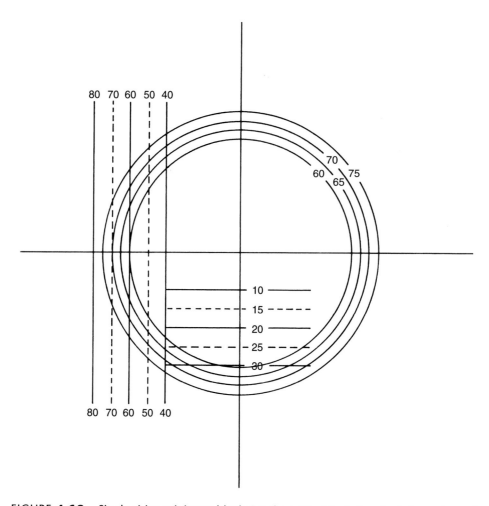

FIGURE **4-18**   Single vision minimum blank size chart. The blank size chart shown is used as follows:
1. The frame is placed front face down in the chart with the right lens opening over the simulated lens circles.
2. The frame bridge is centered over the correct binocular distance PD as indicated by the scale on the left.
3. The practitioner ensures that vertical centration is right. This is done by positioning the lowest point on the inside groove of the lower eyewire on the lower chart scale. The correct lower chart scale level is one half the B dimension of the frame. (If a vertical positioning for the major reference point [MRP] of the lens is specified, use this height instead.)
4. The diameter lens circle that will just enclose the lens opening of the frame, *including* the eyewire groove, is noted. This is the minimum blank size required for a single vision lens without prescribed prism.

result would be for the wearer to gradually become accustomed to the prism. This would contribute to either an outward deviation of the eyes or suppression of one eye with a resultant drop in its visual acuity. Although it is unlikely that the small prismatic amount in the previous example would cause such problems, the degree of difficulty encountered depends on the amount of prism induced and the visual condition of the wearer.

Example 4-8
A lens blank with a power of −0.25 D is too small and won't cut out. What would the consequences be of "pushing" the PD by 2 mm?

Solution
Calculations are done in the same manner as before, but this time the power substituted in the equation is 0.25 instead of 5.00.

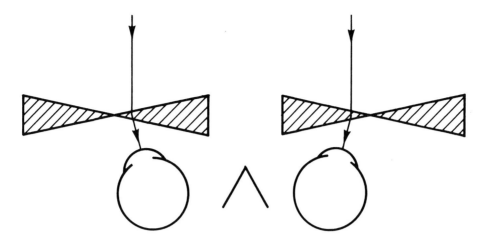

FIGURE **4-19**   Errors in optical center (OC) placement cause objects to appear displaced from their actual location. To compensate for an error in horizontal OC placement, the eyes must turn inward or outward; otherwise the wearer will experience double vision. A minus lens decentered outward results in base in prism.

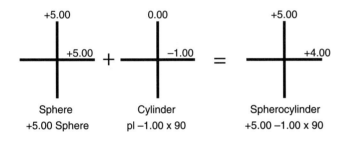

FIGURE **4-20**   The value of a lens in a given meridian often can be better visualized through the use of a power cross system.

$$\Delta = cF$$
$$= (0.2)\ (0.25)$$
$$= 0.05$$

The total prism produced per eye is only 0.05 prism diopters. This amount is hardly measurable. The consequences of pushing the PD outward by 2 mm for a lens of this power are negligible.

Example 4-9

A lens blank is marked for the following prescription:

$$+5.00\ -1.00 \times 90$$

How much prism is induced by pushing the PD 2 mm outward?

Solution

When a lens contains a cylinder, the amount of prism induced depends upon total power in the meridian of decentration. This means that the orientation of the

cylinder axis in relation to the direction of decentration of the lens is important. In this case the lens is being decentered in the horizontal meridian. The practitioner needs to know the power of the lens in the horizontal meridian to calculate prism amount.[8]

Because the cylinder power is at right angles to the axis of the cylinder, the power *(F)* used in Prentice's Rule is +4.00 D (Figure 4-20).

The prism induced by pushing the PD for this lens blank will be as follows:

$$\Delta = cF$$
$$= (0.2)\ (4)$$
$$= 0.80$$

The amount of prism induced is 0.80Δ of prism base out.

Warning: Combining Oblique Cylinder and Incorrect Interpupillary Distances

Whenever a cylinder or spherocylinder lens having an oblique axis direction is decentered horizontally, a certain amount of vertical prism always is induced. The amount of vertical prism induced increases as the following occur:

1. The cylinder power increases
2. The cylinder axis approaches the 45- or 135-degree position

In other words, moving an oblique spherocylinder horizontally would require a compensating vertical movement to counteract the vertical prismatic effect

---

[8]To find the power of a lens in a given meridian, it is helpful to use a power cross. For more on power crosses, see Chapter 16 in Brooks CW, Borish I: *System for ophthalmic dispensing*, ed 2, Boston, 1996, Butterworth-Heinemann.

being induced. The amount of vertical compensation depends upon the cylinder power and axis direction. In short, when oblique cylinder is present, pushing the PD horizontally will result in some degree of vertical prism. This prism will not show up at the optical centers of the incorrectly placed lenses but will show up if the lens is checked at the location of the wearer's PD.

AMOUNT OF REQUIRED ACCURACY

Accuracy required for the location of the OC may be specified either as millimeters of deviation from the ordered PD, or as the amount of prism induced by the incorrectly located OC, or both.

Low-powered lenses can have their OC off location by a relatively large amount before the prismatic effect becomes significant. However, as lens power increases, even small errors can cause a major prismatic effect. The American National Standards Institute (ANSI) has published agreed-upon Recommendations for Prescription Ophthalmic Lenses. These include prismatic effect and PD accuracy. (ANSI Z80.1 Prescription Ophthalmic Lens Recommendations may be found in Appendix B at the back of this book.)

Published standards are recommendations only; the practitioner may demand higher or accept lower standards. The supplying laboratory may remind an account of the generally accepted standards but should not attempt to hide behind them, as more precision in certain specified parameters is not an impossible task. If the practitioner and supplying laboratory cannot come to an acceptable agreement, then other sources of supply should be sought. Wearers of low refractive powers are often more sensitive to deviations from the absolutes required than wearers of high prescriptions, making higher standards well within reason in certain circumstances.

Standards for Interpupillary Distance and Unwanted Prism

The ANSI Recommendations for Prescription Ophthalmic Lenses (Z80.1) tries to balance unwanted prism amounts with what is realistically feasible. More than two thirds of a prism diopter of horizontal prism is undesirable. However, as in Prentice's Rule, as the power of the lens increases, the amount of prism that is induced with a small movement of the lens center location also increases. The ANSI committee determined that for prescriptions of above plus or minus 2.75 D, it was realistically possible to require that the PD be within 2.5 mm of what was ordered. Unfortunately for high prescriptions this will induce more than two thirds of a prism diopter.

For unwanted vertical prism the ANSI Z80.1 standards state that no more than one-third prism diopter should be induced by any differences between left and right MRP heights. However, if the prescription is above plus or minus 3.375 D, the MRPs should be kept to within 1 mm of vertical difference for lens pairs or 1 mm of what was ordered for one lens only. This means that more than one-third prism diopter of vertical prism may result, even though the lens centers are vertically within 1 mm of each other. For these lenses, ANSI standards for vertical prism are still met.

ETHICAL FACTORS IN PRESCRIPTION ACCURACY

Because published prescription eyewear standards are recommendations only, in some instances a laboratory may be tempted to supply an account with prescription materials that fall outside the normally accepted standards when no one raises an objection. The laboratory supplying prescribed materials has an ethical responsibility to supply materials according to standard. Failure on the part of the account to check adequately for accuracy does not release the supplier from this responsibility. If anything, it places the ethical responsibility for the welfare of the wearer more directly on the laboratory.

Ophthalmic frames and lenses cannot be regarded as a commodity for which the consumer is the ultimate judge of acceptability. The laboratory that accepts materials that fall outside of normally accepted standards does not suffer from incorrect power or prism that was not prescribed. Wearers, who must trust in the judiciousness of those supplying their needs, are the ones who bear the consequences of dispenser and/or laboratory negligence.

Proficiency Test Questions

Horizontal Decentration

1. What is the distance between centers (DBC) for a frame with the following dimensions?

    A = 47
    B = 39
    DBL = 20
    ED = 48

2. How much decentration, and in which direction, is required for each of the following?
    (*Note:* 50 □ 20 means the 50 mm eyesize and 20 mm bridge size is measured according to the boxing system.)

    a. PD 66, 50 □ 20
    b. PD 60, 50 □ 18
    c. PD 59, 44 □ 16

3. How much decentration per lens is required to correctly position the following lenses for edging?

    R: +1.00 −1.00 × 70
    L: +1.00 −1.00 × 100
    A = 52
    B = 49
    DBL = 16
    PD = 70

    a. 1 mm in
    b. 1 mm out
    c. 1.5 mm in
    d. 2.0 mm in
    e. None of the above

4. How much decentration per lens is required for a prescription having the following specifications?

    A = 52
    B = 43
    ED = 54
    DBL = 18
    R monocular PD = 32
    L monocular PD = 33.5

5. How much decentration per lens is required for a prescription with the following specifications?

    A = 48
    B = 38
    ED = 48
    DBL = 18
    R monocular PD = 31.5
    L monocular PD = 31.0

6. How much decentration per lens is required for the following prescription if it is to be used for reading glasses only?

    R: +3.25 −0.50 × 90
    L: +3.00 −0.25 × 90
    A = 52
    B = 47
    ED = 57
    DBL = 20
    PD = 65/61

    a. 6 mm
    b. 4 mm
    c. 4.5 mm
    d. 3.5 mm
    e. 5.5 mm

7. How much decentration per lens is required if the person wearing these glasses will be wearing them for reading only?

    R: +3.25 −0.50 × 90 1Δ base down
    L: +3.00 −0.25 × 90 1Δ base up
    A = 52
    B = 47
    ED = 57
    DBL = 20
    PD = 65/61

    a. 6 mm
    b. 4 mm
    c. 4.5 mm
    d. 3.5 mm
    e. 5.5 mm

Vertical Decentration

8. The optical laboratory receives an order for a frame and lenses. The wearer's PD is the same size as the (A) + (DBL) of the spectacle frame. The order specifies an MRP height of 23 mm for both lenses. If the frame has a vertical (B) dimension of 40 mm, how much vertical decentration is needed?

9. How much vertical and horizontal decentration per lens is required for the following single vision prescription?

   > R: −1.25 −0.75 × 15
   > L: −1.00 −1.00 × 162
   > Height of MRPs: 26 mm
   > PD = 66
   > A = 53
   > B = 48
   > ED = 57
   > DBL = 17

10. How much vertical and horizontal decentration of the major reference points (MRPs) of the lenses are required for the lenses that are to be placed in the following frame?

    > R: +3.00 sphere with 2Δ base in
    > L: +3.00 sphere with 2Δ base in
    > MRP height = 21 mm
    > Wearer's PD = 61 mm
    > A = 47
    > B = 33
    > DBL = 17

Minimum Blank Size

11. For the following frame and the wearer's PD, which of the choices describes the minimum blank size required if 2 mm is allowed for lens chipping?

    > A = 49
    > B = 40
    > ED = 54
    > DBL = 20
    > PD = 61

    a. 57
    b. 66
    c. 59
    d. 64
    e. None of the above

12. What would the finished, single vision, minimum blank size be for a frame with an A dimension of 53 mm, a DBL of 18 mm, and an ED of 56 mm if the person who will be wearing these frames has a PD of 68 mm? (*Note:* Allow 2 mm for lens chipping.)

    a. 58 mm
    b. 61 mm
    c. 65 mm
    d. 69 mm
    e. 73 mm

13. An order for the same frame as in the question above is received, but it is for someone with a PD of 60. Which of the following lists the minimum blank size for this order if a finished, single vision lens blank is to be used? (*Note:* Allow 2 mm for lens chipping.)

    a. 58 mm
    b. 61 mm
    c. 65 mm
    d. 69 mm
    e. 73 mm

Z80 Standards

American National Standards Institute (ANSI) standards for prescription ophthalmic lenses have several different aspects. One of those is for the amount of unwanted horizontal prism that may be considered acceptable. Because lenses positioned for a wrong PD will induce horizontal prism, this is part of the standard as well.

14. A lens pair has a power of −5.25 D sphere for both right and left lenses. The wearer's distance PD is 64 mm, but the glasses are made with a geometrical center distance of 62 mm. This will cause a total unwanted prismatic effect of 1.05Δ for both right and left eyes combined. Is this prescription acceptable according to ANSI standards in regards to PD/horizontal prism?

    a. Yes
    b. No
    c. Not enough information given

15. A lens pair has a power of –0.75 D sphere for both right and left lenses. The wearer's distance PD is 60 mm, but the glasses are made with a distance of 66 mm between the optical centers. This will cause a total unwanted prismatic effect of 0.45Δ for both right and left eyes combined. Is this prescription acceptable according to ANSI standards in regard to PD/horizontal prism?

    a. Yes
    b. No
    c. Not enough information given

16. A lens pair has a power of –7.25 D sphere for both right and left lenses. The right lens optical center is higher than the left lens optical center, but the vertical difference between the two optical center heights is just less than 1 mm. However, there is 0.5Δ of vertical prism that results. Is this prescription acceptable according to ANSI standards in regards to vertical prism/vertical MRP placement?

    a. Yes
    b. No
    c. Not enough information given

Pushing the Interpupillary Distances

17. If the PD were "pushed" outward 1.5 mm per lens, what would be the total horizontal prismatic effect (right and left lenses combined) for each of the following prescriptions?

    a. R: +2.00 D sphere
       L: +2.00 D sphere
    b. R: $-4.00 -1.00 \times 90$
       L: $-4.00 -1.00 \times 90$
    c. $+5.25 -1.00 \times 180$
       $+6.25 -1.00 \times 180$

General Questions

18. A right lens has a power of $+5.00 -2.00 \times 30$. The frame chosen has dimensions of 52 □ 20. The patient's PD is 66. Assume that the uncut lens blank is facing up *(convex side up)*. The OC is at the geometrical center of the blank. Which of the following represents where on the lens the center of the lens block would be located?

    a. 6 mm to the right of the geometrical center of the lens blank
    b. 6 mm to the left of the geometrical center of the lens blank
    c. 3 mm to the right of the geometrical center of the lens blank
    d. 3 mm to the left of the geometrical center of the lens blank
    e. None of the above

19. Tony and Julie work at the same place. Both verify prescriptions. When a question exists about whether the prescription is acceptable, they both check the same one and compare notes. Tony checked the following prescription:

    R: $-2.00 - 3.50 \times 45$
    L: $-2.00 - 3.50 \times 45$

    The PD was supposed to be 58 mm. He found the PD to be 66 mm and also found unwanted horizontal prism, but no vertical prism. He told Julie to check it as well. Julie found the same thing for PD and horizontal prism but said that she found unwanted vertical prism, too. Julie was right. Why?

    a. Julie checked for vertical prism at the 66 mm location, and Tony checked at the 58 mm location. Because of the oblique cylinder, this made a difference.
    b. Julie checked for vertical prism at the 58 mm location, and Tony checked at the 66 mm location. Because of the oblique cylinder, this made a difference.
    c. Julie checked at both locations and averaged the difference.
    d. It is impossible to tell why Julie found the unwanted vertical prism from the information given. Julie was obviously just better.

20. Off-Center Optical Dispensers sent a prescription to Futile Vision Optical Laboratory. When the prescription was completed Randy from Futile Vision Optical verified their work and found that the PD was outside of standards and caused 1.5 Δ of unwanted base in horizontal prism. A small amount of unwanted vertical prism also existed. Randy asked his manager what to do and mentioned that the prescription was for Off-Center Optical, to which his manager replied: "They never verify the work we send 'em. Send it out like it is." Sure enough, the job is sent out and never comes back. The wearer has difficulty in keeping her place when reading and has frequent headaches when doing extended near work. She attributes the headaches to stress. Which or who of the following is responsible?

   a. Off-Center Optical and its employees and owners
   b. Futile Vision Optical and its employees and owners
   c. Both Off-Center Optical and Futile Vision and their owners and employees
   d. The wearer, who did not follow up

Challenge Questions

21. For the following prescription lens, how far from the center of the lens block on the uncut lens (i.e., the location of the geometrical center of the edged lens) will the optical center be located?

    +4.00 D sphere 2Δ base out
    A = 50
    B = 48
    ED = 56
    DBL = 18
    PD = 60

22. A left lens has a power of −4.00 −1.00 × 180. The frame chosen has dimensions of 50 □ 18. The patient's PD is 60 mm. The prescription calls for 1.0Δ base down prism for the left eye. The OC is at the geometrical center of the lens blank. The uncut lens blank is *convex side up* (facing up). How far horizontally and vertically is the lens block center from the OC of the lens?

5 Centration of Progressive Addition Lenses

Single vision lenses are lenses that have the same prescription power over the whole lens. That power can be a sphere power, a cylinder power, or a spherocylinder power. The prescription also may call for prism. A single vision lens works well as long as the wearer still has a sufficiently full range of accommodation.

Accommodation is the ability to change the power of the eye's inner crystalline lens. Changing this power enables a person to see objects clearly at a near viewing distance. *Presbyopia* is the loss of this ability to focus well enough to see clearly and comfortably at near viewing distances.

To correct for presbyopia, a person must have either more than one pair of single vision lenses or a pair of glasses with lenses having more than one power. Lenses with more than one power are called *multifocal lenses* or *multifocals*.

Two Major Categories

Multifocal lenses are divided into the following two major categories:

1. Segmented multifocal lenses
2. Progressive addition lenses

Segmented multifocal lenses are lenses that have two or more distinctly divided areas of power. These areas of different powers are demarcated clearly by a visible bordering line[1] (see Figure 1-3).

---

[1]The exception here is the blended bifocal that has two areas of different powers, with a blended, nearly invisible border between the two.

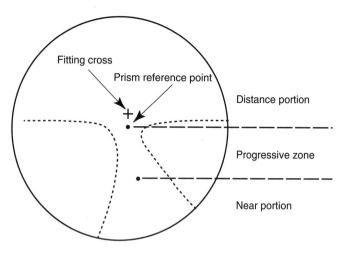

FIGURE **5-1** Progressive addition lenses leave the upper distance portion of the lens relatively undisturbed. The power begins to change at the prism reference point (which is also the major reference point of the lens) and increases in plus along a central corridor. The spin-off of a gradually increasing power in combination with the invisible near section is a peripheral area with varying cylinder power. This area varies in optical clarity to the wearer, depending upon the width of the progressive corridor and the power the near addition.

Progressive addition lenses also have different viewing areas—a distance viewing area and a near viewing area. In between those two areas is a progressive zone where the power of the lens gradually changes. Power increases in a plus direction from the distance viewing area to the near viewing area (Figure 5-1).

Because the progressive addition lens is processed more like a single vision lens it will be considered in this chapter; segmented multifocals will be addressed in Chapter 6. However, the order in which these two types of lenses are presented is not critical. Readers who would prefer to begin with multifocal lenses may skip to the next chapter and return later to consider the progressive lens.

Progressive Addition Lens

The progressive addition lens attempts a gradual increase in power from distance to near portions of the lens so that the wearer may see an object clearly at any distance with only a slight repositioning of the head. As stated previously, although the progressive addition lens looks more like a complicated lens than a segmented or multifocal, it is treated much the same as a single vision lens in preparation for edging.

REFERENCE POINTS ON THE PROGRESSIVE LENS

Certain key reference points are found on the progressive addition lens. None are seen on first glance. There are only a few permanently marked references, and these are visible only under optimal viewing conditions. Because of their importance, this discussion begins with the lightly marked, nearly invisible reference points.

The upper areas of the lens are for distance vision. Like other lenses, a progressive addition lens has a major reference point (MRP). When no prism is prescribed, the optical center (OC) and the MRP are one and the same.

The power of the lens begins changing at the major reference point of the lens. It increases in plus power within a progressive corridor below the MRP until the full near addition power is reached (see Figure 5-1). This corridor varies in length from approximately 12 to 17 mm,[2] depending on design.

The MRP may be found on a progressive lens in the same manner as the MRP on a single vision lens is found. When no prescribed (Rx) prism is present, the MRP is the OC. With use of the lensmeter, this is the location where the prismatic effect is zero. Refractive power begins changing at the MRP of a progressive lens, which makes it hard to measure distance power at the MRP. Therefore the distance power is measured far enough above the MRP to eliminate the possibility of measuring part of the progressive corridor by mistake.

PRP, DRP, and NRP

To differentiate the two places where the prism and the distance powers are measured, with progressive lenses the MRP is referred to as the *prism reference point* or *PRP*.

The place where distance power is measured is called the *distance reference point* (DRP). The lens manufacturer chooses the location of the DRP. When the semifinished lens comes from the manufacturer, an incomplete circle has been stamped on the lens. This circle surrounds the location of the DRP (Figure 5-2).

The lens manufacturer also chooses the point in the near viewing area where the full near power of the lens should be measured. On the semifinished lens this area sometimes comes surrounded by a full circle. It is called the *near reference point* (NRP).

Fitting Cross

Because of gradual power change and the lack of any distinct viewing area lines on the lens, a segment height

---

[2]It should be noted that corridor length and minimum fitting height are not the same thing.

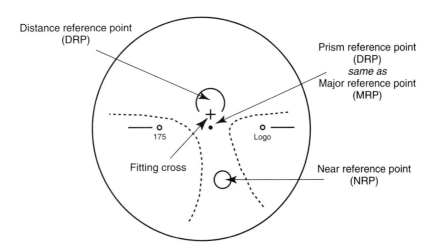

FIGURE **5-2**   In verifying a progressive addition lens, the practitioner verifies the distance power higher up on the lens than it would be on any other type of lens. The manufacturer determines where distance power should be verified, calls this location the distance reference point, and marks its location with a semicircle. Prism is verified at the MRP, which, for progressive addition lenses is sometimes called the *prism reference point*. (Note: the fitting cross where the pupil center is located is not the same as the MRP. Nevertheless, many dispensers erroneously use the terms *fitting cross height* and *MRP height* interchangeably.) The add power is verified at the location set by the manufacturer, calling it the *near reference point*. No power or prismatic verification is done at the fitting cross. (Modified from Brooks CW, Borish IM: *System for ophthalmic dispensing,* ed 2, Boston, 1996, Butterworth-Heinemann.)

with a progressive addition lens does not exist. Instead, the dispenser fitting the lenses denotes vertical placement with a *fitting cross*. The fitting cross is a reference point on the lens usually 2 to 4 mm above the MRP, depending upon lens design.

When progressive addition lenses first entered the market, fitting crosses did not exist. Instead the lens was to be positioned vertically so that the MRP was a certain number of millimeters below the center of the pupil. However, many dispensers were fitting the lenses too low. Too many unsuccessful cases resulted. Out of self-defense the lens manufacturers developed a way around the problem. Knowing where the MRP should be relative to the pupil center, they measured up from the MRP and named that point the *fitting cross*. From then on the fitting cross always was positioned exactly at pupil center and the progressive zone ended up where it needed to be.

CONVENTIONAL CENTRATION OF THE PROGRESSIVE LENS

The fitting cross is to be positioned exactly in front of the wearer's pupil and comes visibly marked on the lens. It is the only reference point for both horizontal and vertical lens positioning for the dispenser. It is also the primary reference point for both horizontal and vertical lens positioning for the edging laboratory.[3]

In simplest terms, centration of a progressive add lens is done as if the lens were a single vision lens. For single vision lenses, the MRP is placed at the correct monocular or binocular PD, depending upon how it is ordered. For a progressive lens, the fitting cross is placed at the correct monocular PD.

For a single vision lens, the MRP is placed on the horizontal midline of the lens or at the specified MRP height, if one is ordered. For a progressive lens the fitting cross is placed at the specified fitting cross height.

Example 5-1
A progressive addition lens is ordered as follows:

R: +3.00 −1.00 × 70
L: +3.00 −1.00 × 110
Add: +1.50
Monocular PDs—R: 33; L: 31

Vertical fitting cross heights are as follows:

R: 25
L: 23

---

[3]The fitting cross is not the most important reference point for the surfacing lab. For the surfacing laboratory the MRP remains paramount.

Frame dimensions are as follows:

A = 50
B = 40
DBL = 20

The reader should answer the following questions:

- How much horizontal decentration is required per lens?
- How much fitting cross raise or drop is needed per lens?
- How will the right lens appear on a centration device when correctly centered for blocking?

Solution

First the lens is verified to make sure it has the power needed. Distance power is checked at the DRP (Figure 5-3). Near add is measured as the difference between distance and near powers. Near power is measured at the NRP (Figure 5-4). If distance or add powers are high, the glasses are turned around in the lensmeter and the add power is measured as the difference between front vertex distance and near powers.

It should be noted that the add power appears as a hidden marking on the front surface of the lens and is generally reliable. (For additional information see Chapters 6 and 11 in Brooks CW, Borish IM: *System for Ophthalmic Dispensing*, ed 2, Boston, 1996, Butterworth-Heinemann.)

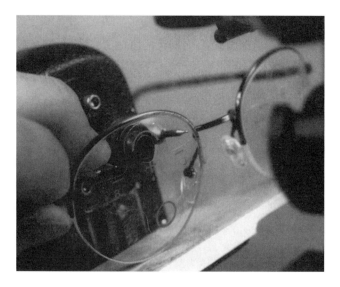

FIGURE **5-3** To verify distance power on a progressive addition lens, the lens must be positioned with the incomplete circle around the lensmeter aperture as shown. This ensures that the power reading will not be affected by the changing power in the progressive zone. (From Brooks CW, Borish IM: *System for ophthalmic dispensing*, ed 2, Boston, 1996, Butterworth-Heinemann.)

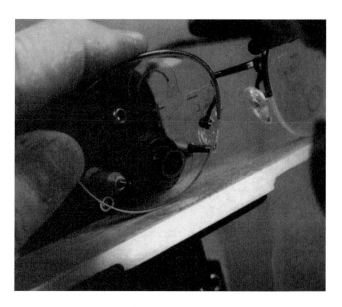

FIGURE **5-4** When distance and near powers are low, the near power may be verified with the use of the back vertex power as shown in the figure. In any case, the near power must be read through the near circle. (The more correct method, however, is to find the near add using front vertex powers.) (From Brooks CW, Borish IM: *System for ophthalmic dispensing*, ed 2, Boston, 1996, Butterworth-Heinemann.)

Vertical prism in progressives. The accuracy of Rx prism or freedom from unwanted prism is measured at the PRP as shown in Figure 5-5. Key words here are *unwanted prism.* Up to this point, *any* unprescribed prism at the MRP (vis-à-vis, PRP) has been considered unwanted prism. With progressives, this is an exception.

Progressive lenses that are plus in power, or even low minus in power, are thicker than single vision lenses in those same powers. This is because the progressive surface cuts into the front of the lens to achieve the needed plus power change (Figure 5-6, *A*). The lens must have more center thickness to keep the bottom of the lens from getting too thin.

To overcome this problem, the surfacing laboratory can grind base down[4] prism into right and left lenses. This allows the lenses to be made thinner (Figure 5-6, *B* through *E*). If both lenses have "small" (less the 4Δ[5]) and equal amounts of base down prism, the wearer's vision and comfort is undisturbed.

Equal amounts of base down prism (called *yoked* base down prism) found at the PRPs are not considered unwanted vertical prism. This applies only to vertical

---

[4]In some instances equal amounts of base up prism may be appropriate. (See Meister D: Understanding prism-thinning, *Lens Talk* 26(35), 1998.)
[5]Sheedy JE, Parsons SD: Vertical yoked prism—patient acceptance and postural adjustment, *Ophthal Physiol Optics* 7:255, 1987.

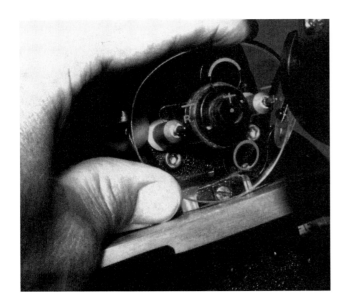

FIGURE **5-5** To verify prismatic effect, the lens is verified at the prism reference point (PRP) located by the central dot directly below the fitting cross. (For other lenses, the PRP is referred to as the *major reference point*, or MRP.) (From Brooks CW, Borish IM: *System for ophthalmic dispensing*, ed 2, Boston, 1996, Butterworth-Heinemann.)

prism and is acceptable only when right and left lenses have the same amount of vertical prism in the same base direction.

Calculating horizontal decentration. Horizontal decentration per lens must be calculated using monocular PDs. PDs are specified monocularly because the progressive corridor must begin directly below the eye. If the corridor is not centered exactly, the eye will be too far to one side of the corridor. This means the wearer will not be able to use the intermediate viewing area contained within the progressive corridor.

For a progressive lens, the horizontal decentration for a monocular PD is calculated in the same way as it is for a single vision lens.

$$\text{Decentration} = \frac{A + DBL}{2} - \text{Monocular PD}$$
$$= \frac{50 + 20}{2} - 33$$
$$= 2 \text{ mm}$$

Therefore horizontal decentration for the right lens is 2 mm. Horizontal decentration for the left lens is calculated as follows:

$$\text{Decentration} = \frac{A + DBL}{2} - \text{Monocular PD}$$
$$= \frac{50 + 20}{2} - 31$$
$$= 4 \text{ mm}$$

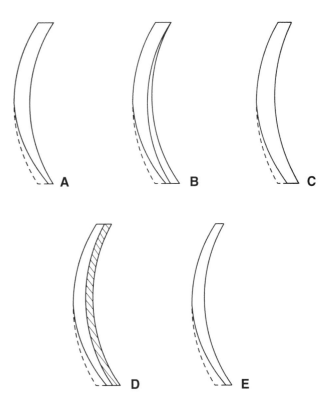

FIGURE **5-6** This figure shows how base down prism may be used to thin plus- and low-minus-powered lenses. **A,** A progressive lens with no power in the distance portion in cross-section. The *dotted line* shows where the lens would have been without the progressive zone of the lens cutting into the lower thickness of the lens. The lens must be made thicker overall to allow for thinning in the lower half by the progressive section. **B,** By adding base down prism to the lens, the bottom gains thickness, but not the top. **C,** The lens with base down prism added. The whole lens is thicker than it needs to be. **D,** Now the lens can be thinned without changing the power of the lens. The hatched area is the lens thickness that may be removed without affecting lens optics or without over-thinning the lens. **E,** The lens when finished. It is significantly thinner that it was as seen in **A.** (From Brooks CW, Borish IM: *System for ophthalmic dispensing*, ed 2, Boston, 1996, Butterworth-Heinemann.)

Even through progressive lenses have a near area of viewing, the near PD is not specified. Most progressive addition lenses have a standard inset for the near zone. The amount of inset may be constant or may increase slightly with higher add powers.[6] Either way it will not affect centration for edging when monocular distance PDs are used.

---

[6]Practitioners normally do not specify an inset for the near zone of a progressive addition lens. When inset is specified it may be achieved by rotation of the semifinished lens blank. This is normally done in the surfacing process. Spherocylinder lenses *must* be rotated *before* surfacing. However, if a sphere lens already has been surfaced, it may be rotated in a manner similar to the method used to rotate round-segment lenses to increase or decrease segment inset.

Calculating the vertical position of the lens. After horizontal lens positioning has been determined, the vertical position of the lens must be calculated. For the right lens the fitting cross raise or drop above or below the horizontal midline is calculated as follows:

$$\text{Raise or drop} = \text{Fitting cross height} - \frac{B}{2}$$

$$= 25 - \frac{40}{2}$$

$$= 25 - 20$$

$$= +5 \text{ mm}$$

Therefore the fitting cross raise for the right lens is 5 mm. For the left lens the fitting cross height is as follows:

$$\text{Raise or drop} = \text{Fitting cross height} - \frac{B}{2}$$

$$= 23 - \frac{40}{2}$$

$$= 23 - 20$$

$$= +3 \text{ mm}$$

Therefore the fitting cross raise for the left lens is 3 mm.

Positioning the lens in the centration device. The right lens is placed face up in the centration device. Because decentration is inward, this right lens is moved to the right. On the centration device the movable line is shifted 2 mm to the right. The fitting cross is placed on the movable line. It is then raised 5 mm above the horizontal line. Care should be taken to make certain that the 180 line marked on the lens is still exactly horizontal. Figure 5-7 shows the right lens correctly positioned on the centration device.

For a summary of how progressive addition lenses are positioned for edging, see Box 5-1.

CENTRATION OF THE PROGRESSIVE LENS USING HIDDEN 'CIRCLES'

Progressive addition lenses come from the surfacing laboratory with brightly colored, non–water-soluble marks that are stamped on the front surface of the lens. These marks are used to indicate locations of the fitting cross, distance reference point, prism reference point, and near reference point. These marks may have been on the semifinished lens blank when the surfacing laboratory received the lens. Or they may have worn off during surfacing and been re-marked by the surfacing laboratory. In either case, because of human error these marks may not be exact.

So that the accuracy of these marks may be verified, the lens comes with two hidden circles on the front surface of the lens. These marks are usually circles, although they may be triangles, squares, or other forms

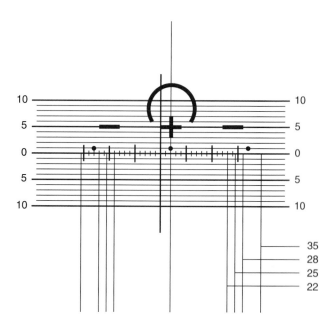

FIGURE 5-7 Progressive lenses using a fitting cross system require that the fitting cross be used for reference in centration for edging instead of the prism reference point (PRP). In the right-eye example shown, a 5-mm raise and a 2-mm inset are required. The near portion should automatically fall into place.

of markings, depending upon manufacturer. This author refers to them simply as *circles*. These circles may be found by viewing the front surface carefully. Once located, the centers of these circles should be dotted with a marking pen.

Each manufacturer provides a lens blank chart that is drawn to scale and shows the location of each of the points on the progressive lens (Figure 5-8). Using that chart, the lens is placed on the chart with the dotted hidden circles on the hidden circles shown in the drawing. The accuracy of the lens markings is verified, especially the location of the fitting cross. If they are wrong, the old markings are removed and the marks redrawn on the lens.

The lens is verified as the following are checked: distance power at the DRP, prism power at the PRP, and near power at the NRP.

Positioning the Progressive Lens for Blocking Using Hidden Circles

Because the fitting cross location is based on the location of the hidden circles, a more accurate way to position a lens for blocking is to use the hidden circles instead. Most of the procedure using hidden circles is the same as the conventional method using the fitting cross. However, two main differences exist.

The first difference is that the two circles are used to horizontally center the lens. To do this, the movable line is first set for the distance decentration. Then the practitioner pretends that the dotted hidden circles are the outer edge of a bifocal segment. These hidden circles are generally about 34 mm apart. Knowing this, it is possible to position these two circles so that they are centered using the 35-mm bifocal segment bordering lines to the left and right of the movable vertical line. If no set of lines has the same width as these hidden circles, then they are spaced evenly from each line.

The second difference is in the vertical positioning of the lens. The hidden circle is used for raise or drop instead of the fitting cross.

To find the hidden circle raise or drop, the practitioner determines the distance from the PRP up to the fitting cross. This may be done by measuring the distance from the PRP up to the fitting cross on the manufacturer's lens blank chart. This distance is subtracted from the fitting cross raise. This is the hidden circle raise or drop. The two hidden circles are positioned at this level (Box 5-2).

Example 5-2

The following is an order for a lens and frame:

R: -1.00 –0.50 × 5
L: -1.00 –0.50 × 175

Add: +2.25
Monocular PDs—R:32; L: 32

Vertical fitting cross heights are as follows:

R: 24
L: 24

The frame dimensions are as follows:

A = 48
B = 38
DBL = 20

The progressive addition lens to be used has a 4 mm distance from the PRP to the fitting cross. Using the hidden circles instead of the fitting cross, the right lens is positioned for blocking.

Solution

The hidden circles are located and the prescription verified as accurate.

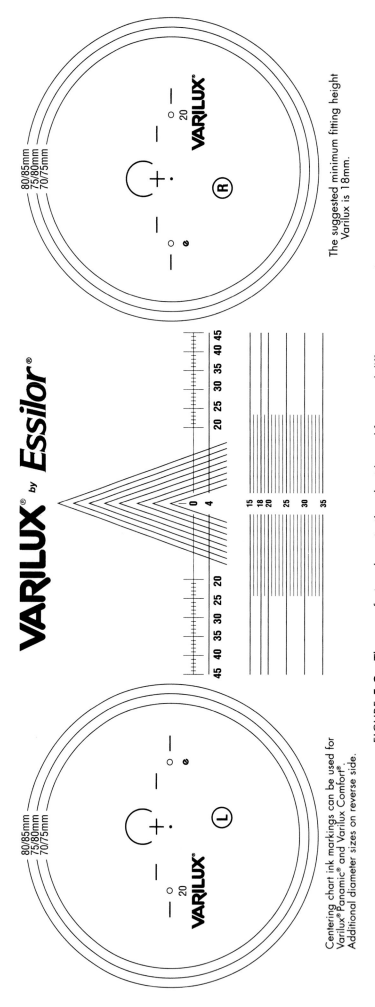

FIGURE **5-8** The manufacturer's centration chart is used for several different purposes. A laboratory may use it to mark the location of the fitting cross, prism reference point, distance reference point and near reference point with ink or by using a decal. It also may be used to find out if the lens blank is large enough for the frame chosen.

The distance decentration for the right lens is as follows:

$$\text{Decentration} = \frac{A + DBL}{2} - \text{Monocular PD}$$
$$= \frac{48 + 20}{2} - 32$$
$$= \frac{68}{2} - 32$$
$$= 34 - 32$$
$$= 2 \text{ mm}$$

The fitting cross raise for the right lens is as follows:

$$\text{Raise or drop} = \text{Fitting cross height} - \frac{B}{2}$$
$$= 24 - \frac{38}{2}$$
$$= 24 - 19$$
$$= +5 \text{ mm}$$

Next the raise or drop of the hidden circles is found by subtraction of the PRP/fitting cross distance from the fitting cross raise, calculated as follows:

$$\text{Hidden circle raise} = \text{Fitting cross raise}$$
$$- \frac{PRP}{\text{Fitting cross distance}}$$

or

$$\text{Hidden circle raise} = 5 - 4 = +1 \text{ mm}$$

The movable line is set for 2 mm and the hidden circles are centered between the appropriate bifocal border line. Then the dotted hidden circles are moved up 1 mm from the horizontal line (Figure 5-9).

Specialty Progressive Addition Lenses

PROGRESSIVES FOR IMMEDIATE AND NEAR WORKING DISTANCES

People who work for extended periods of time at intermediate and near distances appreciate having a larger viewing area in their eyeglasses than is afforded with standard progressive add lenses. Progressives designed with a longer progressive zone and lower "add" also can be made with less unwanted peripheral astigmatism and a resulting wider field of view. Some refer to these lenses as *"variable focus lenses"* to distinguish them from other progressive addition lenses. The following is how these lenses work.

For example, a person needs the following prescription:

R: plano
L: plano
Add: +2.50

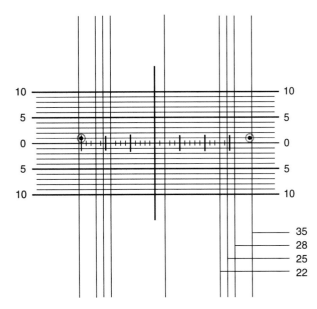

FIGURE **5-9** Progressive addition lenses can be centered for blocking by using the hidden circles instead of the fitting cross. The fitting cross may be mismarked accidentally and might introduce error. The hidden circles are molded onto the lens surface. Their location never changes. To use the hidden circles, the practitioner finds them and puts a dot in the center of each. These dots are used for reference. The dots are aligned in the centration device using the 35-mm segment reference lines.

The +2.50 add gives good vision at near (40 cm working distance). A bifocal lens would provide good vision at distance and at near. If sharp vision at an intermediate viewing distance were required, a trifocal lens could be chosen. For this prescription, a trifocal lens with a 50% intermediate would have a +1.25 D power through the intermediate portion. (Of a +2.50 add power, 50% is +1.25 D.) Some people want clear working vision at intermediate and near but would wear other glasses or no glasses for distance viewing. In this case, the intermediate lens power of +1.25 is placed in the upper portion of a bifocal lens and a +1.25 D add is used.

Because

(+1.25 "Distance" power) + (+1.25 Add power) = +2.50 Total near power

the net power at near still ends up being +2.50 D.

Advantages of an Intermediate/Near Progressive over a Regular Progressive

Should not the practitioner just use a regular progressive lens instead of specialty lens? In the above example, why not just put +1.25 D of power in the distance portion of a regular progressive and give a +1.25 add power? The total power at near will still end up being +2.50 D for either lens.

The answer is no. A regular progressive should not have the prescription changed for intermediate and near use. A regular progressive lens designed for general purpose wear has a different corridor position and length of corridor between distance and near viewing areas than does an intermediate/near design (Figure 5-10, *A*). An intermediate/near design increases the length of the corridor so that it covers more of the lens (Figure 5-10, *B*).

Because the practitioner wants +1.25 D of power in the straight-ahead position for intermediate viewing, the long progressive corridor allows the progressive zone to be made much wider. This results in more usable lens area for intermediate and near, which is desirable. Therefore the specialty lens is great for an office environment but inappropriate for walking around or driving. Although the general purpose progressive is great for walking around or driving, it is not optimized for many close- and intermediate-environment working situations.

Now a large variety of these types of "occupational" progressives are available for intermediate and near use. Each brand of lens varies somewhat to avoid patent infringements and meet different design philosophy goals. Table 5-1 shows a number of designs. All lenses are intended to result in a near viewing power equivalent to the near viewing power the wearer's normal presbyopia-correcting prescription would have.

Originally Marketed as 'Reader Replacements'

Originally these designs were thought of as "reader replacements." The intention was to find a product that would be an attractive alternative for individuals who wore single-vision reading glasses and no distance prescription at all. Although this is still a prime target market for the lens, it fills an important need for anyone who wants a wider and higher intermediate viewing area and a wider near portion.

Ordering these Lenses

Lens manufacturers recommend ordering the intermediate/near style progressive lens in a variety of ways. Some recommend using monocular PDs; others say that binocular PDs are sufficient. Some ask for near power (meaning the sum of the distance power plus the add power); others ask for the standard distance power/near add prescription. Some request a fitting height; others require none at all.

In reality, no matter what the recommendation, the laboratory will be expected to take whatever information it is given and change it into the format required for the brand of lens ordered.

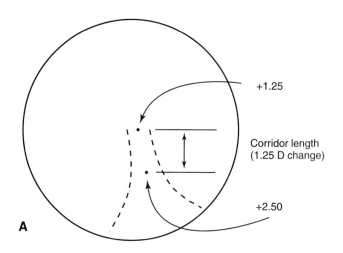

Standard progressive

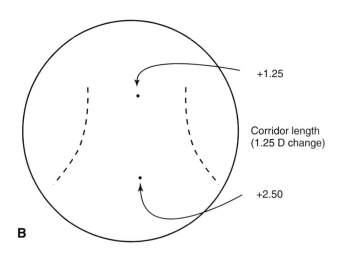

Intermediate/near specialty progressive

FIGURE **5-10** This is a simplified comparison of a standard progressive **(A)** and an intermediate/near specialty progressive **(B)**, both with a 1.25 D power change along the length of the progressive corridor. By lengthening the progressive corridor and/or maintaining a low add power, the manufacturer can design the corridor considerably larger. This increases the area of clear, useable vision for intermediate and near viewing. (These lenses are not a representation of any particular existing lens design.)

Layout for Intermediate/Near Progressives

Layout for edging of intermediate/near-style progressives varies between that of a single vision lens and a progressive lens.

If the brand of lenses ordered requires only distance PDs and no fitting height, the lens is treated as if it were a single vision lens. The only difference is that instead

TABLE 5-1
Variations in Intermediate/Near Specialty Progressives*

LENS	POWERS USED TO ORDER LENS	REQUIRED PDs	POWER CHANGE(S) FROM TOP TO BOTTOM OF LENS	RECOMMENDED FITTING REFERENCE POINT
Sola Access[a]	Near	Binocular near	0.75 D for adds of +1.50 and below 1.25 D for adds of +1.75 and above	On midline
Rodenstock Office[b]	Distance and add powers	Monocular distance	1.00 D for adds of +1.75 and below 1.75 D for adds of +2.00 and above	Pupil center
Zeiss RD[c]	Distance and add powers	Monocular distance	0.50 D less power change than the normal add	Pupil center
Essilor Interview[d]	Near	Monocular near	0.80 for all add powers	Lower lid
Hoya Desktop[e]	Distance and add powers	Monocular distance and below	0.75 D for adds of +1.50 1.25 D for adds of +1.75 and +2.00 1.75 D for adds of +2.25 and above	Pupil center
AO Technica[f]	Distance and add powers	Monocular distance	Full add power	Pupil center or 2-3 mm below

*These are examples of specialty progressives available at the time of writing. They are intended as examples only. New lens designs will continue to appear and availability will change rapidly.
[a]Sola Access, AOSola, Petaluma, Calif.
[b]Rodenstock Office, Rodenstock North America, Inc., Lockbourne, Ohio.
[c]Zeiss RD, Carl Zeiss Optical, Inc., Chester, Va.
[d]Essilor Interview, Essilor of America, St. Petersburg, Fla.
[e]Hoya Desktop, Hoya Lens of America, Bethel, Conn.
[f]AO Technica, American Optical, Southbridge, Mass.

of spotting the optical centers and using these to lay out the lens, fitting crosses are used. Fitting crosses will be present already on the lens when it arrives from the surfacing laboratory. If the fitting cross is not on the lens, its position may be located by using the hidden circles on the lens surface and the manufacturer's lens blank chart, just as with ordinary progressive lenses.

Other designs may ask for monocular PDs and fitting heights. The fitting height may be based on the location of the lower lid, as with bifocals, or the pupil center, as with progressives. In both cases, fitting height is changed to raise or drop because centration for edging requires raise or drop.

Some lens designs come in only one power range between upper and lower portions: +1.00 D, for example. Others may have two, such as the Sola Access lens (AOSola, Petaluma, Calif.) with +0.75 and 1.25. The higher range is for higher adds. Still others have a variable range that changes based on add power.

The following text provides some examples of how some intermediate/near-style specialty progressives are ordered.

Example 5-3
A Sola Access lens is ordered. The order comes to the laboratory with the following information:

R: +0.75 −0.50 × 180
L: +0.75 −0.50 × 180
Add: +2.25
PD = 66/62
Frame:
    A = 48 mm
    B = 36 mm
    DBL = 20

The Sola Access lens comes with two possible power ranges; +0.75 D and +1.25 D. With the help of Table 5-1, the reader should answer the following questions:

- What power should be used for the Sola Access lens?
- Power range has not been specified by the prescriber. Which power range is appropriate?
- How would the lens be laid out for edging?
- What power will there be in the top part of the lens?

Solution

1. The Sola Access lens is ordered using the near power, just like reading glasses. The near power for this prescription is found as follows:

| +0.75 −0.50 × 180 | (Distance) |
+2.25 D sphere	+(Add)
= +3.00 −0.50 × 180	=(Near power)

2. According to the manufacturer recommendations, people with add powers of +1.75 D or more should use the +1.25 D power range. This means that for a prescription with a +2.25 add, the +1.25 D power range lens is chosen.
3. The lens does not need a fitting height and the near PD is used. The lenses are spotted with the lensmeter after finding the MRPs. The lens is decentered using the following equation:

$$Decentration = \frac{A + DBL - Near\ PD}{2}$$
$$= \frac{48 + 20 - 62}{2}$$
$$= 3\ mm$$

Because the lenses were not ordered with an MRP height, nor were they required to be, no vertical decentration exists.

4. Because the power range of the lens is 1.25 D, the power in the upper part of the lens is 1.25 D less than the near power. The near power is +3.00 −0.50 × 180. Therefore the power in the upper portion is as follows:

| +3.00 −0.50 × 180 | (Near power) |
−1.25 D	− (Power range)
= +1.75 −0.50 × 180	= (Power in the upper portion of the lens)

This is shown and further explained in Figure 5-11.

Example 5-4

A Rodenstock Cosmolit Office lens (Rodenstock North America, Inc., Lockbourne, Ohio) is ordered for the following prescription and frame:

+1.25 -0.75 × 90
+1.25 -0.75 × 90
Add: +1.00
Monocular distance PDs—R: 33 L: 34
Fitting heights to pupil center—R: 24 L: 24
Frame:
    A = 50
    B = 38
    DBL = 19

With the help of Table 5-1, the reader should answer the following questions about this order:

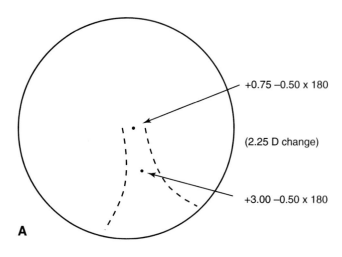

Standard progressive

+0.75 −0.50 × 180

(2.25 D change)

+3.00 −0.50 x 180

A

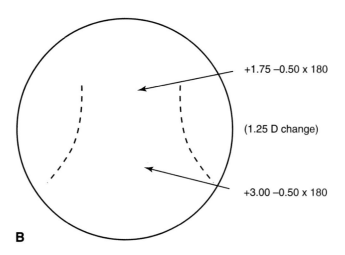

Intermediate/near specialty progressive

+1.75 −0.50 x 180

(1.25 D change)

+3.00 −0.50 x 180

B

FIGURE 5-11 This schematically compares a standard progressive (A) and the Sola Access intermediate/near specialty progressive (B; AOSola, Petaluma, Calif.) in the text example. Both lenses are for the same individual, and both are derived from the same lens prescription. A, General-purpose-wear lens. B, Lens for intermediate and near use only.

- Because the power range has not been specified by the prescriber, what power range is chosen?
- What will the powers in the lower and upper portions of the lens be?
- How will the right lens be laid out for edging?

Solution

1. (Which power range is chosen?) The Rodenstock Office lens comes in two power ranges: 1.00 D and 1.75 D. The add power prescribed is +1.00 D.

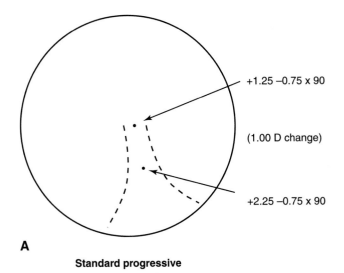

A

Standard progressive

+1.25 –0.75 x 90

(1.00 D change)

+2.25 –0.75 x 90

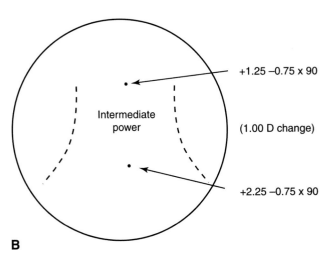

B

Intermediate/near specialty progressive

Intermediate power

+1.25 –0.75 x 90

(1.00 D change)

+2.25 –0.75 x 90

FIGURE **5-12** This simplified diagram shows the example problem that compares a standard progressive **(A)** to a Rodenstock Office intermediate/near design specialty progressive lens **(B;** Rodenstock North America, Inc., Lockbourne, Ohio) with a 1.00 D power range. The specialty lens is inappropriate for all-purpose use such as driving, even though the power in the upper area is identical to the distance power. In too many situations the overplussed straight-ahead gaze through lens **B** hinders normal distance vision. Distance viewing is overplussed because straight-ahead gaze, with the head erect, will be through the progressive zone, where power is more than called for in the distance prescription. Straight-ahead viewing in lens **A** will not be overplussed.

According to Rodenstock, adds of +1.50 and below normally use a power range of +1.00 D. Therefore the power range chosen is +1.00 D.

2. (Identify upper and lower lens powers.) The power in the lower portion of the lens is equal to the near

power of the prescription. This is as follows:

| +1.25 –0.75 × 90 | (Distance power) |
+1.00	+(Add power)
+2.25 –0.75 × 90	=(Near power)

Now, which power is expected in the upper portion of the lens? To find the expected power in the upper portion of the lens, knowing near power is +2.50 –0.75 × 90, and a range of 1.00 D, the practitioner can work backward from the near power.

| +2.25 –0.75 × 90 | (Near power) |
–1.00	–(Power range)
+1.25 –0.75 × 90	=(Power in the upper portion of the lens)

This concept is demonstrated and further explained in Figure 5-12.

3. (How will the right lens be laid out for edging?) The Office lens is fit like a regular progressive. The lens uses a fitting cross that is above the MRP[7] and based on the distance PD. The near position of the lens is inset from the fitting cross so that the near optics are properly positioned for near viewing even when using the distance PD. This fitting procedure is the same as is used for regular progressive lenses.

The lens comes from the surfacing laboratory with the fitting cross marked. (If the lens is not marked, the hidden circles are found on the front surface of the lens and the fitting cross and 180 line are re-marked using the manufacturer's centration chart, which will be similar to the centration chart that is shown in Figure 5-8.) For the right lens, the practitioner must find the distance decentration and fitting cross raise.

Distance decentration is calculated as follows:

$$\text{Distance decentration} = \frac{A + DBL}{2} - \text{Monocular PD}$$
$$= \frac{50 + 19}{2} - 33$$
$$= \frac{69}{2} - 33$$
$$= 34.5 - 33$$
$$= 1.5 \text{ mm inset}$$

Fitting cross raise is as follows:

$$\text{Raise or drop} = \text{Fitting cross height} - \frac{B}{2}$$
$$= 24 - \frac{38}{2}$$
$$= 24 - 19$$
$$= +5 \text{ mm raise}$$

[7]Major reference point (MRP) and prism reference point (PRP) are identical.

Using the Full Range of Available Intermediate/Near Lenses

Not every wearer's intermediate and near working situations are identical. Some people may work only with a computer in an enclosed environment. Others may work at a control panel with longer intermediate distances than the computer user would require.

For this reason a specialty progressive lens may be ordered with a power range that does not correspond to the add power normally recommended for that prescription. A skilled practitioner who knows the variations in power ranges available from different manufacturers can tailor the selected lens to the needs of the wearer and choose the brand according to the needed power range.

SPECIALTY COMPUTER LENSES

Intermediate/near-type specialty lenses often are recommended for computer users. But if the computer user still has a need to see distant objects clearly, the AO Technica lens is an option. This lens has an extended (lengthened) progressive corridor to allow an intermediate viewing area that is deeper and wider than standard progressives. This moves the distance portion into the very top of the lens (Figure 5-13).

Layout for edging is done in exactly the same manner as for conventional progressive lenses. Prescription information is also the same: distance power, add power, fitting cross heights, and monocular PDs. Because this lens has a long progressive corridor, the manufacturer recommends a 23-mm fitting cross height. The manu-

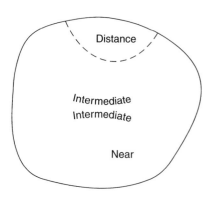

FIGURE **5-13** The Technica lens (American Optical, Southbridge, Mass.) is designed for computer use while a small distance viewing area is preserved in the upper part of the lens. The frame must have a large enough vertical size or much of the distance portion may be cut away during edging. (From Brooks CW, Borish IM: *System for ophthalmic dispensing,* ed 2, Boston, 1996, Butterworth-Heinemann.)

facturer also recommends a minimum of 19 mm between the fitting cross and the top of the frame. Reducing this 19 mm distance results in an unintended reduction in the distance viewing area. If the laboratory notes a significant reduction in these recommended minimums, the account should be contacted with appropriate recommendations for solving the problem.[8]

---

[8]For more information on specialty progressives related to fitting and dispensing, see Chapter 11 of Brooks CW, Borish I: *System for ophthalmic dispensing,* ed 2, Boston, 1996, Butterworth-Heinemann.

Proficiency Test Questions

1. Which of the following points on a progressive addition lens is a synonym for the MRP (major reference point)?

    a. Fitting cross
    b. DRP
    c. NRP
    d. PRP
    e. None of the above

2. True or False? Binocular PDs always work fine for progressive addition lenses.

3. Which of the following reference points is used for lens layout of progressive addition lenses during centration?

    a. The fitting cross
    b. The major reference point
    c. The center of the near progressive zone

4. True or False? In the simplest terms, the centration of progressive add lenses is done as if the lens were a single vision lens.

5. A progressive lens is to be marked for edging. The frame and PD dimensions are as follows:

   Frame: A = 51
           B = 42
           DBL = 17
   Monocular PDs—R: 31; L: 33
   Fitting cross heights—R: 27; L: 26

   How much raise and decentration are required for each lens?

6. A progressive lens is ordered with the following parameters:

   Frame: A = 47
           B = 39
           DBL = 20
   Monocular PDs—R: 29.5; L: 31.0
   Fitting cross heights—R: 24 mm; L: 24 mm

   How much raise and decentration are required for each lens?

7. Use the hidden circles on this progressive addition lens to lay the lens out for edging.

   Frame: A = 48
           B = 38
           DBL = 19
   Monocular PDs—R: 31.5 mm; L: 32.0 mm
   Fitting cross heights—R: 22 mm; L: 23 mm

   If the lens fitting cross is 4 mm above the lens PRP, what *hidden circle* raise or drop is required for each lens? What distance decentration is needed?

8. Use the hidden circles on this progressive addition lens to lay the following lens out for edging:

   Frame: A = 46
           B = 33
           DBL= 18
   Monocular PDs—R: 29.5 mm; L: 28.5 mm
   Fitting cross heights—R: 20 mm; L: 21 mm

   If the lens fitting cross is 2.5 mm above the lens PRP, what *hidden circle* raise or drop is required for each lens? What distance decentration is needed?

9. True or False? An intermediate/near specialty progressive can be worn for general purposes if these conditions are met: The power in the upper half of the specialty lens must be made equal to the distance power of the general-purpose progressive without changing the total near power of the lens.

10. True or False? All intermediate/near specialty progressives have close to the same intermediate/near power range options.

11. A Zeiss RD lens (Carl Zeiss Optical, Inc., Chester, Va.) is ordered. Following is the regular lens prescription:

    R: −050 −0.50 × 170
    L: −0.25 −0.75 × 5
    Add: +2.50

    Identify the powers in the lower and upper portions of the Zeiss RD lens.

12. The prescription in question 11 is now ordered for a Sola Access lens. Identify the powers in the lower and upper portions of the Sola Access lens.

13. An order for an AO Technica lens (American Optical, Southbridge, Mass.) has right and left fitting cross heights of 23 mm. The B dimension of the frame is 35 mm. Which of the following statements is true?

    a. There will not be enough reading area, but the distance viewing portion will be fine.
    b. There will not be enough area for distance viewing, but reading will be fine.
    c. There will not be enough area for either reading or distance viewing.
    d. There will be sufficient viewing area for both distance and near viewing.

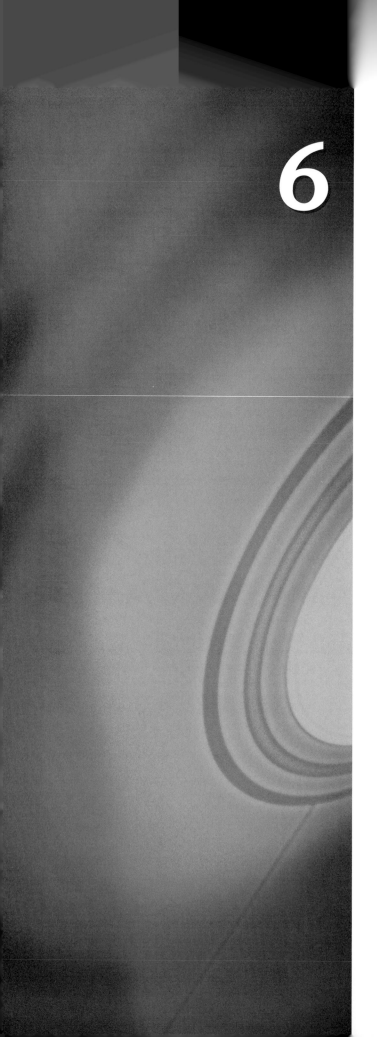

6

Centration of Segmented Multifocal Lenses

Segmented Multifocals

The near viewing segment area in conventional multifocal lenses has a clearly demarcated line that borders it. This can be used as a stable, convenient reference when positioning the lens for blocking.

The vertical location of the segment is measured for each wearer. The dispenser gives this vertical location in terms of segment height. The optical laboratory must convert segment height to segment raise or drop.

The dispenser gives the horizontal location of the segment in terms of the wearer's distance and near PDs. The laboratory must convert to segment inset relative to the boxing center of the edged lens.

SEGMENT HEIGHT

The dispenser specifies vertical segment location as segment height. Segment height is the vertical distance from the lowest position on the boxed lens shape to the level of the top of the bifocal or trifocal (Figure 6-1). This is the most logical method for measuring in the dispensary. It is not the measurement the laboratory personnel must use in making the lens.

SEGMENT DROP OR RAISE

In the laboratory, segment height must be specified as *segment drop* or *segment raise*. The two definitions of segment drop or raise are as follows:

Definition 1: The vertical distance from the major reference point (MRP) to the level of the segment top.

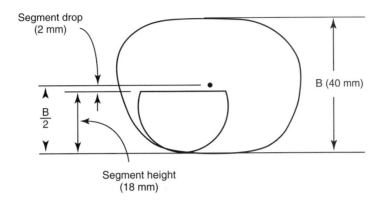

Segment drop
(2 mm)

B (40 mm)

$\dfrac{B}{2}$

Segment height
(18 mm)

FIGURE **6-1** The vertical position of the segment top can be expressed either as *segment drop* or *segment height*.

Definition 2: The vertical distance from the horizontal midline of the edged lens shape to the level of the segment top. This is the definition commonly used in U.S. optical laboratory practice.

Normally these measurements end up being at the same location because the MRP usually falls on the horizontal midline of the edged lens anyway. In the following two instances these two measurements would not be the same:

1. When a specific MRP height is specified on the order
2. When the segment top is above the middle of the edged lens and the surfacing laboratory personnel place the MRP above the line so that it may be found when the lenses are verified

For this discussion, the author assumes that the MRP is positioned on the horizontal midline. Therefore it does not matter which definition is used because both answers will be the same.

CONVERTING FROM SEGMENT HEIGHT TO SEGMENT DROP (OR RAISE)

To convert from segment height to segment drop, the same procedure is used as described for calculation of vertical positioning of the major reference point for single vision lenses, and for fitting cross height for progressive addition lenses.

First the vertical dimension of the frame's lens opening is determined. This is the B dimension. Half this measurement is then subtracted from the segment height. If the direction from the midline to the segment top is down, the resulting number will be negative. This is *segment drop*. If the number is positive, the segment top is above the horizontal midline. This is called *segment raise* and is expressed in the following formula:

$$\text{Segment drop (or raise)} = \text{Segment height} - \frac{B}{2}$$

Example 6-1

A frame has the following dimensions:

A (eyesize) = 52 mm
B = 40 mm
DBL = 20 mm

The segment height specified on the order is 18 mm. What is the segment drop or raise?

Solution

Only the vertical frame measure is important for segment drop. In this example the following calculation is applied:

$$
\begin{aligned}
\text{Segment drop} &= \text{Segment height} - \frac{B}{2} \\
&= 18 - \frac{40}{2} \\
&= 18 - 20 \\
&= -2 \text{ mm}
\end{aligned}
$$

Because the number is negative the answer is 2 mm of segment drop (Figure 6-1).

SEGMENT INSET

The near segment is moved nasally or *inset* from the position of the major reference point to allow for convergence of the eyes while a person is reading or working up close. (Convergence is the inward turning of the eyes that occurs when viewing objects close up.) The amount that the segment is nasally inset from the MRP is known as *segment inset*. Written as an equation, segment inset is defined as half the distance between distance and near PDs.

$$\text{Segment inset} = \frac{\text{Distance PD} - \text{Near PD}}{2}$$

Example 6-2

How much would segment inset be for a bifocal lens worn by a person with a distance PD of 69 and a near PD of 66?

Solution

Because segment inset is the difference between distance PD and near PD, divided by 2, the segment inset would be equal to the following:

$$\begin{aligned}\text{Segment inset} &= \frac{69 - 66}{2} \\ &= \frac{3}{2} \\ &= 1.5 \text{ mm}\end{aligned}$$

making segment inset equal to 1.5 mm.

TOTAL INSET

When a single vision lens is laid out for blocking, the reference point on the lens used for decentration is the MRP. When laying out a segmented multifocal lens for blocking, the practitioner uses the center of the lens segment as a reference for decentration.

The distance between the centers of the left and right multifocal segments is equal to the wearer's near PD. So when the multifocal order is written, the dispenser specifies the desired distance between segment centers as the wearer's near PD. For the dispenser, near PD is the most convenient and logical measure to use.

The optical laboratory uses the near PD to find needed measurements. To specify horizontal segment placement for edging purposes, the correct position for the segment is the horizontal distance from the boxing center of the lens.

Decentration of the MRP for single vision was figured in terms of distance PD.

$$\text{Decentration} = \frac{(A + DBL) - \text{Distance PD}}{2}$$

But segmented multifocals are positioned in terms of the near segment (Figure 6-2). Segment decentration is calculated using near PD. This segment decentration per lens is called *total segment inset* or simply *total inset*.

$$\text{Total inset} = \frac{(A + DBL) - \text{Near PD}}{2}$$

(*Note:* The amount of near segment displacement also can be thought of as distance decentration plus segment inset. This probably is why the name is *total* inset.)

Example 6-3

A frame has the following dimensions:

A = 52 mm
B = 40 mm
DBL = 20 mm

The wearer's PD equals 66/62. What is the total inset?

Solution

$$\begin{aligned}\text{Total inset} &= \frac{(A + DBL) - \text{Near PD}}{2} \\ &= \frac{(50 + 20) - 62}{2} \\ &= \frac{10}{2} \\ &= 5 \text{ mm}\end{aligned}$$

Therefore the total segment inset per lens is 5 mm.

Flat-Top Multifocals

HISTORICAL BACKGROUND: CENTRATION USING A LENS PROTRACTOR

To help in understanding the mechanics of multifocal lens positioning, the process can be described initially for hand marking with the aid of a lens protractor. This process is seldom used, but an understanding of it can be helpful in visualization of the different points on the lens.

The intersection of the main horizontal and vertical lines on the protractor denotes the location of the boxing center of the edged lens. The lens is positioned with use of the center of the multifocal segment as a reference. The midpoint on the top of the widest part of the segment is found and dotted. With practice this can be done visually. Until then, the protractor has a grid upon which the segment may be centered.

Now the lens is placed face down on the lens protractor. It is moved laterally until the centrally

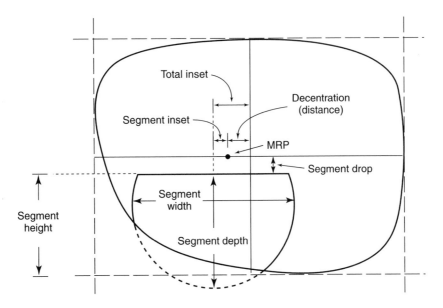

FIGURE **6-2** Decentration is sometimes referred to as *inset*. This must not be confused with segment inset or total inset. These are difference measures.

placed segment dot is displaced from the intersection by an amount equal to the total inset. With the segment center at the correct total inset, the segment top may be moved up or down to the correct distance above or below the horizontal reference line.[1] The amount above or below corresponds to the segment raise or drop. When this positioning is complete, the segment will be at the correct height and inset. As a result the previously spotted MRP also should be properly inset and will be on the horizontal reference line.

A long horizontal line and a short vertical line are drawn on the lens corresponding to the location of the center of the lens protractor. This denotes the location of the boxing center of the edged lens (Box 6-1).

Example 6-4

An order has the following specifications:

R: +1.00 −0.75 × 175
L: +1.00 −0.75 × 5
Add: +2.00
PD: 67/63
Flat-top 28 bifocal, segment height 18 mm
Frame: A = 55
       B = 42
       DBL = 18

How would the *left* lens be marked for blocking with use of a lens protractor?

---

[1]This horizontal reference line indicates the position of the horizontal midline on the edged lens if the pattern is made according to accepted practices.

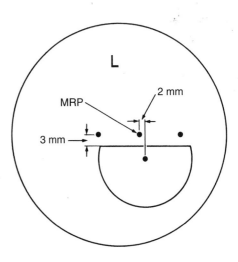

FIGURE **6-3** The back view of the left lens shows the relationship between major reference point (MRP) and segment positions. The MRP will not necessarily fall in the center of the lens.

Solution

The surfacing process already has positioned the major reference point and the cylinder axis orientation relative to the segment. The MRP and the 180-degree reference dots have been marked on the lens during the "spotting" process. As in Figure 6-3, these three dots should be parallel to the top of the segment.

The lens is placed *face down* on the lens protractor. The segment center must be inset. To find out how much, the practitioner must find the amount of total segment inset:

$$\text{Total inset} = \frac{(A + DBL) - \text{Near PD}}{2}$$

Therefore when the calculation is applied to this example, the following equation results:

$$\begin{aligned}\text{Total inset} &= \frac{(55 + 18) - 63}{2}\\[4pt] &= \frac{73 - 63}{2}\\[4pt] &= \frac{10}{5}\\[4pt] &= 5\text{ mm}\end{aligned}$$

The vertical position of the segment line can be simultaneously positioned and is calculated as follows:

BOX 6-1
Using a Lens Protractor in the Centration of Flat-Top Multifocals

1. Verify the lens for power accuracy and spot it in the same manner described in Chapter 2 for a single vision lens.
2. Calculate the total segment inset per lens, as follows:

$$\text{Total segment inset per lens} = \frac{(A + DBL) - \text{Near PD}}{2}$$

3. Calculate the segment drop or raise as follows:

$$\text{Segment drop (or raise)} = \text{Segment height} - \frac{B}{2}$$

4. Locate and dot the segment center, or dot the center of the segment top.
5. Determine whether the lens must be decentered to the right or to the left. If the lens is facing downward, a right lens will be decentered to the left and a left lens will be decentered to the right. Normally, a lens is placed face down (front surface down) on the protractor.
6. Place the lens face down on the lens protractor and move it laterally until the centrally placed segment dot is displaced from the intersection by an amount equal to the total inset.
7. With the segment center at the correct total inset, move the segment top up or down to the correct distance above or below the horizontal reference line to the correct segment drop or raise.
8. Draw a long horizontal line and a short vertical line on the lens corresponding to the location of the center of the lens protractor.

$$\text{Segment drop} = \text{Segment height} - \frac{B}{2}$$
$$= 18 - \frac{42}{2}$$
$$= 18 - 21$$
$$= -3\text{ mm}$$

The negative number indicates a segment drop. Therefore the segment drop is 3 mm below the horizontal midline.

Figure 6-4 demonstrates the way in which the lens would be positioned for marking. Because the lens is *face down* on the protractor and is a *left* lens, the segment center is moved 5 mm to the *right*. The segment top is moved 3 mm down. (Because of exactness in surfacing, the MRP is exactly where it should be. It is 3 mm inward. This is right where it should be when decentered for the distance PD. It is also exactly on the 180-degree line, where it belongs.[2])

To mark the lens by hand, a longer horizontal line would be drawn along the main horizontal reference line of the protractor and a short vertical line where the main vertical protractor line crosses the horizontal. (This was shown previously in the marking of single vision lenses in Figure 4-6.)

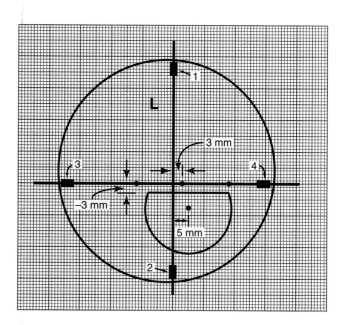

FIGURE 6-4 The center of the segment may be used for horizontal reference and the segment top for vertical reference. The four marks at the edge of the lens become reference points for placing the standard cross mark on the lens surface when the lens is being marked by hand.

---

[2]Although not the recommended procedure, in this case centration could have been accomplished using only the three dots marked by the lensmeter.

USING A CENTRATION INSTRUMENT WITH FLAT-TOP MULTIFOCALS

The process for centration of flat-top multifocals is done in about the same way with a centration instrument as it was done with a lens protractor, but it is easier. An example problem may help explain the process.

Example 6-5

A prescription for a flat-top lens reads as follows:

R: –2.50 –1.75 × 10
L: –2.75 –1.50 × 171
Add: +1.25
PD: 63/60
Segment height = 15 mm
Frame: A = 50
        B = 38
        DBL = 18

How would the *left* lens be centered and marked for edging?

Solution

Step 1. The practitioner verifies the lens for power and MRP location. The location of the MRP is spotted with the lensmeter. (Even though the lens has been spotted, these dots are ignored until the lens has been centered with reference to the segment. After this has been completed, the location of the dots is checked for accuracy.)

Step 2. If the instrument has blocking capabilities, a double-sided adhesive blocking pad is placed on a lens block and the block is mounted on the instrument. The paper is peeled away from the pad on the block to expose the adhesive.

Step 3. The total segment inset required is determined. In the example, total inset is as follows:

$$\text{Total inset} = \frac{(A + DBL) - \text{Near PD}}{2}$$
$$= \frac{(50 + 18) - 60}{2}$$
$$= \frac{68 - 60}{2}$$
$$= \frac{8}{2}$$
$$= 4 \text{ mm}$$

Step 4. The practitioner determines whether the lens must be decentered to the right or to the left. Because the lens is to be placed in the centering device face up and is a left lens, the lens must be decentered to the left (see Figure 4-3, *B*, and Box 4-1).

Step 5. The vertical reference line in the instrument is moved to the right or left by the amount of decentration calculated. In this example the vertical reference line would be moved 4 mm to the left.

Step 6. The amount of segment drop or raise required is calculated. In this case, the following calculation applies:

$$\text{Segment drop} = \text{Segment height} - \frac{B}{2}$$
$$= 15 - \frac{38}{2}$$
$$= 15 - 19$$
$$= -4 \text{ mm}$$

Because the number is negative, the vertical movement of the segment top is downward, indicating a segment drop.

Step 7. The lens is placed face up in the instrument and the segment is aligned between the segment border lines. Centration instruments have a variety of methods for bordering the outer edges of the segment so that the segment center will not have to be located by hand.

In this example, the left lens has been placed face up for blocking. The nasal, segment side will be to the left. The movable vertical line has been positioned 4 mm to the left of center. Marking the center of the segment is not necessary because boundary lines spaced equally to the left and right of the movable vertical line border the segment. The segment is centered horizontally when symmetrically enclosed by bordering lines. This is shown in Figure 6-5.

Step 8. The lens is moved up or down so that the segment top is at the appropriate segment drop or raise. In the example this is 4 mm below the main horizontal reference line.

Step 9. The handle of the instrument is grasped and swung into place, or the button or footswitch is pressed. This blocks the lens.

These steps are summarized in Box 6-2.

Catching Errors before the Lens is Edged

Laying out a segmented multifocal is possible using only the segment for reference. If everything in lens centration has been done correctly, the near PD and the segment height should come out exactly right when the lens is edged and placed in the frame. However, the

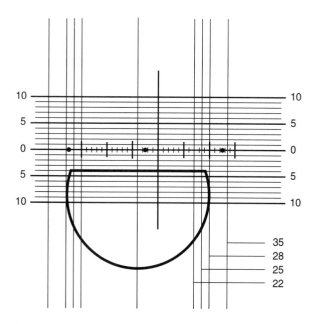

FIGURE **6-5**   This left lens, placed convex side up, has a 2.5-mm distance decentration, a 1.5-mm segment inset, a 4-mm total inset, and a segment drop of 4 mm.

completed spectacles may still be unacceptable. There are several reasons why they might be rejected. The following are a few:

- The MRPs of the distance portion of the lenses may be either too high or too low.
- The MRPs of the distance portion of the lenses may not be at the same height. This most likely will cause unwanted vertical prism.
- The distance PD may be too wide or too narrow and cause unwanted horizontal prism. This happens because the segment inset has not been surfaced correctly.
- The cylinder may be at the wrong axis.

If the lens has not been properly surfaced, any or all of these errors can occur. They may occur even if the lens segment is positioned properly during centration. The primary reason errors occur is the relationship between the distance MRP and the segment have not been proofed. The following section outlines how these errors happen and how they may be prevented.

CHECKING MAJOR REFERENCE POINT HEIGHT IN THE DISTANCE PORTION

Before edging a lens, the practitioner checks the distance power. Sphere and cylinder powers should be correct. With the segment line horizontally straight in the lensmeter, the cylinder axis should be as ordered. Now the lens is spotted.

BOX 6-2
Using a Centration Device for Flat-Top Multifocals

1. Verify the lens for power and MRP location. Spot the location of the MRP with the lensmeter.
2. Place the lens block in the instrument.
3. Determine the total segment inset required:

$$\text{Total inset} = \frac{(A + DBL) - \text{Near PD}}{2}$$

4. Determine whether the lens must be decentered to the right or to the left. If the lens is convex side up, for a right lens decenter to the right; for a left lens, to the left.
5. Position the movable vertical line in the instrument to the right or left by the amount of decentration calculated.
6. Calculate the amount of segment drop or raise required:

$$\text{Segment drop} = \text{Segment height} - \frac{B}{2}$$

7. Place the lens face up in the instrument and align the segment between the segment border lines.
8. Move the lens up or down so that the segment top is at the indicated segment drop or raise.
9. Grasp the handle of the instrument and swing into place, or press the button or footswitch. This blocks the lens.

MRP, Major reference point; *DBL,* distance between lenses; *PD,* interpupillary distance.

During the centration process the vertical location of the MRP is checked. When the segment drop or raise is correct in the centration instrument, the MRP should be on the main horizontal line. If it is, the MRP height has been placed correctly. This assumes that no specific MRP height has been ordered. If the segment height is especially high or low, an MRP that is not on the main horizontal line may also be correct. The box on p. 119 MRP Placement provides an explanation of this idea.

If after centering a lens with a flat-top bifocal segment, the practitioner discovers that the MRP is 2 mm above the horizontal midline as shown in Figure 6-6, is this a problem? In some cases this may be inconsequential, even normal. But in other instances the lens will almost certainly cause the prescription to be unsuitable and should be rejected or returned before more time is wasted. These two factors are critical in the decision whether to accept or reject the lens:

FACTOR 1: *Is the second lens in the pair identically surfaced?*

If the second lens in the pair also has its

MRP Placement

In theory, the dispensary should specify the location of the major reference point for all single vision and multifocal lenses. In practice they do not. Therefore some choices that perhaps would better be made in the dispensary must be made in the optical laboratory.

When a specific MRP height is not given, the surfacing laboratory must make the decision on where to place it. The software program used by the surfacing laboratory provides the following two options:

1. The MRP always is placed on the 180-degree line, regardless of where the top of the segment happens to be.
2. The MRP is placed on the 180-degree line unless the segment is either high and will approach or cross the 180-degree line or especially low.

With the second option the surfacing laboratory sets maximum and minimum distances the MRP can be from the top of the segment.

Following are some typical maximum and minimum distances:

	MAXIMUM ALLOWABLE DISTANCE OF MRP FROM SEGMENT LINE	MINIMUM ALLOWABLE DISTANCE OF MRP FROM SEGMENT LINE
Bifocals	5 mm	2 mm
Trifocals	1.5 mm	3 mm

Example
A frame has a B dimension of 38 mm, and the lens has a bifocal segment height of 20 mm. Where would the distance MRP end up being for option 1 and option 2?

Solution
For option 1, the MRP would be directly on the horizontal midline of the lens, halfway between the top and bottom. Half of 38 mm is 19 mm, so the MRP is at 19 mm. This is found in the segment, 1 mm below the segment line.

For option 2, the typical measurements shown above will be used. The minimum allowable distance from the MRP down to the top of the segment is 2 mm. This means that if the bifocal segment is 20 mm high, then the MRP must be 20 mm plus 2 mm, or 22 mm, high.

MRP, Major reference point.

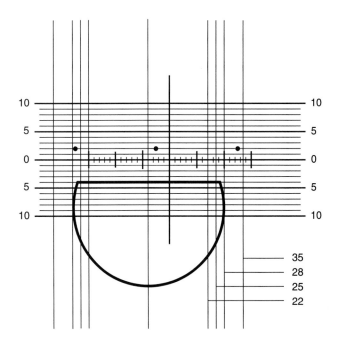

FIGURE 6-6 This figure has one potential problem: The inset is correct; the axis should also be correct because the 180-degree line marked by the lensmeter is parallel to the horizontal; but the major reference point will fall above the 180 line if fabricated. This may or may not be a problem, depending on the other lens.

FACTOR 2: *Are the left and right MRPs at different vertical heights?* The practitioner should note how much farther the MRP is from the segment line in one lens than it is in the other lens. If the difference in heights is more than 1 mm when the power of the weaker lens is greater than or equal to ±3.375 D, the lens pair will not pass ANSI standards.

This should emphasize the importance of care in measuring lens parameters for the duplication or replacement of a single lens in a pair of lenses.

If the power of the weaker lens is less than ±3.375 D and the two MRP locations are more than 1 mm apart vertically, a problem may still exist. To find out whether a problem still exists, the two spotted lenses are placed front-to-front so that the segments are superimposed. (The practitioner should not actually touch the front surfaces of the lenses against each other, or the surfaces may get scratched.) The strongest lens should be facing outward. The center spot of the stronger lens is viewed through the weaker lens and the weaker lens is dotted at that location.

Now the newly spotted point is placed on the weaker lens in the center of the lensmeter aperture. Read the prismatic effect. If it is greater than or equal to one-

MRP 2 mm above the horizontal midline, then no differential vertical prism will result between the two eyes. In fact, if no vertical MRP height was specified, then with both MRPs at the same vertical height (within reasonable limits) no error has occurred.

third prism diopter, the lens will not pass ANSI Z80.1 standards. (Without actually using a lensmeter, this prismatic effect can be predicted using Prentice's Rule. This is done by multiplying the difference in vertical MRP heights in centimeters by the power of the weaker lens in the 90-degree meridian.)

Example 6-6

The following prescription is fabricated:

R: –7.00 D sphere
L: –5.00 D sphere
Add: +1.50

The two lenses are spotted. The right MRP is 2 mm higher than it should be. The left MRP is exactly on the horizontal midline. Is this acceptable?

Solution

Because both lenses are greater than ±3.375 D and the two MRP locations more than 1 mm apart vertically, the lens pair will be unacceptable. Unwanted vertical prism will be beyond what is tolerable. The right lens should be remade.

Example 6-7

Following is another example that is a bit more complex:

R: +1.00
L: +1.50 –1.25 × 180
Add: +2.00

In checking for correct vertical MRP placement during the centration process, the practitioner sees that the right lens is 3 mm above the horizontal midline. However, the MRP of the left lens is right on the line.

Will the lens pair prove suitable after edging? (In thinking through the question, the reader should look carefully at the prescription when considering which lens is stronger in the vertical meridian.)

Solution

The reader should look at the powers of both lenses in their 90-degree meridians (Figure 6-7). As can be seen, two different results will be obtained depending upon whether point A on the right lens or point B on the left is considered. So which lens is used to evaluate prismatic effect?

(*Hint:* When evaluating a lens pair for unwanted vertical prism, the practitioner uses the lens with the weakest power. It would not be "fair" to use the lens with the stronger power. What would happen if one lens has no power and the other lens has –7.00 D of power? If the zero-powered lens is spotted first, no prismatic effect will be detected, no matter where on the lens a measurement is taken. Sliding the lens pair over to the –7.00 D lens could show a great deal of vertical prism at any distance above or below the center of the lens.)

The power of the left lens is +1.50 –1.25 × 180. To make it easier to visualize, the lens powers are placed on a power cross. This is shown in Figure 6-7 and tells us that the lens with the least power in the 90-degree meridian is the left lens. This is the lens used to determine how much vertical prismatic effect is caused by the lens pair.

What is the prismatic effect for the left lens? Prentice's Rule is used to evaluate the prismatic effect on the decentered point of the weaker lens. The formula for Prentice's Rule is $\Delta = cF$. The values for c and F must be determined.

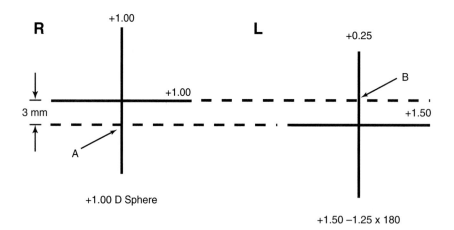

FIGURE **6-7** Evaluated in terms of point A, the vertical prism would be 0.30Δ base up. In terms of point B, however, the prismatic effect is only 0.075Δ base down.

The reference point on that lens is 3 mm (or 0.3 cm) away from its center. Therefore the following is true:

$$c = 0.3 \text{ cm}$$

The power manifested in the vertical (90-degree) meridian is +0.25 D. Therefore the following is true:

$$\begin{aligned} \Delta &= cF \\ &= (.3)(0.25) \\ &= 0.075\Delta \end{aligned}$$

In this case the unwanted vertical prism is 0.075Δ.

What is the allowable amount of vertical prism? According to ANSI Z80.1 standards, the allowable amount of prism is a maximum of one-third prism diopter. The 0.075Δ prism amount is definitely less than the 0.33Δ allowable. This is sufficiently below the maximum allowable tolerance to make the lens pair acceptable and not cause discomfort for the wearer.

CHECKING FOR INCORRECT SEGMENT INSET

Naturally the practitioner wants the distance PD and the near PD to be right once the lenses are edged. To predict whether this will happen or not, the practitioner needs to know whether the MRP is at the right position horizontally relative to the center of the segment. The correct distance between the two is equal to the segment inset. The segment inset was defined as follows:

$$\text{Segment inset} = \frac{\text{Distance PD} - \text{Near PD}}{2}$$

Checking to see whether segment inset will be correct is really done at the same time the lens is being positioned in the centration instrument for blocking. After the lens is positioned for blocking, the practitioner looks for the previously spotted MRP. It should be temporal to the movable vertical line by an amount equal to the segment inset.[3] (The movable vertical line marks the location of the center of the segment top.)

For example, if the distance PD is 65 and the near PD 62, then the MRP should be 1.5 mm outward from the movable vertical line that goes through the center of the segment.

---

[3]Another way of checking correct MRP location is to see whether it is at the correct distance decentration. The MRP should be nasal from the stationary vertical line in the centration instrument by an amount equal to the distance decentration. This is the case because of the following equation:

Total segment inset = Distance decentration + Segment inset

INCORRECT SEGMENT INSET

If the MRP is found to be horizontally off compared to the segment, the practitioner needs to know whether the problem is bad enough to reject the lens. Sometimes the way the lens is centered for edging determines whether it is usable.

If the MRP is horizontally off, the lenses can be edged so that *either* the distance PD *or* the near PD will be correct, but not both. However, producing a perfectly acceptable pair of lenses still may be possible. So if it is determined that the segment inset is wrong before the lenses are edged, the practitioner may choose one of the following four options:

1. To reject the lens and have it remade
2. To elect to have a correct *near* PD, but an incorrect distance PD
3. To elect to have a correct *distance* PD, but an incorrect near PD
4. To elect to position the lens midway between near and distance, altering both PDs slightly. This may be done only if the prismatic effects resulting from this choice are insignificant.

This discussion is not about how to get by with an unacceptable lens, which should not be tolerated. Any of these choices are possible only if the resulting pair of spectacles is comfortably within ANSI prescription standards. Sometimes more than one option will allow this. How does the practitioner decide which option is best?

The Factor that Favors an Accurate Distance Interpupillary Distance

When the relationship between distance PD and near PD is affected by a segment inset that is slightly off, the centration process allows the practitioner to favor either distance or near PD accuracy. The factor that especially favors a high exactness in the distance PD is the power is the distance lens. If the distance lens has a high refractive power, any slight variation in optical center placement will cause unwanted horizontal prism.

Factors that Favor an Accurate Near Interpupillary Distance

Just as a high-powered distance prescription favors an accurate distance PD, so does a high near addition favor an accurate near PD. Even though it is easier for the eyes to tolerate horizontal prism at near power because the eyes already are converging and diverging with changes in viewing distances, high addition powers do cause unintended horizontal prism when not properly positioned.

Compensating for Small MRP Placement Errors

Factors Favoring Maintenance of Distance PD, Alteration of Near PD
1. A high-powered distance prescription (in 180-degree) meridian
2. A low near addition power
3. A very wide segment

Factors Favoring Alteration of Distance PD, Maintenance of Near PD
1. A low-powered distance prescription (in 180-degree meridian)
2. An especially high near addition power
3. An especially small segment

MRP, Major reference point; *PD*, interpupillary distance.

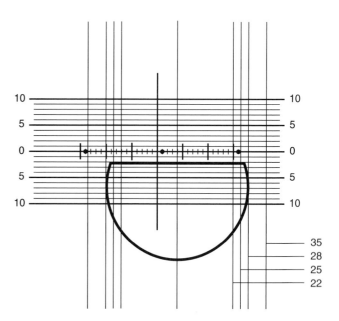

FIGURE 6-8 After the near segment is centered as indicated by the prescription, the position of the major reference point (MRP) should be checked to assume accuracy of the finished interpupillary distance (PD). In this instance, the required total inset is 4 mm, which is correct. Yet the MRP is incorrect because a 2 mm decentration per lens is indicated and only 1 mm appears. Correcting the position of the MRP to achieve the correct distance PD will throw off the near PD.

With segmented multifocals a limited viewing area exists for near vision. If the segment is small, the viewing area is small. Moving the segment away from its intended location takes off viewing space from one side or the other. If the near PD is off it will cut down that viewing area either temporally or nasally. So, if the segment is small, it should be accurately placed with a correct near PD. Box 6-3 summarizes factors that favor either the distance or the near PD.

Favoring Distance or Near Interpupillary Distance?
The following examples help the reader understand the logic used to decide whether to favor the distance PD or the near PD, or whether to split the difference.

Example 6-8
The following is prescribed:

R: +5.50 sphere
L: +5.50 sphere
PD: 69/65
Add: +1.00
Flat-top 28 segment: segment height 19 mm
Frame: A = 53
       B = 42
       DBL = 20

The right lens is positioned for blocking as shown in Figure 6-8. Although the segment height and total segment inset is correctly positioned so that the lens will cut out with the near PD correct, the MRP is incorrectly positioned. Is the lens usable? If so, should distance or near PD be favored?

Solution
To answer the question, the practitioner must know how far off the MRP is from where it should be in relation to the segment. In the example, the distance decentration should be as follows:

$$\text{Distance decentration} = \frac{(A + DBL) - PD}{2}$$

$$= \frac{(53 + 20) - 69}{2}$$

$$= \frac{73 - 69}{2}$$

$$= \frac{4}{2}$$

$$= 2 \text{ mm per lens}$$

For the distance PD to equal 69 mm, the center dot of the right lens should have a 2-mm distance decentration. Unfortunately this lens shows only 1 mm. So even if the left lens is accurate, the distance PD will be off 1 mm. It will end up being 70 mm instead of 69 mm. Left this way, the near PD will be a correct 65 mm. Which is more important in this prescription, distance or near PD accuracy?

The distance power in this prescription is high. If the distance PD is wrong, unwanted horizontal prism occurs at distance. The amount of unwanted prism will be as follows:

$$\Delta = cF$$
$$= (0.1)(5.5)$$
$$= 0.55\Delta \text{ base out}$$

Now what would happen if the practitioner decided to make the distance PD correct at the expense of throwing off the near PD? To do this the near PD would have to be decreased by 1 mm. If the near PD is intentionally decreased to 1 mm less than it should be, this will decrease the distance PD back to the required 69 mm. Doing this will eliminate unwanted horizontal prism in the distance portion. But what will happen if the near PD is 64 mm instead of 65 mm?

If the near PD is off by 1 mm, two optical effects will be produced at near, as follows:

1. The prismatic effect will change. But because of the low add power, that amount of change is small. The exact amount is found with Prentice's Rule ($\Delta = cF$), where c is the distance the segment has been moved from its proper location and F is the power of the add. Therefore the prism produced by intentionally making the near PD too small is only as follows:

$$\Delta = (0.1)(1)$$
$$= 0.10 \text{ base in}$$

2. The other effect from allowing the near PD to be wrong is that the temporal field of view through the near segment will be slightly reduced at near. However, this point becomes less significant with sufficiently large segment sizes because still plenty of room exists for near viewing through the segment.

Therefore which option should the practitioner choose in this case: correct distance PD or correct near PD? In making the final choice, the practitioner should look at ANSI Standards for prescription lenses. The ANSI tolerance for near PD for multifocals is ± 2.5 mm. For an ordered near PD of 65 mm, anything between 62.5 mm and 67.5 mm is considered acceptable.

ANSI tolerances for the distance PD are also ± 2.5 mm. But in this prescription, the unwanted prismatic effect produced by a wrong distance PD is more than that produced by a wrong near PD. Therefore the best choice would be to modify the near PD so that the distance PD will come out right.

Example 6-9

In another example, a pair of glasses is ordered using the same frame as before. This time the prescription is somewhat different:

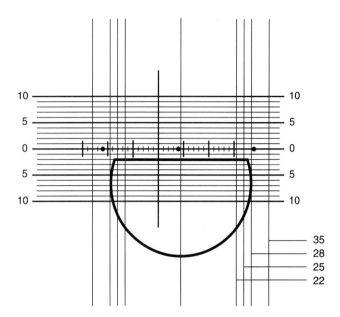

FIGURE **6-9** This high near addition lens was supposed to be made for a 70/64 interpupillary distance. But after positioning the segment, the spotted major reference point location is checked for accuracy. Distance decentration should have been 1.5 mm per lens. Instead it is 4 mm per lens.

R: +0.75 −0.50 × 90
L: +0.75 −0.50 × 90
PD: 70/64
Add: +4.00
Flat-top 28: segment height 19 mm
Frame: A = 53 mm
       B = 42 mm
       DBL = 20 mm

The practitioner lays out the right lens for edging. The total segment inset is 4.5 mm. However, checking the position of the MRP for the distance unearths an error. Instead of getting the needed distance decentration of 1.5 mm, the decentration is 4.0 mm (Figure 6-9). This is 2.5 mm different from what was ordered. Is the lens usable? If it is, either the distance or the near PD (or both) will have to be slightly off. Which should it be?

Solution

In evaluating what to do, the practitioner first should look at unwanted prism. Because the error occurs in the horizontal meridian alone, the power of the lens in that meridian causes unwanted prism. What would the lens look like in front of the eye if it were edged this way? See Figure 6-10. Because the distance PD will be wrong, the eye looks through a point 2.5 mm away from the MRP. But according to Prentice's Rule the amount of unwanted prism that occurs is only as follows:

$$\Delta = cF$$
$$= (0.25 \text{ cm})(0.25 \text{ D})$$
$$= 0.0625\Delta \text{ base in}$$

This is a small prismatic effect. But displacing the near portion changes the prismatic effect at near by the following:

$$\Delta = (0.25 \text{ cm})(4.00 \text{ D})$$
$$= 1.00\Delta \text{ base out}$$

It also narrows the near field of view. Therefore the best choice is to alter the distance PD so that the near PD will be correct. Even though the distance PD appears to be off considerably because distance power is small, unwanted prism is very low. It is well within ANSI standards.

In the previous examples, one example favored altering the near PD. The other favored the distance PD. Not all examples are clear cut. Many times the answer lies in between the two, with both being altered somewhat.

In evaluating lens pairs like this, the practitioner is trying to make lenses work that will not in any way compromise vision for the wearer. The point is not to try to sneak a reject lens through the system and use it.

Preventing Expensive Mistakes

The accurate spotting of lenses is of extreme importance. When any doubt exists as to the correctness of the original spotting, it should be double-checked.

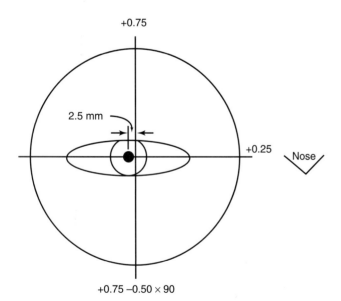

FIGURE **6-10** Imagining or sketching out a power cross on an eye can help in understanding how prism is figured using Prentice's Rule. The horizontal meridian of the lens containing the +0.25 D lens power is used for calculations.

During the centration process, the practitioner takes notice of the location of the spotted MRP. The two previous examples were instances in which the prescription looked like it might fail, but because of giving attention to MRP location, failure was prevented. However, when the MRP is not where it should be, the glasses are likely to fail ANSI standards. Edging a pair of lenses that were surfaced incorrectly wastes time and may disqualify the finishing laboratory from credit for the cost of the surfaced lenses.

TILTED 180-DEGREE LINE

After centration the segment may be positioned properly, but the previously spotted 180-degree line is tilted. Following are some factors that indicate how serious a problem this might be.

If the lens is a sphere and the central MRP dot is located at the proper vertical height and inset, no problem exists. An example of this is shown in Figure 6-11. A spherical lens has the same power in all meridians. Because no cylinder exists, any rotation of the lens has no effect on refractive power.

If the lens is a cylinder or spherocylinder, rotation is important. The cylinder axis will be correct only if the 180-degree line is at 180 degrees. For example, in

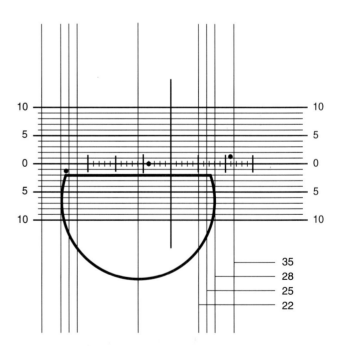

FIGURE **6-11** In the lens spotting process, the correct axis is set in the lensmeter. Afterward, the lens is rotated until it conforms to the specified axis, then spotted along the 180-degree line. While centering this lens, the practitioner discovers that when centration is "complete," the spotted 180-degree line is no longer on the 180. This indicates an axis error during surfacing.

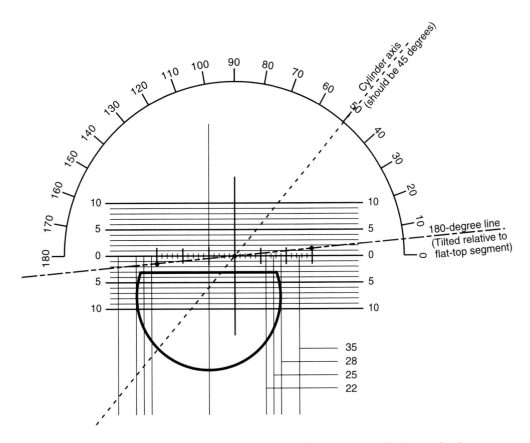

FIGURE **6-12** In the figure, the required cylinder axis is 45 degrees. The lens was oriented in the lensmeter during spotting—it correctly reads 45 degrees. The 180-degree line has been marked. If the 180-degree line is tilted in relationship to the segment top, the cylinder was surfaced off axis. The amount in degrees that the lens is off axis equals the degree of tilt of the 180-degree line.

Figure 6-12, a tilt of 5 degrees in the 180-degree line results in an error of the cylinder axis of 5 degrees. The amount of error considered to be within tolerance depends upon the power of the cylinder (see Appendix B for these tolerances). Because a flat-top bifocal segment cannot be rotated to allow for correction of the cylinder axis, the 180-degree line must not be at an angle that exceeds accepted standards.

POSITIONING FLAT-TOP TRIFOCALS

No difference exists between the basic procedure for centration of trifocals and that of bifocals. Remembering the following points helps prevent confusion.

Only the *top* line of the trifocal is used in segment positioning. (The lower line can be ignored.) Therefore if a segment height is 19 mm, the uppermost line will be at 19 mm.

The top of the trifocal is much more likely to be above the horizontal midline than the top of a bifocal. For a segment raise, the major reference point may fall within the segment, depending on how the surfacing laboratory ground the lens. If this is the case, spotting

of the MRP will not be accurate, because of the prismatic effect exerted by the segment add power.

If the lens has a segment raise and there is no MRP height given by the practitioner, the surfacing laboratory automatically may raise the MRP above the trifocal segment top (see MRP Placement box on p. 119). If this is the case, the dot indicating MRP positioning should still have the correct horizontal inset. However, it will be vertically higher by an amount equal to the segment raise plus this laboratory-determined amount. Both lenses will have MRPs of equal vertical height.

Curve-Top Segment Lenses

Curve-top segments are positioned nearly identical to that of flat-top segments. Following are the differences:

1. Segment height is judged from the highest point of the curved upper portion.
2. Horizontal orientation is gauged by aligning both corners of the segment top with the same horizontal reference line.

The following problem illustrates this procedure.

CURVED-TOP SEGMENT CENTRATION

Example 6-10
The reader should correctly center a left lens for the following order:

R: +1.00 +1.75 × 78
L: +0.75 +2.00 × 109
PD: 62/59
Add: +2.25
Curve-top 25 segment; segment height 17 mm
Frame: A = 48
       B = 39
       DBL = 18

Solution
Before placing the lens in the marking device, the practitioner should figure distance decentration, total inset, and segment drop. (Distance decentration is used to check for accuracy of MRP placement in surfacing.)

Total inset will be used to preset the centration device and can be figured two ways:

(1)
$$\text{Total inset} = \frac{(A + DBL) - \text{Near PD}}{2}$$
$$= \frac{(48 + 18) - 59}{2}$$
$$= \frac{66 - 59}{2}$$
$$= \frac{5}{2}$$
$$= 3.5 \text{ mm per lens}$$

(2)
$$\text{Total inset} = \text{Distance decentration per lens} + \text{Segment inset}$$

$$\text{Distance decentration} = \frac{(A + DBL) - \text{Distance PD}}{2}$$
$$= \frac{(48 + 18) - 62}{2}$$
$$= \frac{66 - 62}{2}$$
$$= \frac{4}{2}$$
$$= 2 \text{ mm per lens}$$

$$\text{Segment inset} = \frac{\text{Distance PD} - \text{Near PD}}{2}$$
$$= \frac{62 - 59}{2}$$
$$= \frac{3}{2}$$
$$= 1.5 \text{ mm per lens}$$

Therefore
$$\text{Total inset} = 2 \text{ mm} + 1.5 \text{ mm}$$
$$= 3.5 \text{ mm per lens}$$

Both methods yield the same results.

Now the movable vertical line in the marking device is moved 3.5 mm to the left. The line is moved to the left because the lens is placed face up in the unit and blocked on the front side. This is shown in Figure 6-13.

The grounds for acceptance or rejection of a curve-top multifocal blank are the same as those for flat-tops.

Round-Segment Lenses

Some bifocal lenses have segments that are perfectly round. The segment diameters may vary from 22 to 38 mm. These lenses were popular many years ago but have steadily decreased in popularity. They are a versatile segment style because they are not restricted in orientation. They may be rotated without making the segment appear tilted like a flat-top segment would appear if it were rotated.

Round-segment lenses also are used less now because at first, they are harder to process. The person doing centration for edging or surfacing must have more of an understanding of the optical properties of the lens.

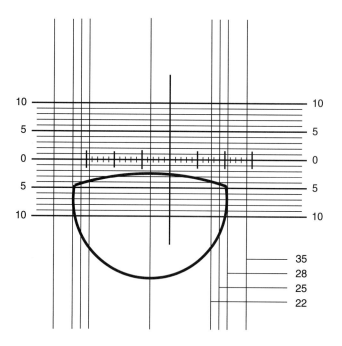

FIGURE **6-13** For a curved-top segment, the lateral corners of the curved upper segment border are equidistant from the horizontal reference line. They both must be at the same level.

With flat-top multifocals positioning the lens for blocking is possible using only the segment area for reference. However, for round-segment lenses, reliance solely upon the segment for positioning is not possible. This is because a round-segment lens offers no visible horizontal reference. A flat-top lens is easier because it has the top of the segment as a visible horizontal reference.

CENTRATION OF ROUND-SEGMENT LENSES WITH A CENTRATION INSTRUMENT

The centration of round-segment lenses starts with the MRP. After spotting the MRP, the lens blank is positioned so that the centrally dotted MRP falls at the calculated distance decentration. This may be done with the aid of the movable vertical line. All three dots should be horizontal.

Once the MRP and 180-degree line are set correctly, the moveable vertical line is repositioned, this time to the total inset position. For spherocylinder lenses the round-segment should now be positioned at its correct height and inset.

For spherical lenses, however, aligning the three dots horizontally does not mean that the segment will be located where it should be located. This is because only the center dot of the three dots means anything. The 180-degree line indicated by the other two dots is merely arbitrary. Therefore in the case of spherical lenses with no prescribed prism, the only point of importance is the dotted MRP.[4] Once this MRP is positioned, the lens may be rotated around the MRP until the correct segment inset and/or the correct segment height is achieved.

The following example outlines the procedure as described, again step by step.

Step 1

The lensmeter is set for the correct sphere power and cylinder axis. The practitioner rotates the lens clockwise or counterclockwise to the correct cylinder axis. The lens is verified for power, and the location of the MRP is found with the lensmeter, then spotted.

Step 2

If the distance portion of the lens is spherical and the prescription contains neither cylinder nor prescribed prism, the outer two lensmeter dots are removed. They are not needed. If they are left on the lens and are at an angle during lens layout, they only cause confusion.

---

[4]For lenses having no prescribed prism, the optical center and the major reference point are one and the same point.

Step 3

The total segment inset required is determined. The total inset is as follows:

$$\text{Total inset} = \frac{(A + DBL) - \text{Near PD}}{2}$$

Step 4

The location of the movable vertical line is changed to the location of the total segment inset. The segment is positioned so that it is bordered by the appropriate segment guide lines. (These guide lines move concurrently with the movable vertical line in the centration instrument.)

Step 5

The needed segment drop or raise is found, as follows:

$$\text{Segment drop} = \text{Segment height} - \frac{B}{2}$$

Drop is negative; raise is positive.

Step 6

The lens is moved upward or downward until the segment drop or raise is positioned correctly.

Step 7

The distance decentration is found, as follows:

$$\text{Distance decentration per lens} = \frac{(A + DBL) - \text{Distance PD}}{2}$$

Step 8

Without moving the segment either up and down or sideways, the practitioner rotates the lens around the segment center until the center lensmeter dot is at the correct distance decentration. The dot also should be on the 180-degree line. (If a specific MRP height is specified, the center dot should be at that height.) The following points should be checked:

- If the lens has cylinder, all three dots are on or parallel to the 180 line. If the three dots are not parallel with the 180-degree line, the cylinder is off axis.
- Sometimes the center MRP dot may too high or too low. If the other lens has the MRP equally positioned above or below the 180 line, no induced vertical prism occurred. (In addition, no vertical prism exists without power in the vertical meridian of the distance lens prescription.)

Step 9

When satisfied that the lens is ready, the practitioner should block the lens.

As practitioners gain experience, some of the above steps may be combined. These steps on round-segment lens centration are summarized in Box 6-4.

MRP, Major reference point.

Example 6-11

How is the *right* lens in the following prescription centered for edging?

R: +3.00 sphere
L: +3.25 −0.50 × 175
PD: 65/62
Add: +2.00
22 mm round-segment; segment height = 16 mm
Frame: A = 50 mm
       B = 40 mm
       DBL = 18 mm

Solution

The right lens is verified for power and spotted. The two outer spots on the lens are removed because this is the right lens and is a sphere.

Next the total segment inset is calculated using the following equation:

$$\text{Total segment inset} = \frac{(A + DBL) - \text{Near PD}}{2}$$
$$= \frac{(50 + 18) - 62}{2}$$
$$= \frac{68 - 62}{2}$$
$$= \frac{6}{2}$$
$$= 3 \text{ mm}$$

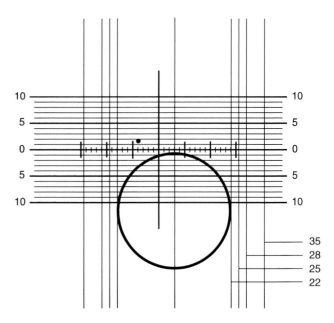

FIGURE 6-14 For this right round-segment lens, the total decentration of the segment is 3 mm. The process begins by positioning the lens between the segment bordering lines.

The movable vertical line is then positioned. Because the calculated total inset is 3 mm, the movable vertical line is moved to the right 3 mm. The bifocal segment is centered between these two lines (Figure 6-14).

Next the segment drop is calculated as follows:

$$\text{Segment raise or drop} = \text{Segment height} - \frac{B}{2}$$
$$= 16 - \frac{40}{2}$$
$$= 16 - 20$$
$$= -4 \text{ mm}$$

Because drop is a negative number, the segment should be 4 mm below the 180-degree line. The segment is moved to a 4-mm drop (Figure 6-15).

Now the distance decentration is calculated as follows:

$$\text{Distance decentration per lens} = \frac{(A + DBL) - \text{Distance PD}}{2}$$
$$= \frac{(50 + 18) - 65}{2}$$
$$= \frac{68 - 65}{2}$$
$$= \frac{3}{2}$$
$$= 1.5 \text{ mm}$$

Without the horizontal or vertical position of the segment moving, the lens is rotated around the center

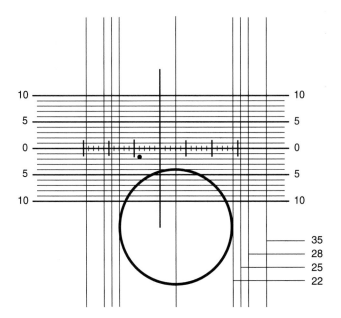

FIGURE **6-15** Next the segment is moved to the calculated segment drop position of 4 mm below the 180 line. The major reference point looks as if it is hopelessly misplaced.

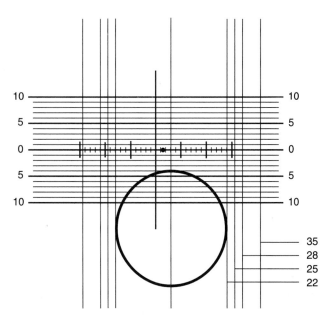

FIGURE **6-16** Finally, without moving the segment horizontally or vertically, the lens is rotated around the center of the segment until the MRP dot is positioned for the correct distance decentration. In this case distance decentration is 1.5 mm inward.

of the segment until the MRP dot is positioned for a 1.5-mm distance decentration. If everything is in order, the MRP dot should also be on the 180-degree line (Figure 6-16).

Blended Bifocals

Blended bifocals are invisible to the observer but are not progressive addition lenses. Blended bifocals are really just another form of a round-segment bifocal. They have two sections of refractive power: distance and near. However, to make the bifocal demarcation line invisible, the line is blurred out or blended. Because the demarcation line is blurred out, different methods of lens centration must be used.

CENTRATION OF BLENDED BIFOCALS USING THE DOTTED SEGMENT BORDER

Because all presently available blended bifocals are round, the procedure is basically the same as for conventional, round-segment bifocals. Some blended bifocals come with the center of the segment marked; some come with the border of the segment spotted (Figure 6-17). These marks are usually not water soluble. After edging they may be removed with acetone or left in place for the dispenser's convenience.

As mentioned previously, some blended bifocal lenses come with the circumference of the segment dotted. When marking such a lens on a centering device, the segment may be positioned with the use of the bordering dots for reference. These dots are most generally in the middle or toward the outside edge of this blurred out or blended zone. Centration of the lens is done exactly like that of a normal round-segment. The dots are taken to be the segment border.

If, by chance, all markings have been removed, they may be reapplied by holding the lens up in front of a textured, illuminated background. The blurred outline of the segment immediately becomes visible, and the blended zone may be hand-dotted (Figure 6-18).

CENTRATION USING THE SEGMENT CENTER

Many blended bifocals have an "invisible" small circle at the very center of the segment for finding the segment center. This circle is the same as the hidden markings on progressive addition lenses. It is possible to use this central segment dot in lens centration. Because the size of the blended segment is known, the central segment dot will be exactly half the segment diameter from the segment top. Therefore the segment may be positioned using only the center segment dot and the distance MRP.

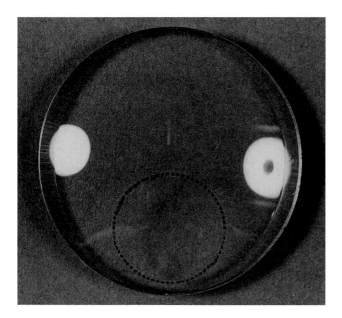

FIGURE **6-17** This factory-marked blended bifocal outlines the segment around the outermost borders of the blended zone. The optically usable portion of the segment is of a smaller diameter than the circle shown.

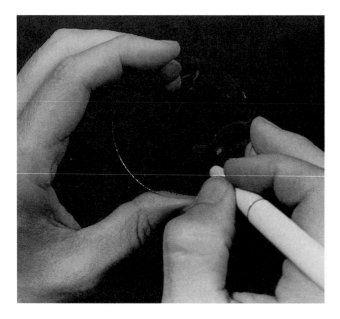

FIGURE **6-18** To re-mark a blended bifocal border, it is held against a background that will make distortion easy to see. The circular area of distortion outlining the segment is dotted.

Example 6-12

A blended bifocal has a segment diameter of 25 mm. The order calls for a distance decentration of 3 mm and a segment inset of 2 mm. The segment drop required is 2 mm. If the lens in question is a right lens and is

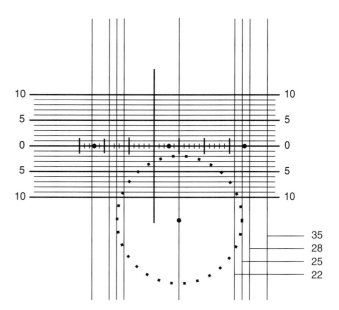

FIGURE **6-19** Blended bifocal centration is done the same way that round-segment centration is done. It is also possible to use the center of the segment for reference. The grid on the layout marker shown does not go down far enough to allow segment height to be done using just the segment center, although many devices do.

spherical in power, how would the lens be centered for blocking?

Solution

If the border of the segment is not marked, the practitioner finds the hidden segment center and dots it with a marking pen.

The MRP is used to position the distance portion at its 3-mm distance decentration. The dot in the center of the segment is rotated until it reaches the total segment inset. The lateral position of the dot is an additional 2 mm in from the OC, as shown in Figure 6-19. (The total segment inset equals the distance decentration plus the segment inset.)

The lens must also be positioned for segment drop. If the lens were already marked with a circle of dots that fall on the *border* of the circular blended zone, it would be positioned for centration in a manner identical to that of a conventional round-segment. This is the situation illustrated in Figure 6-19. If no circle of dots is present on the lens, the following text describes how the lens can be set for a correct drop using the segment center.

Because the segment dot is in the center of the segment, it will be half the segment diameter below the segment "line." The vertical position of the segment center will be below the horizontal reference line by the following amount:

$$\text{Vertical segment center position} = \frac{\text{Segment diameter}}{2} + |\text{Segment drop}|$$

(Because segment drop is a negative number, the absolute value is taken.) So in this instance the vertical position will be as follows:

$$\text{Vertical segment center position} = \frac{25}{2} + |-2|$$
$$= 12.5 + 2$$
$$= 14.5 \text{ mm}$$

(*Note:* In Figure 6-19, the vertical scale of the drawn centration device screen does not go beyond 10 mm. Most actual scales do, however.}

Franklin-Style Multifocals

The Franklin-style lens is made from one piece of lens material. The entire lower half of the lens is devoted to near vision. It is divided from the upper half by a horizontal ledge running the entire width of the lens. This lens design also is known commonly by the name *Executive*, although this is a trade name.

Because no lateral border exists other than the edge of the lens for a Franklin-style segment, inset is accomplished using the dotted MRP. The top border of the segment is used for segment height. But segment inset, when specified, must be accomplished during the surfacing process. Even then proper inset may not always be possible, depending upon constraints produced by the size of the lens blank.[5]

CENTRATION OF FRANKLIN-STYLE LENSES

The step-by-step procedure for Franklin-style lens centration is as follows:

1. The movable vertical reference line is set for the distance decentration.
2. The marked MRP is placed on this reference line.
3. The lens is moved up or down until the segment line is at the correct height.
4. The practitioner ensures that the segment line is horizontal. (If the lens is spherocylindrical, the three lensmeter dots must be parallel to horizontal.)
5. The lens is marked or blocked.

Example 6-13

A lens order for a Franklin-style lens is specified as follows:

[5]For more information see Chapter 6 in Brooks CW: *Understanding lens surfacing*, Boston, 1992, Butterworth-Heinemann.

R: +1.25 −0.50 × 70
L: +1.25 − 0.50 × 115
PD: 66/62
Add: +1.25
Segment height 16 mm
Frame: A = 48
       B = 38
       DBL = 20

How would the left lens be positioned for blocking using a centration instrument?

Solution

Lens power is verified and the MRP of the lens is spotted. Distance decentration is calculated as follows:

$$\text{Distance decentration} = \frac{(A + DBL) - \text{Distance PD}}{2}$$
$$= \frac{(48 + 20) - 66}{2}$$
$$= \frac{68 - 66}{2}$$
$$= \frac{2}{2}$$
$$= 1 \text{ mm}$$

Segment drop is calculated as follows:

$$\text{Segment drop} = \text{Segment height} - \frac{B}{2}$$
$$= 16 - \frac{38}{2}$$
$$= 16 - 19$$
$$= -3 \text{ mm}$$

The movable vertical line in the centration device is positioned for distance decentration for the left lens. This is 1 mm to the left. The MRP is placed on this line. The segment line is moved to the segment drop position 3 mm below the 180-degree line (Figure 6-20). The lens may now be blocked for edging.

The near PD was never used in the centration process for Franklin-style multifocals.

Double-Segment Lenses

Most wearers who need a prescription with a near addition for close work need mainly to be able to see up close for significant lengths of time when looking at objects in the lower half of their viewing area. Some individuals, however, need regularly to see objects at close range in the upper area of the lens clearly. An example is an automobile mechanic who works under cars.

To overcome this problem some lenses are made with two near viewing areas. These lenses have a near addition in the lower half of the lens and a second

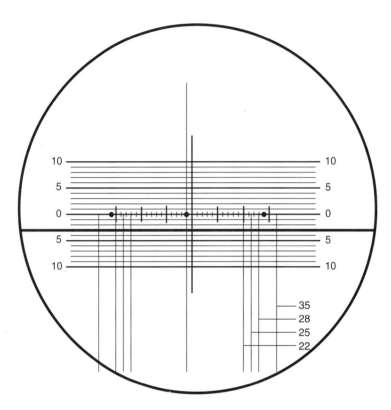

FIGURE **6-20** Centration for Franklin-style lenses uses the major reference point for horizontal alignment and the segment top for vertical alignment.

segment area in the upper half of the lens. These are called *double-segment lenses*. Such lenses allow freedom for wearers to work comfortably and to clearly see near objects if they are looking upward.

Styles of segments used for double-segment lenses are the same as those used for conventional bifocal or trifocal lenses. The most common types are flat-top, small round, and Franklin-style segments.

CENTRATION OF DOUBLE-SEGMENT LENSES

A standard distance of 13 or 14 mm usually separates the upper and lower segment areas. Because segment separation is known, both segments can and should be positioned by specifying only the location of the lower segment.

Lower-segment specifications are given in exactly the same manner as for the regular bifocal. Therefore lens centration procedures are identical to those previously described. When the lower segment is correct, the upper segment positions itself automatically.

The final location of the upper segment should be checked before edging. Following are three ways the practitioner may check this location:

1. Superimposing the image of the lens pattern on the lens during centration will do this (Figure 6-21). The location of the upper segment is noted in reference to the top of the edged lens. If there is less than 7 mm of upper segment showing below the upper rim of the frame, it is likely that an error was made in fitting. The practitioner should verify accuracy.
2. A second way to check for adequate upper segment viewing area is to hold the lens over the frame before edging. The lower segment is placed at the appropriate height. Is there still at least a full 7 mm of usable space in the upper segment? If not, the lenses should not be edged before talking to the practitioner.
3. An adequate viewing area can be checked by use of the segment height and B dimension of the frame. This is done with the addition of the upper and lower segment separation distance to the segment height, followed by subtraction of that number from the B dimension. This provides the viewing area through the upper segment, as follows:

Upper segment viewing area = B − (Segment height + 13)

The distance from the lower to upper segment is taken to be 13. If this distance is 14 mm, the number 14 should be used in place of 13.

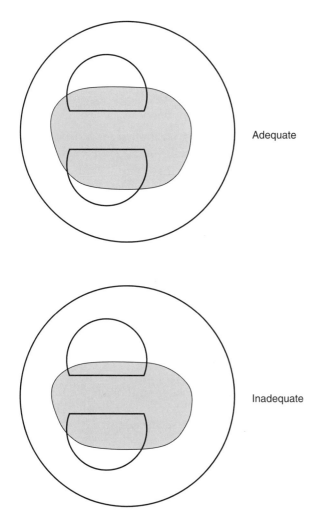

Adequate

Inadequate

FIGURE **6-21**   A double segment lens must have sufficient vertical lens area to allow the upper segment to be useful.

Example 6-14
How much vertical viewing area will be present in the upper segment of a double-segment lens that is to be placed in a frame with a 35-mm B dimension? The segment height is specified as 17 mm. Will this be enough vertical viewing area?

Solution
Using the formula described previously, the following equation is developed:

$$\begin{aligned}
\text{Vertical upper segment viewing area} &= 35 - (17 + 13) \\
&= 35 - 30 \\
&= 5 \text{ mm}
\end{aligned}$$

Only 5 mm of vertical viewing area will remain if this prescription is filled. This distance is too small, and there would be no point to edging the lenses.

Whenever the making of a prescription would provide unsatisfactory results, the dispensing practitioner should be called. The best policy is to always provide possible solutions for the problem. In Example 6-14, for instance, a good suggestion would be to either select a frame with a larger B dimension or keep the frame that was originally chosen and lower the segment height 2 mm. Lowering the lower segment from 17 mm to 15 mm would also lower the upper segment, providing the additional 2 mm needed in the upper viewing area.

Proficiency Test Questions

1. If the segment height is 20 mm, which of the choices indicates the segment drop or raise with reference to the horizontal midline for a frame with the following dimensions?

   A = 42
   B = 38
   DBL = 16

   a. 0
   b. -1 mm (drop)
   c. +1 mm (raise)
   d. −2 mm (drop)
   e. +2 mm (raise)

2. Which of the choices describes the segment inset for the following frame and PD measurements?

   Frame: A = 51
   B = 44
   DBL = 17
   PD: 64/61

   a. 1.5 mm
   b. 2 mm
   c. 3 mm
   d. 4 mm
   e. 8 mm

3. For the following prescription, how far in is the segment positioned for blocking the lens? How is the segment positioned vertically?

> R: –1.75 –1.00 × 180
> L: –1.50 –1.25 × 180
> Frame: A = 46
>   B = 42
>   DBL = 16
> PD: 59/56
> Segment height = 18

4. For a flat-top 28 lens, how far vertically and laterally will the MRP of each lens be from the center of its segment top line? The lens and frame have the following parameters:

> R: +2.00 –0.25 × 15   2Δ base out
> L: +4.25 –0.25 × 165   2Δ base out
> Add: +1.50
> Frame: A = 52
>   B = 47
>   DBL = 17
> PD: 64/61
> Segment height = 21

5. A frame has the following dimensions:

> A = 50
> B = 44
> DBL = 20

Given a wearer with a PD of 66/62, for which of the following is "4 mm per lens" the correct measure?

a. Segment drop
b. Segment inset
c. Total segment inset
d. Distance decentration

6. A bifocal for the right eye is placed convex side up on the centration device so that it may be blocked directly. If A = 47, DBL = 16, and PD = 61/57, which of the following denotes the location of the center of the segment in reference to the center (origin) of the grid?

a. To the left
b. To the right
c. Exactly in the middle

7. If a lens were being marked using a lens protractor, in which of the following positions would it be placed?

a. Convex side up
b. Convex side down

8. If a lens were being positioned for blocking using a centration device, in which of the following positions would it be placed?

a. Convex side up
b. Convex side down

9. A left lens calls for a total segment inset of 5 mm. If it were placed on a lens protractor for marking, in which of the following directions would the segment be moved?

a. Right
b. Left

10. A left lens calls for a total segment inset of 5 mm. If it were placed on a centration device for layout and blocking, in which of the following directions would the segment be moved?

a. Right
b. Left

A pair of lenses is supposed to have a 3 mm segment drop for both right and left lenses. Instead, the right lens has a 3 mm drop, but the left lens has a 5 mm drop. Indicate whether this is acceptable or unacceptable for each of the following lens prescription situations according to ANSI Z80.1 standards.

11. –6.50 sphere
–4.75 sphere

a. Acceptable
b. Unacceptable

12. +5.00 sphere
+3.00 sphere

a. Acceptable
b. Unacceptable

13. +3.00 sphere
+1.00 sphere

a. Acceptable
b. Unacceptable

14. +1.00 sphere
+3.00 sphere

a. Acceptable
b. Unacceptable

15. −1.00 −1.00 × 180
−1.00 −1.00 × 180

a. Acceptable
b. Unacceptable

16. −1.00 −1.00 × 90
−1.00 −1.00 × 90

a. Acceptable
b. Unacceptable

17. A bifocal prescription is received from surfacing with the right MRP 4 mm above the segment line and the left lens MRP 2.5 mm above the segment line. For the following prescription, which choice indicates the amount of vertical prism that could be manifested, assuming equal segment heights?

R: +2.75 −1.00 × 180
L: +0.50 sphere

a. 0.26Δ
b. 0.08Δ
c. 0.19Δ
d. 0.41Δ

18. If a 2.5-mm variation in near PD is considered within accepted standards for segmented multifocals, which of the following indicates the largest and smallest near PDs that fall within these standards for a wearer with a PD equal to 59/56?

a. 61.5 − 56.5
b. 61.5 − 53.5
c. 58.5 − 53.5
d. The correct answer depends on the distance power.

19. A prescription calls for a segment inset of 2 mm (per lens). During centration it is noticed that the lateral distance from the segment center to the distance OC is actually 4 mm for each lens. Which choice describes the amount of lateral prism that will be induced in the distance portion if the near PD is set correctly? The distance prescription is as follows:

R: +5.00 −1.00 × 180
L: +5.00 −1.50 × 180

a. 1.4Δ
b. 1.5Δ
c. 1.6Δ
d. 2.0Δ
e. None of the above

20. For the prescription described in the preceding question, which of the following will be the base direction of the induced prism?

a. Left
b. Right
c. In
d. Out
e. Down

21. When a segment inset is incorrect after surfacing and it is decided that the lens is nevertheless within normal limits of quality, which factor(s) would favor altering the near PD and maintaining distance PD?

a. An especially small segment
b. A low near addition power
c. A high-powered distance prescription in the 180 meridian

A pair of surfaced but unedged lenses should have a segment inset of 2 mm for the right lens and 2 mm for the left lens. Instead, they both have segment insets of 4 mm each. These surfaced uncut lenses are edged using the near PD for reference. In other words after edging, the near PD comes out right and the distance PD ends up being wrong. Which of the following lens pairs would still pass ANSI standards for distance PD and horizontal prism?

22. −6.00 sphere
    −5.00 sphere

    a. Acceptable
    b. Unacceptable

23. +3.00 sphere
    +3.00 sphere

    a. Acceptable
    b. Unacceptable

24. +1.00 sphere
    +1.00 sphere

    a. Acceptable
    b. Unacceptable

25. −1.00 −1.00 × 180
    −1.00 −1.00 × 180

    a. Acceptable
    b. Unacceptable

26. −1.00 −1.00 × 90
    −1.00 −1.00 × 90

    a. Acceptable
    b. Unacceptable

27. During centration of a flat-top bifocal, you notice that the spots made by the lensmeter are tilted 10 degrees in reference to the segment line. The central dot is correctly placed. In which of the following cases would this be of no consequence?

    a. It would always be of consequence.
    b. In the case of a plano cylinder
    c. When oblique prism is prescribed
    d. When the decentration is small
    e. When the lens is spherical

28. A flat-top, 7 × 28 trifocal calls for a segment height of 23 mm. If the frame B dimension was 46, which of the following describes the segment drop (or raise) for correct centration?

    a. 0
    b. −7 mm (drop)
    c. +7 mm (raise)
    d. −2 mm (drop)
    e. +2 mm (raise)

29. For a curve-top segment lens, the segment height is based on which of the following?

    a. The center of the segment top
    b. The upper outer corners of the segment
    c. The optical center of the segment

30. True or False? A round-segment spherocylinder lens is spotted for edging. During layout it is apparent that the segment inset is wrong. This is of no consequence. Round-segments can be rotated and the segment top will not look any different after edging.

31. From a lens flexibility standpoint, round-segment lenses are considered to be which of the following?

    a. More versatile than flat-top segments
    b. Less versatile than flat-top segments

32. In lens layout, a blended bifocal lens is centered in a manner most similar to which of the following?

    a. A progressive addition lens
    b. A trifocal lens
    c. A flat-top segment lens
    d. A round-segment lens
    e. A curve-top segment lens

33. Which of the following lenses cannot be centered correctly using only the segment for reference? (*Hint:* More than one response may be correct.)

    a. Curve-top bifocals
    b. Round-segment bifocals
    c. Flat-top bifocals
    d. Executive (Franklin-style) bifocals
    e. Progressive addition lenses

34. Franklin-style bifocals are horizontally decentered for edging using which of the following?

    a. Distance decentration
    b. Segment inset
    c. Total segment inset

35. To center an occupational double segment exactly as indicated on the order during the layout process, which of the following steps should be taken?

    a. Center first the lower segment and mark the lens. Then center the upper segment and re-mark. Block the lens exactly between the two marks.
    b. Center the upper segment first. Before marking, note whether the lower segment is in the prescribed location.
    c. Center the lower segment as indicated. Ignore the upper segment.

36. A double-segment flat-top bifocal (double D) has an ordered segment height of 18 mm. Which of the following frames has a vertical depth that is suitable for this segment style?
    (*Hint:* More than one response may be correct.)

    a. B = 30
    b. B = 35
    c. B = 40
    d. B = 45
    e. None of the above

37. Which bifocal(s) can be marked for blocking without first spotting?

    a. Executive bifocals
    b. Flat-top bifocals
    c. Round-segment bifocals
    d. Curve-top bifocals

38. You would like to alter the segment inset of an already-surfaced lens before edging it. Which of the following lenses listed can you slightly rotate around the distance OC to alter the lens as described?

    a. A flat-top 25 segment with a power of -2.00 D sphere
    b. A 22-mm round segment with a power of -2.00 -2.50×15
    c. An executive or Franklin-style segment with a power of $+1.25$ -0.25×30
    d. An Ultex A segment (38-mm semicircular segment) with a power of -7.25 D sphere

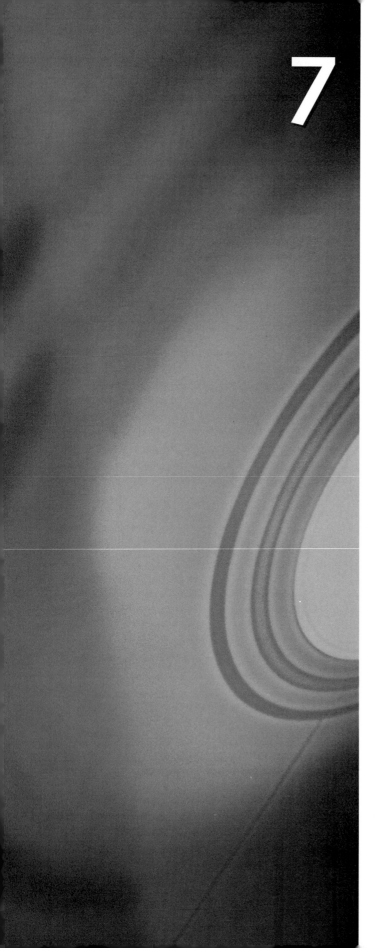

7

Blocking of Lenses

For a lens to be edged to its proper shape, it must be clamped securely in the lens edger. This positioning holds the axis, decentration, and segment location as intended. A "block" is placed on the lens as a handle so that the lens may be held in place during edging.

Types of Blocking

Five basic methods have been used to block a lens, as follows:

1. *Pressure blocking:* The lens is held in place between felt pads.
2. *Suction blocking:* A small suction cup is pressed onto the lens.
3. *Metal alloy blocking:* A low melting temperature metal alloy is molded onto the protected surface of the lens.
4. *Precast FreeBlock blocking:* A recyclable waxlike material is molded onto the surface of the lens.
5. *Adhesive pad blocking:* A thin pad, which is adhesive on both sides, is applied to a block. Then the block is applied to the lens.

The blocking method most commonly used in the United States is adhesive pad blocking.

Pressure Blocking

Those who used the early method for "blocking" a lens held it in place by pressure alone. The lens was squeezed between two felt pads in the edger. Because no block was used, it was never really "blocked" in the true sense of the word. Hand positioning the lens between the felt pads is an impractical method for ensuring accuracy of edged lens parameters. Instead the lens is pre-positioned in a centering fork.

With the lens properly aligned in the centering fork, the adapter is slipped into the accepting portion of the edger. The second felt pad might then be pressed into place and tightened. Then the centering fork may be removed as the lens is clamped in at the correctly centered cutting line orientation.

The pressure blocking system has fallen into disuse. Besides the danger of lens slippage, such a system does not allow for periodic removal of a lens from the edger to check for size. Once the lens is removed, it is practically impossible to put back in the edger in its exact previous position.

Blocking with Suction

Another method of holding the lens in place is by means of a small suction cup (Figure 7-1). This suction cup is constructed with an adapter on the back surface that allows it to fit into the spindle assembly within the lens edger.

The advantage of a section cup system is that it may be used with no preparation. Although it is not often used for mass production purposes, it lends itself to smaller facilities where lenses are edged on a more periodic basis. In Europe, where most of the edging is done on location at the dispensary, this system was more widely used than in the United States.

The holding surface of the suction cup must be kept free of oil or foreign substances. Suction cups must be applied dry to a dry lens to prevent slippage and a corkscrewing effect. These cups may be reused often but must be inspected regularly for cracks in the material caused by drying.

Metal Alloy Blocking

A metal alloy blocking system is another system that enjoyed widespread usage in the past. It is practically out of use now. In this system a metal alloy with a low melting point is heated and molded to the lens. The metal cools and forms a small metal block that adheres to the lens (Figure 7-2).

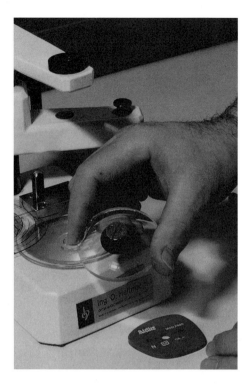

FIGURE **7-1**   The adapter attached to the suction cup may vary in its configuration, depending on the edger manufacturer's design.

Metal alloy will not adhere directly to a lens surface and withstand the edging process. The surface must first be precoated. The coating was applied to the front surface of the lens in the form of a spray or with a brush or dab-on applicator.

Alloy blocking has the major disadvantage of using heavy metals in the alloy such as lead and cadmium. The environmental problems associated with heavy metals are a growing disincentive for working with a metal alloy blocking system.

Precast FreeBlock Blocking

This system of blocking uses a precast waxlike lens block that adheres to the surface of the lens when heated. The adhesion of these blocks is excellent as they conform nicely to the lens surface and prevent slippage. FreeBlocks are used in Gerber-Coburn Step Two blocking. The Step Two system incorporates centration and blocking in one "Step Two Finish

Blocker" that heats and presses the block against the lens. Reuse of the blocks is not recommended.

Adhesive Pad Blocking

Another method for blocking lenses utilizes adhesive pads.[1] A block made of metal or plastic is fastened to the lens by means of a double-sided adhesive pad (Figure 7-3).

---

[1]Adhesive pad blocking is sometimes referred to as *LEAP blocking*. 3M was the first company to introduce this type of system, which is known as the *3M LEAP System*.

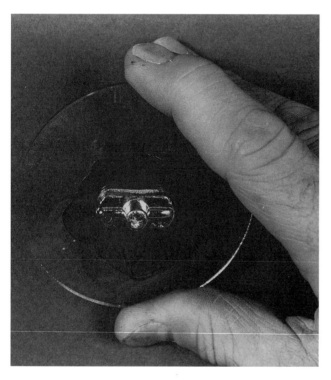

FIGURE **7-2** The shape of the metal block can be molded to any one of several different chucking systems.

BLOCKS

Block designs vary according to shape of the chuck used to hold the lens in the edger. In other words, the back of the block may be available in a variety of shapes to adapt to the chuck of the edger being used. This could be a problem for laboratories with edgers from different manufacturers. With only a few exceptions, most edger manufacturers are able to supply a variety of chuck designs so that chucks may be interchanged. This way the same block design may be used throughout the laboratory.

Metal Blocks

When the block is *metal*, the side contacting the adhesive pad must approximate the front curve of the lens. Blocks can be classified as low, regular, and high base, depending upon the steepness of curvature. They are color coded. A common color is black for low base blocks, gray for regular base blocks, and gold for high base blocks (Figure 7-4). Low base blocks are for lenses with base curves from approximately 0.00 to 4.25 D, regular base from 4.50 to 8.00 D, and high base above 8.50 D. These numbers are front surface base curve numbers. They are not lens refractive powers.

The front curve of a lens steepens as lenses increase in plus power and flattens as the power moves toward the minus direction. For lenses of equal refractive powers, aspherics are generally flatter than regular lenses. So aspheric plus lenses will not require a high base lens block as quickly as a nonaspheric lens of equal refractive power.

Plastic Blocks

Some blocks are made from either semirigid or flexible plastic material. These types of blocks are designed to conform to the front curvature of the lens because the flange of the block is designed to take on the lens shape (Figure 7-5). Plastic blocks sometimes require a larger adhesive pad.

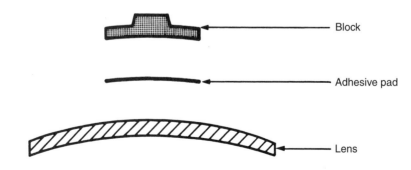

Block

Adhesive pad

Lens

FIGURE **7-3** Adhesive pad blocking consists of a block applied to the lens by means of double-sided tape.

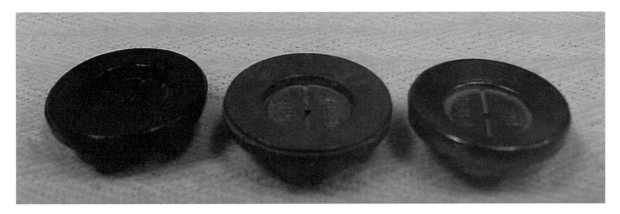

FIGURE **7-4** Metal blocks come in three color-coded types: high base, regular base, and low base.

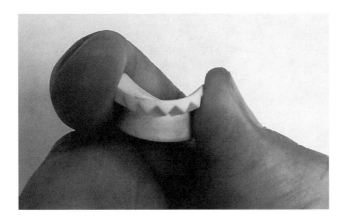

FIGURE **7-5** Flexible plastic lens blocks offer the advantage of conforming well to the front surface of the lens, regardless of how steep or flat the surface is.

Plastic blocks continue to appear in new designs and are rapidly replacing metal blocks.

BLOCKS FOR HALF-EYE LENSES AND NARROW B FRAMES

Frames that are small in their vertical dimension, such as some children's frames and half-eye glasses, can be troublesome during edging. An ordinary lens block is larger than the edged lens will be. When this happens, the edger begins grinding the block and the lens. To prevent it, the lens block has to be cut off in the vertical dimension and used just for these types of frames (Figure 7-6). Switching the chucks being used in the lens edger is also necessary because these are also too large.

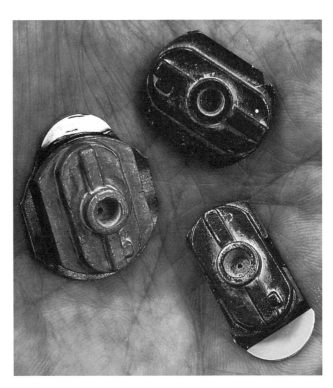

FIGURE **7-6** These three half-eye blocks are regular lens blocks with the top and bottom edges removed to allow for a very narrow lens. If a smaller half-eye block is needed, it is likely that a smaller chuck in the edger will also be required.

PREVENTING BLOCK SLIPPAGE

If slippage occurs during edging, the first thing to check for is an incorrect base block. If a high minus lens is edged on a regular base block, the lens adheres tightly only at the edges (Figure 7-7, *A*). If a high plus lens is edged on a regular base block, the lens holds

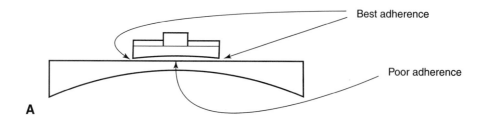

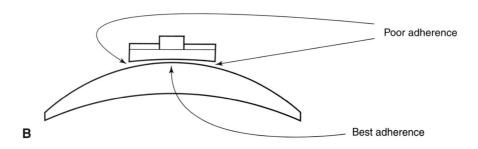

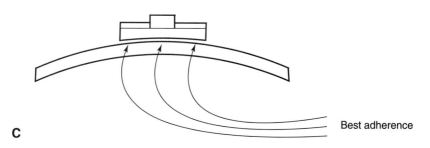

FIGURE **7-7** Metal blocks should be chosen to match the front base curve of the lens. **A,** The front curve of this minus-powered lens is too flat for a regular-base block. The only good area of adherence is around the periphery of the block. **B,** This high plus lens has a base curve that is too steep for a regular base block. The only good adherence is in the middle of the block. When the curve of the lens matches the curve of the block, as shown in **C,** an even, tight adherence exists across the whole area of the block. When metal blocks are used, the block must match the front lens curve.

well only in the center of the block (Figure 7-7, *B*). The lens block should parallel the curve of the lens surface for maximum adhesion (Figure 7-7, *C*).

If the lens is on the correct base block, the next most likely problem is incomplete cleaning. The lens and the block should be cleaned thoroughly before blocking occurs. A dirty or oily surface prevents tight adhesion. Extreme torque is on the lens during edging. Without maximum adhesion, the lens may twist or slip. Then, even if the shape is right, the prescription will be incorrect.

Methods of cleaning vary. Some people find that only minimal cleaning of the blocks is necessary; others soak recycled metal blocks in solvent or place blocks in an ultrasonic cleaner to remove all grease and oils before reusing.

If more thorough cleaning does not alleviate the situation, it may indicate that the roll of adhesive pads has been exposed to excess heat or humidity. Excess humidity decreases the adhesion of the pads and also can result in slippage (Box 7-1).

FIGURE **7-9**   Some efficiency may be gained by placing a number of lens blocks on a strip of adhesive pads ahead of time.

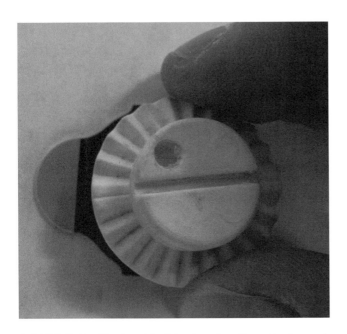

FIGURE **7-8**   The lens block is placed on the adhesive pad.

ADHESIVE PAD BLOCKING PROCESS

In preparation for blocking, a pad is peeled from the roll and placed against the lens block (Figure 7-8). The fingers should not touch the surface of the adhesive. This introduces oil onto the surface and keeps the pad from sticking to the block as tightly as it should.

Maintaining consistency in how the tab is placed on the block may be helpful. This way when picking up the block to mount it in the blocking device, no uncertainty exists regarding whether the block is right side up or upside-down. *The protective paper is not peeled from the pad.* The pad is pressed firmly against the block.

Alternatively the block may be mounted on a strip of pads. The backing is peeled from the pad while it is still on the roll. The block is placed on the pad. In this way a whole strip of pads is neatly prepared and ready (Figure 7-9). When removing the pad and block from the roll, the practitioner should be careful to avoid touching the exposed adhesive.

Next the block is placed in the centration device in preparation for blocking. It is mounted on a movable arm that may be manually or automatically swung into place over the lens and pressed onto the lens surface. The protective paper may be removed from the block.

The lens is now placed on the centration device and decentered as required. This was previously described in earlier chapters on centration of lenses. Once the operator is assured that the alignment is correct, the block is swung into place and pressed against the lens (Figure 7-10).

The blocked lens is removed from the instrument and the block pressed against the lens to ensure maximum contact between the adhesive pad, lens, and block (Figures 7-11 and 7-12).

High Adds and Wide Segments

Plastic flat-top bifocal lenses have their segment area on the front surface of the lens. The segment gets its additional plus power because it has a steeper curvature than the rest of the lens (Figure 7-13). With regular plus lenses, the larger the size of the lens, the thicker the lens will be. And again, with regular plus lenses, the higher the power of the lens, the thicker the lens will be. The same is true for the segment area of a plastic

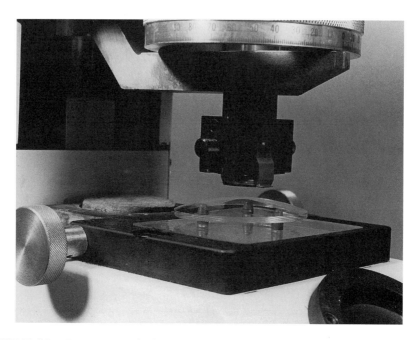

FIGURE **7-10**   By centering the lens convex side up in the centration device, a pretaped lens block can be lowered directly onto the lens. This eliminates one step in the production process.

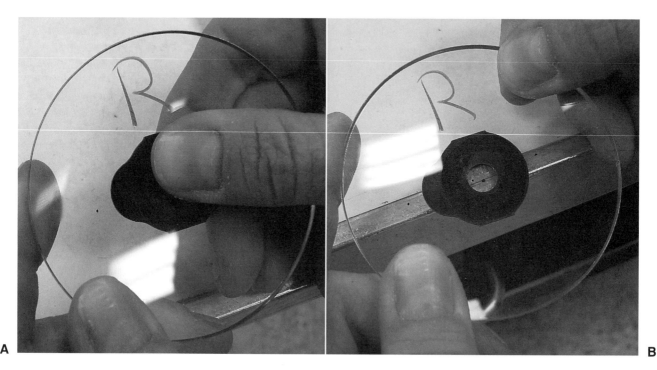

A   B

FIGURE **7-11**   **A,** The lens block should be pressed onto the lens to get good adherence. **B,** It may also be pressed against a solid object instead of just squeezed between the fingers.

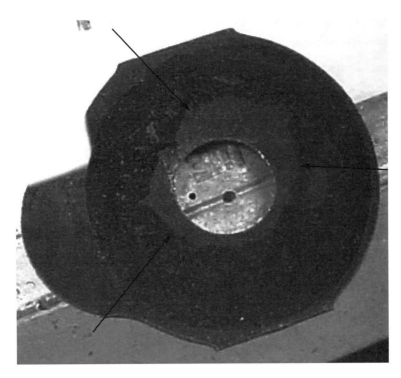

FIGURE **7-12** The technician should check the way the pad looks against the lens surface. The lighter area indicated by the *arrows* shows no contact between the lens and the pad and thus no adherence toward the center of the pad.

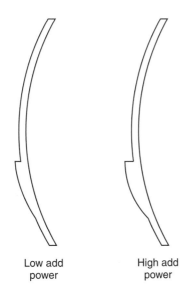

Low add power   High add power

FIGURE **7-13** Two flat-top bifocal lenses with the same bifocal segment size. One has a low add power, the other a high add power. When the two lenses are edged, the higher add power lens is more likely to crack along the segment line or have the segment line indented or chipped because of chucking pressure unless precautions are taken.

bifocal lens. The wider the bifocal segment, the thicker the ledge will be on the flat-top bifocal. Flat-top 35 segment ledges will stick out farther from the lens surface than will flat-top 28s of the same power.

A flat-top 28 with a +1.25 add has a much thinner ledge than a flat-top 28 with a +3.50 add.

If a thick bifocal ledge is left unprotected during edging, the lens can be damaged because of the pressure exerted when the lens is chucked for edging. The following may happen:

• A thin lens can split along the bifocal line.
• The segment line can be slightly indented or can chip.

To prevent such problems, an adhesive pad is cut into two. The half pad is placed against the lens just above the segment as shown in Figure 7-14. The half pad should be just far enough above the line to make the segment line visible during lay out. The hole in the pad should be placed so that it allows the center lensmeter dot to show clearly.

Next the lens is blocked normally. (The back must be peeled off the half-pad first.) The half pad completes the circle of the bifocal segment and allows the block to hold the lens along the segment line evenly.

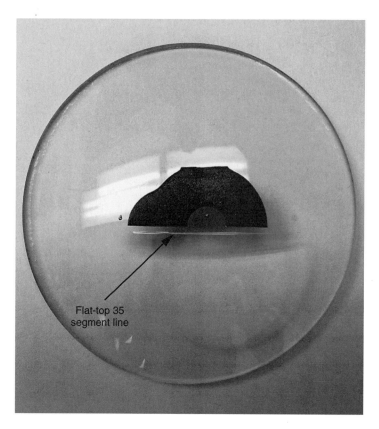

Flat-top 35
segment line

FIGURE **7-14**   Plastic flat-top lenses that have either a large segment or a high add power are more susceptible to damage during the edging process. This flat-top 35 segment lens has a half pad above the segment to help even out the pressure during chucking.

Protective Tape

All currently used blocking systems adhere well when directly mounted on the surface of the lens. (A notable exception is the seldom-used metal blocking system, which requires that the lens be spray-coated ahead of time.) However, in some instances using protective tape on the lens may be advisable.

Formerly the primary concern was to protect a plastic lens surface from scratching. With most plastic lenses coming with scratch-resistant coatings, concern about scratching the lens itself may be reduced. However, concern remains for protection of the coating.

A large variety of lens coatings are possible: scratch-resistant, antireflective, and mirror, for example. When the edger holds the lens tightly in the chuck during the edging process, excess pressure on small areas of the lens can damage the coating, which causes it to crack or peel. To reduce the likelihood of this happening, many use a protective tape disc, such as the 3M Blue Chip lens protector, on the back surface of the lens (Figure 7-15). These discs come precut in 35-mm circles on a large dispensing roll with nonadhesive tab areas for easy application and removal.

These tape discs protect the surface and are also said to help in reducing excessive, localized pressure during edging. That pressure may be the result of too many pounds per square inch of chucking pressure. Reducing the chuck pressure somewhat may help. But excess localized pressure results from use of the wrong base block for the lens being edged. Selection of the correct base block is important.

For extra protection from pressure on thin, antireflection coated lenses, it may be helpful to use the tape disc and an extra adhesive pad. First the tape disc is placed on the back side of the lens. Next an adhesive blocking pad is placed on the back side of the lens on top of the tape disc. The protective paper backing from the adhesive pad should not be removed. When the lens is placed in the edger, the pad further cushions the lens against points of localized pressure.

Lensmeter/Blockers

To increase efficiency, a natural evolution of any process is to combine steps. Blocking may be done as a step

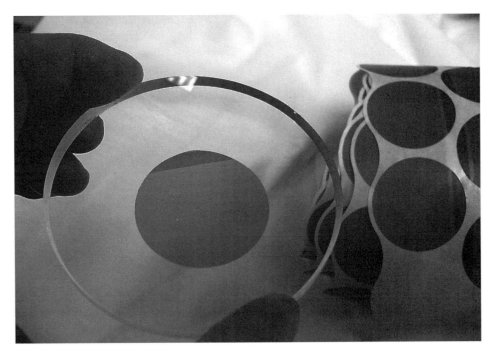

FIGURE **7-15**   These easy-peel lens protector discs often are applied to the back surface of an antireflection coated lens to keep the coating from cracking when squeezed by the lens chucking device in the edger. Chucking pressure should be kept as low as feasible when edging such lenses.

totally independent of any other step in the edging process. However, that is now the exception, rather than the norm. The most logical first combination of steps was to combine the blocking process with the centration process, which already has been described. Some blockers now include the centration device and the lensmeter. Although this may be accomplished in different ways, one existing instrument recognizes the optical center of the lens and reads the location of the cylinder axis. By inputting frame and lens prescription information, the required location of the 180-degree line and inset are calculated. The instrument rotates the block to the correct orientation and moves it to the location needed for proper lens decentration.

Proficiency Test Questions

1. Which of the following system(s) does/do not allow lenses to be removed from the edger to check for correct size, and then put back in the edger again?

   a. Pressure blocking
   b. Suction blocking
   c. Metal alloy blocking
   d. Adhesive pad blocking
   e. Molded resin blocking

2. Coating of the lens surface is *required* for which of the following blocking systems?

   a. Molded resin blocking
   b. Suction blocking
   c. Metal blocking
   d. Adhesive pad blocking

3. Of the following blocking systems, which is considered to be the least environmentally friendly?

   a. Molded resin blocking
   b. Suction blocking
   c. Metal blocking
   d. Adhesive pad blocking

4. When adhesive pad blocking is used with metal lens blocks, a high minus lens is most likely to require which of the following?

   a. A high-base block
   b. A regular-base block
   c. A low-base block
   d. Lens power has nothing to do with which base blocks are used.

5. An aspheric lens generally has which of the following characteristics?

   a. A steeper base curve than a regular spherically based lens of equal refractive power
   b. The same base curve as a regular spherically-based lens of equal refractive power
   c. A flatter base curve than a regular spherically-based lens of equal refractive power

6. True or False? Flexible plastic lens blocks used in adhesive pad blocking may be used with any powered lens, regardless of base curve.

7. Which of the following kinds of frame can cause problems during edging if the adhesive pad–type lens block is not modified?

   a. Metal
   b. Plastic
   c. Rimless
   d. Nylon cord
   e. Half-eye

8. Which of the following is not a possible cause of a lens slipping on the block during the edging process when adhesive pad blocking is used?

   a. A lens that has not been thoroughly cleaned
   b. An improperly chosen metal base block
   c. Adhesive pads that have been exposed to high humidity
   d. A lens block with an oily film or other foreign material on the surface
   e. An edger that has insufficient coolant flow during edging
   f. All the above may cause a lens to slip during edging.

9. With some lenses it may be advisable to place protective tape on the back surface of a lens before edging. In which of the following situations might this be appropriate?

   a. When the lens is a thin glass lens, to keep it from breaking
   b. When the lens is AR coated, to keep from damaging the coating
   c. When the lens is thin and made from polycarbonate, to keep from throwing the bevel placement off
   d. When the lens is tinted, to keep the tint from looking splotchy
   e. None of the above are helpful.

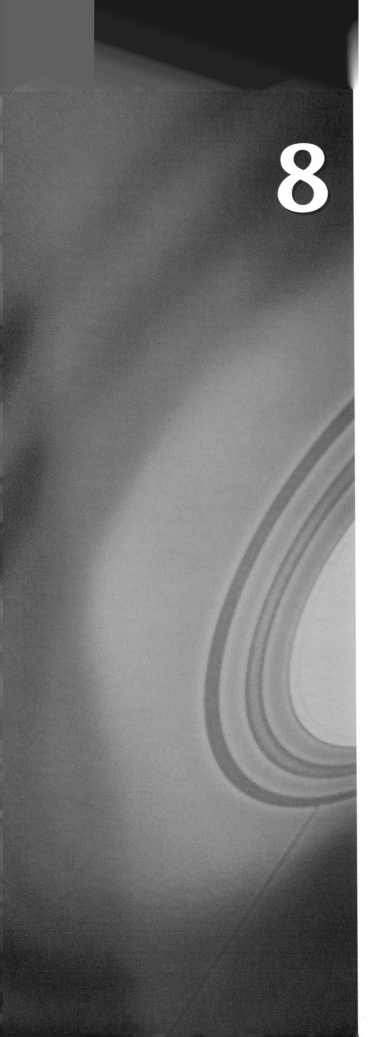

8

Edging

Patterned and Patternless Edging

For an edger to produce a lens of the right shape for the frame, it has to have some sort of a template to guide it. That template can be a visible template, usually plastic, and the same shape as that of the desired lens. This template is called a *pattern*. Edgers that require a physical pattern to guide the edger often are referred to as *patterned edgers*.

However, the template to produce a lens shape does not have to be something tangible like a plastic pattern. It can be a shape that is stored digitally. That electronic version also can guide the lens edger. This type of an edger works without a physical pattern and therefore is referred to as a *patternless edger*.

The first part of this chapter addresses patterned edgers; the next part, patternless. Much of what is covered in the information about patterned edging is needed for understanding patternless edging. Even if the reader is using or will be using a patternless edger, the material in the Edging with Patterns section of the chapter should be read.

EDGING WITH PATTERNS

Historical Background

The process of lens edging involved more steps than placement of an entire lens blank in an automatic edger and cutting the lens to finished form in one operation. In the past, a lot more of the process was done by hand.

Cutting and Chipping

In the past the cutting and chipping process involved the glass cutter outlining the desired lens shape on the glass lens with an appropriate marking instrument. The shape was then cut into the lens surface using a glass cutter (Figures 8-1 through 8-3). The glass cutter did not cut through the glass but simply scored the surface so that the outermost unwanted portions of the lens would break away clean along the scored line.

Then a more refined system was developed that made use of the lens pattern, as Figure 8-4 shows; this method allowed the lens to be scored in the exact outline of the desired shape. In both freehand or guided scoring, the lens was cut several millimeters larger than required to allow room for some inaccuracy in chipping the lens and for an even lens edge finish.

After lens cutting, the outermost areas of glass were removed using chipping pliers that were, and still are, available in a variety of designs (Figure 8-5). The outer lens areas may be removed by loosely grasping the lens near the scored section, as Figure 8-6, A, shows, and breaking it away with a twist, as in Figure 8-6, B.

Lenses also may be chipped to size without being scored. Chipping pliers are used to "nibble" away the glass a little at a time from the edge, while the pliers are slightly squeezed, combined with the twist of the hand via the forearm in a rotational movement away from the

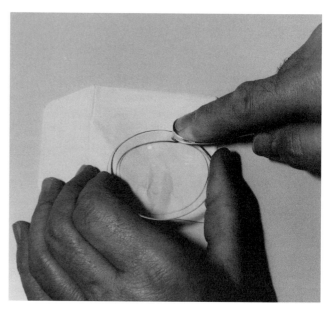

FIGURE **8-2** A premarked line is scored as the practitioner traces around the shape a single time.

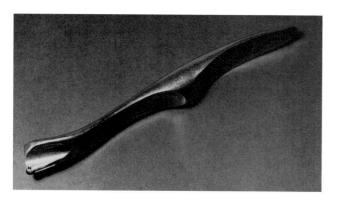

FIGURE **8-1** A "cutting spoon" has a small cutting wheel that cuts and rolls across a surface to create a scored line.

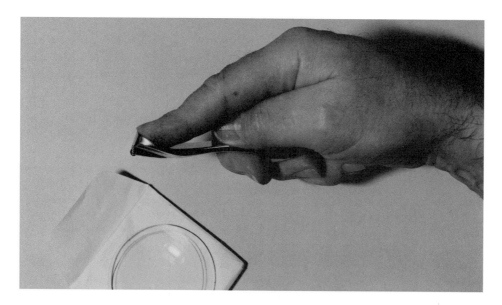

FIGURE **8-3** Holding the cutting spoon for optimum control.

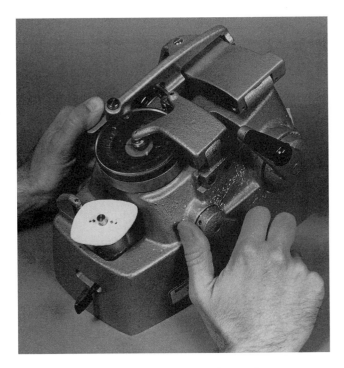

FIGURE **8-4** The same function as the cutting spoon was later performed on a lens cutter with the help of a pattern.

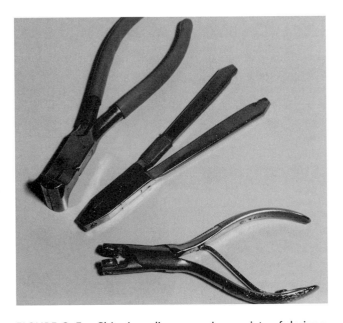

FIGURE **8-5** Chipping pliers come in a variety of designs, allowing for the preference of the individual and the thickness of the lens being chipped or broken away.

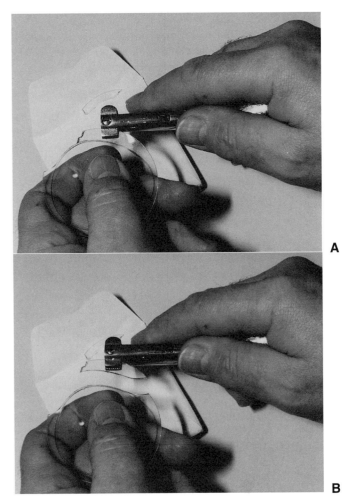

FIGURE **8-6** **A,** The lens is grasped near the scored section for support as sections are snapped off. **B,** Scored lenses that are not excessively thick break off in fairly large pieces even if very little force is exerted.

individual. The other hand holds the lens near the edge being chipped, as in Figure 8-7. After chipping to shape, the lens can be hand edged to size using a ceramic wheel. All scoring and chipping procedures are applicable only to glass lenses.

Automatic Edging with Ceramic Wheels

The first automatic edgers were the automatic rimless edgers with ceramic wheels. These edgers put a flat edge on the lenses and were sufficient for the majority of prescription work done at the time. If any other type of edge was needed, such as a beveled edge, it had to be done by hand.

The ceramic wheel itself is composed of grit and a bonding agent that is cast to shape, fired in a kiln, then machined to proper specifications.[1]

---

[1]Hirschhorn H: Modern edging methods. Part I. *The Optical Index* 55(4):93, 1980.

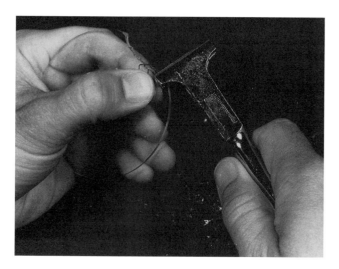

FIGURE **8-7** Lenses may be chipped without scoring as the practitioner nibbles away at the edge with a turning motion of the pliers.

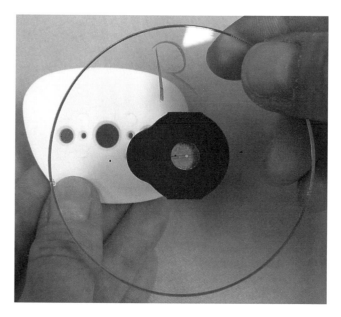

FIGURE **8-8** When a lens is placed into the edger, the pattern must be turned to cut a right eye shape for the right lens. Fortunately most lens blocks are made to prohibit the lens from being placed in the edger upside down. (The back surface of the lens is toward the reader.)

When the abrasive material wears and loses its cutting ability, the bonding agent dissolves, which allows the worn grit to fall away and exposes fresh, sharp material. Ceramic wheels give an excellent, smooth finish and are still used occasionally for hand edging. Ceramic wheels have a long life because, with the exception of the central hub, they are composed entirely of abrasive grit and bonding material.

Edging Process

Since automatic ceramic edgers were first developed, vast improvements in edger cutting technique, automatic cycling, bevel style, and bevel placement have occurred.

For a patterned edger, the edging process begins when the operator places the pattern on the edger so that it is properly oriented to cut either a left or right lens. (By convention, most operators begin with the right lens.) As long as the front surface of the lens is facing left, the pattern will, in most cases, be right side up with the nasal half in the direction of the operator (Figure 8-8). The lens must then also be oriented right side up. Fortunately most blocking systems are now constructed so that fitting the blocked lens into the edger chuck is difficult if it is oriented upside down.

For the left lens, the pattern must be removed and turned around so that the nasal side is away from the operator. Then the edger must be set so that it will cut the lens to the required size.

SETTING THE EDGER SIZE

If all lens patterns were exactly the same size as the required finished lens, then no size setting would be required. The edger could duplicate the pattern exactly in a one-to-one relationship. However, this would mean that instead of one pattern for each frame shape, a separate pattern would be required for every available size.

This raises the question of pattern size. When patterns were first used with rimless edgers, far fewer shapes were available. So that the operator would know how to set the machine, all patterns had to have one standard size. The "standard size" was set by the manufacturer such that American Optical patterns, for instance, were 37 mm in their A dimension, Shuron patterns were 36.5 mm, and some European types were standardized at 40 mm.

This meant that, if an instrument was calibrated for a 37-mm pattern, when a 42-mm eyesize lens was required, the instrument dial could be set for 42 mm, and the lens would cut out to have an A dimension of exactly 42 mm. This assumes, of course, that the necessary 37-mm pattern was used. Eventually, within the United States, a standard pattern size of 36.5 mm evolved.

Any of these small standard pattern sizes was appropriate when most eyewear was being fit in very conservative sizes. With the advent of major frame style changes, lenses began to be edged for sizes significantly larger than the pattern, which created problems of "pattern distortion."

USING LARGER PATTERNS TO PREVENT PATTERN DISTORTION

When a lens is edged to a shape that is 2 mm larger than the size of the pattern, the edger makes the lens a millimeter larger in every direction: nasally, temporally, upward, and downward. But in adding an equal amount of lens size to the original shape in every direction, the integrity of the original shape starts to be lost. (This is explained in Chapter 3 and can be seen in Figure 3-15.) To keep the shape from being distorted the only feasible solution was to produce a pattern for larger style frames that was closer in size to the actual lens size being edged.

LARGER-THAN-STANDARD PATTERNS

If the pattern is made larger than the standard 36.5 mm size, the lens will be too large. Without compensation, the lens will be edged larger than the frame eyesize.

Example 8-1

A pattern is supplied for a certain frame. This pattern measures 46.5 mm in its A dimension. For example, a lens is to be edged for a 50-mm eyesize. If the edger is calibrated for a pattern size standard of 36.5 mm, what size lens will be edged if the edger-sizing dial is set for 50 mm?

Solution

For this edger, a 36.5-mm pattern will produce the lens size at which the dial is set. If a 50-mm lens is desired, the dial is set at 50 mm. However, because the pattern is 10 mm too large, the lens produced also will be 10 mm too large. Setting the edger at 50 mm in conjunction with this pattern will produce a lens with a 60-mm eyesize.

Example 8-2

In the previous example, what would the edger setting have to be to produce a 50-mm lens.

Solution

That pattern is 46.5 mm. This is 10 mm larger than the standard and produces lenses 10 mm too big. Therefore 10 mm must be subtracted from the required eyesize:

$$50\ mm - 10\ mm = 40\ mm$$

To arrive at a 50-mm lens, the edger must be set for 40 mm.

SET NUMBERS

To make it easier to know how to compensate for a pattern that is larger than the 36.5-mm standard pattern size, frame manufacturers put a compensation number on the pattern. This compensating number is called the *set number*. Because patterns are almost always larger than the standard this difference must be subtracted from the eyesize. For this reason, set numbers are seen as negative numbers.

Patterns that accompany a manufacturer's frame in most cases have a set number stamped directly on the pattern. Knowing the eyesize and pattern set number means the edger setting can be determined without having to measure the pattern.

Example 8-3

A lens is to be edged for a frame having an A dimension of 53 mm. The pattern is stamped *set –15*.

1. What is the proper edger setting?
2. If measured, what would the expected A dimension of the pattern be?

Solution

1. *Set –15* means that the edger must be set 15 mm less than the desired lens size. Therefore to find the edger setting the following equation is used:

$$Edger\ setting = Eyesize + (Set\ number)$$

In this case that number equals the following:

$$Edger\ setting = 53 + (-15)$$
$$= 38\ mm$$

Therefore the edger is set for 38 mm.
2. Now, what would be the size of the pattern? Set number is the difference between the standard sized pattern and the actual sized pattern, as follows:

$$Set\ number = Standard\ pattern\ size - Actual\ pattern\ size$$
$$= 36.5 - Actual\ pattern\ size$$

In this case the set number is known but not the pattern size. Therefore changing the formula around algebraically results in the following equation:

$$Actual\ pattern\ size = 36.5 - (Set\ number)$$

In this example, the numbers are as follows:

$$Actual\ pattern\ size = 36.5 - (-15)$$
$$= 36.5 + 15$$
$$= 51.5\ mm$$

The pattern in this example can be expected to have an A dimension of 51.5 mm.

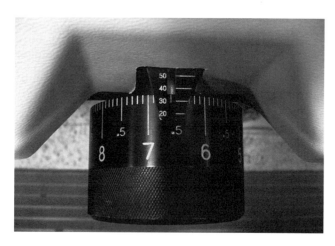

FIGURE **8-9** When an edger is set for 36.5 mm, the lens will be the same size as the pattern after edging is completed.

MARKING EDGER DIALS

Generally, edger dials are marked in one of the following three ways:

1. Mark the dial according to eyesize.
2. Mark the dial with a zero, plus-minus scale.
3. Mark the dial with both options.

Dials Marked According to Eyesize

The first way is a direct eyesize reading as shown in Figure 8-9. The edger is set for lens size with pattern set numbers being subtracted from the frame's eyesize to obtain the correct edger setting. When such an edger is calibrated for a standard size pattern whose A dimension is 36.5 mm, setting the edger at 36.5 mm always produces a lens that is exactly the same size as the pattern. So if a pattern is made directly from a frame and duplicates the frame's eyesize, then a 36.5-mm setting will give the correct lens size.

Example 8-4

A frame has a 55-mm eyesize. A pattern is made on a one-to-one ratio so that it is the same size as the frame and measures 55 mm.

1. What is the set number for the pattern?
2. What must the edger setting be?

Solution

1. Pattern set number is equal to the following:

$$Set\ number = Standard\ pattern\ size - Actual\ pattern\ size$$
$$= 36.5 - Actual\ pattern\ size$$

In this example the equation is applied as follows:

$$Set\ number = 36.5 - 55$$
$$= 18.5\ mm$$

Therefore the pattern set number is −18.5.

2. To find the edger setting the edger is set less than the actual eyesize by an amount equal to the set number. In other words, the following equation is true:

$$Edger\ setting = Eyesize + (Set\ number)$$

For this example the edger setting is as follows:

$$Edger\ setting = 55 - 18.5$$
$$= 36.5$$

Now it is evident why an edger is always set for 36.5 mm when the pattern size equals the eyesize.

A Second Dial Configuration: Zero, Plus-Minus Scale

Some edger dials are marked so that the difference between eyesize and pattern size may be used to set the edger. To introduce this second edger dial configuration is another example.

Example 8-5

A 55-mm pattern like the one in the previous example has been made. Now it must be used for a frame with a 53-mm eyesize.

1. What would the normal edger setting be?
2. The zero, plus-minus scale uses zero instead of 36.5 mm. How far from the 36.5-mm (zero) setting must the edger dial be moved in order to achieve the correct lens size for the 53 mm frame? Is this in a plus or a minus direction?
3. Can this be found without calculating an eyesize edger setting?

Solution

1. To make a lens 2 mm smaller than the previous one, set the edger 2 mm less than it was before, or at 34.5 mm. Calculating edger setting in the traditional manner gives these results:

$$Edger\ setting = 53 - 18.5$$
$$= 34.5\ mm$$

Therefore the edger would normally be set at 34.5 mm.

2. To find how far from 36.5 mm we would move the edger setting, one setting is subtracted from the other. The first setting was 36.5. The second setting was 34.5 mm.

$$Setting\ difference = 36.5 - 34.5$$
$$= 2\ mm$$

Because the second setting is smaller than the first (34.5 is smaller than 36.5), the second setting is minus compared to the first. In other words, if 36.5 were written as 0, then 34.5 would be a minus 2.

3. This setting can be found more easily by noting that because 53 mm is 2 mm less than 55, the edger setting for a 53 mm eyesize is –2.

When patterns are made to fit exactly the size of the frame, an edger can have a 0 where the 36.5 mm reading would otherwise be. If the frame is larger than the pattern, the edger is set that much larger. If the frame is smaller than the pattern, the edger is set for the difference in a minus direction. The dial is still marked off in millimeters, but it is numbered above and below the zero (Figure 8-10).

The operator simply dials in the difference in millimeters between the pattern size and the desired lens size. With this type of system the following equation applies:

$$\text{Edger setting} = \text{Lens size} - \text{Pattern size}$$

Taking the previous example in this second system of edger setting, a 55-mm pattern is used and a 53-mm edged lens is desired, as follows:

$$\text{Edger setting} = 53\,\text{mm} - 55\,\text{mm}$$
$$= -2\,\text{mm}$$

This means the dial is turned to a –2 reading.

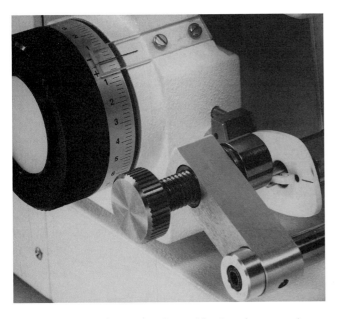

FIGURE **8-10** If a pattern is used having the same size as the lens to be ground, a plus-minus scale would require a zero setting. If the pattern is not the same size as the lens, then the size difference is added or subtracted by means of a dial. (Courtesy Essilor, Paris.)

There are advantages to both systems. The eyesize setting dial works best when premanufactured patterns with printed set numbers are used. However, when patterns are made for every frame, many operators prefer the second system.

Combination System

The third system is really a combination of the previous two. In a combination system, both types of scales are printed on the dial. If the standard size chosen for the pattern is 36.5 mm, the zero mark is printed adjacent to that size number.

When an edger is equipped with more than two grinding wheels, more than one complete set of scales may be on the edger dial, as Figure 8-9 illustrates. Each scale may be recalibrated independently for grinding wheel wear, because groove depth in each wheel may vary, influencing the final lens size.

INCREASING ACCURACY IN EDGER SETTINGS

Unfortunately not all frames have the same A dimension as the eyesize that may be marked on the frame. This may be because the marked eyesize is intentionally different from the A dimension, or simply because certain frames run somewhat larger or smaller than their marked value. Relying totally on the marked frame size to set the edger means that the lens may not fit the frame.

The most accurate method is to use a frame tracer in conjunction with a patternless edger. However, with patterned edgers in most cases it means measurement of the frame. With use of the boxing system the A dimension is the distance between two parallel vertical lines enclosing the lens or lens opening in the frame and not necessarily the width of the lens across the middle.

When a millimeter rule is used, as shown in Figure 8-11, *A*, a high degree of accuracy cannot be expected. The locations of the far left and right points on the imaginary box surrounding the "lens" are only visually estimated. An improvement is to use a device such as the "T-seg" shown in Figure 8-11, *B*. The top of the T part of the ruler allows a more accurate positioning of the ruler.

For frames made from certain materials, the lenses often are edged somewhat larger to ensure a secure fit. The nature of the material dictates how much larger the lenses are edged; the amounts given as guidelines are shown in Table 8-1.

Generally, conventional plastic frames made from cellulose acetate material can be stretched somewhat. This assures a snug, secure-fitting lens. Depending upon the individual frame, lenses for frames made from this

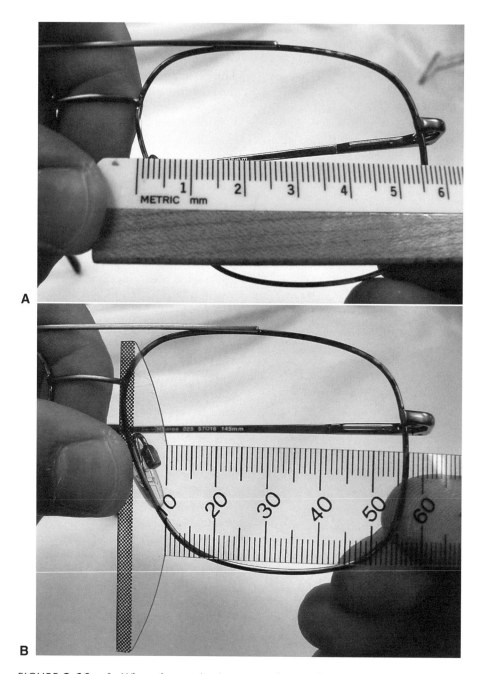

FIGURE **8-11** **A**, When the eyesize is measured according to the boxing system, the ruler is held horizontally with the zero as far left as the most left-hand edge of the lens groove. The reading corresponds to the farthest right-hand lens groove location. **B**, The "T-seg" style ruler shown allows a better alignment of the outermost portion of the lens area. The ruler-wide markings on the body of the ruler help in accurately locating the outermost portion of the lens area on the opposite side.

material are edged approximately 0.5 mm larger than the actual frame size.

Many of the newer plastic materials do not stretch when heated. In fact some materials actually shrink when heated. As a result, lenses for these frames must be made exactly to size, assuming the exact size is known.

When the exact size is not known, it is better to error on the larger side, because lenses may be checked for size after edging and before the block is removed. If the lens is too large it may be re-edged to a slightly smaller size. But if it were edged and found to be too small, it would be ruined.

TABLE **8-1**	
Size Compensation Used to Edge Frames of Various Materials	
FRAME MATERIAL USED	SIZE AFTER EDGING
Cellulose acetate	0.5 mm larger than the measured size
Nylon	0.2 mm larger than the measured size
Optyl	0.6 to 1.0 mm larger than the measured size
Metal	On size
Carbon fiber	
Polyamide	

Plastic frame materials requiring on-size edging are carbon fiber, polyamide, polycarbonate, and other similar materials. Generally speaking, if a plastic frame is very thin, the material is probably not the more conventional, acetate-type of frame material and falls into this category.

Lenses are mounted into these frames, not by heating the material, but by "snapping" the lenses into the frame while the frame is "cold." In this instance, cold means normal room temperature. This technique is referred to as "cold-snapping" the lenses in place.

INCREASING ACCURACY WITH A CIRCUMFERENCE GAUGE AND CHART

One of the ways to increase edging size accuracy is to use the circumference of the lens in addition to the eyesize or A dimension. The circumference is both longer and more accurately measured, giving a closer comparison between two identical shapes having different sizes.

The most obvious way to use circumference is to measure the circumference of the wearer's old lens and carefully match the circumference of the new lens to it. An accurate fit is then ensured. This is more of a trial-and-error process of starting large and slowly reducing edger setting size, each time remeasuring the circumference of the edged lens until the exact match is reached. However, another way exists to use circumference to help choose the correct edger setting and avoid the trial-and-error process.

The "standard" pattern size is 36.5 mm. The circumference of a round pattern with a diameter of 36.5 mm may be found by multiplying the diameter by π.

$$\begin{aligned} \text{Circumference} &= \pi(\text{Diameter}) \\ &= \pi(36.5) \\ &= 114.7 \text{ mm} \end{aligned}$$

The circumference chart developed for edging purposes actually uses 36.6 as the basic number because 36.6 comes out with a circumference of almost exactly 115; an even number.

The following procedure ensures accuracy when a pattern is not the same size as the frame to be used:

1. Using the circumference gauge, measure the size of the pattern to be used. This is pattern circumference (PC).
2. Measure the size of the wearer's existing lens or the demonstration lens from the selected frame. This is lens circumference (LC).
3. Subtract the pattern circumference from the lens circumference, or (LC) – (PC).
4. If the difference is a plus number, add this amount to 115. The lens is bigger than the pattern and the edger setting must be increased. If the difference is a minus number the lens is smaller, and it is subtracted from 115.
5. Look up the new number on the circumference chart (or divide it by π) to find the required edger setting (Table 8-2).
6. Edge the lens and measure it for circumference. It should match the lens circumference of the wearer's lens or demonstration lens.

This chart works best when comparing pattern and lens sizes that are not miles apart from each other. Obviously the circumferences cited in the chart are for circles. Edged lenses are seldom circles. Yet the relative proportionality of two identical shapes is strong enough to make the chart effective for what it is intended.

Example 8-6

A "lenses only" order has been placed. It is for a metal frame. The pattern for the frame is given but not the frame. The account has sent an eyesize and has measured the circumference of the lens. The circumference of the lens is 141.5 mm. How would you set the edger?

Solution

These steps are used to find the needed edger setting for this "lenses only" order using circumferences for increased accuracy.

1. Measure the circumference of the pattern on hand. The pattern circumference is 138.5 mm.
2. The order states that the lens circumference is 141.5 mm.
3. Subtract pattern circumference from lens circumference, as follows:

TABLE 8-2
Lens Edging Circumference Chart

1. Measure the circumference of the pattern to be used (PC).
2. Measure the circumference of the wearer's existing lens or the demonstration lens from the selected frame (LC).
3. Perform the following calculation: (LC) – (PC)
4. Add this amount to 115. The result may be a positive or a negative number.
5. Look up the new number on the circumference chart (or divide it by π) to find the required edger setting.
6. Edge the lens and measure it for circumference. It should match the lens circumference of the wearer's lens or demo lens.

CIRCUMFERENCE	EDGER SETTING	CIRCUMFERENCE	EDGER SETTING	CIRCUMFERENCE	EDGER SETTING
90	28.6	117	37.2	144	45.8
91	29.0	118	37.6	145	46.2
92	29.3	119	37.9	146	46.5
93	29.6	120	38.2	147	46.8
94	29.9	121	38.5	148	47.1
95	30.2	122	38.8	149	47.4
96	30.6	123	39.2	150	47.7
97	30.9	124	39.5	151	48.1
98	31.2	125	39.8	152	48.4
99	31.5	126	40.1	153	48.7
100	31.8	127	40.4	154	49.0
101	32.1	128	40.7	155	49.3
102	32.5	129	41.1	156	49.7
103	32.8	130	41.4	157	50.0
104	33.1	131	41.7	158	50.3
105	33.4	132	42.0	159	50.6
106	33.7	133	42.3	160	50.9
107	34.1	134	42.7	161	51.2
108	34.4	135	43.0	162	51.6
109	34.7	136	43.3	163	51.9
110	35.0	137	43.6	164	52.5
111	35.3	138	43.9	165	52.5
112	35.7	139	44.2	166	52.8
113	36.0	140	44.6	167	53.2
114	36.3	141	44.9	168	53.5
115	36.6	142	45.2	169	53.8
116	36.9	143	45.5	170	54.1

$$141.5 - 138.5 = +3.0$$

4. Add this difference to 115 to get the following:

$$115 + 3 = 118$$

5. Looking up 118 (or dividing it by π) results in an edger setting of 37.6.
6. Edge the lens and measure the circumference of the edged lens for accuracy.

Example 8-7
An order for a frame has been received. The frame comes with well-fitting demonstration lenses. The practitioner has a presumably on-size pattern for that frame. However, she would like to match the size of the new lens to that of the demonstration lens. She tries to measure the A dimension of both pattern and demonstration lens but finds it is too difficult and she cannot be sure her measurements are correct. Using a circumference gauge, she measures the pattern circumference as 157 mm. Then she measures the circumference of the demo lens. This she measures as 157.8 mm. What would she set the edger for to get a correctly sized lens?

Solution
To find the answer, first the pattern circumference is subtracted from the lens circumference. This is 157.8 – 157 = 0.8. Next 0.8 is added to 115 to get 115.8, the circumference needed to find the edger setting. Looking up 115.8 on the chart, the practitioner finds that the closest edger setting would be close to 36.8 mm.

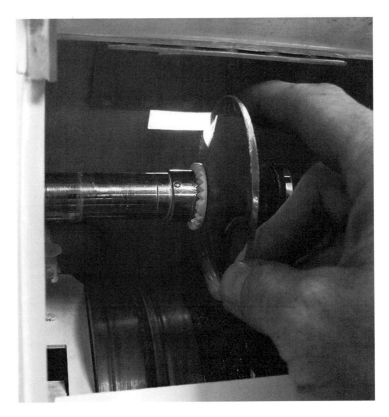

FIGURE **8-12**   Chucking a lens for edging.

LENS CHUCKING

After a final determination of correct edger setting is made, the lens block is slipped into the edger chuck (Figure 8-12) and clamped in place. This process is referred to as *lens chucking* and may be done manually, with compressed air, or electronically.

A general rule in chucking lenses is to use the largest block feasible. This distributes pressure better and holds the lens more securely but may make it necessary to change the chuck size on some edgers.

Small finished lenses, as in the case of lenses for half-eye frames, frames with small B dimensions, and some children's frames, may pose a problem. The edger wheel grinds the block and sometimes the lens-holding assembly, which damages both assembly and wheel. For small children's frames or half-eyes a smaller device is required (Figure 8-13).

Manual Chucking

For manual chucking, the lens should be clamped firmly, but not with excessive pressure, and the handle should be locked in place. Too little pressure can cause lens slippage on the block, whereas too much pressure contributes to lens breakage during edging.

The material used for the pad that holds the lens in place is compressible but has resilience. Because of the nature of the pad, the lens may be squeezed in place regardless of variations in curvature that naturally occur with different lens powers.

Air Chucking

Although manual lens chucking is not difficult, when a large number of lenses are being run through the edger daily, *air chucking* or *pneumatic chucking* may be advisable. An air line is run from a compressor to the specially adapted edger so that when activated, the lens holding assembly is pressed against the lens and held in place by the force of the compressed air.

Electric Chucking

With electric chucking a drive motor presses the lens holding assembly together to hold the lens in place. This allows pressure to be individually controlled for different lens material needs, including AR-coated lenses.

BEVEL PLACEMENT

How the bevel is placed on the lens makes a great deal of difference in the appearance of the finished eyewear.

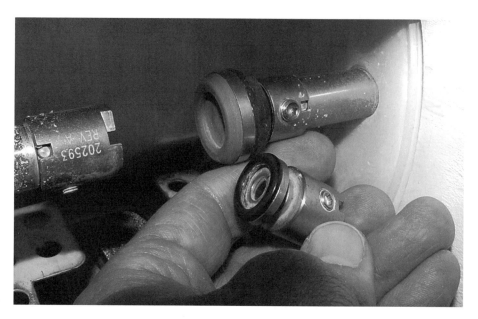

FIGURE **8-13** For most lenses the standard, larger pad holds the lens well. The larger the pad, the larger the holding area will be. However, for small lenses a smaller pad is required, as shown here.

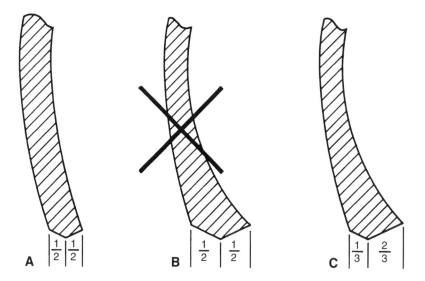

FIGURE **8-14** **A,** For thin lenses, the bevel apex is placed approximately in the middle of the edge. **B,** When the lens is thick, a center bevel placement gives a poor cosmetic result because the bevel shows too much. **C,** As the lens becomes thicker, and *if* the bevel is to occupy the entire lens edge, it should be moved toward the front. When the bevel occupies the entire lens edge, a one third:two thirds ratio is correct.

Placement of Apex for Hand-Beveled Lenses

In the past, when lenses were hand-beveled, the main requirement for achieving a good cosmetic effect was the placement of the bevel apex. Figure 8-14, *A,* illustrates that for low-powered lenses with relatively thin edges, the apex was best positioned at the center of the lens edge. However, when lens edges become thicker because of high-minus power, the center bevel positioning was not as cosmetically suitable (Figure 8-14, *B*).

Positioning the bevel apex right in the center of the lens with a thick edge makes the lens "spill out" the front of the frame. The wearer knows the lenses are thick, and everybody else does too. Therefore, to correct this problem, the apex of the bevel was pushed forward such that it was one third of the edge thickness from the front, as the right-hand lens in Figure 8-14, *C,* shows. When this was done, the major portion of the lens was behind the frontal plane of the spectacles and less of the lens bevel was seen from the front. Although reflections from the larger beveled surface on the posterior lens edge still were seen as a concentric ring effect, the overall appearance was better.

Placement of Apex by Automatic Edger Wheels

The quality of edge design was vastly improved with the development of a grooved automatic edger wheel. This wheel allowed a bevel to be placed on a thick lens edge at any position while the remainder of the bevel was edged flat, as in Figure 8-15.

American Optical Company referred to the resulting bevel as a *Hide-a-Bevel.* When the lens with this style bevel is inserted into a spectacle frame, the finished prescription appears considerably better cosmetically. The bevel often completely disappears into the frame groove. Because of forward placement, the front of the lens does not protrude, and the concentric ring effect, although still present, is reduced by the more favorable edge angle.

OVERALL PROCESS

Roughing Wheels

To replace the troublesome and risky process of chipping a lens down to a slightly larger preedging size, edgers have a roughing cycle.

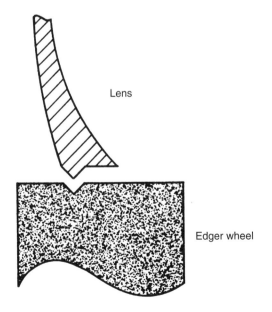

Lens

Edger wheel

FIGURE 8-15 Much cosmetic advantage was gained with the introduction of the so-called "hidden bevel."

The complete blank either received from the surfacing laboratory or pulled from stock is placed in the edger. As the cycle begins, the lens blank is brought into contact with a coarse diamond wheel called a *roughing wheel,* which cuts it down rapidly (Figure 8-16). When the roughing cycle is complete, the lens will have the correct shape as dictated by the pattern but will be slightly large. The lens may then pass to the second phase of edging, in which a finer *finishing wheel* puts the correct edge on the lens while cutting it to its final size.

Two basic types of roughing wheels exist; those for plastic and those for glass.

- *Electroplated* roughing wheels for plastics and polycarbonate are coated with larger, more coarsely spaced diamond particles. This allows for cutting lens material away without clogging the diamonds.
- *Bonded* roughing wheels are used primarily for glass lenses. The bonding of the diamond to the wheel is tight and withstands the relative hardness of a glass lens.

Although roughing wheels designed for glass may be used intermittently for conventional plastic lenses, roughing wheels designed for plastic should *never* be used for glass. (For more on roughing wheels, see Chapter 17 on diamond wheels and cutter blades.)

Finishing Wheels

Once a lens is rough-edged to shape, it must be beveled on a finishing wheel. There are a large variety of finishing wheel designs available. Selection of the best wheel for a particular laboratory depends on several factors.

Flat edges for rimless. The simplest design in bevels is not a bevel but a *flat edge.* The flat edge is appropriate for rimless style eyewear. Seldom is a flat edge produced on a special flat wheel; they usually are ground on the flat portion of a grooved wheel used for another style of bevel as well. If the edger does not have a program that places and keeps the lens on the flat portion automatically, it may be necessary to prevent the lens from slipping into the groove manually.

In the case of a manual operation for rimless lenses, compensation for the lack of a bevel in setting the eyesize is necessary. The eyesize should be set larger by an amount equal to twice the wheel groove depth. If the groove is 1 mm deep this will total 2 mm. Therefore for a 48-mm lens size the edger is set for 50 mm.[2]

---

[2]Another method used is to change the set number on the pattern so that the computation is automatically done with the initial edger setting. For example, a rimless pattern is marked *set −15.* Normally for a 54-mm eyesize, a 39-mm setting is selected and then increased by twice the groove depth to approximately 41 mm. If, however, the pattern were re-marked to a *set −13,* the operator simply could subtract (54 − 13 = 41) to obtain the correct setting. With selection of this option, every rimless pattern should be checked before adding it to the pattern file to prevent costly mistakes.

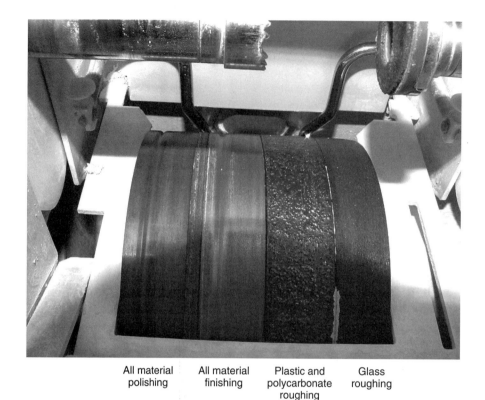

| All material
polishing | All material
finishing | Plastic and
polycarbonate
roughing | Glass
roughing |

FIGURE **8-16** Diamond particles are more widely spaced on wheels used in the edging of polycarbonate lenses. The wheel used in the roughing of polycarbonate lenses is the second wheel from the right.

V-bevels. The V-bevel wheel is the most elementary design and duplicates results that could be accomplished by hand. The wheel is shaped like a V and, as a general rule, *standard V-bevel wheels* are used with a free-floating carriage or head system. That is to say, the lens is allowed to position itself in the groove and will "float," or gravitate to the middle of the groove itself. Because of the free-floating situation, a 50-50 bevel results with the groove apex in the middle of the lens. This system is seldom used today.

Hide-a-Bevels. A finishing wheel capable of producing a flat or slightly angled edge either in front of or behind the bevel of the lens is referred to as a *Hide-a-Bevel* (American Optical; Figure 8-17). Although many term this type of bevel a *hidden bevel*, the expression "hidden bevel" has become a more general term that may refer to most any type of edge that has some type of ledge instead of being a conventional V-bevel configuration.

Mini-bevels. Some hidden-bevel finishing wheels have an angled ledge. The wheel shape causes the lens edge to angle out a bit both on the front and back (Figure 8-18). The current general usage term for this edge configuration is a *mini-bevel*. The meaning of the term *mini-bevel* has varied. It has also been referred to as a *special-V bevel*.

Free-Float Bevel System

One method of guiding the bevel is simply to allow a "free-float" situation for the lens on the edger wheel. When V-bevels were the norm, free-float systems worked well. The lens dropped into the V-shaped wheel edge and gravitated to the center.

Guided Bevel Systems

When the edge of the lens changed from only a V to a V with a ledge, it became necessary to guide the location of the bevel on the edge on the lens. Two methods, *mechanically controlled* and *electronically controlled,* exist for positioning a bevel on the edge of a lens without relying on a free-float system.

One method of mechanically guiding the location of the bevel is to restrict how far across the wheel groove the lens edge is permitted to float. One system uses a small guide wheel that tracks along the front surface of the lens as the lens rotates in the edger (Figure 8-19).

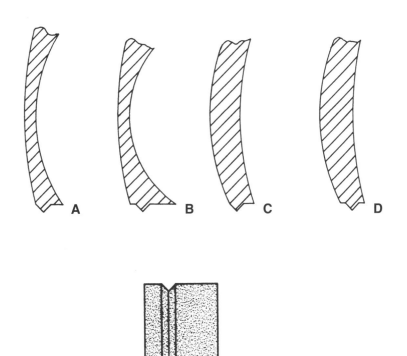

FIGURE **8-17** Hide-a-Bevels should not automatically be placed at the front edge of all lenses, as shown in **A**. High-minus lenses are often better edged with the bevel slightly back from the front surface, as seen in **B**. This keeps the back edge from touching the wearer's face, and with plastic frames may better hide thickness. Moderately thick-edged plus lenses, as shown in **C**, are edged in a manner similar to that of moderately powered minus lenses. Thick-edged plus lenses often do well with the bevel more toward the midline, as in **D**. However, when edges are excessively thick on plus lenses, the thickness may be due to having selected too large a lens blank for the eyesize.

The guide wheel rolls, which reduces the chance of marring the front surface of the lens.

If the front surface were always flat, the lens could just be locked in position and edged. Only vertical movement would happen as the pattern and lens rotates on the wheel. But few lenses are flat. Most lenses are curved. If a curved lens does not move left and right as it turns, its edge will completely leave the groove and not have a bevel.

The front curvature of a lens changes as its power changes. This means that how much the lens must move left or right with a guided bevel system will change with lens curvature (Figure 8-20).

Any guided bevel system requires the control of two variables. The first allows for lens steepness (base curve) so that the bevel does not travel off the lens edge because the frame shape has "long corners." The second variable positions the bevel closer to the front or back of the lens. This allows the bevel to be placed according to the optical or cosmetic needs of the frame and prescription.

Using a guided bevel system becomes especially important when the frame has stiff rims that are curved for a lens with a more commonly used base curve. The most common base curves are found on low-powered lenses. Unfortunately, a high-minus lens has a front surface that is practically flat. To overcome this problem, the edger must not allow the lens to float freely. Instead it must guide the lens as it turns in the edger.

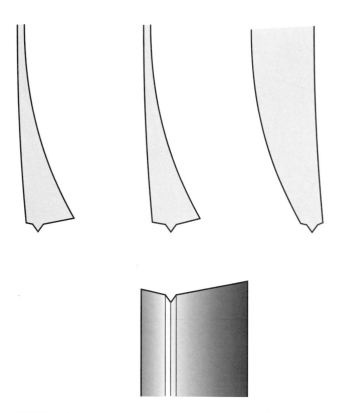

FIGURE **8-18** Examples of how the mini-bevel may produce edges on minus lenses are shown on the two left lenses. The lens on the right is a high-plus lens showing how one of the thicker edge locations on the lens might look.

It is advantageous to make the bevel fit the frame rather than the lens. This is shown in Figure 8-21. In these cases only a nonfloating, guided bevel system works. (Most patternless edgers have the capacity to take all these factors into consideration and allow the operator to choose the appropriate process.)

Dry Cut Edgers

Instead of using diamond wheels, some edgers use a spinning blade to edge the lens (Figure 8-22). These edgers use no coolants and cut the lens dry. They are suitable for polycarbonate and plastic but not for glass. They cut the lens to size using a small, rapidly rotating *blade* similar to a router blade used in woodworking (Figure 8-23).

When a lens is edged with a blade, no coolant is required. Small chips of lens are removed with a slicing action. Because no coolant is present, chips are sucked out of the edging chamber with a vacuum system. With a blade, speed of edging is increased considerably, which reduces the actual cutting cycle to anywhere from 13 to 35 seconds.

Special blades are available that, instead of beveling the edge, groove it. These are for frames that hold the lens in place with a nylon cord.

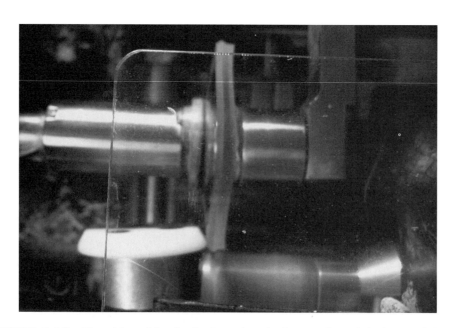

FIGURE **8-19** The white guide wheel rolls against the front surface of the lens and allows the bevel to be positioned at a given distance from the front of the lens edge. This same edger allows the wheel to be easily switched to an assembly that positions the bevel by desired base curve, then back again.

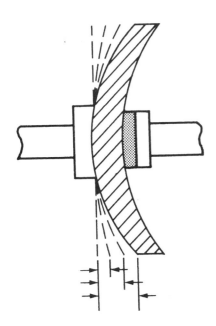

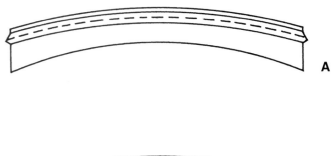

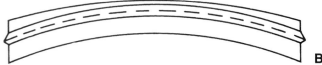

A

B

FIGURE **8-20** Lens base curves vary. The higher the curve is and the larger the lens, the farther back from the chucked central portion the edge is placed. *Dotted lines* indicate where the front surface base curve would be for lenses with increasingly steeper base curves. Were the lens to be locked in a stationary horizontal location and only allowed to move up and down during edging, the bevel would move completely off the edge on long corners. *Arrows* demonstrate how far the lens must move at this diameter to ensure that the bevel will be placed properly.

FIGURE **8-21** These lenses are seen from the top and have been edged using a guided bevel system. The frame to be used was manufactured to accept a lens with an average front curve (usually +6.00 D). The eyewires of the frame front are made to fit this curve and are not easily bent to a new conformation. Because the front curve of the lens is flatter than the curve of the frame, the bevel on lens **A** will not fit properly. However, if the lens is edged using a guided bevel system, the bevel can be made to fit the frame, rather than simply follow the front curve of the lens. The bevel shown in **B** will conform to the curve of the frame.

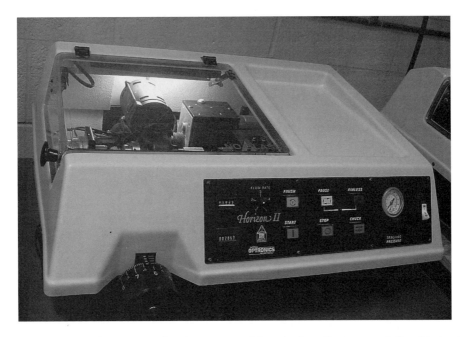

FIGURE **8-22** This is example of a patterned bevel edger that uses rotating blades to edge the lenses. This technology is also available in patternless edging systems.

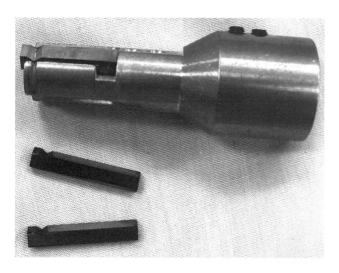

FIGURE **8-23** Plastic and polycarbonate lenses can be edged using cutter blades and no coolant. Blades may be resharpened.

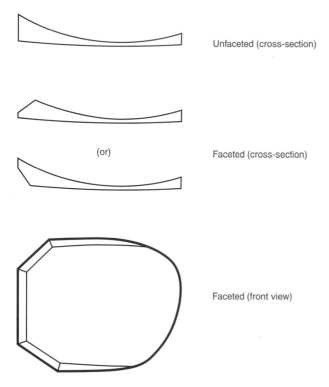

Unfaceted (cross-section)

(or)

Faceted (cross-section)

Faceted (front view)

FIGURE **8-24** A faceted edge is intended for a minus lens. Placing a faceted edge on a plus lens requires intentionally increasing lens thickness and is counterproductive. Faceted edges can be made to feature a variety of different looks when finished.

Facet

A facet is an edge shape used with rimless, grooved, and in some cases, thin metal frame eyewear. It resembles the beveled edge on custom-ground mirrors.

A relatively steep bevel is ground onto the front or back edge of the lens, then highly polished (Figure 8-24). Instead of making the lenses look awkward because of thickness, such lenses look almost as if the edge was designed thicker to accommodate the beveled glass effect.

The beveling can be done by hand with patience and skill, or in conjunction with an edger wheel or blade designed especially for the purpose. In either case the edges must afterward be polished. Frame and lens fashion changes cause facets to go in and out of style.

Rolled Edges

Another edge configuration that may be done either by hand or with a special edger wheel or blade is a rolled edge. The rolled edge reduces minus lens edge thickness by rounding out the back surface edge of the lens. This is shown in Figure 8-25. Even plus lenses with nasal thickness and high prism lenses are good candidates for rolled edges. The rolled edge is polished to match the high degree of polish present on the surface of the lens.

Polished Edges

Some edgers polish the edges of the lens. This may mean that the edge is truly polished or that the last finishing wheel on the edger has a fine grit, which gives the lens edge an especially smooth appearance. (For more on polished edges, see Chapter 10.)

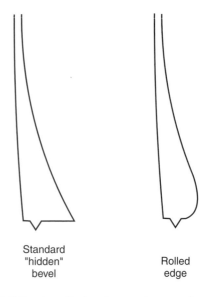

Standard "hidden" bevel

Rolled edge

FIGURE **8-25** A rolled edge reduces edge thickness without resulting in any visible demarcation line.

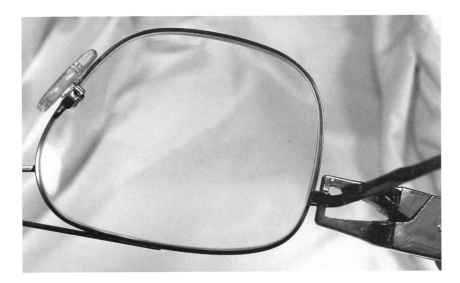

FIGURE **8-26**   A lens may be checked for size accuracy with a pair of closure pliers. With the lens in place, the barrels are simply squeezed together, eliminating continuous insertion and removal of the eyewire screw.

Emergency Stops

As with any type of equipment, occasionally stopping the operation in midcycle becomes necessary. Edgers have some system to stop the cycle and lift the lens off the wheel, resetting the machine to start.

Checking Size Accuracy

Once a lens has been edged, the block should not be removed until it is certain that the lens fits into the frame exactly. This is especially true for metal frames, in which small size increments determine the difference between ill- and well-fitting lenses.

To check lens size accuracy for a metal frame, the lens is placed in the eyewire with the block still on. Then, using eyewire closure pliers, the two sections of the eyewire are squeezed together, as in Figure 8-26. This draws the eyewire around the lens. If the upper and lower halves of the barrel fail to come together, the lens is still too large. The eyewire should close fully and leave no gaps between the lens and the eyewire, yet without putting undue stress on a lens.

Undue stress from a metal eyewire causes a plastic lens to warp and a glass lens to exhibit stress when viewed with the aid of a colmascope.[3] Figure 8-27 shows how the strain appears with a colmascope.

While the block remains on the lens, an operator may make slight steps in size reduction by running the lens through the finishing cycle again. However, once

the block is removed, it is extremely difficult to reblock the lens accurately enough to allow an even removal of only a few tenths of a millimeter.

Because plastic frames stretch upon lens insertion, some variation in lens size is possible without serious consequences. Such lens size variation is not possible when using a metal frame because the frame will not expand or contract. It is best to have the frame in the laboratory when the lenses are edged, but if this is not the case, a more accurate indication of size than a ruler or a Box-o-Graph (Kosh Manufacturing Co., Ft. Lauderdale, Fla.) can be obtained using a circumference gauge (Figures 8-28 and 8-29). By knowing the circumference necessary for each eyesize of a given metal frame, precision in duplication is possible. Therefore for metal frames that are uniformly manufactured to precisely repeatable sizes, an exact fit can be obtained without the frame being in the laboratory. (*Note:* Patternless edging combined with a remote tracer placed on location at the dispensary ensure an accurate fit even without having the frame in the laboratory, especially if used in conjunction with circumference measurements.)

Variations in Edging Lenses of Different Materials

Although the edging process remains approximately the same in spite of differences in lens materials, some aspects require special attention. These are discussed separately on the basis of the lens material used.

---

[3]A colmascope consists of a light source behind two crossed polaroids. When a lens is placed between two polaroids, internal lens stress becomes visually apparent.

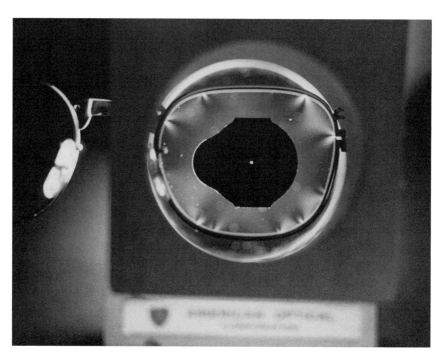

FIGURE **8-27**   A lens may be checked for stress with back-lighted, crossed polaroids (a colmascope). In this figure the adhesive pad block is still on the lens so that it may be re-edged easily. The bright marks around the periphery of the lens will show up with a rainbow effect and indicate entirely too much strain. Were such a lens to be dispensed, it could chip or flake along the edge at one or more of these strain points, especially if the lens is glass and the spectacles are dropped or knocked against an object.

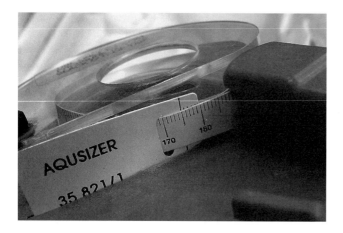

FIGURE **8-28**   Knowing the desired circumference of the lens and then edging the new lens size to match this desired circumference will provide more accurate results than edging using only eyesize measurements.

CROWN GLASS

Crown glass lenses are considered to be the standard for glass ophthalmic lenses. Lens fabrication equipment ordered for glass assumes crown glass lenses as the standard glass lens. Crown glass for ophthalmic use has

an index of 1.523. Glass lenses are also referred to as *mineral lenses.*

PHOTOCHROMIC GLASS

Photochromic glass, which darkens as light intensity increases, is treated almost the same as crown glass during the edging process. Because of its composition the photochromic lens generates more heat when being edged and is harder on edger wheels. As a result, some wheels have been designed for use in situations in which a high percentage of photochromic lenses are used.

When a large proportion of photochromic lenses are edged, the coolant must be of good quality and of sufficient concentration to produce the desired effect. Failure to maintain a clean, efficient coolant flow causes unnecessarily rough lens edges and a reduced abrasive wheel life.

HIGH-INDEX GLASS

Some clear glass lenses are made from materials that result in a higher refractive index than the standard crown glass lens. Common refractive indices for these so-called high-index lenses are 1.60, 1.70, and 1.80.

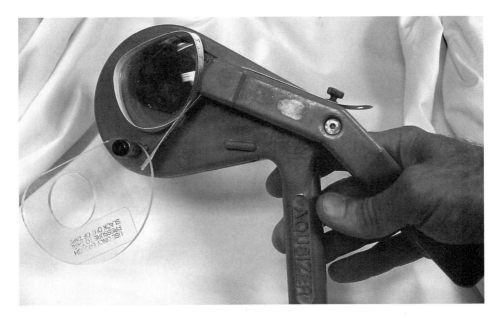

FIGURE **8-29** The lens is placed in the circumference gauge and the tape lightly tightened around the circumference of the lens. The clear plastic cover may be swung into position over the lens for more stability.

Because of basic property differences in the material, high-index lenses should be edged with less pressure than standard crown lenses.

It is advisable to avoid large temperature shocks with high-index glass, as when a hot lens is rinsed with cold water. A standard crown lens can generally withstand a 70° C difference in temperature, whereas a 50° C maximum difference is average for high index.[4]

High-index lenses should not be notched or drilled because these processes reduce impact resistance.

LENSES MADE FROM PLASTIC

Edging of plastic CR-39[5] lenses can be performed on the same equipment and with the same edger wheels as are used for glass *if* relatively few of the lenses are plastic. Because most lenses are plastic and not glass, this is impractical. When the percentage of plastic lenses increases, the plastic begins to glaze the wheel. *Glaze* means that the spaces between abrasive diamond cutting edges become clogged with plastic, preventing good, clean cutting.

A glazed wheel results in increased cutting time for lenses being edged. An extremely glazed wheel can even cause the edges of a glass lens to chip to a depth of 4 to 5 mm into the lens surface, ruining the lens. This does not occur when only a few plastic lenses are

interspersed with glass because the wheel is cleaned by the glass before plastic can build up to a glaze.

The solution to the problem of glazing can be handled in one of two ways. The first is to use two edgers—one for glass, the other for plastic. The second solution is an edger with three or more cutting wheels. Most three-wheel edgers made to handle two different lens materials are designed with one finishing and two roughing wheels. One roughing wheel may then be used for glass, and the second for plastic. All lenses may use the same finishing wheel because the same kind of finishing wheel is often used for both plastic and glass. Glass lenses must not inadvertently be allowed to rough on the wheel designed for plastic because wheel damage will occur.

HIGH-INDEX PLASTIC

With the exception of polycarbonate, lenses made from high-index plastic material are edged in essentially the same manner as are CR-39 plastic lenses. Some high-index lenses emit a sulfurous odor when edged. Although not considered hazardous, ventilation should be considered, especially if the laboratory is within proximity to a retail dispensary.

POLYCARBONATE LENSES

Polycarbonate lenses are highly impact resistant and are excellent for regular wear and as protective lenses in industrial situations. Although of a higher refractive index (1.586) than CR-39 plastic, polycarbonate is a

---

[4]High-Lite, S-1005 High Index, Low Density, Schott Optical Glass, Inc., Duryea, Pa., 1979.
[5]Columbia Resin 39, a trademark of Pittsburgh Plate Glass Co.

softer material and easily scratched unless coated. A protective coating is standard.

Care should be taken to ensure that all surfaces or points that come into contact with the lens are free from rough edges or burrs. Lensmeter marking points should not be overlooked.

Lens surfaces should be free of dirt and oils in order to prevent slippage during edging. For this reason, it is best to hold the lenses by their edges.

Wet or Dry?

Even though the edging process for polycarbonate lenses can be performed either wet or dry, a combination of both processes yields a cosmetically better, more stress-free lens. In this combination process, the lens is rough edged with no coolant. Halfway through the finishing cycle the coolant pump is activated and the edging process completed with coolant.

Polycarbonate lenses are also edged on dry-cut, rotating blade edgers. Although this system gives nicely configured edges, National Optronics (Charlottesville, Va.) makes an edger that first dry-cut edges the lens, then shifts the lens to a diamond polishing hub. During polishing this hub is misted with water to produce a clear edge finish.

Stress in Polycarbonate Lenses Resulting from Edging

If the speed of the diamond wheel or rotating blade is too slow, stress develops in a lens. Although stressed, lenses may still edge rapidly and look acceptable from a cosmetic viewpoint. Stress also can develop when cutting with a dull cutter. Over a period of time, this lens stress is released in the form of cracking or surface crazing.

Completing the Polycarbonate Process

Like other lenses, polycarbonate lenses should be safety beveled. Variations in this process are discussed in Chapter 10 on hand edging.

The lens must be edged and mounted stress-free to prevent future cracking or surface crazing. Although improper edging techniques can be the greatest source of stress in a polycarbonate lens, mounting the lenses too tightly also yields significant stress.

Cleaning of polycarbonate lenses may not employ harsh chemicals. Acetone damages the exposed edge of a polycarbonate lens. A mild detergent should prove sufficient. Alcohol is used to remove progressive lens manufacturer's markings.

ANTIREFLECTION-COATED LENSES

Antireflection (AR) coated lenses present some challenges in edging. A number of factors cause the coating to develop microcracks over the surface called *crazing*. Heat, pressure, and lens flexing can cause the coating to craze. With these things in mind, reducing the possibility of subjecting the lens to these factors also reduces the possibility of lens spoilage. The following list provides some ways to reduce AR spoilage.[6] Although not all are directly involved with edging, they are included together for convenience, as follows:

- Hold the lenses by the edges, not the surfaces.
- Edge AR lenses on an edger not used for glass. If glass lenses have been edged, or if the edger has not been cleaned recently, clean the edger so that debris will not recirculate over the AR-coated lens.
- Use surface-saver tape or surface-saver discs on the lens. This will protect it from scratching and will cushion the lens when it is chucked in the edger. If more cushioning is needed, use an adhesive blocking pad on the back surface of the lens.
- Reduce the chuck pressure on the edger, especially if the lens is also a high-minus, high-index plastic lens.
- Use the largest block and chuck possible to spread the pressure over a greater area.
- Do not use an edger with a bevel guide that touches the front of the lens.[7] (If this type of edger is used, then surface-saver tape also should be used to protect the surface.)
- Many of today's patternless edgers have self-adjusting features that keep chucking pressure and other stress forces to a minimum. They also are often able to get the lens exact the first time and pin-bevel it simultaneously so that the lens is handled less. For best results, use one of these.
- Do not leave the lenses blocked for long periods of time before edging them.
- Deblock the lens carefully.
- Rinse the lens after edging to remove any debris.

LAMINATED LENSES

When lenses are composed of two or more materials laminated together, the lens must be edged on a wheel that is compatible with both materials.

Special Edging Situations

EDGING LENSES FOR WRAP-AROUND FRAMES

Some sunglass frames are made primarily for plano sunglasses that are made with a high base curve to give

---

[6]Herrick T: The A-R upgrade: you're ready to sell S-R coated lenses, but can you finish them? *20/20* January:54-56, 2000.
[7]Edging instructions for Reflection Free Plus stock lenses, undated.

a wrap-around effect, which adds to protection from the sun and fashion appeal. One of the problems encountered is that prescription lenses are made on a variety of base curves, depending upon lens power. When a lens with a low base curve (flatter front curve) is edged for one of these frames, they do not always want to fit in and stay in the frame. There are two ways that may be tried to make the lens fit into the frame.

A Steeper Base Curve

The first method for making the lenses fit better in a wrap-around frame is to use a lens with a steeper base curve. This means ordering a lens with a base curve of about 8.00 D. The average prescription has a base curve of about 5 or 6 D. For lenses of low power this may not interfere significantly with the overall optical performance of the lens. However, each lens power has a specific base curve that is optically correct. Changing the base curve will decrease the optical performance when viewing objects in the periphery of the lens.[8] Therefore caution should be taken when changing base curves. The higher the lens power, the more significant will be the effect optically.

An Edger with a Guided Bevel System

The best way to edge a lens for a wrap-around frame is to use an edger with a guided bevel system. It is possible to use a lens with the correct base curve for the power of the prescription. To get the lens to fit properly, use an edger that allows any base curve configuration to be placed on the lens. In other words, a lens with a +6.00 D base curve can be edged with an 8.00 D bevel, which will better fit the curvature of the wrap-around frame (see Figure 8-21). The main drawback is that the edge of the lens must be thick enough to prevent the bevel from going off the lens edge completely.

WHEN THE BEVEL LEAVES THE LENS

Some types of lenses are notorious for causing the bevel to leave the edge of the lens, which makes it difficult to get the lens to stay in the frame or requires that the lens be re-edged completely. This often occurs on Franklin-style (Executive) lenses (Figure 8-30) and on lenses with high base curves. The following discussion presents some solutions.

A Guided Bevel System

When edging "Executive" lenses or high base curve lenses, the bevel may run off the lens edge. This is

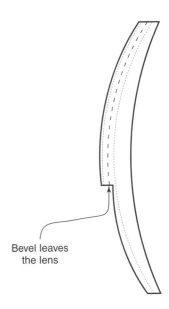

Bevel leaves
the lens

FIGURE **8-30** A bevel tracking around the lens a certain distance from the front surface often leaves the lens when it reaches the ledge of an Executive bifocal. This ruins the lens.

especially the case for long corners of the lens farthest from the center.

The best answer is to go to an edger that allows for manually guided bevel placement. Good results may be obtained on some lenses using a patternless edger that is auto-guided. These systems "feel" the thickness of the lens where the bevel will go and often show on-screen exactly where the bevel should appear on the lens after it is edged. Best results are obtained when this information may be actively used by the operator by allowing for manual adjustment for optimum bevel guidance all the way around the lens.

MAKING A PATTERN FROM AN EXISTING LENS

Some edgers have a kit that will allow the edger to cut a pattern from an existing lens. The wearer's lens or a coquille[9] is blocked with an adhesive pad so that the special block is exactly in the middle of the lens. The blocked lens is mounted where the pattern would normally be placed and a pattern blank is blocked and chucked in the edger as if it were a lens. The edger is set as if it were edging a lens for a rimless frame with no bevel.

---

[8]Changing the base curve of a lens successfully without affecting peripheral lens optics is possible if the lens is redesigned in aspheric form for that particular base curve.

---

[9]A coquille is the dummy lens that comes in the frame for frame display purposes.

PATTERNLESS EDGING

Patternless edgers and patterned edgers work in basically the same way. There are two main differences.

1. The patternless edger does not use a physical pattern. Instead it uses a digitized shape.
2. The patternless edger is already electronically sophisticated, so it builds in many more computer-controlled options. This makes it considerably easier to get a more refined end result.

Electronic Shape

A patternless edger is like a regular edger, except that it accepts frame shape information electronically instead of mechanically. This means that a patternless edger must work together with a frame tracer. The frame tracer creates a pattern shape electronically. (Frame tracers are explained in Chapter 3.)

Frame tracers can be a separate piece of equipment, hooked by cable to the patternless edger (Figure 8-31). Or the frame tracer can be a part of the edger, built right in to save space (Figure 8-32). Some patternless edgers are even more self-contained and have the layout blocker built into the housing of the edger (Figures 8-33 through 8-36).

Because each frame is traced individually, it is as if the electronic pattern is the same size as the edged lens will be.

Patternless Possibilities

What are some of the extras that can go along with a patternless edger? Not all of the options listed in this chapter's section on patternless edging are on every patternless edger. Each edger is unique in what it offers and will vary in how effectively and skillfully it is able to carry out that option.

USING PATTERNS WITH SOME PATTERNLESS EDGERS

Most patternless edgers cannot use patterns. Yet from time to time it is easier to use a pattern. For this reason, some patternless edgers are made to also run with a pattern. They are more the exception than the rule.

'FEELING' THE LENS FOR EDGE THICKNESS

One of the better options on a patternless edger is the ability to "feel" the lens where the edge will be located after edging. Many edgers use two "measuring arms,"

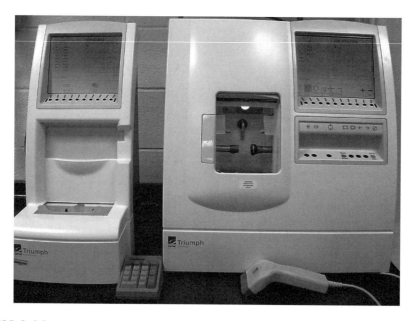

FIGURE **8-31** A tracer and a patternless edger can be two separate units that are electronically linked together.

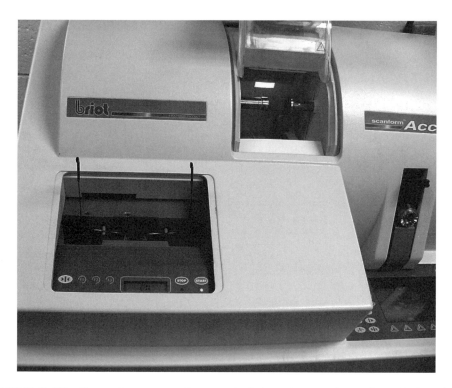

FIGURE **8-32** Frame tracers may be a part of the edger as shown here. In fact this particular edger also includes a blocker, visible at the lower right, as part of the same piece of equipment.

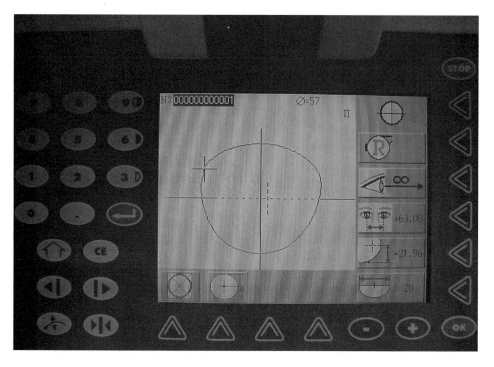

FIGURE **8-33** Information such as lens size, bridge size, segment or fitting cross height and wearer's PD is already input into many patternless edging systems. In this photograph the blocker viewing screen has the decentered lens location already preset.

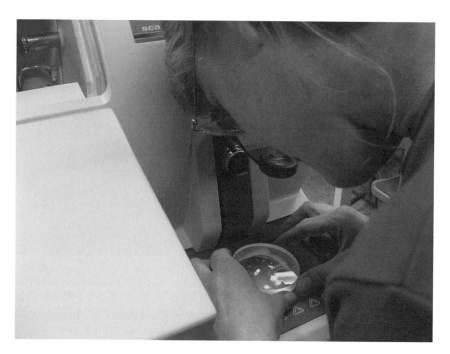

FIGURE **8-34** The lens is positioned for blocking. In this photograph the blocker and edger are part of the same machine shown in Figure 8-32.

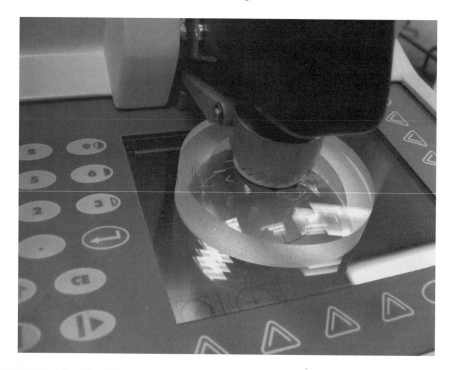

FIGURE **8-35** The block is either automatically or manually pressed against the lens.

one on the front of the lens and the other on the back. Before the lens is actually edged, the edger turns the uncut lens in the edger. These two measuring arms touch the front and back surfaces of the lens (Figure 8-37). As the lens turns, the arms trace the future shape of the edged lens at the exact lens size dictated. This tells the edger how thick the lens is at each point on the edge. The edger uses this information to decide an optimum bevel position. How well the edger makes this decision depends on the sophistication of the computer software. (Other ways exist for measurement of lens thickness besides use of measuring arms.)

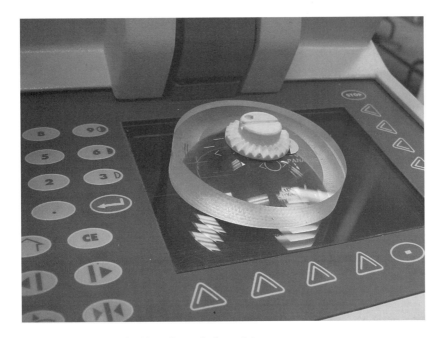

FIGURE **8-36**   The blocked lens is ready for edging.

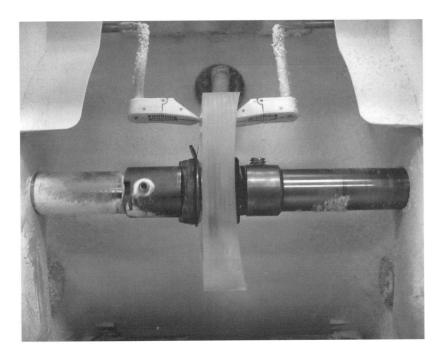

FIGURE **8-37**   To make the best judgment on where to place the bevel, an exact measure of edged lens thickness all the way around the lens is needed. To find this thickness, many edgers use measuring arms that touch the front and back of lens surfaces at the exact place where the lens edge will be when edging is complete. In this image the measuring arms are seen resting on front and back lens surfaces.

REQUIRED LENS AND FRAME MATERIALS

Patternless edgers often have a prompt that asks for the lens and frame material being used (Figure 8-38). The edger needs to know which *lens material* is used for the following reasons:

* The edger will rough the lens on the correct roughing wheel. The correct roughing wheel for

glass is not the correct roughing wheel for plastic or polycarbonate.
* If the lens is polycarbonate, the coolant flow will cycle on and off at different times. Other materials have a continuous coolant flow.
* The edger presses the lens against the wheel with the appropriate pressure.

Knowing the *frame material/bevel style* is important for the following reasons:

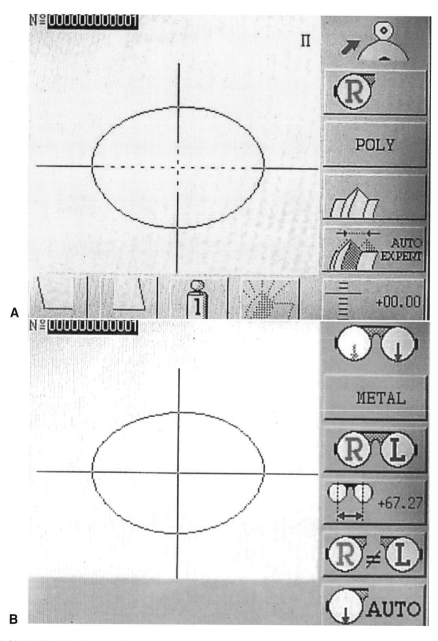

FIGURE **8-38** Patternless edgers commonly ask for not only the lens material, as shown in screen **A,** but also the frame material being used, as seen in screen **B**. In this image the screen shown in **B** indicates a metal frame. If the frame is not metal, the edger operator will press a triangular button adjacent to the word *METAL* until the appropriate frame material appears on the screen.

- To determine the way the edge will be finished, as when rimless lenses are needed
- To help determine if the lens is to be edged exactly on size, or will be edged slightly larger, as with certain plastic frames. Overriding the traced size and edging the lens slightly larger or smaller is possible. Size difference may be set at the discretion of the operator.

Newer edgers that receive information from previous data entry points in the laboratory will not need to prompt for lens and frame material. They will already have obtained that information.

PATTERNLESS EDGER VIEWING SCREENS

The viewing screen shows what the lens will look like when finished. A viewing screen can allow a number of options. The following are some of those options.

Viewing Screen that Shows the Lens Shape

The most basic screen type shows the shape of the lens as it appears when viewed from the front (Figure 8-39). This is important for several reasons, as follow:

- If the lens tracer has hit an irregularity in the frame eyewire, this will show up on the screen.
- If the frame has become deformed while being traced,

the operator may be able to pick it up by looking at the traced shape.

- The shape may not match the frame. Sometimes someone else scans the shape. This could have been either at order entry or off-site with a remote tracer. In either case the shape on the screen needs to be compared with the frame. If the frame and the traced shape on the screen do not match, the error will be caught and the lenses will not be ruined.

Screens that Show the Edge of the Lens

Edgers that show the edge thickness and shape will, of necessity, have the capacity to "feel" the front and back surface of the lens as described above. However, what is possible from this point on varies considerably.

If the edger can show the way the lens edge will look after edging, it usually allows some operator discretion on bevel placement, otherwise there would be no point in showing the edge.

Edgers should allow the operator to move the bevel forward and backward. In other words, the bevel may be moved closer to the front or closer to the back of the lens edge. But, for maximum control, the bevel should be able to move forward or backward different distances for different points around the rims of the frame. This may be done on the screen first to see what it will look like before being edged as shown in Figures 8-40 and 8-41.

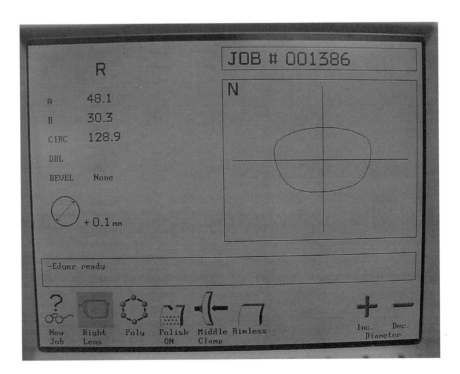

FIGURE **8-39** Being able to see the shape of a lens on the viewing screen of a patternless edger allows a quick check to be certain that the correct lens shape is being edged.

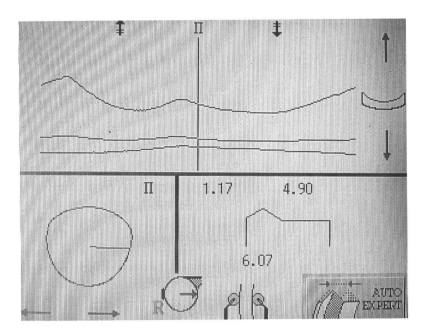

FIGURE **8-40**   The lower right quadrant of this screen shows the way in which the lens edge will look in cross-section on the temporal side. The upper half of the screen shows where the bevel apex is located relative to the front and back edges of the lens all the way around the lens. (It is as if this thick minus lens edge were removed from the lens and spread out flat on the screen.) The vertical line at II (lower-left area) shows where the cross-section in the lower right hand quadrant of the screen is located.

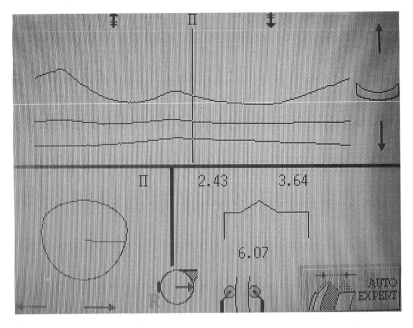

FIGURE **8-41**   The bevel on the same thick lens pictured in Figure 8-40 has been moved back on the lens edge. It is possible to leave bevel placement to the preprogrammed settings, or to override these settings with what the operator feels is most appropriate for the prescription.

Taking Advantage of the Third Dimension

Frame tracers will either trace in two dimensions or three dimensions. If the tracer traces in two dimensions, it only gives basic lens shape, exactly like a pattern would. If it traces in three dimensions, it tracks forward and backward and finds how the frame is curved (Figure 8-42).

Figure 8-43 shows a frame front with an eyewire curvature made for lenses with moderately curved front surfaces. If a lens has a very flat or a very steep front surface, either the frame will have to be reshaped or the lens bevel modified. It can no longer simply follow the front edge of the lens.

Figure 8-44 shows a high-minus lens with a flat front curve. This flat-front lens will not fit into a curved-rim frame without modifying either the frame or the lens bevel position. If the lens is edged with bevel positioning based on the front edge of the lens (Figure 8-45), then the frame must be reshaped.

For example, what if this frame were traced with a frame tracer capable of tracing in three dimensions? Knowing this information, the edger is set to follow the

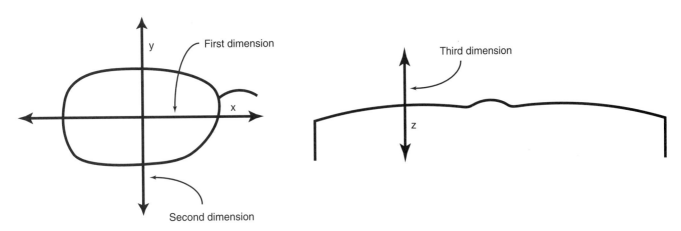

FIGURE **8-42** This drawing shows the three dimensions referred to for tracing and edging lenses. The first and second dimensions correspond to x and y coordinates in mathematics and correspond to horizontal and vertical measurements on a flat piece of paper. They resemble a flat screen television. The third dimension corresponds to the z coordinate in mathematics. This dimension is the out and in direction, in front and in back of the paper. If television were in three dimensions, the viewer would feel like the action was happening in the room.

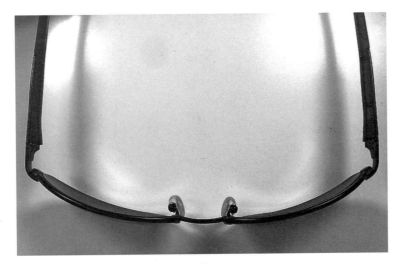

FIGURE **8-43** This frame is made for lenses that have a moderately curved front surface, as do most lenses that are neither high-plus nor high-minus in power.

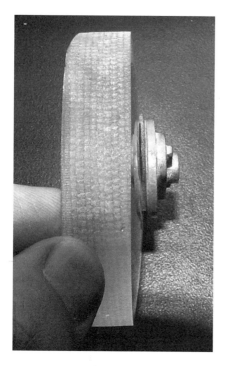

FIGURE **8-44**   This lens is high minus in power. The front surface has little curve. It is almost flat.

However, a frame tracer may trace in three dimensions but the patternless edger may not be able to use that information. The edger must be capable of interpreting the information given to it by the tracer and capable of edging in three dimensions.

LENS DRILLING AS AN OPTION

WECO makes an edger that has a drilling option (see Figure 13-53). The edger will drill holes, blind holes, and slots and blind slots. Blind holes and blind slots are holes and slots that go only halfway into the lens. A part of the rimless mounting presses into the blind hole or slot to give the finished spectacles more stability.

OPTIONS AVAILABLE ON PATTERNLESS AND PATTERNED EDGERS

Some options on patternless edgers are also options on patterned edgers. These include, but are not limited to, edge polishing, safety beveling, and edge grooving.

SELF-DIAGNOSTICS WITH EASY CALIBRATION

When a piece of equipment becomes computer controlled, it should include some level of self-diagnostic ability. At start-up it should be able to run through a program of self-check that will set up needed standards and check the various system components to ensure that they are functioning as they should. If they are not, the faulty system should be displayed.

frame (Figure 8-46). This moves the bevel to conform to the curvature of the frame as shown in Figure 8-47. (This is not a good frame choice for this particular lens prescription, but it is used in this discussion for demonstration purposes only.)

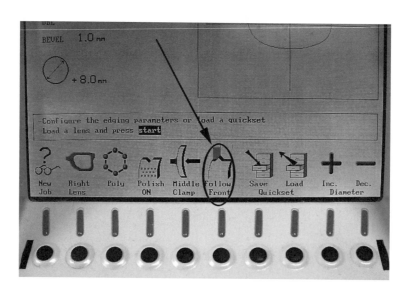

FIGURE **8-45**   A lens can be edged so that the bevel follows the front edge of the lens. In this image the edger is set to follow the front of the lens, maintaining a constant distance from the front edge.

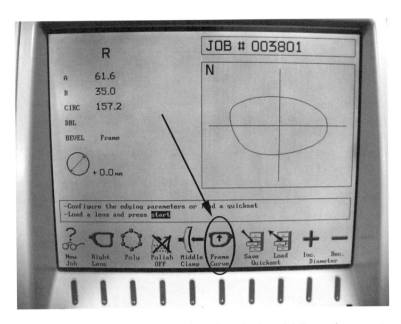

FIGURE **8-46** A lens also can be edged so that the bevel follows the curvature of the frame, instead of the lens. This edger is set to follow the frame curve. If this option is chosen, the bevel will not always be an even distance from the front of the lens.

Patternless edgers should have some kind of system for easy calibration. This would include things such as wheel differential, eyesize, and axis. Some edgers dress the grinding wheels when they become worn and are not cutting as crisply as they should be. The extent of the calibration and diagnostics for patternless edgers varies considerably.

DECENTRATION CALCULATIONS

Patternless edgers may calculate decentration for the edger operator, but require the operator to decenter the lens in the layout/blocking process. Other edgers do not require the operator to physically decenter the lens. These edgers are made to work with the layout blocker. If a direct interface exists between blocker and edger, the lens does not have to be physically decentered nasally by the operator. The operator just positions the spotted lens so that the optical center (or major reference point) is in the middle of the blocker grid as if no decentration existed at all. Then one of the following two things happens:

1. The blocker moves the lens block over to where it would normally be positioned.
2. The lens is blocked right in the middle and the edger takes that factor into consideration when it is edging the lens.

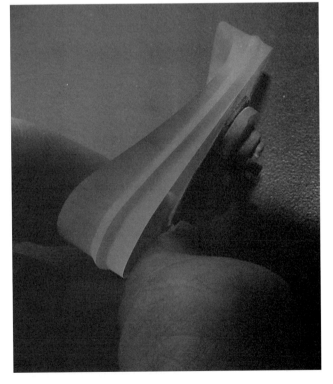

FIGURE **8-47** The bevel's appearance when the lens in Figure 8-44 is edged for the frame in Figure 8-43. Notice that the bevel is close to the front of the lens at the top but is farther back from the edge on both temporal and nasal sides of the lens. (*Note:* This lens/frame combination is not a good one but is chosen only for the purpose of clearly illustrating the way in which bevel location can be made to follow the curve of the frame instead of the curve of the lens.)

ABILITY TO INTERFACE WITH THE REST OF THE LABORATORY

A feature of growing importance for patternless edgers is the ability to interface with the rest of the laboratory. Patternless edgers are only one part of an optical laboratory. Increasingly optical laboratory equipment is being interconnected, tied together with laboratory management software programs.

A patternless edger may be completely self-contained, including frame tracing, blocking, edging, safety beveling, and edge polishing. It will prompt for frame dimensions and the wearer's PD measurement. However, what if the order has been sent to the laboratory electronically with all of that information already entered? By having the capacity to accept frame tracings, frame dimensions, and PD from a laboratory software program it is no longer necessary to reenter all of the information. This saves time and eliminates one more source of human error that can occur by reentering existing information.

Using a bar code reader, the operator may scan a job tray (Figure 8-48). This tells the edger which job to call up. Any missing information may be entered and the job processed. It also tells the software program where the job is located. If any questions about the job arise, the tray may be located easily.

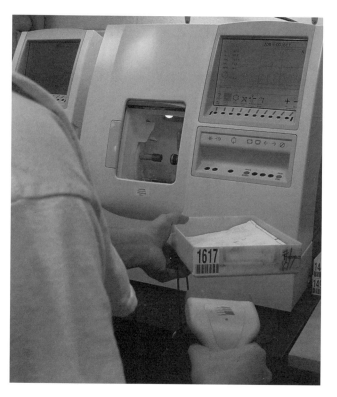

FIGURE **8-48** Bar coding each job allows information to be downloaded into the edger and at the same time keep track of the exact location of the job in the laboratory.

Proficiency Test Questions

1. Definite relationships exist between pattern size and edger setting. Assuming a "standard pattern size" of 36.5 mm, fill in the missing information for each of the following lens size/pattern size combinations.

EYESIZE	PATTERN SIZE	SET NUMBER	EDGER SETTING
50	50	a	b
48	c	−10	d
45	e	f	37
g	44.5	h	44
50	36.5	i	j
k	l	−5	57
50	51.5	m	n
52	50	o	p

2. If a pattern is marked, "set −5," which of the following is the pattern's A dimension?

   a. 37.5
   b. 41
   c. 45
   d. 41.5
   e. Cannot be determined from information given

3. A pattern measures 56 mm. If the frame to be used is a 58 □ 20, which of the following edger settings will result in a correctly edged lens, assuming a correctly calibrated edger?

   a. Set at 36.5 mm
   b. Set at 38.5 mm
   c. Set at 54 mm
   d. Set at 56 mm
   e. Set at 58 mm

4. A pattern has a B dimension of 47 and a pattern difference of 4. Which of the following is the pattern set number?

   a. −14.5
   b. −4
   c. −6.5
   d. −40.5
   e. None of the above

5. Suppose a pattern has a size of 36.5 mm and has a "pattern difference" of 6. If the edger is correctly calibrated and set for 52 mm, which of the following is the measurement for the B dimension of the edged lens?

   a. 42.5 mm
   b. 30.5 mm
   c. 46 mm
   d. 58 mm
   e. None of the above

6. An edger has a setting dial with a zero, plus-minus scale. A pattern has an A dimension of 53. The frame has an A dimension of 49. Which of the following indicates the edger setting?

   a. −2 mm
   b. −12.5 mm
   c. −16.5 mm
   d. −4 mm
   e. None of the above

7. An edger has a setting dial with a zero, plus-minus scale. The pattern is marked "set −10." The frame has an A dimension of 52. To which of the following is the edger dial set?

   a. −10
   b. +5.5
   c. 62
   d. −15.6
   e. None of the above

8. A "lenses only" order comes with the name of the frame, an A, a distance between lenses, and the lens circumference. The circumference measurement is 151.4 mm. You have the pattern. The pattern has a circumference of 146 mm. Which of the following would you use for an edger setting?

   a. 34.9
   b. 36.5
   c. 38.3
   d. 41.9
   e. Not enough information given

9. An order comes with the patient's old glasses, including the lenses. You are to put new lenses in the old frame. To be sure you get the right size, you measure the circumference of the old lenses. The circumference is 157 mm. You have the pattern and measure it. The pattern measures 161.8. Which of the following edger settings would you use?

   a. 35.1
   b. 36.5
   c. 38.1
   d. 41.3
   e. Not enough information given

10. True or False? The groove for a nylon cord lens retention system can be produced on some edgers.

11. Which of the following statements about faceted lenses is true?

   a. When the facet is used, high-minus lens edge thickness is reduced.
   b. When the facet is used, high-minus lens center thickness increases.
   c. When the facet is used, plus lens center thickness decreases.
   d. When the facet is used, plus lens edge thickness decreases.

12. True or False? The term *polished edges* always means the edge has the same high luster as is found on the surface of the lens.

13. Which of the following pliers is helpful in the process of determining whether a lens is the correct size for a metal frame?

   a. Fingerpiece plier
   b. Endpiece plier
   c. Half-padded plier
   d. Eyewire closure plier
   e. Lens rotation plier

14. "Mineral lens" is another name for which of the following?

   a. High-index plastic
   b. Polycarbonate
   c. Glass
   d. CR-39

15. Which of the following lenses are said to emit a sulfurous odor when edged?

    a. Glass
    b. High-index glass
    c. CR-39 plastic
    d. Polycarbonate
    e. High-index plastic

16. Which of the following is/are some possible reason(s) for a bevel coming out incorrectly on a thin, high-index lens? (*Note:* More than one answer may be correct.)

    a. A flexible plastic lens block was used instead of a stable, metal block.
    b. A metal block was used instead of a flexible plastic block.
    c. The wrong base block was chosen for the base curve of the lens being edged.
    d. The lens was edged on a patternless edger equipped with measuring arms. As the thin, flexible lens was cut down, the curvature of the lens changed and caused the bevel to be misplaced.

17. Which of the following actions will not help prevent a high-index plastic lens from cracking during edging?

    a. Using the edger's reverse rotation option
    b. Blocking the lens on a steeper base block
    c. Reducing edger clamping pressure
    d. Reducing the head pressure the edger exerts on the lens

18. Which of the following edging methods and/or a similar variation to this method yields a more stress-free polycarbonate lens?

    a. Edging the lens wet
    b. Edging the lens dry
    c. Edging the lens wet until partway through the finishing cycle, after which the coolant is turned off and the cycle finished dry
    d. Edging the lens dry until partway through the finishing cycle, after which the coolant is turned on and the cycle finished wet

19. Match the refractive indices to the correct lens material.
    crown glass _____
    polycarbonate _____
    CR-39 _____
    high-lite glass _____

    a. 1.425   e. 1.586
    b. 1.498   f. 1.621
    c. 1.523   g. 1.70
    d. 1.530

20. Which of the following is not a way that may reduce spoilage of antireflection-coated lenses? (*Note:* Not every response may be necessary in every instance but should at least be considered helpful in some instances.)

    a. Use surface-saver tape or discs on the lens.
    b. Reduce chuck pressure on the edger.
    c. Avoid heat on the lens when heating the frame and lenses together.
    d. Leave the lenses blocked overnight before edging to allow initial stress to subside.

21. True or False? It is always best to increase the base curve to approximately +8.00 D when using prescription lenses in a wrap-around frame.

22. Which of the following is *not* a workable suggestion for keeping the bevel on the edge of an Executive lens?

    a. Instead of a free-float bevel placement system, use a guided bevel system.
    b. Use a patternless edger with measuring arms that "feel" lens thickness at the proposed location of the lens edge.
    c. Edge the lens a bit large. Bring the final lens size down by hand to control bevel placement.
    d. All of the above are workable suggestions.

23. True or False? Some patternless edgers are still capable of directly edging a lens from a pattern.

24. True or False? A patternless edger may ask for the frame material being used. Frame material will determine which roughing wheel should be used.

25. True or False? If a patternless edger viewing screen shows the proposed location of the bevel on the lens, that bevel position can be moved uniformly forward or backward on the lens edge.

26. True or False? If a patternless edger viewing screen shows the proposed location of the bevel on the lens, it may be possible to move the bevel selectively (e.g., moving the bevel back on the nasal and temporal sides while leaving the bevel toward the front of the lens at the top and bottom).

27. True or False? All frame tracers trace in three dimensions and send three-dimensional frame information to the patternless edger.

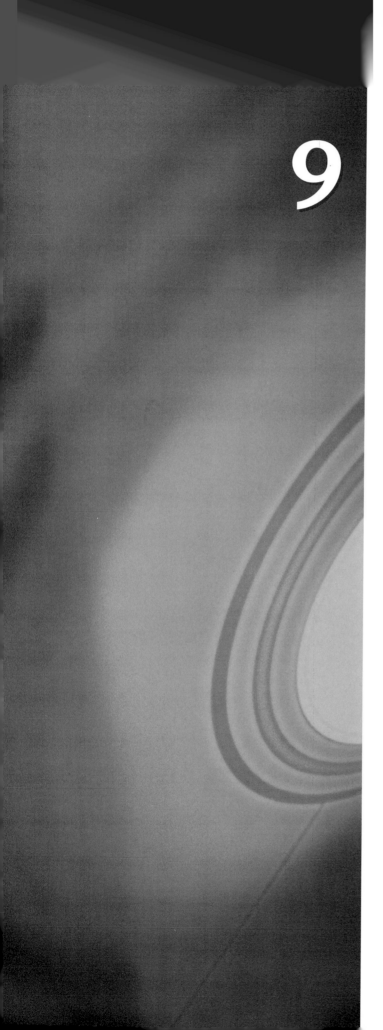

9 *Deblocking*

The method used to deblock a lens depends on the type of blocking. Each is explained by blocking method used.

Deblocking Lenses Blocked by Suction

The method used for deblocking a suction-blocked lens is self-evident. When the suction cup seal is broken by lifting the edge of the suction cup, the lens deblocks easily. Grasping it with a plier and twisting it off also removes the lens.

Deblocking Metal Alloy–Blocked Lenses

As mentioned in Chapter 7 ("Blocking of Lenses"), metal blocking of lenses is used rarely. It is not as environmentally friendly and has disadvantages when used with certain types of lenses.

Only two ways exist to deblock plastic lenses. The first is to twist or torque the lens to pop off the block (Figure 9-1). Unfortunately this is appropriate only for uncoated lenses. Flexing coated lenses should be avoided because this can damage the coating.

The second is to use a hot water system of deblocking. The blocked lens is placed in hot water and the block melts off and sinks to the bottom. If this method is used, the water must then be processed before it can be

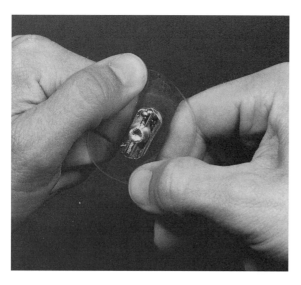

FIGURE **9-1**   If a plastic lens is twisted slightly, adhesion is broken and the alloy block drops off.

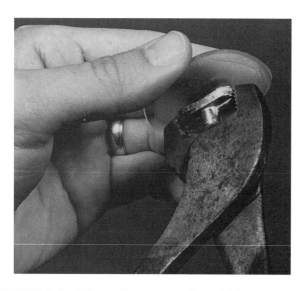

FIGURE **9-2**   When pliers are used to deblock an alloy-blocked lens, the long axis of the block is squeezed to deblock, not pulled.

poured down the drain because it contains heavy metals. This method works for glass lenses.

Metal blocks also may be removed from glass lenses using a large-jawed plier. The jaws are oriented so that they span the longest axis of the block, as in Figure 9-2. Deblocking is *not* accomplished by pulling the block off but rather by squeezing. As pressure is applied to the longer axis, slight flexing of the metal occurs, which breaks the seal between lens and alloy. The pliers never touch the lens. This method does not work well on plastic lenses because the plastic lens flexes with the block and does not release.

Deblocking 'Wax'-Blocked Lenses

Deblocking the waxlike blocks used in the Gerber-Coburn Step Two blocking system is done with deblocking pliers. The block is grasped with the pliers and twisted from the lens.

Deblocking Adhesive Pad–Blocked Lenses

Lenses blocked with adhesive pads use either metal or plastic blocks. Deblocking differences between metal blocks and plastic blocks are slight.

DEBLOCKING ADHESIVE-PADDED METAL BLOCKS

To deblock an adhesive pad–blocked lens, the lens is held firmly with a tool and twisted off. The "classic" type of deblocking tool is shown in Figure 9-3. It is shaped to accept the block in the same manner the edger chuck does.

The lens is held with a laboratory towel when twisting it off. If the lens is held without a towel the technician

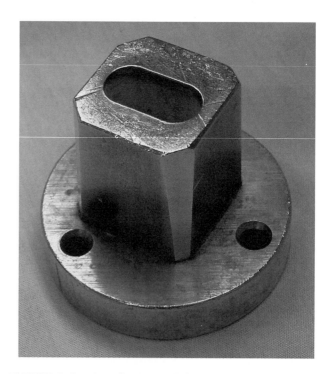

FIGURE **9-3**   An adhesive pad deblocker is simply a holding mechanism for the block. Deblocking occurs when the lens is twisted off the block. (This deblocker resembles the "classic-type" deblocker but is an "in-house" constructed model.)

can get small surface cuts on the hand when sharp edges have not been removed by safety beveling the lens.

Most people think that turning force is most important when removing a block, such as when a person tries to remove the lid from a pickle jar. However, the technician can remove the lens from the block easier by pressing the block harder into the deblocker while twisting.

If the lens is small and hard to get off the block, the towel being used to grasp the lens should be dampened to increase the grip on the lens. Figure 9-4 shows a lens being deblocked with a deblocking tool.

Many layout-blockers come with a deblocker fastened to the side of the unit (Figures 9-5 and 9-6). These are

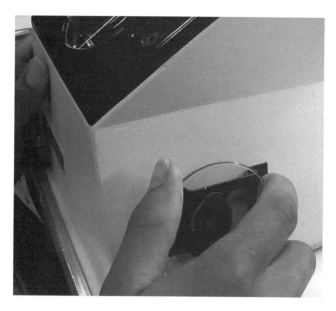

FIGURE **9-6** Twisting a lens off the lens block with the deblocker on the side of a layout-blocker has the advantage of having the deblocker mounted on a solid, heavy object. Because it is sometimes necessary to deblock and reblock a lens during layout before it has been edged, the location is handy.

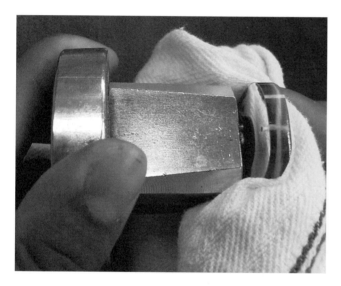

FIGURE **9-4** Although many practitioners deblock lenses without the use of a laboratory towel, small cuts can be prevented by padding the edges of the lenses.

simply wide slots with rounded ends that are cut into stainless steel. They work just as well as the classic-type deblocking tool.

DEBLOCKING ADHESIVE-PADDED PLASTIC BLOCKS

Plastic blocks are usually deblocked using a plier shaped to fit the block. The block is grasped with the plier and removed by tilting the pliers, rather than twisting the block (Figure 9-7).

Reminder

A lens should not be deblocked until the technician is certain it will fit exactly into the frame. Once a lens is deblocked, reblocking the lens exactly as it was blocked before is almost impossible. Attempting to reblock the lens and then re-edge it will probably result in a poor fit with a slight gap or misshape to the lens. It is much easier to take a lens down in size on an edger than to hand edge it to size.

Table 9-1 summarizes the deblocking methods discussed in this chapter.

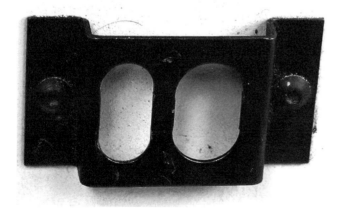

FIGURE **9-5** A lens deblocker that comes mounted on the side of a lens layout-blocker. The large slot fits nicely around the raised section of a metal lens block.

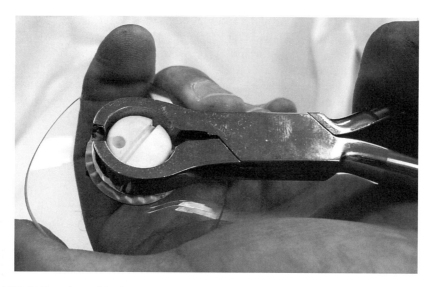

FIGURE **9-7** Plastic blocks may be removed with a plier designed for that purpose. The lens is held along the longest meridian and the pliers tilted away from the technician, who pulls the block from the lens, rather than twists if off.

TABLE **9-1** *Deblocking Methods*	
BLOCKING METHOD	BLOCK REMOVAL TECHNIQUES
Pressure blocking	Remove lens from edger.
Suction blocking	Break seal by lifting edge of suction cup with fingernail. Twist off.
Metal alloy blocking	For glass lenses, use: • Plier pressure • Hot water For plastic lenses, use: • Lens torquing (uncoated lenses only) • Hot water
Blocking with a waxlike material	Twist off.
Adhesive-padded blocking	Twist or tilt off.

Proficiency Test Questions

1. Which of the following method(s) is/are appropriate for deblocking of a lens that has been blocked with a waxlike material?

   a. Just remove the lens from the edger.
   b. Break the seal on the edge of the block.
   c. Grasp the lens by the block with a plierlike deblocking tool and twist it off.
   d. Peel the pad off with the fingernail.

2. True or False? Deblocking of metal alloy–blocked glass lenses is accomplished by grasping the block across the short dimension and pulling it off.

3. True or False? Using a classic-type deblocking tool is unequivocally the best method for deblocking lenses from a metal block with adhesive pads.

4. How may an adhesive-padded blocked lens be deblocked?

    a. Just remove the lens from the edger.
    b. Break the seal on the edge of the block.
    c. Grasp the lens by the block with a plier or deblocking tool and twist it off.
    d. Torque the lens.
    e. Peel the pad off with the fingernail.
    f. Use hot water.

5. True or False? Regardless of blocking methods, the safest way to deblock a plastic lens is with hot water.

6. True or False? It works out well to deblock a lens before checking lens size. The lens is easily reblocked if the size needs to be slightly reduced.

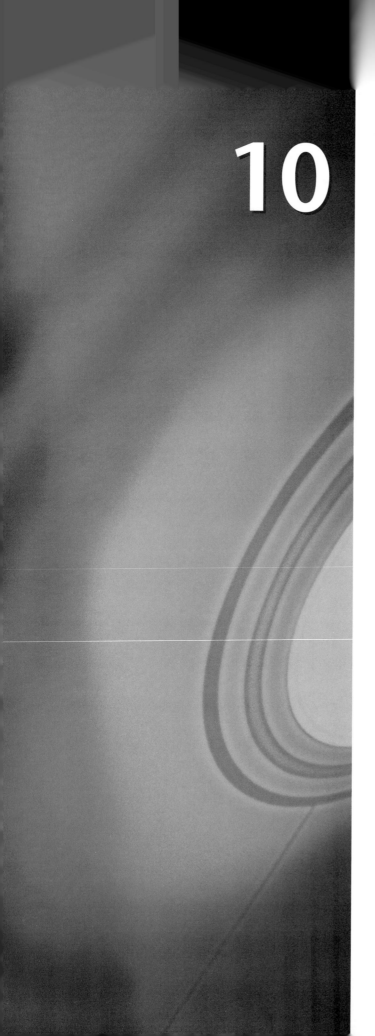

10 Hand Edging

Rationale for Hand Edging

In hand edging the lens is held in the hand and its edge pressed against a rotating smoothing surface. Hand edging is used for the following tasks:

1. Smoothing edge surfaces *(edge smoothing)*
2. Removing sharp edges from a lens after it has been machine edged *(safety or pin beveling)*
3. Reducing a lens in size
4. Reshaping the lens

Types of Hand Edgers

Described in simplest terms, a *hand edger* is an abrasive wheel mounted so that the edges may be ground by hand.

CERAMIC WHEEL HAND EDGERS

The older style of hand edger was a large diameter wheel with a wide edge as shown in Figure 10-1. The wheel is ceramic and may be retrued often to remove surface irregularities. Because the wheel is ceramic down to the hub it has a long life.

DIAMOND WHEEL HAND EDGERS

A commonly occurring design for diamond hand edgers is the *face-type hand edger* (Figure 10-2). This uses the face rather than the edge of a rotating wheel for grinding. Such a design does not allow use of the corner of the wheel for hard-to-reach sections on the

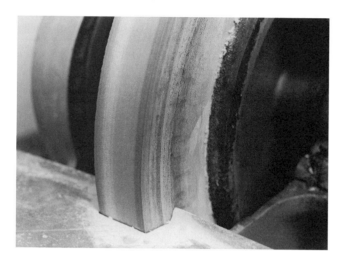

FIGURE **10-1** Although it requires occasional retruing, a ceramic hand-edging wheel has an exceptionally long life because of its depth.

back bevel. In compensation, a central curved hub is provided. Some manufacturers still maintain the basic design of a ceramic wheel but have reduced either the wheel diameter (Figure 10-3) or the edge width.

Hand Edgers with V-Bevel Grooves

One option available in selection of a hand edger is the kind of V-grooved wheel shown in Figure 10-4. This groove allows the size of an edged, hidden-bevel lens to

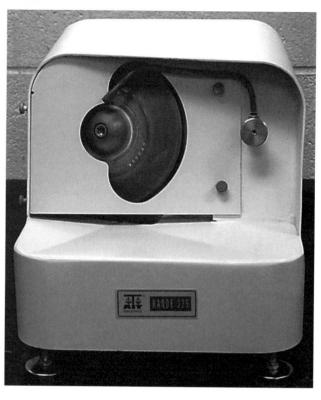

FIGURE **10-2** A face-type hand edger reduces the amount of diamond required by placing the abrasive on the side of the wheel.

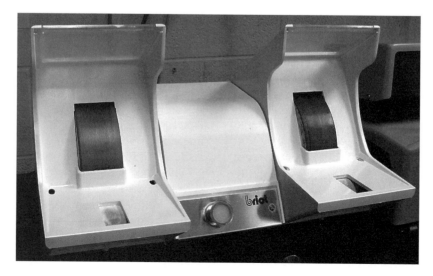

FIGURE **10-3** Smaller diamond wheels with a wide surface area offer versatility and resemble the older ceramic wheel hand edgers.

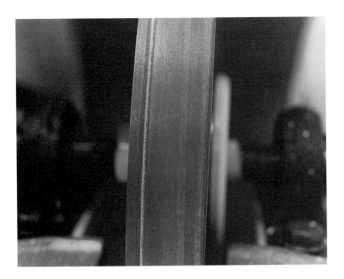

FIGURE **10-4** A grooved wheel is not primarily designed to smooth both bevel surfaces of normal lenses simultaneously. It allows lenses with hidden bevel edge shapes to be reduced in size without destroying the edge configuration.

be reduced. Unless this option is available, a size reduction or shape modification by hand is possible only if the hidden bevel is changed to a standard V.

A V-bevel groove may be useful for dispensary situations in which inexperienced personnel are required to change the size of a lens. Maintaining an attractive bevel during hand edging without practice is difficult.

WHEEL GRITS

Using different types of diamond wheels allows versatility. As would be expected, those wheels with extra-fine grit are excellent for pin beveling, whereas rough grit is used for rapid removal of lens edge substance.

Grit types and their purposes are listed in Table 10-1. If only one wheel must be chosen for all purposes, the fine-grit wheel is the most versatile. It allows smooth pin beveling yet can still be used to reduce size. A super-fine wheel is for pin beveling and edge smoothing only. In contrast, rough wheels are excellent for rapid shape reduction or alteration but cannot be expected to adequately perform smoothing tasks. For maximum efficiency, two wheels of different grits are used next to one another.

Two Parts to Hand Edging

Hand edging includes the following two parts:

1. Edge smoothing
2. Pin or safety beveling

TABLE **10-1** *Hand-Edger Wheel Grit Types and Their Purposes*	
TYPE	PRIMARY PURPOSE(S)
Rough	Removing edge stock rapidly
Medium	Removing edge stock
Fine	Pin beveling and edge smoothing; also, removing edge stock moderately well
Extra-fine	Pin beveling and edge smoothing

Edge smoothing once was used to improve the coarse, frosted look of a lens after it had been edged. All lenses had to have their edges smoothed to make the lens look decent. This is no longer necessary. However, the technique used in edge smoothing is the same as that required to reshape a lens or to reduce a lens in size by hand. Learning the basic technique of edge smoothing is the first step in learning to resize or reshape a lens.

Pin or *safety beveling* is used to remove the sharp interface between the lens bevel and the front and back surfaces of the lens. Another name for pin beveling is *chamfering*. Pin beveling by hand is still used but will be used less often as more edgers come equipped with a pin-beveling option. This, too, still will be needed when the size or shape of an existing lens is changed, such as when someone breaks a frame and needs his or her lenses put in another frame. If the lenses are not pin beveled after reshaping, they are subject to chipping.

Edge Smoothing

Edge smoothing is done with the needed angle of the bevel on the lens edge in mind. At the same time the smoothing process is being carried out, the quality of bevel is checked for both angle and apex position.

The angle of the bevel apex is greater than would be expected. It is normally a 115-degree angle and should not be larger than 130 degrees. This was shown in Chapter 8 (see Figure 8-14). The lens bevel angle is larger than the angle of groove in the frame. The most common mistake in beveling the lens is to make the bevel too pointed.

The apex of the bevel should be placed centrally for thin lenses. For thicker-edged lenses the apex is placed a third of the way from the front (see Figure 8-14).

PREPARING THE WHEEL

With the exception of polycarbonate lenses, before the hand edger is used, the wheel must be wet. Some hand edgers have a coolant recycling system with a pump and coolant tank below the unit. Others use tap water that does not recirculate but simply drains out. In either case, a steady drip on the wheel is required. Because of the smoothness of most wheels, the thumb may be drawn across the face of the spinning wheel to ensure that the entire surface is wetted; this method is illustrated in Figure 10-5.

Some wheels use a sponge to prevent splashing and to spread the water evenly over the surface. The sponge should be wetted and positioned before the unit is turned on. It also must be removed whenever the unit is turned off. If this is not done, ceramic wheels absorb water from the sponge and swell, which creates a lump on the wheel.

HOLDING THE LENS PROPERLY

Edge smoothing begins with the back surface of the bevel. The left hand[1] is rested on the hand rest and the lens is grasped between thumb and forefinger with both hands. The right thumb and forefinger act as a pivotal point, while the left thumb and forefinger guide the lens.

---

[1]The sequence is explained from the right-handed point of view. Those who are left-handed should substitute left for right and right for left. Pictures visualized in mirror image give the left-handed perspective. (Holding the book in front of a large mirror will show correct left hand positioning.)

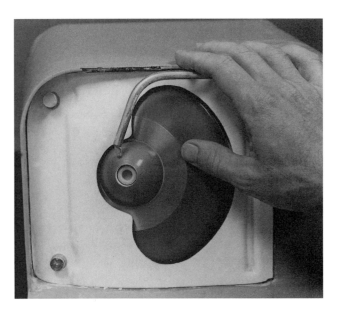

FIGURE **10-5** Drawing the thumb across the hand wheel ensures even wetting before grinding begins.

Assuming that the angle on the bevel is correct, the lens is held with the back surface of the lens bevel flat against the cutting plane of the wheel. Figure 10-6 shows this in cross-section from the side. When viewed from this perspective, the lens makes about a 41-degree angle with the cutting plane of the wheel.

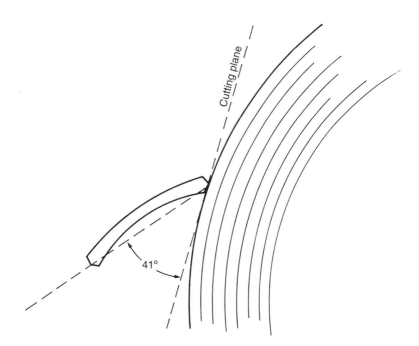

FIGURE **10-6** During edge smoothing, the back bevel surface is smoothed first. This helps to position the apex. The lens is held somewhere near a 41-degree angle with the cutting plane. It is angled downward considerably more than it will be when the front bevel surface is smoothed.

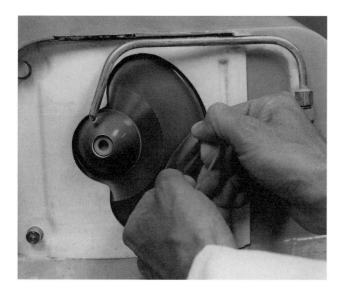

FIGURE **10**-7 By tilting the lens to approximately 60 degrees and rotating it clockwise, the upward pull of the wheel can be used to advantage. (Those who are left-handed tilt to the mirror image and rotate the lens counterclockwise.)

If the lens is viewed from the front, the angle that the lens makes with the horizontal plane can vary considerably. The personal preference of the practitioner determines how the lens is held. An angle of approximately 60 degrees works well because it allows a good view of the lens without having to lean sideways. It also still takes advantage of the upward pull of the wheel for a smoother, steady lens rotation.

To start out, the lens is held on its 180-degree cutting line, as shown in Figure 10-7. Lens rotation will be clockwise.[2] The hand edger wheel surface is spinning upward. When the lens is rotated in a clockwise direction, the edge contacting the wheel will also move upward. This way the lens is moving with the direction of wheel rotation instead of against it. When the lens turns with the wheel, it is easier to control the speed of stock removal[3], angle, and movement of the lens.

As Figure 10-8 demonstrates, the best spot on the lens to place the edge on the wheel is just past a lens corner.

The lens is held tightly between right thumb and forefinger. This point on the lens becomes the pivotal point. Figure 10-9 shows how the left thumb and forefinger (primarily the thumb) guide the lens across the surface of the wheel. As the lens turns 180 degrees, the left forefinger is removed from the lens and the

thumb guides it on around. This is shown in Figure 10-10.

POSITIONING THE BEVEL APEX

As stated earlier, the edge-smoothing process begins with the back surface of the bevel. During the process of smoothing the back bevel surface, the apex of the bevel can be repositioned toward the front of the lens. Applying extra pressure to the back bevel surface moves the bevel apex forward more.

Once the bevel apex is in its desired location, the front bevel surface can be smoothed. (For thin-edged lenses, the bevel apex is centered. As the lens edge thickens, the bevel apex should be moved toward the one-third/two-thirds position.)

EDGE SMOOTHING THE FRONT BEVEL SURFACE

When the bevel apex has been properly placed, the front surface of the bevel is smoothed. Because of bevel configuration, however, the angle between the cutting plane of the wheel and the lens is considerably greater than it was for the front surface. As Figure 10-11 shows, the actual angle is approximately 74 degrees, but the lens appears to be almost at right angles to the wheel, depending upon where the wheel is contacted. Compared with back bevel smoothing, front bevel smoothing is done lightly. It is done with less pressure to prevent alteration of bevel positioning.

Basic Rules for Better Results

The following sections describe some basic hints for getting better results during the hand-edging process and some suggestions on how to practice.

MONITORING PRESSURE AND LENS ROTATION SPEED

The finer the grit of the hand-edger wheel is, the more pressure may be applied. However, several variables affect just how much pressure is appropriate.

The thicker the edge of the lens, the greater the pressure that may be applied. This is true primarily for the backside of the bevel. The backside of the bevel contains more surface area than the front.

Pressure on the lens against the wheel must be slackened as the corners are smoothed. As lens/wheel contact area reduces, if the overall force being applied is not reduced, pressure per square inch increases dramatically. Corners grind down faster.

---

[2]Left-hand practitioners rotate counterclockwise with the lens at 120 degrees instead of 60 degrees.
[3]Stock removal means removal of lens material.

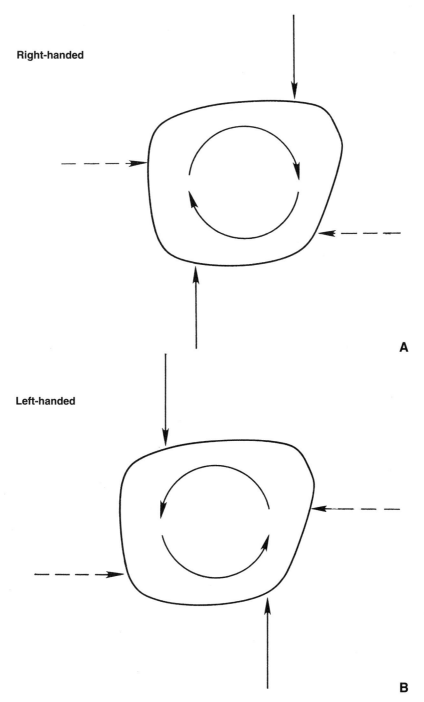

Right-handed

Left-handed

A

B

FIGURE **10-8** It is best to start edging a lens from a point just past a lens corner. These places are indicated by the *straight arrows; curved arrows* indicate lens rotation direction.

An alternative to reducing pressure against the lens as corners are rounded is to increase the speed of rotation. Because less time is spent in contact with the wheel, cutting is reduced. In practice, speed of rotation and force against the wheel are varied simultaneously (Box 10-1).

LISTENING TO THE WHEEL

A great deal can be learned about the edge quality of the finished lens by listening to the sound of the wheel during hand edging. *The wheel should make a constant, unbroken sound.* For several reasons the wheel may emit

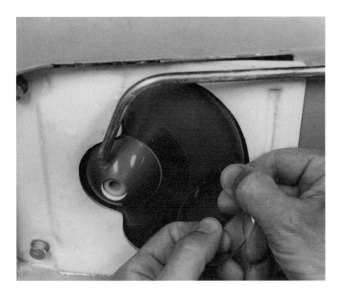

FIGURE **10-9**   To begin hand edging hold the lens with thumb and forefinger as shown. The right thumb and forefinger serve as a pivotal point. The left thumb and forefinger guide the lens onto the wheel, controlling speed. The lens will be rotated clockwise.

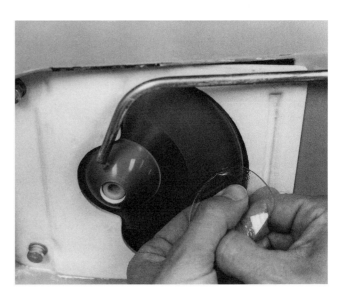

FIGURE **10-10**   The lens is not removed from the wheel surface often. In the figure, the lens has been rotated clockwise a full 180 degrees. The right hand still functions as a pivotal point and the left as a guide. If the left finger is moved out from under the lens, further uninterrupted clockwise rotation may be accomplished, guiding the lens with the thumb of the left hand.

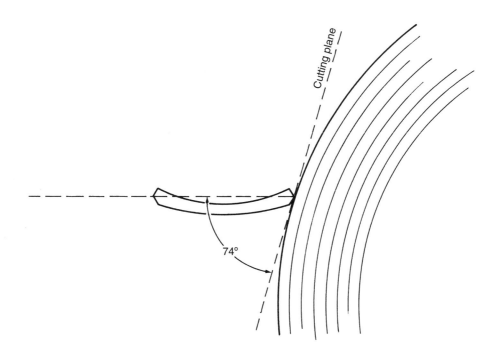

FIGURE **10-11**   A common mistake in hand edging is to make the lens bevel too sharp. The near horizontal position of the lens shown in the figure is correct but invariably seems wrong to the novice.

> **BOX 10-1**
>
> *Factors Affecting Cutting Speed in Hand Edging*
>
> - If pressure against the wheel increases
> - If speed of rotation decreases
> - If a rougher grit wheel is used
> - At a corner of the lens shape
> - As lens edge thickness decreases
>
> *Cutting Speed Will Decrease...*
>
> - If pressure against the wheel decreases
> - If speed of rotation increases
> - If a finer grit wheel is used
> - Along a straight side of the lens shape
> - As lens edge thickness increases

a wavy, irregular tone, all of which relate to faulty technique:

- *A wavy sound.* A wavy sound occurs if the angle of lens *tilt* is being altered. This results in a wavy bevel apex and an uneven, irregular appearance of the face of the bevel.
- *Variations in sound volume.* Changes in sound volume indicate that *pressure* on the lens is uneven. An uneven, wavy bevel results and the lens may not have the same shape as before. Applying too much pressure on corners causes corner gaps that will show up after the lens is inserted into the frame.
- *Short, choppy sounds.* Short, choppy sounds indicate that the lens is being lifted from the wheel too often. This can cause the surface of the bevel to lose its smoothness. Smooth, long motions result in smooth bevel surfaces.
- *A smooth sound interrupted by periodic wavy sounds.* A smooth sound interrupted by periodic wavy sounds indicates an attempt to regrip the lens without first lifting it from the wheel. Each time the grip is changed, the lens must first be lifted from the wheel. Maintaining a correct wheel/lens relationship is impossible while simultaneously shifting the grip on the lens.

SUMMARIZING A FEW BASIC HAND-EDGING RULES

The following rules apply generally, not just for edge smoothing:

1. Maintain a constant angle between the wheel face and lens.

2. Never reposition a grip on the lens while the lens is against the wheel.
3. Travel as far around the bevel as possible before lifting the lens from the wheel.
4. Listen to the sound of the lens on the wheel.

PRACTICING EDGE SMOOTHING

Practicing proper smoothing begins with choosing a lens large enough to permit an easy grip. A low-minus lens has an optimum edge configuration. Before advances were made in edger wheel quality, lenses would leave the edger with a "frosted" appearance. That frosted surface had to be removed by edge smoothing. A lens with an edge that is as "frosted looking" as possible should be used so that it is easier to see what has been accomplished.

After each major "pass" around the lens, the lens edge is wiped dry and the "frosted" area checked. If translucent-like "frosted" area is being removed near just the apex, for example, the lens is being held at the wrong angle and should be tilted so that the lens is closer to the wheel. The hands are too unsteady if the translucence that remains is scattered here and there on the bevel. Resting the hands firmly on the hand rest and maintaining a consistent angle of tilt helps solves this problem.

Pin Beveling

Lenses need to be pin beveled. It does not matter if the lens has been just edged or edged then edge smoothed by hand. The only reason not to pin bevel is if the edger includes the pin beveling process.

REASONS FOR PIN BEVELING

Three primary reasons exist for pin beveling, as follows:

1. *Breakage prevention:* If the intersection is allowed to remain as a sharp corner, the risk of chipping or flaking at the interface between the two surfaces is considerably higher. Hence the alternative term, *safety bevels.*
2. *Cosmetic considerations:* Pin beveling removes microchips or "stars" left as the abrasive wheel grinds away lens material. Microchips are seen by holding the lens up to a light source and turning it slightly. Starlike reflections on the edge indicate their presence.
3. *Wearer safety:* Pin bevels may reduce the risk of injury to the wearer's face if the glasses are struck and then impact the wearer's face. For this reason some

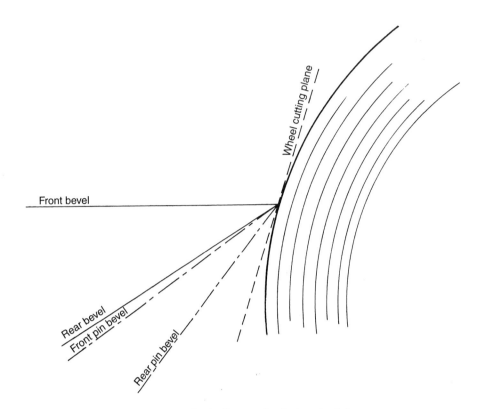

FIGURE **10-12**   A comparison of grinding angles in hand edging.

suggest that safety lenses should have a greater-than-normal pin bevel.

PIN BEVELING A LENS

The basic procedure for pin beveling uses much the same technique as is used for edge smoothing. For pin beveling the front and rear surfaces, the lens is held in basically the same manner as it was for edge smoothing. The difference is in the angle the lens makes with the cutting plane. This needed angle for pin beveling is only half of what it was for edge smoothing. Figure 10-12 compares the angles used for edge smoothing and pin beveling.

To pin bevel the apex, the lens is held vertically with the right hand. The lens may be guided with the left hand but should be held loosely enough to allow free rotation (Figure 10-13). Some people safety bevel the apex with only one hand.

The following are some key points in the pin-beveling process:

- Little pressure should be applied in pin beveling. The lens is permitted to rotate almost from the upward pull of the wheel alone.
- Speed of rotation is much faster than for edge smoothing.

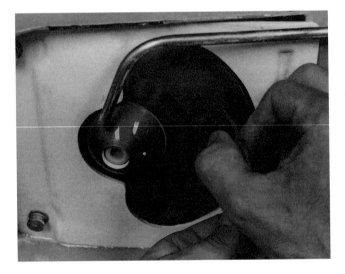

FIGURE **10-13**   Pin beveling the bevel apex is done with very little pressure.

- When completed, the pin bevel should be noticed only by the absence of edge sharpness and microchips. It does not need to be visible.

Table 10-2 summarizes the sequence of steps in the edge-smoothing and pin-beveling process.

TABLE 10-2
Order of Steps in Hand Edging of a Lens

AREA FOR HAND EDGING	APPROXIMATE ANGLE-TO-WHEEL CUTTING PLANE
Rear face of bevel (and rimless rear pin bevel)	41 degrees
Front face of bevel (and rimless front pin bevel)	74 degrees
Front pin bevel	37 degrees
Rear pin bevel	21 degrees
Apex pin bevel	Held vertically at right angles

Pin Beveling the Rear Surface of a High-Minus Lens

Back-surface pin beveling may prove difficult if a lens has a high-minus back curve. It is made even more difficult when the frame being used has a narrow B dimension. This happens because the center of the back bevel spans the surface of the wheel and cannot be reached (Figure 10-14). The only way to reach the center is by use of either the edge of the wheel or a curved hub. Figure 10-15 demonstrates how to pin bevel the rear surface of a high-minus lens using the rounded edge of a traditionally shaped hand-edger wheel.

Face-type hand edgers do not have an exposed edge, but they usually have a curved central hub area. This curved central hub portion is used for pin beveling the back surface of the lens. Figure 10-16 shows how this is done.

Pin Beveling for Rimless Lenses

A pin bevel has an angle that is halfway between the two surfaces it separates. For beveled lenses the pin bevel is light. For glass, flat-beveled lenses the pin bevel may be a bit heavier (Figure 10-17). Rimless pin bevels are more obvious than regular pin bevels and for plastic lenses should be done very lightly (see Figure 10-17).

Reducing Lens Size by Hand

Reducing the size of a lens by hand is easier when it is to go into a plastic frame. Metal frames are harder to do. One of the most difficult tasks in hand edging is to reduce the size of an edged lens for a metal frame and have it fit right. Much skill is required to maintain the integrity of the lens shape during the process. The following list outlines the steps used to reduce a lens size by hand:

1. **Apply pressure to the rear bevel** surface and rotate the lens exactly as was done during the edge-smoothing process.
2. **Continue edge smoothing** with more pressure than usual until the apex of the bevel moves toward the front of the edge.
3. Next, **edge smooth the front bevel** until the apex of the lens bevel returns to its proper position.

If only a slight size reduction is required, just repeating the edge-smoothing process without attempting to move the bevel position may be sufficient.

CHECKING METAL FRAME LENS SIZE

Even a small lens size reduction can make a large difference in how well a lens fits. If the frame is available, the lens should be checked often; it is placed in the frame and the eyewire closed. The best way to check eyesize is to remove the screw and squeeze the eyewire barrels together with a pair of eyewire closure

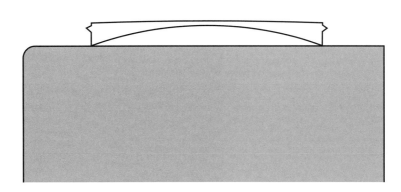

FIGURE **10-14** For lenses with high-minus back curves, a flat hand edger surface will not reach all the sections where the back pin bevel belongs. (The lens shows a top view in cross-section.)

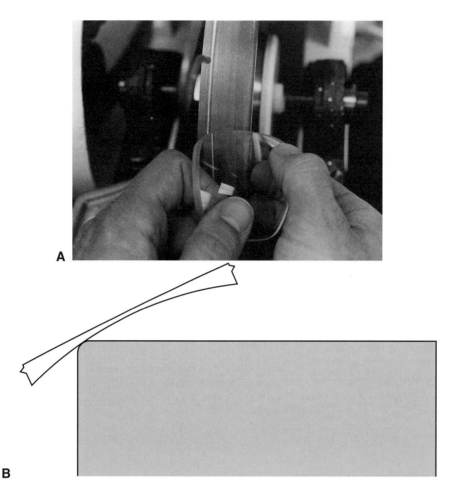

FIGURE **10-15**   **A,** When pin beveling the back edge of the lens on the rounded corner of the wheel, care must be taken to reduce pressure. The small lens/wheel contact area quickly raises the pressure per unit area. **B,** Hand-edger wheels with flat surfaces may have one rounded corner that allows the back pin bevel of a high-minus lens to be applied. (The lens shows a top view in cross-section.)

pliers. This was shown in Chapter 8 (see Figure 8-26). Backing the eyewire screw out just far enough to allow the lens to be removed and reinserted may seem easier. Unfortunately, the edge of the lens often flakes when being shoved back into the eyewire. It is better to just remove the screw.

Simply being able to screw the eyewire barrels flush together does not indicate a good fit. The eyewire may exert undue pressure on the lens. In plastic lenses this causes the lens to warp, and in glass lenses a stress pattern is set up within the lens. If nothing is done to relieve the stress, edge flaking will occur when the rims receive even a slight blow. (Edge flaking is surface chipping at the lens edge.)

Stress also may result when the curve of the lens edge does not match the curve of the frame's rim. In this case, either the rim must be shaped to match the lens curve, or the lens bevel must conform to the same base curve for which the frame was designed.

The practitioner checks the lens for stress by placing it in a colmascope,[4] as would be done to check for a heat-hardened glass lens. Viewing the lens in this state shows a zigzag color-fringed pattern around the lens edge wherever a stress buildup occurs. If this encompasses the lens completely, as was shown in Figure 8-27, the lens is still too large. It should be taken down evenly all the way around the lens. If, however, the stress pattern occurs only in one place, note that place. The edge should be made to better conform to the frame in that area.

_____
[4]A colmascope consists of two polarizing films, illuminated from below. The lens is placed between the two for viewing.

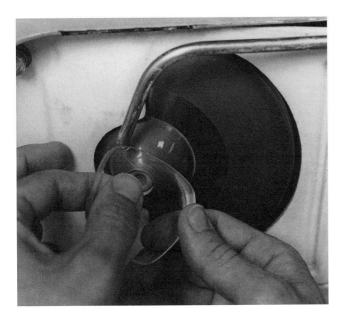

FIGURE **10-16** The spherical section of the face hand edger is designed to pin bevel the hard-to-reach back edge of high-minus lenses.

REDUCING LENS SIZE FOR HIDDEN-BEVEL LENSES

To reduce lens size for a lens having a hidden bevel, a hand-edger wheel with a V-groove is helpful. The lens is held perpendicular to the wheel with its bevel in the V-groove (Figure 10-18).

HAND EDGING FOR FRANKLIN-STYLE LENSES

The Franklin-style (Executive) lens is ruined easily in inexperienced hands. Because of lens design, a large portion of the front bevel ends abruptly where it meets with the segment ledge on both the temporal and nasal sides of the lens. Ledge corners form small points. In smoothing the front bevel surface near these corners, little pressure should be used. Lens material is removed extremely rapidly. This same precaution is necessary during safety beveling. A poor job of safety beveling will look worse than if the lens had never been safety beveled.

HAND EDGING OF POLYCARBONATE

After edging, sometimes a polycarbonate lens may have a residue of plastic material clinging to the lens bevel. This buildup is known as *flash* or *swarf* and has been described as looking like white shredded wheat. (The amount of swarf remaining on the lens can be

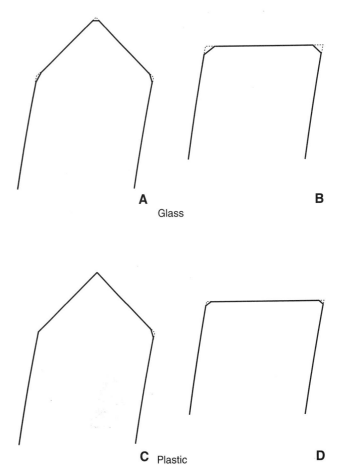

FIGURE **10-17** Glass lenses have a pin bevel that is a bit heavier than the pin bevels on plastics lenses will be, since glass lenses are more likely to chip along any sharp edge. **A** and **B** show approximately what the size of glass pin bevels are for regular and flat-beveled lenses. Plastic lenses with a regular bevel (**C**) will have less of a safety bevel. The back surface interface with the bevel will have more of a safety bevel than the front surface interface or the apex. Before pin beveling this is generally the sharpest edge, especially for lenses with minus lens power. Plastic flat-beveled lenses (**D**) have sharper angles and have minimally more of a safety bevel.

reduced by increasing edger head pressure.) The polycarbonate lens should be pin beveled dry. Dry means the coolant to the hand edger is turned off. Pin beveling must be done lightly because the wheel cuts faster when it is dry.

Two exceptions exist. One is for rimless bevels and the other is for antireflection (AR)-coated lenses. These are pin beveled wet. Wet pin beveling of polycarbonate gives a smaller, less noticeable pin bevel and a polished appearance. After pin beveling, any remaining swarf is removed by scraping the lens edge with a razor or knife blade held perpendicular to the lens surface (Figure 10-19).

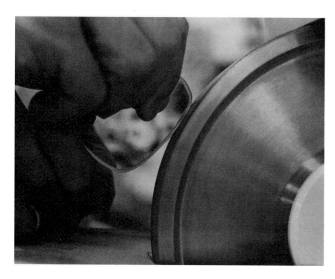

FIGURE **10-18** It is helpful to brace one hand on the tray while reducing size or reshaping a lens with a hidden bevel edge configuration on a grooved wheel.

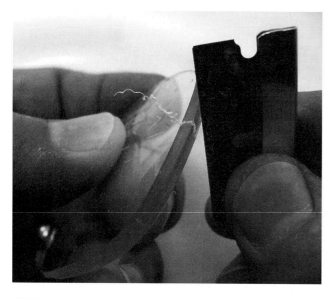

FIGURE **10-19** After a lens has been hand edged, it will have curled threads of polycarbonate material clinging to the edges. This is removed by scraping it with a single-edged razor blade held perpendicular to the edge.

HAND EDGING ANTIREFLECTION-COATED LENSES

Some AR coatings are more sensitive to heat, pressure, and flexing. Any of these may cause some coatings to craze.

In hand edging of lenses with an AR coating, the practitioner should not press too hard or too long against the wheel. Pressing the lens hard against the

hand-edger wheel causes a plastic lens to flex. A wet hand-edger wheel should always be used.

Re-edging a Lens for a Different Frame

Most wearers just assume that putting their old lenses into a new frame is a simple matter. It is not. Several factors must be considered before deciding to try it. The following are a few:

- *The distance between optical centers needs to remain the same.* Even if old lenses do fit into the new frame without re-edging, the new PD may not be correct. If the distance between lenses (DBL) of the new frame differs from that of the old, the PD will no longer be correct. The lens major reference point (MRP) must be located close enough to the wearer's PD to prevent prism that would exceed ANSI Z80 standards for prescription ophthalmic lenses.
- *The lenses must be large enough.* The old lenses have to be large enough for the new frame. If the new frame is metal, then the old lens must be big enough so that the entire lens opening is covered.
- *Rotating the old lens so it fits the new frame may not work.* Lenses that have a cylinder component to the prescription may not be turned from their prescribed axis, nor may most segmented multifocals and progressive addition lenses.
- *Glass lenses need to be rehardened.* If the lens has been heat-treated it must be dehardened[5] before re-edging. Fortunately heat treating of glass lenses is now rare. Chemically hardened lenses may be re-edged as they are. However, both types need to be rehardened before dispensing.

If all these factors have been considered, the lens may be reshaped.

Lenses are not re-edged if the chosen frame is plastic and can be stretched to accept the old lenses. Stretching the frame's eyewire usually eliminates unwanted air spaces between the lens and the eyewire.

HAND EDGING A LENS FOR A DIFFERENT FRAME

If possible, the lenses are blocked and re-edged with an edger. If this is not possible, the following is one method for hand edging the lenses for a new frame:

[5]Dehardening is done by placing the lens in the heat-treating unit for the same length of time as is required for hardening. As the lens is removed from the furnace area, instead of fast cooling with forced airto create internal stress, the air is turned off and the lens is allowed to cool slowly.

1. Spot the lenses in the lensmeter according to the wearer's prescription.
2. Measure on the frame from the center of the frame bridge to half the wearer's prescribed PD.
3. Hold the lens over the frame with its dotted MRP at the wearer's PD. The lens opening must still be completely covered by the lens. (If the lens does not cover the opening, and moving it left or right slightly[6] will not cover the gap, do not go any further.)
4. Note those places where the lens is too big and must be edged away.
5. Reshape the lens on a hand edger.
6. Once the first lens has been satisfactorily shaped, use it as a model for the second to ensure left-right symmetry.

Changing a Frame's Lens Shape

Sometimes practitioners request that a lens be made to a different shape than the shape of the chosen frame. The purpose for substitution of a different lens shape may be simply cosmetic. Some frame shapes may compliment a particular facial shape. Or a shape change may be requested to obtain either a better bridge fit or a slightly larger B dimension. Commonly requested shape alterations are for nasal cuts, nasal adds, and increases in the B dimension. These requested changes work primarily for plastic or rimless frames.

NASAL CUT

A *nasal cut* is requested when the wearer's nose broadens more toward the nostril area than the frame does. When this happens, the frame rests on the lower nasal corners of the rims rather than on the bridge area of the frame. The amount of nasal cut desired is specified in millimeters or with a tracing or drawing, as Figure 10-20 shows.

If the frame specified is rimless, the matter is simple. Assuming an extra pattern is available, the pattern is marked for a nasal cut and the marked area filed away. Figure 10-21 is an example of this method. The lens is edged normally on the modified pattern.

If the lens is for a plastic frame, this procedure will not work. Filing the pattern with no other compensation only causes an inferior nasal gap between lens and frame groove. Following is a list of some alternative possibilities.

---

[6]The lens is moved only to the left or right from where it should be if certain that the prismatic effect created will not exceed ANSI standards.

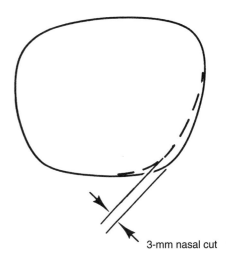

3-mm nasal cut

FIGURE 10-20 This lens will have lens material removed to the point where the dotted line appears. The person wearing the lens has a nose that flares out at the bottom. If the lens shape were not given this "nasal cut," the lower nasal rim of the frame would rest on the wearer's cheeks. If the lens were for a rimless frame, the lens itself might otherwise touch the cheek.

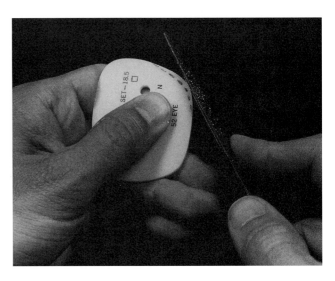

FIGURE 10-21 A simple method used to achieve a symmetrical nasal cut on both lenses is to reshape the pattern.

Method 1

If the lens is plastic, the frame is heated and reshaped. Then either the frame is traced to create an electronic pattern or a new pattern is made for the shape.

Method 2

The frame's existing pattern is modified for a nasal cut by filing. If the nasal cut is extreme, the lenses are edged somewhat larger to take up slack in the rim. Any time a change in eyesize is made, decentration must be recalculated.

Example 10-1

The frame to be used has an A dimension of 50 and a DBL of 18. The wearer has a 65-mm PD. If the lenses are edged to a 51-mm eyesize, what is the change in the amount of decentration required?

Solution

With a 50-mm eyesize, the decentration per eye is as follows:

$$\frac{50 + 18 - 65}{2} = 1.5 \text{ mm}$$

However, if the lenses are edged to a 51-mm eyesize to allow for a nasal cut, decentration per lens is as follows:

$$\frac{51 + 18 - 65}{2} = 2 \text{ mm}$$

or 2 mm per lens.

Method 3

The lenses are edged slightly large using the normal pattern and the nasal cut is done on the hand edger. The practitioner determines whether enough lens stock has been removed by comparison of the lens to the frame and the paired lens. When results are satisfactory, the other lens is hand edged to conform to the new shape.

NASAL ADD

The nasal cut technique just described was used to reshape the lens to better fit a wide nose. The reverse modification is to add more lens area to the inferior nasal portion of the lens shape. The purpose is to achieve a better fit for wearers who have less than the normal amount of nasal flare. Figure 10-22 illustrates how a lens is edged to create a *nasal add*. Results are somewhat less predictable than with the nasal cut from both a cosmetic and fitting viewpoint. If a lens were to be ordered with nasal add, the amount of nasal add also is specified in millimeters. The following are some different methods of producing a nasal add.

Method 1

Best results are obtained by finding a pattern that almost duplicates the desired shape. If an exact pattern cannot be found, a closely related shape can be used and the lenses modified on the hand edger to conform to the shape desired.

Method 2

When only a small amount of add is required, the lenses can be first edged large without compensating the decentration. The lens is then reduced to size on

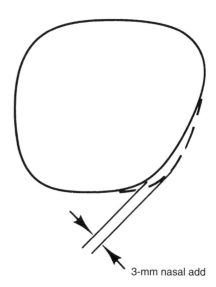

FIGURE **10-22**   If a suitable alternative pattern cannot be located, nasal add is more difficult to achieve by hand. The lens must be edged large, then reduced everywhere except in the nasal-add area.

the hand edger on all sides, skipping only the area of the requested nasal add.

INCREASING THE B DIMENSION OF THE FRAME

When frame styles are large, seldom does a need exist for requesting an increase in the B dimension. Narrow frame styles, though, may prevent effective use of trifocals and progressive addition lenses. By far the best solution is to select an appropriately shaped frame so that modifications are not needed. However, a frame may be fine in every aspect but one: it is too narrow vertically. In other words the B dimension of the frame is too small. If this is the case, the following method details how to increase vertical lens size.

Method 1

The easiest way to increase the B dimension is to find a pattern that is nearly the same as the chosen frame, except with a larger B dimension.

Method 2

To increase the B dimension of the shape, this method is done best using the frame's original pattern[7] and graph paper to perform the following steps:

---

[7]If no pattern is available, it is possible to use the coquille (dummy lens) that comes with the new frame or to trace the inside of the frame's lens opening.

1. Place the pattern on the graph paper and trace the shape. The pattern must be correctly oriented along the 180-degree line and must not be tilted.
2. Slide the pattern downward by the amount the B dimension is to be increased. Take care not to tilt the pattern away from the 180-degree line.
3. Retrace the lower half of the pattern. This vertically increased shape represents the new shape needed.
4. Take a pair of scissors and cut out the new shape.
5. Make a new pattern from this cut-out shape. (See Chapter 3 for instructions on how this is done.)

This method permits the upper half of the lens to fit into the frame exactly as it should, even if a nylon cord–style frame is used.

The method also may be used to decrease the B dimension of a frame. The only difference is that after the original pattern is traced, the pattern is moved upward —instead of downward—by the amount the B dimension is to be decreased. The lower half of the lens is retraced, and this trace becomes the lower edge of the new shape.

Note: Whenever the B dimension of the frame is altered, care must be taken to ensure that any ordered multifocal segment or progressive addition fitting-cross heights have been measured with the new vertical depth taken into account. The new vertical depth is used to determine segment or fitting-cross drop or raise.

Correctional Modifications

After learning how to edge smooth and pin bevel, it is easier to do other things on a hand edger. The following are some possible corrections and lens modifications. For most single vision lenses, it is more costly to modify the lens than to simply replace it. These modifications should be done only for lenses especially worth salvaging.

REMOVING CHIPS

A large chip should not be ground out at the lens surface/lens bevel border with a heavy pin bevel. This creates a double-bevel appearance clearly visible to both wearer and observer. If the lens can be salvaged, the procedure is to steepen the rear bevel angle in the area of the chip. In other words, without moving the bevel apex forward, the rear bevel surface is smoothed in the chip area until it disappears. This area must be approached gradually and the bevel angle changed gradually from either side of the chip. This ensures that the bevel still looks normal. (In extreme cases, duplication of this bevel shape change on the other lens may be necessary to maintain prescription symmetry.) Afterwards the lens can be pin beveled lightly. This

will work only for V-beveled lenses, not for lenses with hidden bevels.

SALVAGING AN OFF-AXIS LENS

After a lens is mounted in a plastic frame it is determined that the axis of the cylinder is off. If the lens shape is rounded, it may be possible to twist the lens slightly with lens rotating pliers without disturbing the appearance of the frame.

Shapes having distinct corners do not allow a lens that has actually been edged off axis to be twisted much. Rotated corners cause unusual humping. The best policy is to replace the lenses. Unless the lens pair is very expensive, replacement may be cheaper. Spending the additional time may not yield results that are successful anyway. However, an attempted correction should be conducted as follows:

1. Trace the lens on a piece of paper as it would appear were the axis correct (Figure 10-23, *A* and *B*).
2. Turn the lens on the tracing to the correct axis (Figure 10-23, *C*).
3. Note the areas of the lens that are outside the tracing and mark them, taking into consideration the overall lens shape (Figure 10-23, *D*).
4. Remove the marked areas by hand edging them away.

If the integrity of the lens shape is restored and the lens still fits snugly in the frame, it may be used. With experience, it will no longer be necessary to trace the lens out on a piece of paper.

This practice is limited to plastic frames. Metal frames do not have the elasticity required.

CORRECTING FOR UNWANTED VERTICAL PRISM

When a high-powered pair of lenses is edged, a small amount of error in vertical positioning can induce vertical prism. Assuming that the prescription is for a plastic frame, it may be possible to hand edge the lenses as follows to reduce the unwanted vertical prism to zero:

1. Remove the lenses from the frame and respot on their MRPs.
2. Hold the lenses front to front[8] so that their shapes exactly overlap each other. Take care to keep the lenses from touching each other so that they are not scratched. With lenses so aligned, as in Figure 10-24, *A*, the spotted MRPs will be seen one above the other. (If both lens meter spots and lens shapes overlap

---

[8]Lenses are held front to front to prevent parallax. When lenses are held back to back, it is more difficult to determine when the marks are truly aligned.

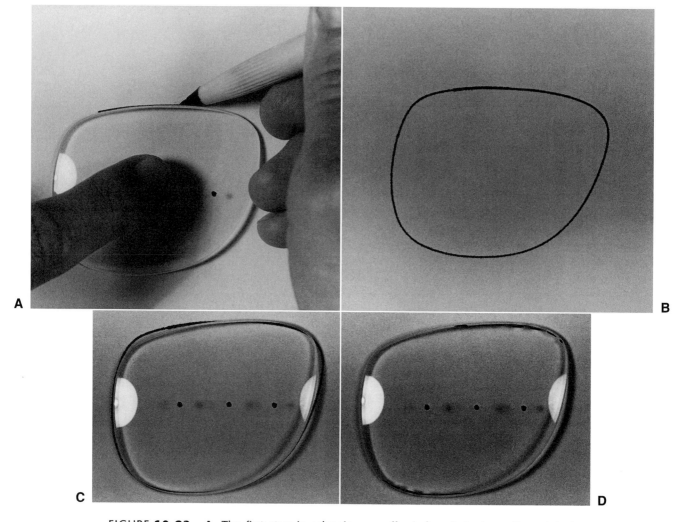

FIGURE **10-23   A**, The first step in salvaging an off-axis lens is to trace the original shape. **B**, Once the shape has been traced, a better idea of where to modify the lens is possible. **C**, The lens is placed on the tracing and the 180-degree cutting line oriented until perfectly horizontal. The lens will be "trimmed" wherever the traced line shows through the lens. The areas to be removed should be outlined with a non–water-soluble pen. **D**, Once marked, the indicated areas of the lens can be removed by hand edging. The lens then fits into the frame without causing the frame to hump up or be distorted.

exactly, then the measured imbalance was due to a frame irregularity. The lenses are not the problem.)

3. Slide one lens up or down until the two MRPs overlap, as in Figure 10-24, *B*.
4. Remove extra lens material that extends above and below[9] the areas of overlap, as marked in Figure 10-24, *C*.

---

[9]Simply removing extra lens material from the top or bottom of one lens eliminates the lensmeter-measured imbalance because the lower rim will shrink up around the lens and allow the frame to drop on that side. However, if the glasses were turned upside-down and measured for vertical imbalance, the distances from the often thicker upper rim will have remained unchanged. Part or all of the unwanted vertical prism may still remain. Because the upper rim is more of a reference for frame straightness on the face, this measure is more definitive.

The total B dimension reduction will equal the amount that the two MRPs were separated initially. If edging away the overhanging material reduces the overall B dimension too much, then the lenses must be remade.

Edge Polishing

The term *edge polishing* can have different definitions, depending upon the material being described.

EDGE POLISHING GLASS LENSES

In relation to glass lenses, *edge polishing* refers to the edge-smoothing process carried out on a fine or extra-

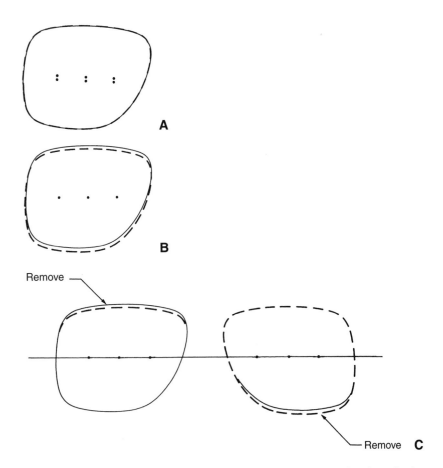

FIGURE **10-24** **A**, This lens pair has been edged, then respotted. When the lenses are held "front-to-front," the dots should exactly overlap one another. If they do not, vertical prism will be manifested in the mounted prescription. **B**, To salvage a lens pair with manifested vertical prism, the result must be an overlapping set of lensmeter dots. By sliding one lens up until an overlap is achieved, it is now possible to visualize which lens area must be "trimmed" away. The left lens is represented by dotted lines, the right by a solid line. **C**, By removing the upper portion of the wearer's right lens and the lower portion of the left, the B dimension of each lens is reduced equally. The amount of material to be removed from each lens equals the amount of separation between the two sets of dots, as first noted in **A**.

fine grit wheel. This can be produced in an edger with an extra-fine grit wheel or by hand edging. The hand edging was described previously in this chapter (see section on Edge Smoothing). This process is not edge polishing but is generally the highest degree of polish that glass lens edgers will allow. This method permits further increase in edge gloss on glass lenses by buffing the edges with a rotating drum tool while using the same type of polishing compound as for lens surfacing. This proves extremely time consuming and is currently neither cost effective nor in demand.

EDGE POLISHING PLASTIC LENSES

When speaking of plastic CR-39 lenses, people may use the term *edge polishing* to refer to edge smoothing or to

indicate that the edges have truly been brought to a high degree of luster.

Polishing on the Edger

The easiest method for edge polishing of plastic lenses is use of an edger with "polishing" capability. But as mentioned earlier, the amount of polish on the finished lens edge may vary. Newer edgers give excellent results for plastic lenses and yield a high luster edge.

Polishing with a Rag Wheel

A second method does not require a grooved wheel. Initially the edge is buffed on a rag wheel with a white buffing compound. Figure 10-25 illustrates this procedure. (If the edges are especially rough or heavily frosted, hold the lens edge against the side surface of the rag

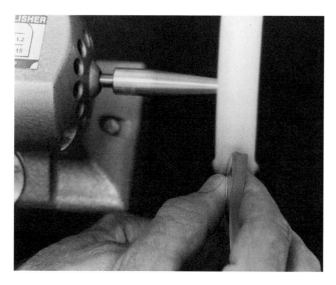

FIGURE **10-25** Using buffing compound on a rag wheel can help ensure a smooth luster on plastic lens edges.

wheel for a preliminary first buff.) A hand buffing may tend to round the bevel apex. To restore a distinct bevel apex the *front* bevel surface is smoothed on an extra-fine hand-edger wheel.

Polishing on a Drum Tool

A third method works only for rimless. This method makes use of a flat rotating drum tool. The felt surface of the tool is prepared with a bar of white polishing compound. The edge surface is then pressed against the rotating tool and a polished edge achieved in approximately 2 minutes. The same unit that was used to facet lens edges also may be used for edge polishing. This unit works like a drum tool but uses liquid lens polishing compound.

Automatic Polishing Machine

Another edge polishing method uses an automatic polishing machine. The lens is not deblocked after edging but is mounted in the unit on its finishing block.

EDGE POLISHING POLYCARBONATE LENSES

Some edge glazes for polycarbonate give a finished appearance. Hand or in-edger polishing may still be the method of choice.

A lighter pressure on the buffing wheel is used to hand polish polycarbonate. Too much pressure results in heat buildup that causes the edge to have a dull appearance instead of a luster. Polycarbonates also can be wet polished like regular plastic lenses.

EDGE POLISHING HIGH-INDEX PLASTIC LENSES

Like polycarbonate, high-index plastic lenses require lighter pressure when being edge polished. Some high-index plastic lenses are sensitive to heat buildup and dull instead of polish when put under too much pressure during edge polishing.

EDGE POLISHING ANTIREFLECTION-COATED LENSES

Some lenses are edged first and then AR-coated. With these, edge polishing should be done before the lens has been AR-coated so that the edges will be coated, too. Many finished single vision lenses come with an AR coating already on the lens. If AR-coated lenses are not edge polished in the edger but polished by hand, they should be wet polished using a liquid lens-polishing compound.

Cleaning Lenses

After the lenses have been deblocked and hand edged, they are almost ready for tinting, coating, drilling, grooving, or hardening. Before further processing, they must be cleaned well and inspected for visible flaws.

GLASS LENS CLEANING

If any non–water-soluble markings are on the lens and must be removed, a solvent such as acetone or alcohol is used on the lens surface. The lens generally is cleaned with use of a tissue or lint-free soft cloth. When no non–water-soluble marks are present, a solution of detergent or a lens cleaner is effective.

Occasionally after cleaning, a small spot remains on the lens. It can, at times, be difficult to tell whether this spot is a surface imperfection or something sticking to the lens. In such cases the best test device may prove to be an ordinary pencil. The pencil point is hard enough to give a good feel for whether the spot is external, yet soft enough not to scratch a glass lens. If foreign material is stuck to the surface, it may be removed simply by the action of the pencil lead. If the spot will not break free with the pencil point, the pencil is turned around to attempt to erase the spot.

If none of the solutions or methods removes the spot, wet pumice rubbing compound (as is used on wood furniture) may be effective. It only should be used gently to prevent abrading the surface.

PLASTIC LENS CLEANING

Acetone or acetone replacers are used extensively for cleaning CR-39 lenses but should not be allowed to come in contact with plastic frame parts. Detergents also clean plastic lenses well.

By far the most effective cleaning method for glass or plastic is an ultrasonic bath. Major manufacturers of uncut lenses use a series of hot ultrasonic baths with different cleaning agents to achieve an extremely clean surface. Ultrasonic cleaners should not be used for AR-coated lenses.

POLYCARBONATE LENS CLEANING

Polycarbonate lenses are coated to make them more scratch resistant. With conventional lenses, lens coatings are more subject to solvent damage than the actual lenses; however, with polycarbonates, the opposite is true. The exposed bevel will show damage before the coated surface. Because of this, a mild, non-citrus liquid dishwashing detergent is recommended. Most alcohols will work but should be considered only secondarily.

Under no circumstances should methylene chloride, methyl ethyl ketone, any of the ketone family, or acetone be used. Highly volatile chlorinated or aromatic hydrocarbons also must be avoided.[10]

WARPAGE

If a plastic lens is warped, it may fixed by placement of the lens in an oven[11] at 200° F for a minimum of 20 minutes. When an oven is unavailable, the lens may be placed in water near the boiling point for an equal amount of time. However, unless the lens is expensive, replacement may be the best choice, especially because lens coatings may be damaged with high heat.

---

[10]Optical Laboratory Marketing Plan, Gentex, Section 4, Finishing and Glazing, 1980.
[11]These are small ovens made especially for lens laboratories. However, regular ovens also work well.

Proficiency Test Questions

1. For a lens with fairly thick edge and a hand-edged bevel, which of the following indicates how far back from the front lens surface the bevel apex should be located?

   a. $\frac{1}{2}$
   b. $\frac{1}{3}$
   c. $\frac{2}{3}$
   d. $\frac{1}{4}$

2. An extra-fine grit hand edger would be least suited for which of the following?

   a. Removing edge stock
   b. Edge smoothing
   c. Pin beveling

3. Which of the following is the correct sequence of steps in hand edging?

   1. Front pin bevel
   2. Smooth front face of bevel
   3. Smooth rear face of bevel
   4. Rear pin bevel
   5. Apex pin bevel

   a. 2, 3, 4, 1, 5
   b. 4, 1, 5, 2, 3
   c. 4, 1, 2, 3, 5
   d. 5, 4, 1, 2, 3
   e. 3, 2, 1, 4, 5

4. True or False? Traveling as far as possible around the periphery of the lens during hand edging before the lens is lifted from the wheel is advantageous.

5. Which of the following is the accepted apical angle that should be produced during the hand-edging process?

   a. 85 degrees
   b. 90 degrees
   c. 100 degrees
   d. 110 degrees
   e. 115 degrees

6. During the hand-edging process, the lens is held at varying angles to the cutting plane of the wheel. Which two hand-edging operations require holding the lens at nearly the same angle?

   1. Front bevel edge smoothing
   2. Rear bevel edge smoothing
   3. Front pin bevel
   4. Rear pin bevel

   a. 1 + 2
   b. 2 + 3
   c. 3 + 4
   d. 1 + 4
   e. 2 + 4

7. Which of the following factors causes hand-edging cutting speed to increase?

    a. Decreasing speed of rotation of lens
    b. Using a finer grit wheel
    c. Approaching a thicker section of the lens
    d. Decreasing pressure against the wheel
    e. All of the above cause cutting speed to decrease.

8. Which of the following is a true statement about pin beveling?

    a. When pin beveling, slightly more pressure should be applied than when edge smoothing.
    b. The speed of rotation for pin beveling is quicker than for edge smoothing.
    c. When pin beveling is completed, it should be visibly noticeable.

9. True or False? During pin beveling of the back surface of a high-minus lens on a face-type hand edger, the central hub area of the wheel should be used.

10. True or False? The process used to reduce the size of a lens by hand is similar to the edge-smoothing process.

11. Which of the following describes a "nasal cut"?

    a. An injury caused by wearing an acetate nose pad with an improper splay angle
    b. Reshaping a lens so that more lens area is in the inferior nasal part of the lens shape than normal for the shape intended by the frame designer
    c. Reshaping a lens so that less lens area is in the inferior nasal part of the lens shape than normal for the shape intended by the frame designer
    d. Reshaping a lens so that more lens area is in the superior nasal part of the lens shape than normal for the shape intended by the frame designer
    e. Reshaping a lens so that less lens area is in the superior nasal part of the lens shape than normal for the shape intended by the frame designer

12. When inserting a lens with an increased B dimension in a plastic frame, which of the following is true?

    a. The whole eyewire should be heated evenly.
    b. The upper eyewire should be heated more than the lower, as it is generally thicker.
    c. The lower portion of the eyewire is heated more than the upper rim.

13. Salvaging a lens that is too far off axis using lens-twisting pliers may be possible. When simply twisting the lens will not work, correction of the problem may be accomplished by hand edging certain parts of the lens. Which of the following frame types would be feasible with this method?

    a. Cellulose acetate frames (plastic frames that stretch when heated)
    b. Metal frames
    c. Any frame is possible to use in combination with this method.

14. Assume that a lens has been found off axis and an attempt to salvage it is made. If the lens reads as axis 5 and should be axis 180, at which of the following locations would lens stock commonly be removed to correct the problem?

    a. Top edge (left half) and bottom edge (right half)
    b. Top edge (right half) and bottom edge (left half)
    c. Top edge (right half) and bottom edge (right half)
    d. Top edge (left half) and right edge (top half)

15. A lens pair manifests vertical prism. It is determined that the right lens optical center (OC) is 1 mm higher than the left lens OC. Which of the following describes the way in which a practitioner should correct the problem?

    a. Take 0.5 mm off the top of the right lens and 0.5 mm off the bottom of the left lens.
    b. Take 0.5 mm off the top of the left lens and 0.5 mm off the bottom of the right lens.
    c. Take 1 mm off the top of the right lens and 1 mm off the bottom of the left lens.
    d. Take 1 mm off the top of the left lens and 1 mm off the bottom of the right lens.

16. Which statement(s) about AR-coated lenses is (are) true?

    a. In some cases lenses are edge polished before being AR-coated.
    b. In some cases lenses are AR-coated before being edge polished.
    c. Lenses should never be AR-coated until they have been edge polished.
    d. Lenses should never be edge polished until they have been AR-coated.

17. True or False? If a small spot remains on a glass lens after cleaning, an attempt may be made to erase it with a pencil eraser.

18. If a plastic lens is warped, which of the following actions should be taken?

    a. Drop ball test it to see if it will be acceptable.
    b. Put it in an oven at 200° F for a minimum of 20 minutes.
    c. Send the lens on anyway, as warpage in plastic lenses is unimportant.

19. True or False? Acetone is a good choice for cleaning polycarbonate lenses.

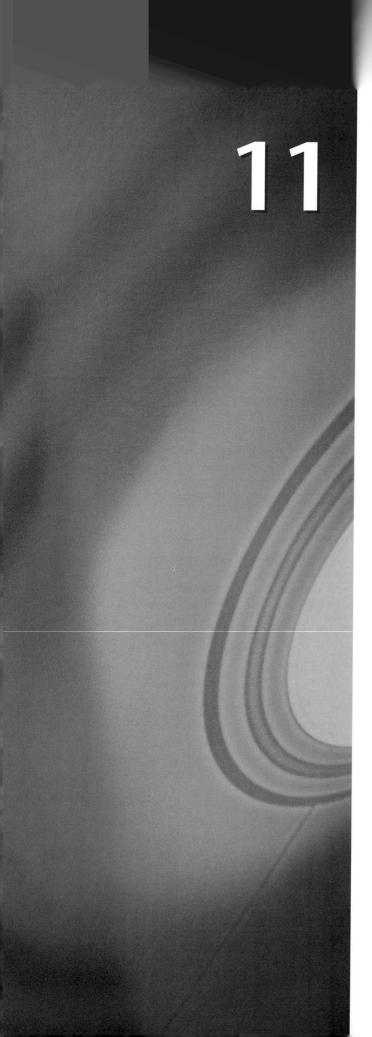

11 Lens Tinting

Ophthalmic lenses may be tinted in the following three main ways:

1. Introducing a coloring substance into the lens material before it becomes a lens
2. Vacuum coating the color onto the surface of the lens in much the same way that antireflection (AR) coatings are applied to lenses
3. Immersing the lens in a liquid dye so that the dye is absorbed into the lens or lens coating

Glass lenses may be tinted with use of only the first two methods. Plastic lenses may be tinted by any of the above methods, but the third method is by far the most common. It is far more versatile and able to be applied in most any optical laboratory setting. This chapter addresses how plastic lenses are tinted by immersion into liquid dye.

How the Process Works

Dyeing plastic lenses is much the same process as dyeing Easter eggs. With eggs a dye tablet or a liquid concentrate is placed in hot water and the eggs dipped in the dye. Lenses are dyed in similar manner. Only with lenses the dye is quality controlled, the temperature of the liquid is much hotter, and care is taken to ensure the lenses are exceptionally clean.

TINT UNIT

In the early days of lens tinting, labs used a variety of methods for heating the lens dye. One of the more common methods was to use kitchen items such as Crock-Pots and deep fryers. Although perhaps still used in some places, such methods have given way to commercially available tint units. These units, sometime called *base units*, allow temperature to be regulated. They are made so that temperature will not change suddenly. A typical unit consists of stainless steel pans called *tint tanks* that are suspended in a bath of heat transfer fluid. Each tank has a different dye and each tank has a lid (Figure 11-1).

Some tint units do not use heat transfer fluid but instead use dry heat or infrared heat. Certain units reportedly are able to reach full operating temperatures within 10 minutes, reduce odors by eliminating heat transfer fluid, and use less electricity.[1] Units that do not use heat transfer fluid also may be able to maintain a stable dye temperature more easily, especially when combined with an automatic stirring device.[2]

DYES

All colors may be produced by mixing primary colors. Mixing blue and yellow makes green. Mixing yellow and red makes orange. Mixing red and blue makes purple.

[1]Underwood W: What's new in lens tinting, *Eyecare Technology* Jan/Feb 1995, p 47.
[2]*BPI Catalog*, Miami, 1999, BPI Incorporated, p 68.

Lens dyes work the same way. Theoretically it therefore would be possible to have only three primary dye colors. A plastic lens would be dipped in first one dye, then in another, to produce any desired color. In practice this is unrealistic. Consequently commercially available dyes come in a large variety of colors. This allows much better color consistency. The availability of colors is ever changing with changing fashion demands.

Dyes are made for different colors. Some dyes are engineered specifically for certain lens materials. Some dyes are made to block certain wavelengths of light; and some dyes are custom made for certain sports. Almost innumerable possibilities exist.

Dyes come as a liquid concentrate in bottles, as a powder, or in tablet form. Many prefer to purchase dyes in single-use bottles or as tablets with just enough concentrate for one tank of dye.

Preparing the Dye

Beginning with a clean tank is important when mixing a batch of dye. Any residue from a previous dye will contaminate the new dye. Any unwanted oil or detergent also will affect the dye.

Distilled or deionized water is used. Tap water or even spring water can present problems. The mineral content of the water binds with some of the dyes in the mixture. Because the minerals do not bind with all of the elements within the dye evenly, the use of anything but distilled or deionized water may cause the color of

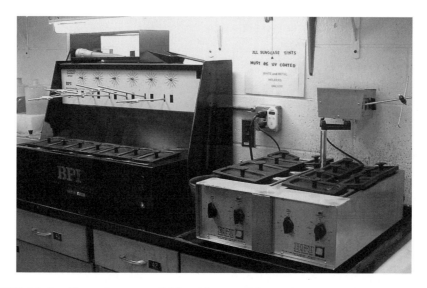

FIGURE **11-1** Tint units are available with a variable number of tint tanks.

the dyed lens to differ from what was intended. And, because water must be added continually to the tank because of evaporation, minerals are introduced continually over time, which bind more of the dye and cause the color to continue to shift.

If tap water is going to be used anyway, it should be drawn the night before and allowed to stand. This removes the chlorine and allows any sediment to settle that may be in the water.[3]

The following is the procedure used to start a new batch of dye.

1. To start a new batch of dye, fill the tank about half full and bring the temperature to 140° F. Having the water too hot when the concentrate is added prevents the new dye from completely dissolving.
2. Shake the bottle well (at least 30 seconds) before adding it to the water.
3. Pour the dye from the bottle into the tank (Figure 11-2).
4. Pour a little water into the bottle, shake the bottle, and pour the rest into the tank. The bottle should be rinsed in this manner three times. The different

pigments in the dye settle to different levels. Failure to get all the tint residue from the bottle is not the same as failure to squeeze the toothpaste tube to get out the last little bit. With tint, not getting all the residue results in obtaining a different color than that anticipated.
5. Fill the tank with distilled water.

Maintaining the Dye

The dye should be stirred when first mixed and restirred occasionally as it heats. The stirring rod should be rinsed each time it is used (Figure 11-3). Once the dye is mixed and heated, it should be stirred periodically to maintain consistency throughout. Some tint units come with magnetic stirrers, which reduce the human element of forgetfulness or neglect.

Because the dye is kept close to the boiling point when dyeing lenses, continual evaporation occurs. Distilled water should be added regularly (Figure 11-4). Waiting too long to add water causes the tank to boil down and leave hardened dye residue on the inner walls of the tank. This affects color and makes it necessary to spend time scrubbing them clean.

---

[3]*The practical guide to coloring all types of plastic lenses*, Miami, 1996, BPI Incorporated, pp 2-3.

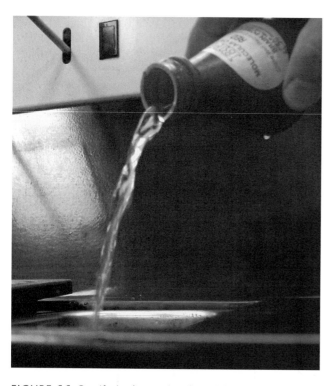

FIGURE **11-2** If single-use bottles of liquid concentrate are used, the dye is poured into a half-full tank of water that has only been heated to 140° F.

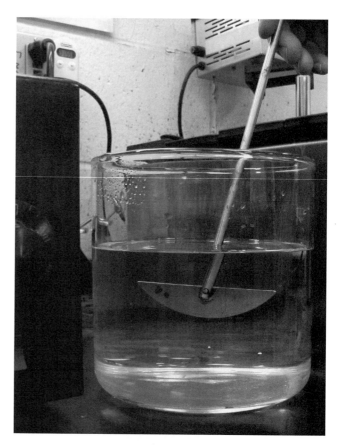

FIGURE **11-3** A stainless-steel stirring rod needs to be rinsed between uses for the sake of cleanliness and to prevent dye contamination.

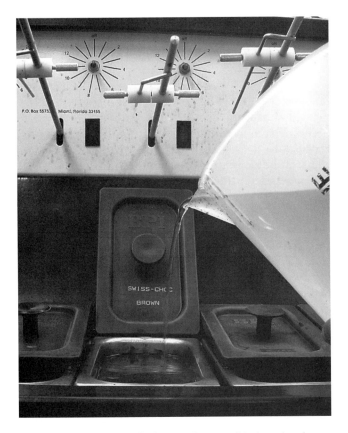

FIGURE 11-4 If distilled water is not added to the dye as it evaporates, the dye will boil down and leave a hardened residue on the walls of the tank.

When a batch of dye is used frequently, the lenses absorb color pigments and remove them from the bath. Except for primary colors, not all pigments may be absorbed equally. After the dye has been used for a while, this leads to a color shift in the lenses being dyed.

Life Span of the Dye

The life of the dye[4] depends upon three things, in the following order:

1. How long has the dye been mixed with water?
2. How hot has the dye temperature been?
3. How many lenses have been tinted?

Even if a dye has never been used it may not be useful if it has been mixed and left in a hot tint unit for a long period of time.

Dye life depends on dye color, too. The dyes that have the shortest life are the grays, browns, and greens. Those that last the longest are the blues, pinks, and yellows.

Tinting Temperatures

Lenses dye best if the dye is kept at the temperature recommended for that particular material. Keeping the tint temperature too low considerably increases the needed time the lens must be in the tint bat. Lens manufacturers are best able to recommend dye temperatures for their own lens materials.

Before the tint unit is first turned on, the dye should be stirred thoroughly. It should not be turned immediately to the full-recommended temperature for the lens material to be dyed. Instead it is better to heat the dye gradually. This allows the individual components within the dye to dissolve well and go into solution. Turning the temperature to 140° F and allowing it to stabilize at that temperature first is advisable. The lids may be left on the tanks while the dye heats up to this temperature and stabilizes.

Next the lids are either fully or partially removed from the tint tanks and the temperature turned up in 10° increments until it reaches 200° to 210° F. Removing or partially removing the lids lessens the chance of boil-over. A kitchen pot with the lid on boils over more easily than one without the lid. Partially removing the lids, instead of full removal, reduces evaporation. Tint temperatures are not far below the boiling point for water (212° F). Having dye tanks boil over gets dye from one dye tank in other dye tanks, down in the heat transfer fluid, over the side of the unit, on the countertop, and maybe even on the floor.

Tint units have temperature dials that can be used to set approximate dye temperature. However, the actual temperature of the dye should be measured directly with a high-quality laboratory thermometer (Figure 11-5).

LENS-CURING FACTOR

The first step in achieving a good, even tint takes place before the order begins its journey through the laboratory. The way that a lens absorbs dye depends upon how that plastic lens was molded and cured. Plastic lenses are made from liquid resin and are cast molded to shape. The process of going from the liquid to the solid state is called *curing*. If a lens is cured slowly, the so-called "lattice structure" of the lens is more impervious to the dye. Dye manufacturers refer to this type of lens as a *hard* lens.[5] Slowly cured, "hard" lenses take a longer time to absorb the dye. Lenses that are cured rapidly are said to have a more open lattice structure. These lenses take on the dye more rapidly.

Because of the differences in curing times, a lens pair with one lens from one manufacturer and the

[4]*The practical guide to coloring all types of plastic lenses,* Miami, 1996, BPI Incorporated, p 2.

[5]*BPI Catalog,* Miami, 1999, BPI Incorporated, p 166.

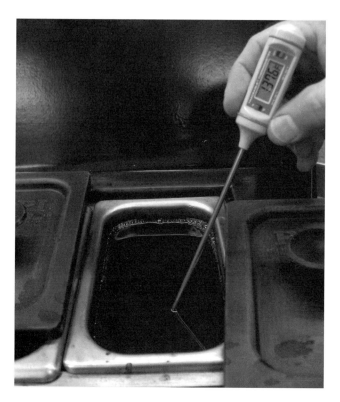

FIGURE **11-5**   Even though the dial on a tint unit is marked with temperature, the actual temperature of the bath should be measured with a high-quality laboratory thermometer.

second lens from another may look different from one another once they are dyed. This may happen even though both lenses were treated exactly the same and left in the same dye for the same length of time. One lens may be darker than the other. Or one lens may take on certain pigments from the dye more rapidly than another lens, which results in slightly different lens colors. Although it is possible to correct for these differences by hand, it will be easier to begin with lenses that are matched by manufacturer (and ideally by purchase date). Using two lenses from two different manufacturers will not make as much difference with light tints as it will for dark tints.

Surfaced Versus Stock Lenses

A lens that is custom surfaced to power is made from a thicker semi-finished lens blank. This lens has been cured differently than a stock lens cast to power. Lenses that are either both surfaced or both pulled from stock produce a better match when tinted than a lens pair where one was a surfaced lens and the other a stock lens.

PREPARING THE LENS FOR TINTING

To get a good quality, even tint, certain preparatory steps must be carried out before actually tinting the lens. Lenses must be thoroughly clean. To remove lensmeter ink, progressive lens identification or layout marks, or remains of grease pencil markings, the lens should be cleaned with alcohol or acetone (or an acetone replacer). (Acetone should not be used on polycarbonate lenses because the acetone will attack the exposed, uncoated edges of the polycarbonate material.) Any grease or oil that remains on the lens will block the transfer of dye and cause a splotchy appearance.

Lens Conditioner

Next, lens conditioner is used to clean the lens. Lens conditioner—known variously as the trade products *Lens Prep* (BPI, Inc., Miami) and *Color Primer* (Seegreen, Bellingham, Wash.)—is a specially formulated solution that "ionizes the lens positively with a special coating that allows it to exhibit a charged interface opposite to that of the tint. This potential difference attracts the tint ions to the lens surface for fast color absorption."[6] The following reminders should be borne in mind when lens conditioner is used:

- Using too much lens conditioner causes streaking because of unevenness of charge.
- The lens should not be rinsed with water or wiped dry after cleaning it with the lens conditioner or it will not work as intended.
- The lens conditioner is changed every 3 or 4 days, depending upon how often it is used. Lens conditioner is not meant to last until it all evaporates.
- Lens conditioner will work without being heated, but it works better if placed in a tint tank and the tank placed in the tint unit.

The lens is mounted in a lens holder that touches only the edges of the lens (Figure 11-6). The lens holder should not be forced down tight on the lens but just enough to keep the lens from moving. Pressure on the lens at tinting temperatures causes the lens to warp. The holder also must be clean so as not to contaminate the dyes.

TINTING THE LENS

The lens is lowered *slowly* into the appropriate lens tint tank. With the tint temperature just below the boiling point, considerable surface tension is present. Breaking the surface tension too rapidly may cause the tint to boil over.

---

[6]*BPI Catalog*, Miami, 1999, BPI Incorporated, p 164.

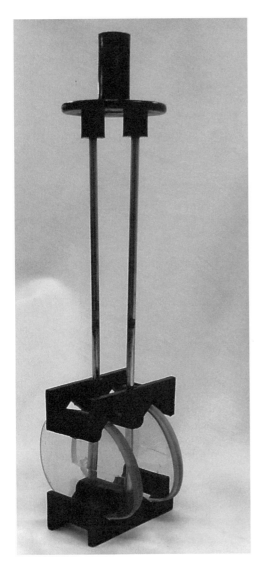

FIGURE **11-6** Lenses should be placed in a lens holder without pressure. Some laboratory managers recommend color coding lens holders so that the same holder is used for the same tint color. This helps prevent the possibility of cross-contamination of colors.

The time that it will take to achieve the darkness required varies and depends on the lens itself and the age and temperature of the dye. When dyes are appropriately strong and heat sufficiently high, normal tinting times range from 5 seconds to 8 minutes. However certain lens material types or lens coatings may increase some tint times considerably. Under less than ideal conditions, times will be increased.

After the lens is removed from the tint, it is rinsed under a faucet in cool tap water. If a sink is not handy, the lens is rinsed in a container of water. The lens is wiped dry with a soft cloth or tissue to prevent water spotting.

Ensuring Accuracy of Transmission and Color

After the lens has been dyed, it is checked to see if it is absorbing the correct amount of light. It is also checked to make sure the color of the finished lens matches the color that was ordered.

MEASURING LENS TRANSMISSION

Transmission can be determined by either visually comparing how one lens looks against a standard sample lens, or by using a *photometer* (transmission gauge) to measure percent transmission. A full *spectrophotometer* measures the transmission of each wavelength of light across the spectrum. A scientific quality spectrophotometer is considerably more than is needed for lens tinting purposes and would be prohibitively expensive. A basic photometer used for this purpose gives an overall percent transmission for visible light and an ultraviolet (UV) percent transmission (Figure 11-7). The visible portion of the spectrum is averaged across the visible color wavelengths. Unfortunately *measured* percent transmission for equally dyed lenses varies, depending upon the power of the lens. Because plus and minus lenses converge and diverge light rays by varying amounts, percent transmission is artificially high or low compared with a plano lens having the same dyed appearance.

Transmission gauges that read the lens and produce a spectral transmission curve are also used in ophthalmic practices. The Humphrey Lens Analyzer (an automated lensmeter) (Zeiss Humphrey Systems, Dublin, Calif.) has an option that reads lens transmission and projects it on the screen of the instrument. Printing out the transmission curve is also possible (Figure 11-8).

For tinting purposes, the two readings that are most important are the percent transmission of the UV light passing through the lens and the overall percent of visible light transmitted. The UV portion is needed to ensure that adequate protection from invisible wavelengths below 400 nm is present.

CHECKING LENS COLOR ACCURACY

The best way to check color accuracy is to visually compare it to a sample lens. Having a sample lens on hand that may be held side-by-side with the newly tinted lens shows how close the color and darkness is to what was ordered. Tint samples will fade over time. In time the lens will become slightly lighter and, perhaps more importantly, will change somewhat in color. If the lens is continually exposed to sunlight or fluorescent light the lens will last from 12 to 18 months before it begins

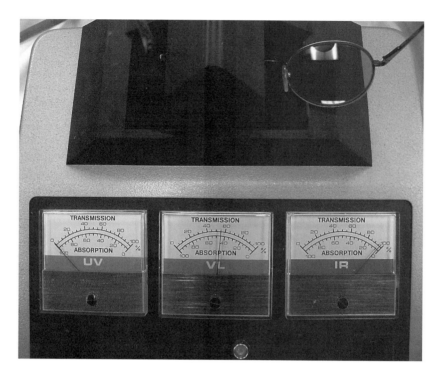

FIGURE **11-7** A basic photometer gives a quantifiable transmission of tinted lenses. This unit shows three areas of transmission. The dial on the left shows that the lens is transmitting no ultraviolet (UV) light. The center dial shows 55% transmission of visible light. This is the averaged percent transmission for visible light. (To see the actual transmission across the visible spectrum for this brown lens, see Figure 11-8.) The dial on the right shows that the lens is transmitting almost all infrared (IR) in the region measured.

to lighten or change in color. If kept in a drawer, they may last up to 5 years before changing.[7]

Fading happens to single lenses in the laboratory or in the dispensary. This can become a source of confusion and misunderstanding when the patient's lens does not match the sample lens in the dispensary.

In examination of a lens for trueness of color, the type of lighting used is important. Artificial indoor light such as fluorescent or incandescent lighting does not give an accurate impression because these light sources do not contain the same spectral balance of colors as does sunlight. Daylight-type bulbs are made to more accurately mimic sunlight. One possibility is to simply replace regular fluorescent bulbs with daylight-type bulbs in the tinting area.

Light Boxes

A convenient device to aide in the comparison of lens colors is a light box. This is a box with a white, translucent piece of plastic on top and a full spectrum bulb inside. The white, illuminated background is the

perfect backdrop for comparing two lens colors (Figure 11-9).

BALANCING LENS COLOR

Sometimes a lens comes out of the dye and is not the exact color expected. If this happens it is still possible to correct the lens color.

By using only three colors, creation of any color is theoretically possible. So if the color is not exactly what it should be, by adding a particular color the overall color may be shifted in the desired direction. For example, if the colors blue and yellow make green, how can a green lens that is too yellowish be corrected? The solution is to dip the yellowish-green lens in the blue dye. This counterbalances the yellowish effect and results in a purer green. Table 11-1 provides a color-correction chart.

MATCHING AN EXISTING LENS COLOR

Sometimes a laboratory is asked to replace one lens, matching the tint of the new lens to that of the original. The first step is to choose the dye that is thought to be

---

[7]Lamperelli K: To dye for: a guide to tints and tinting, *Eyewear* Oct 1998, p 31.

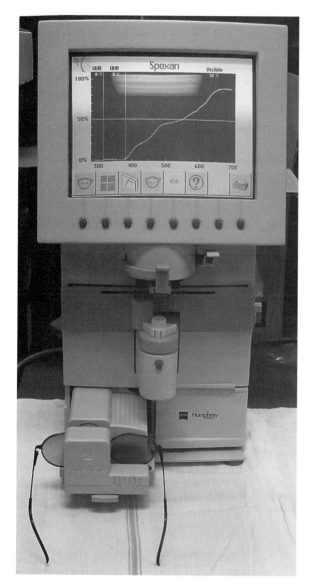

FIGURE **11-8**   The Humphrey Lens Analyzer, an automated lensmeter, has a function that shows and prints a transmission curve of the lens. That transmission curve includes the visible spectrum and ultraviolet region. This lens shows a transmission curve fairly typical for a brown plastic lens.

the closest match. After dyeing the new lens, it may be altered in hue. To change the hue, the color correction chart shown in Table 11-1 can be used.

Forcing a Match

When only one lens in a wearer's old pair of eyeglasses is being replaced, it is sometimes nearly impossible to match the old lens. In an attempt to force a match, sometimes the color is bleached from the wearer's remaining lens and the remaining lens redyed with the new lens.

The risk involved is twofold. The first is that the lenses still may not match because of age and manufacturer differences. The second risk is wearer dissatisfaction. The lenses may match each other but not be a close enough match to the original to satisfy the wearer. Explaining the difficulties and risks to the wearer or to the account before proceeding may be the safer strategy.

REMOVING TINT WITH NEUTRALIZER

To remove color from a previously tinted lens, the lens may be placed in a solution of lens *neutralizer.* Neutralizer works by bleaching some tints and drawing others back out of the lens and into the neutralizer.

Neutralizer can be topped off with more neutralizer as it evaporates. It can continue to be used until it becomes too slow or until it takes on color from bleached lenses and will not clear.

Neutralizer also can be used to lighten the tint of a lens. The lens is left in the neutralizer until it lightens to the desired transmission, then the lens is removed and rinsed clean. For polycarbonate lenses a neutralizer labeled specifically for polycarbonate or a water-based neutralizer must be used.

TINTING AND MATCHING UNCUTS

Whenever possible a lens should be dyed *after* it has been edged, not before. By dyeing the lens after edging, the edges of the lens will be dyed. Dyeing the lens as an uncut, before edging, results in lighter lens edges because the tint does not soak completely into the whole lens thickness.

Yet in certain circumstances a lens is dyed before edging, particularly if a large laboratory is responding to a request from a smaller laboratory. One of these requests may be to match an old lens color from a previously edged lens, then send the new, matched lens to the smaller laboratory for edging.

If a lens is dyed as an uncut, it becomes more difficult to judge a good match because the size of the areas of comparison are unequal. To make the match easier a small black velvet cloth with a hole in the center is used. The size of the hole should be close to the size of the edged lens. Placing the cloth over the uncut lens may make comparison of the two lenses easier and increase the possibility of a more accurate match.[8]

---

[8]Mecteau R: *How to assure maximum quality and productivity in finishing,* Optical Laboratories Association Meeting, Nashville, Tenn, Dec 12, 1995.

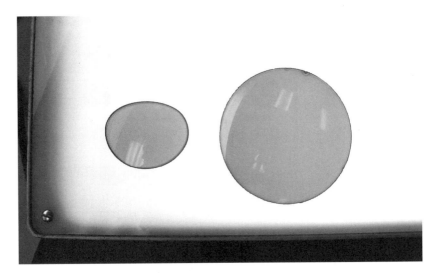

FIGURE **11-9**   A light box is a back-lighted piece of translucent white plastic. It allows easy comparison of two lens colors. The lens on the right is used as the standard sample, against which the newly tinted lens may be compared.

TABLE **11-1** *Color Balancing Table**		
IF THE COLOR IS SUPPOSED TO BE...	BUT THE LENS APPEARS TOO...	THEN TRY TO CORRECT THE PROBLEM BY DIPPING THE LENS IN...
Gray	Red	BPI Red Out
	Blue	Brown
	Green	Pink
	Brown	Blue
	Purple	Yellow
Brown	Red	Gray or blue
	Gray	Yellow
	Purple	Yellow
	Green	First red, then blue
	Blue	First pink, then yellow
Green	Yellow	Blue
	Brown	Blue
	Blue	Brown or yellow
	Gray	Remove the color
Rose	Red	Violet
	Blue	Red
	Brown	Remove the color

From BPI Color Correction Chart, *BPI Catalog*, Miami, 1999, BPI Incorporated, p 172.
*Color balancing recommendations may vary according to dye manufacturer and also according to lens manufacturer, lens material, and lens coating type.

Styles of Tints

SOLIDS

The most common type of lens tint is called a *solid.* A solid is a tint that has the same color and light transmission over the entire lens (Figure 11-10, *A*). This is the easiest tint to produce.

GRADIENT TINTS

Gradients are lenses that vary in transmission over the surface of the lens. A *simple gradient* tint is a lens that has one color but varies in transmission from the top to the bottom of the lens. The lens starts out darker at the top of the lens and gradually lightens toward the bottom (Figure 11-10, *B*). The purpose of a gradient tint is

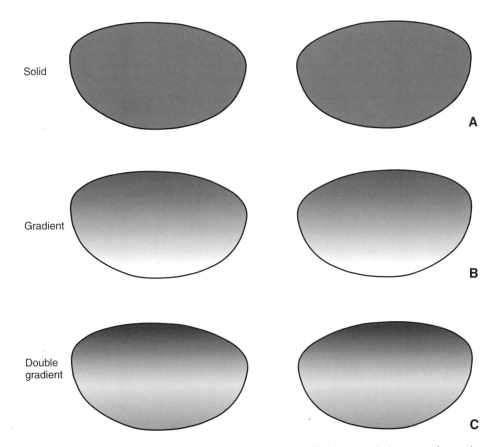

FIGURE **11-10** **A**, A solid tint has the same color and light transmission over the entire lens. **B**, A gradient tint has the same color but is darker at the top of the lens and lightens gradually toward the bottom. **C**, A double gradient usually has two colors, one at the top and a second at the bottom. The color at the top is darkest at the top and fades out toward the middle of the lens. The color at the bottom is most intense at the bottom and lightens toward the middle. An example might be a lens that is blue at the top and pink at the bottom. A triple gradient (not pictured here) is like a double gradient, but with a third, usually light color in the central meridian of the lens.

primarily fashion, although it could be argued that a gradient tint is useful for a pair of eyeglasses in the same way that a windshield with a dark band at the top is useful for driving.

Dyeing a Simple Gradient Lens

To produce a lens with a dark upper half and a clear lower half, the lenses are mounted upside down in the lens holder and the top half immersed in the dye. To achieve a gradual change in transmission, the top half of the lens is dipped in and out of the dye while varying how far into the dye the lens is dipped.

Gradient arms are sold for tint units. These arms mechanically dip the lens in and out of the dye to varying depths (Figure 11-11). With each downward stroke of the gradient arm the lens is lowered deeper into the dye. After the last and deepest stroke in the series, the cycle repeats itself.

A gradient arm does not guarantee a better gradient tint than one done by hand but may save time. Many still prefer to dip the lenses by hand to achieve the effect desired.

Because of the slight pause that the gradient arm makes as it cycles, it is recommended that the tint bath be lowered to between 190° and 200° F. This slows the absorption speed and helps produce a more gradual gradient line instead of a harsh one.

Some gradient arms have a separate setting that allows a solid lens to be lowered into the dye, left there for a predetermined length of time, then automatically lifted from the dye.

Achieving a Level Gradient Line

A gradient should be horizontally straight after the lenses are mounted in the frame. To be sure the gradient is horizontal and not tilted (Figure 11-12),

CHAPTER 11 LENS TINTING

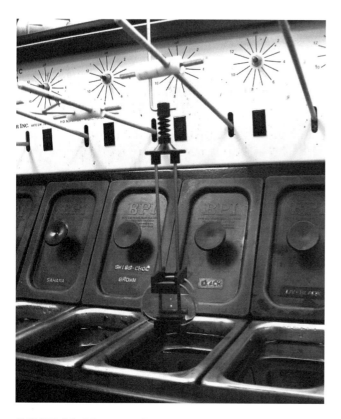

FIGURE **11-11** A gradient arm dips the lens in and out of the dye at varying depths to produce a gradient transmission lens. Note the springlike design at the top of the lens holder. This lens holder, designed especially for use with gradient lenses, is meant to allow the lens to oscillate some as the gradient arm moves, resulting in a more gradual change in transmission over the surface of the lens.

the lenses must be positioned in the holder so that their 180-degree mounting line is exactly horizontal. If the lens has a flat-top bifocal, the flat-top lines give a ready reference, as shown in Figure 11-13. Frames in which the top rim of the frame is straight and level are easiest. However, frames that have perfectly round lenses are hardest (especially if the prescription includes a cylinder component).

One way to ensure straightness of the gradient line is to mount the untinted lenses in the frame correctly and then spot them both on the 180-degree line (Figure 11-14). The edges of the lens are marked along the 180-degree line (Figure 11-15), and the top of the lens is marked with a T (Figure 11-16). Next the apex of the lens bevel is filed lightly on the 180-degree line with a narrow file (Figure 11-17). This mark remains on the lens but is hidden within the frame's groove. This mark works well unless the lenses are rimless.

In fact, the practice of marking the 180-degree line for round frames is a good idea for any round frame where rotation of the lenses may cause optical problems for the wearer. The marks should be barely visible to the wearer. This way the wearer can monitor the position of the lenses and have any problem corrected so that the cylinder axis will remain positioned where it should be.

Creating a Smooth Gradient

When a gradient lens is ordered, it should specify color and transmission(s). If only one transmission is given, this is the transmission of the upper portion. The upper third of the edged gradient lens should have the darkest specified transmission for the lens. The lower third of the lens should be very light or even clear. This lower transmission may or may not be specified in the order. The middle third of the lens should transition evenly between the top and bottom thirds.

If a distinct border appears between the upper and lower sections of a gradient lens with little or no transition, the gradient change is too harsh. This can happen from faulty technique, cleaning solvent still on the lens, or a failure to use lens conditioner. (It also can happen when a gradient arm is used with the dye too hot, as described earlier.)

Removal of harshness from the line and creation of a smoother gradient may not rely on totally bleaching the lenses in lens neutralizer and starting all over again. With the lenses right side up so that the light areas of the lenses are at the bottom, they are dipped part way into the neutralizer until the fade is more appropriate.

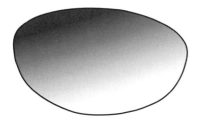
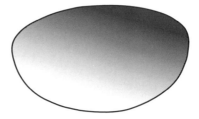

FIGURE **11-12** If lenses are not oriented along the 180-degree meridian when placed in the lens holder, the gradient lines will not be horizontal. These lenses were tipped when placed in the lens holder.

Sometimes it may work better to dip the whole lens in and out of the neutralizer.

DOUBLE GRADIENTS

A gradient lens may be created with one color on the top and another color on the bottom. These two colors fade into one another. This type of lens is called a *double gradient* (see Figure 11-10, *C*). An example of a double gradient would be a lens with a light blue upper gradient area that gives a cosmetic eye-shadow–like appearance to the lid area of the eye combined with a rose-colored lower half that somewhat masks dark circles under the eyes.

To produce a double gradient lens, an upper gradient is created in just the top half of the lens. The bottom half is left clear. Then the lenses are turned over in the lens holder and the gradient process repeated for the lower half in the second color. The second color starts dark at the bottom and fades to the center in "reverse" gradient fashion.

TRIPLE GRADIENTS

Although seldom called for, production of a triple gradient lens is possible. Such a lens has one gradient color in the upper half, a second reverse gradient in the lower half, and a third color in the center.

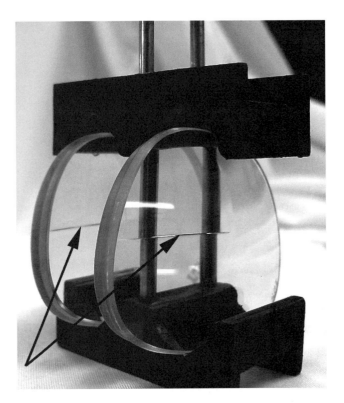

FIGURE **11-13** Flat-top bifocals provide a ready reference for the location of the 180-degree line during tinting of gradient lenses. Remember that the bifocal will be upside down, because the top of the lens must go into the tint first. The top gets more of the tint than the bottom.

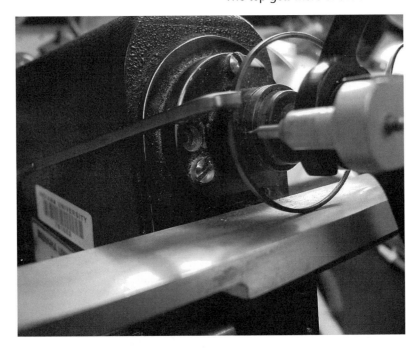

FIGURE **11-14** To ensure a straight gradient line on lens shapes that are either round or close to a round shape, begin by spotting the 180-degree line with the lenses still in the frame. When cylinder is present, the lenses may be placed in the lensmeter without the frame, as long as it is clear which side of the lens is nasal and which is temporal.

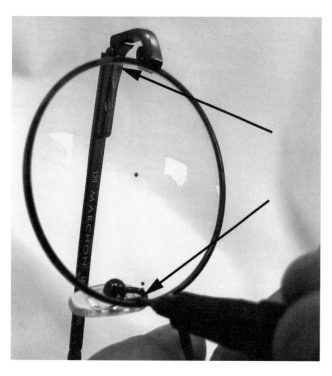

FIGURE **11-15**   The process of making sure a gradient line will be straight began in Figure 11-14. To continue the process, use the lensmeter dots as a guide and mark the 180-degree line at the edge of the lenses.

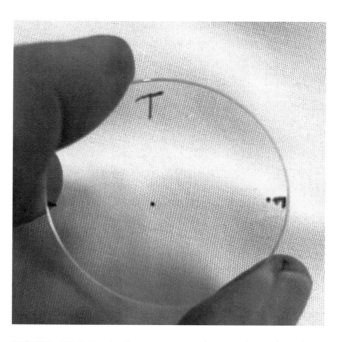

FIGURE **11-16**   In the sequence of preparing a lens for a gradient tint, the top of the lens should be marked so that the lens will not be turned accidentally upside down when placed in the lens holder.

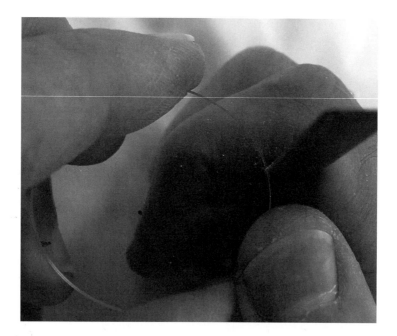

FIGURE **11-17**   With a rimmed frame a small file mark can be made at the edges of the lens along the 180-degree line. (Such marks are inappropriate for rimless lenses.) Once a small file mark is made at each edge, the three lensmeter dots and the "T" are removed. Then the lenses are placed upside down in the lens holder for gradient tinting with the file marks at the horizontal meridian.

This may be created in two ways. The first way is to overlap the upper and lower colors. The third center color will be the result of a combination of upper and lower colors.

The second and most common way to produce a triple gradient is to start with the center color as a solid. The upper and lower colors might be added on top of the solid if they are able to mask it sufficiently. If not, the center color is done as a solid, and then neutralized out of first the top, then the bottom of the lens. The top and bottom gradient colors may then be added without being influenced by the center color.

Ultraviolet Dyeing

Sunglass lens tints that are sufficiently dark may reduce the transmission of visible light, make the eyes more comfortable on bright days, and preserve the eye's ability to fully and rapidly adapt to dark at night.[9] Ultraviolet (UV) radiation is a shorter wavelength light that is not visible but nevertheless can adversely affect the eye. Long-term, low-dose exposure to UV light can increase the incidence of cataracts.[10] UV radiation is present in normal sunlight. The closer to the equator or the higher in altitude one is, the greater the exposure to UV radiation. For this reason those who are exposed to sunlight for significant periods of time should have lenses that block UV rays. This includes both regular dress-wear lenses and prescription sunglass lenses.

When an order includes a UV-blocking component, the UV dye should be applied first, before the application of a colored dye. Otherwise the previously applied color will fade in the UV bath and contaminate the UV dye. How long the lenses must be left in dye depends on the type of dye purchased. Published times for dyes vary. Some are listed from 2 to 10 minutes, others from 30 to 40 minutes.[11] Generally speaking, the less a lens is left in hot dye, the better. This is especially important for a scratch-coated lens or lens that is to be AR-coated.

UV dye should not be allowed to get too old. Because the lens has no actual color after the application of UV, each lens should be checked on a photometer that is capable of measuring UV transmission. Otherwise there is no guarantee that the lens is furnishing adequate protection (Figure 11-18). Over time and with use the UV dye requires longer to produce the required UV absorption. If the dye is not producing adequate UV in the time expected for the dye, the dye should be replaced.

UV dyeing of plastic lenses is a reliable method for providing protection against UV-A and UV-B radiation. Although dyes, including UV dyes, may fade some over time, a 1997 study[12] showed the following. Lenses that were dyed for UV protection in the laboratory and those that were purchased as stock lenses with UV-absorbing monomers incorporated into the polymer of

---

[9]Hecht S, Hendley C, Ross S: The effect of exposure to sunlight on night vision, *Am J Ophthal* 31:1573, 1948.
[10]Brilliant LB et al: Associations among cataract prevalence, sunlight hours, and altitude in the Himalayas, *Am J Epidemiol* 118:239, 1983.

[11]*BPI Catalog*, Miami, 1999, BPI Incorporated, pp 27-34.
[12]Lee DY, Brown WL, Trachimowicz R: Efficacy and durability of ultraviolet tints in CR-39 ophthalmic lenses, *J Am Ophthal Assoc* 68(11):709-714, 1997.

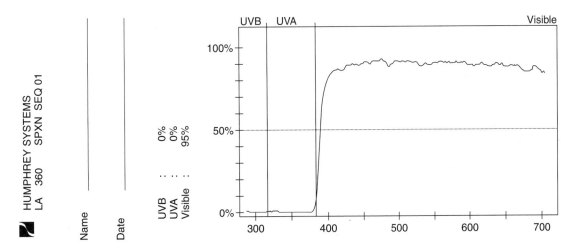

FIGURE **11-18** This lens was measured using a Humphrey Lens Analyzer (autolensmeter) with the ability to read lens transmission. The figure shows that most light below 400 nm has been filtered out by the lens.

the lens material both meet Z87.3-1996 UV standards for nonprescription sunglasses and fashion eyewear. They also maintained that same protection for the life of the study (1 year) under normal daily washing and drying without a significant decrease in the protective effect of the UV tint.

Effects of Lens Material and Lens Coating on the Dyeing Process

DYEING POLYCARBONATE

The process for tinting polycarbonate is basically the same as it is for regular plastic lenses. Only a few differences are listed in this section. As with regular plastic lenses, unevenness in the tint may occur if hard water or contaminated water is used instead of distilled or deionized water. Unevenness of tint also can happen if the dye is not kept mixed well enough, if the dye is overused by trying to tint too many lenses before changing the dye, by incomplete lens cleaning before dyeing, and by attempting to tint the lens with the dye temperature too far above or below 210° F. However, the way the dye is absorbed by the polycarbonate lens does differ from a regular CR-39 plastic lens.

Dye Distribution in Polycarbonates

With regular plastic lenses, the dye is absorbed into the plastic itself. Polycarbonate will not absorb lens dye. Instead the dye is absorbed by the coating on the lens.[13] In the past, the more the coating on the polycarbonate lens resisted scratching, the harder it was to dye. With the changes that have been made in coatings, polycarbonate lenses are not as difficult to dye as they used to be. It is now possible to tint most polycarbonate lenses even to a dark sun lens tint. If a lens will not tint dark enough, at least one manufacturer makes polycarbonate lenses with a number 2 gray tint in the polycarbonate material itself.[14] These number 2 gray lenses can then be dyed to the desired sun lens shade of dark gray.

(*Note:* Polycarbonate lenses already have a UV absorber in the coating and do not have to be UV dyed.)

Heat and Neutralizer Sensitivities

A lens should not be left in the tint longer than 30 minutes. If it has not reached the desired tint, either the dye is too old, too cold, or the lens is already as dark as it is going to get.

The neutralizer should not be hotter than 200° F or it can cause the coating to bubble.[15] Along these same lines, the lens should not be left in hot neutralizer more than 10 minutes. Leaving lenses in the neutralizer too long can cause crazing of the lens surface.[16] (*Crazing* is a microcracking of the coating that makes the surface of the lens look like the surface of dried, cracked mud.) This is the reason some prefer using a capful of noncitrus dishwashing detergent in water for light bleaching of polycarbonate lenses. (Lemon scented detergents may damage the coating.[17]) Even dishwashing detergent needs to be heated to 200° F to be effective.

Box 11-1 provides some additional specific and helpful suggestions from the Polycarbonate Lens Council on tinting polycarbonate lenses.

DYEING HARD-COATED LENSES

A plastic lens that has been hard coated dyes differently than an uncoated plastic lens. It may also take longer to dye. This is because the coating must first absorb the dye before it can get into the lens itself.[18]

A large variety of lens coatings are made. Hence a variety of results also occur when these lenses are tinted. If the lens manufacturer provides recommendations on how to tint their lenses, it is best to follow their advice.

As might be expected, lens coatings cause tint times to change. They also may absorb some pigments better than others. This means that a coated lens may not come out to exactly the same color as an uncoated lens would. It also means that two lenses with two different types of coatings may come out with slightly different shades of the same color, even if they are dyed in the same tank for the same length of time.

DYEING HIGH-INDEX LENSES

Recommendations for high-index plastic lenses vary according to manufacturer. For example, Optima recommends that its 1.66 HyperIndex lenses be tinted at 180° F to 190° F.[19] Optima also recommends leaving 1.66 HyperIndex lenses in the dye for only 10 minutes at a time, alternating between the tint dye and a solution of warm water with three drops of Joy dishwashing liquid. This is only an example and does

---

[13]Polycarbonate Lens Council: *Polycarbonate information for educators: tinting polycarbonate,* accessed May 2001 (http://www.polycarb.org/educ11.htm).
[14]Bruneni JL: Ask the labs, *Eyecare Business* April 1998, p 40.

[15]Breheney ML: Processing tips for polycarbonate, *LabTalk* May 1999, p 30.
[16]*BPI Catalog,* Miami, 1999, BPI Incorporated, p 163.
[17]Grootegoed J (of Walman Optical) as quoted in *Optical Dispensing News,* Nov. 15, 2000.
[18]Bruneni JL: Ask the labs, *Eyecare Business* April 1998, p 40.
[19]*HyperIndex 1.66 Technical Manual,* Stratford, Conn, 1994, Optima Inc, p 5.

- A polycarbonate lens absorbs tint in the coating instead of in the lens material. All tintable coatings absorb moisture from the air and this can cause variations in their ability to absorb tints. For this reason, exposure of the lenses to high humidity should be minimized before tinting.
- Of the maximum tint, 95% will be absorbed within 20 minutes. Tint/neutralizer/tint cycles should not exceed 30 minutes.
- The tint bath should be kept between 205° F and 210° F, using a thermometer for accuracy.
- Too cool a bath will dramatically increase tint times.
- Fresh dyes tint faster and darker. Establish a color sample lens with fresh dye for testing the depth of tint reached within 15 minutes. As the dye ages, lenses dyed for 15 minutes should be checked against that sample. When that level of tint is not reached, it is time to change the dye.
- Some dyes tend to clump causing uneven or blotchy tints. To prevent this, the dye should be stirred regularly. Once blotching starts, it is usually necessary to change the dye.
- For neutralizing, a water-based neutralizer is used.
- For light bleaching, instead of using neutralizer, a capful of noncitrus dish detergent is added to water and heated to 200° F.
- Transfer fluid is maintained at a level where a minimum of half the dye tank is covered.
- Transfer fluid is changed monthly.
- Three drops of noncitrus dish detergent are added to the dye pot to help break up surface tension of coating. This promotes more uniform dyeing.
- To match left and right tints, both lenses should be from the same manufacturer.
- For cleaning of dyed lenses, the lenses are rinsed with clean water. Alcohol is applied to a wipe and both lens surfaces are cleaned.

not apply to other high-index lenses. Procedures for high-index plastic vary. Recommendations likely will change as available lens dyeing products change.

One general recommendation for high-index materials is to use a product such as BPI Spotless solution in the dyes. The purpose is to achieve more uniform colors and prevent spots and blotches.

Another suggestion that may help with high-index lenses is to watch the pH of the lens dye. The pH of lens dyes should be neutral (7; higher than 7 = alkaline; lower than 7 = acidic). Some of the cleaning solutions used to prepare a lens for tinting are carried over in the tint solution in small amounts. This can change the pH of the dye. A hot solution that is not neutral can cause some types of lens coatings to be weakened. To bring the tint bath back to neutral, a stabilizer such as BPI Stabilizer may be helpful.

Some dyes are specifically made for high-index materials. These may be most appropriate for laboratories that work with a large volume of lenses.

DYEING LENSES TO BE ANTIREFLECTION-COATED

AR coatings eliminate the glare that reflects from the surface of a spectacle lens. In eliminating reflections, the net result is an increase in the amount of light that goes through the lens. Normally each surface of a regular plastic lens reflects about 4% of the light. This means that in its "clear" state a CR-39 plastic lens transmits only 92% of the incoming light. When AR-coated, the lens may transmit nearly 99.5% of incoming light, depending upon coating quality. So what does this mean for a lens that is to be first tinted, then AR-coated?

Example 11-1
An order arrives for a lens that calls for a light pink tint with a transmission of 80%. If the lens is tinted so that it transmits 80% of the light in its uncoated state, what percentage of light will it transmit after it has been AR-coated?

Solution
For a normal CR-39 plastic lens, 3.974% of light striking the lens is reflected by the front surface and 3.665% from the back surface. So for a "clear" lens, only 92.36% of the light actually goes through the lens, not 100%.[20]

---

[20]Normally the following describes what happens with a clear, uncoated plastic lens. As light enters a 1.498 index CR-39 lens, 3.974% of the light is reflected from the front surface, leaving 96.026% to travel on to the second surface. There 3.974% of the 96.026% of light that enters the second surface is reflected. This amounts to 3.665% reflection from the second surface. The percent of light that originally enters the lens that gets through is as follows:

$$100 - 3.974 - 3.665 = 92.36\%$$

The exact formula, called the *Fresnel Equation*, is written as follows:

$$I_R = \left[\frac{n' - n}{n' + n} \right]^2 \times I$$

where:

n' = Index of refraction of the second media
n = Index of refraction of the first media
I = Amount of incident light
I_R = Amount of incident light reflected

The equation must be worked twice, once for the first surface and once for the second surface.

So now this "clear" lens is dyed and the transmission measured to be 80%. Next the lens is AR coated. If almost all of the reflected light from front and back surfaces now passes through the lens, the lens transmits slightly more than 7% more light than it did before it was AR-coated. In this case, the lens will transmit 87% of the light. This is measurably more than was ordered.

Lenses that will be dyed to a dark sunglass lens tint will not show a full 7% difference between what the transmission of the lens is before and after AR coating. This is because a dark lens will have less light entering the second surface and therefore less light reflected from the second surface. The following is an example.

Example 11-2

If a CR-39 plastic lens is dyed to a 15% transmission *before* being AR-coated, what percentage transmission will the lens have *after* being AR-coated?

Solution

The first surface of this 1.498 index lens still reflects 3.974% of the incoming light, just like the clear lens. Once the lens is coated, total transmission is increased by this amount. However, the back surface of the lens only reflects 3.974% *of the light it receives*, which is slightly less than 16%. So 3.974% of 16% is just more than 0.6%. This means that for the dark lens, the difference between lens transmission before and after it has been AR-coated is just under 5%.

So what does all this mean in terms of tinting lenses before they are AR-coated? If AR coating were the only factor it would mean that for lightly tinted lenses that are to be lightly tinted, the lens would be dyed 7% darker than the percent transmission ordered. For lenses that are to be darkly tinted, they would be dyed 5% darker than the percent ordered.

However, lenses that are to be AR-coated are subjected to an intensive, multistage cleaning process before they are coated. This can remove some of the dye resident near the outer surface of the lens. When this happens, the lens ends up lighter than it was, even before it is ever AR-coated. To prevent this problem, the lens is dyed too dark. Then it is dipped in neutralizer to lighten it to the needed transmission.

To summarize: CR-39 plastic lenses that are to be lightly AR-coated are dyed 15% darker than ordered, then they are lightened in neutralizer until they are 7% darker than ordered. CR-39 lenses that are to be darkly tinted and AR-coated are dyed 10% darker than ordered and then lightened in neutralizer until they are 5% darker than ordered. This process ensures the requested transmission will come out as requested.

(*Note:* The higher the index of refraction, the more light the surface of the lens will reflect. Both front and back lens surfaces of a 1.66 index lens combined will reflect 12% of total incoming light for a clear lens and 7% of total incoming light for a dark sunglass lens. Consequently, the higher the refractive index a lens has, the greater the compensation required to make the final transmission of an AR-coated lens come out right.)

Dyeing Lenses before AR Coating

If a lens is to be dyed and AR-coated, it must be dyed first. It cannot be AR-coated, then dyed. The AR coating cannot handle the tinting process and prevents the lens from being properly dyed. This means that if a lens is dyed, then AR-coated, it cannot be lightened, darkened, or redyed in any way without first stripping the AR coating off the lens.

An AR-coating stripper may be purchased. The main purpose for this is to remove an old AR coating that is beginning to degrade.

DYEING PLASTIC POLARIZING LENSES

Polarizing lenses reduce the glare of light reflected from water, sand, snow, or pavement. These lenses have a layer of polarizing material sandwiched into the lens. Nevertheless, it is possible to dye a plastic polarizing lens. The process is carried out in the same manner as for normal CR-39 plastic lenses.[21] For best results, the lenses are tinted in uncut form before they are edged.

Polarizing lenses come in a variety of tints already. The only reason to tint a polarizing lens is if the desired lens color is not already available.

DYEING NYLON CORDS

Some frames hold the lens in place by using a nylon cord. These frames are called by a variety of names, including rimlons, nylon supras, nylors, or simply nylon cord frames.

Dyeing the nylon cord that surrounds the lens is possible in the same dye used to tint plastic lenses. Therefore nylon cords may be dyed to match the cord color to the lens or frame color, or just to be different.

Powering Down, Cleaning Up, and Reducing Smells

POWERING DOWN THE TINT UNIT

When lenses are being tinted, the base unit keeps the dye just under the boiling point. The tint tanks need to

---

[21]Frequently asked questions about NuPolar polarized lenses, *LensTalk* January 2000, p 9.

be monitored continually to keep the contents from evaporating too fast. While the unit is running at full temperature, water must be added constantly or the tint in the tanks evaporates and leaves a pigment residue on the sides of the tanks. (Some units even have warning systems that sound if the tint level is too low.[22])

If the tint unit will not be used for a while, it should be turned down. If the dial is turned down *and* the temperature of the dye reaches 130° F, the lids may be put on to reduce evaporation. The *tint* temperature should reach 130° F before putting the lids on. Simply turning the dial to 130° F and putting the lids on will make the temperature rise rapidly and cause the tints to boil over.

CLEANING TINT TANKS AND LENS HOLDERS

Tanks should be cleaned thoroughly every time the tint is changed. This may be done with a mild detergent. The inside of the tank must not be contaminated with the heat transfer fluid that is on the outside of the tank. (To be sure the inside of the tank is free of transfer fluids, after washing, the inside of the tank is rinsed for 10 minutes with running water.)

The inside of the tank should be free from scratches. Scratches serve as a magnet for dye residues. For this reason, the unit should not be cleaned with scouring pads, powders, chemicals, solvents, or steel wool. A cleaning agent purchased from the tint manufacturer,

---

[22]Lamperelli K: To dye for: a guide to tints and tinting, *Eyewear* Oct 1998, p 30.

or ordinary dishwashing detergent (without citrus) is sufficient. If scrubbing is required, only a plastic or nylon pad that is not impregnated with cleaning agent should be used. Lens holders should be cleaned in the same manner as are tint tanks.

REDUCING DYE SMELLS IN THE LABORATORY

Certain characteristic smells accompany lens tinting. This factor must first be considered before adding a tinting facility. Even though these smells are not considered to be hazardous, certain steps may reduce them, as follows:

1. Locate the tint unit in a well-ventilated area.
2. If needed, use a hood over the unit that is vented to the outside.
3. If a hood is needed and it cannot be vented outside, use a hood or alternative fan unit, which draws air through a charcoal filter before returning it to the room.
4. Use odor-absorbing tint tank lids.

Troubleshooting

Any process has problems. The most effective solution for problems is to avoid them. However, despite the most careful procedures, sometimes problems do arise. Table 11-2 lists several problems, their cause, and how to correct them. The list is not inclusive and does not try to address all of the issues already discussed in the chapter.

TABLE 11-2
Troubleshooting for Tinting

PROBLEM	PROBABLE CAUSE(S)	CORRECTION
Why does the lens appear blotchy?	The lens was not properly cleaned.	Put the lens in neutralizer to remove the color, and then thoroughly clean it and start over.
	The lens cured unevenly during manufacture.	Some practitioners recommend placing the lens in a 240° F oven for 15-20 minutes after removing the dye with neutralizer and before retinting. (Dye manufacturers sell small ovens for this and other purposes.)
Why does the lens have a circlelike variation in the tint?	The lens cured unevenly during manufacture.	Use the same corrective procedure provided above for uneven curing.
Why are my colors "off?"	Minerals or contaminants are in the dye water.	Use distilled or deionized water when dyes are mixed.
	Someone keeps using hard tap water in the dyes.	Obtain a product such as BPI Water Soft and add a few drops to the tint solution. It will bind some of the contaminants in the water so that the contaminants will not bind with the dye.

Continued

TABLE **11-2** *Troubleshooting for Tinting—cont'd*		
PROBLEM	PROBABLE CAUSE(S)	CORRECTION
	If tap water is being used regularly...	...put the tap water into a container and let it stand 24 hours before it is to be used. This will allow some of the chlorine, fluoride, and other chemicals to evaporate before the water is used.*
	Some heat transfer fluid got into the dye. This could have happened when the dye tank was removed from the unit. The heat transfer fluid from the bottom of the tank being moved may have dripped into an open dye tank. It could also be that transfer fluid got inside the tank when the tank was being washed.	Thoroughly wash the tint tank. Begin by first completely rinsing the outside. After washing the entire tank, rinse the inside 10 minutes under running water.
Why do my lenses appear too purplish?[†]	The tint hue has been mixed and in the tank too long, causing some of the tint pigment to react with the oxygen in the water.	Add a bit of yellow dye to the tank.
Why do my lenses appear too reddish?[†]	The tint concentrate did not all get into the tank.	When using large bottles of concentrate intended for more than one tank of dye, thoroughly shake the bottle before pouring the tint concentrate. (*Hint:* To make mixing easier, place a marble in the bottle.) When using a single-use, small bottle, shake the bottle well and rinse it at least three times, pouring the rinse water into the tank. Ensure that all the tint pigment empties into the tank.
	You may be trying to tint the lens darker than was intended for the dye you are using.	For dark tints, use a dye intended for dark tints.
Why does the lens appear streaked?	That particular tint has not been used for awhile, and some of the pigment has begun to clump together.	From time to time, heat and stir those tints that are not being actively used. (Laboratories often have more mixed tints in tint tanks than places in the base unit in which to keep them. These tints may not get heated and stirred often enough.) Preventively add a drop or more of a solution designed to prevent clumping, such as BPI Color Developer. It resuspends pigment and breaks up clumping.
	The lens was cured unevenly.	Use better-quality lenses.
	The lens holders contain dried tint pigment.	Clean the holders regularly.
	The dye was contaminated with heat transfer fluid.	Thoroughly wash the tint tank. Begin by first completely rinsing the outside. After washing the entire tank, rinse the inside 10 minutes under running water.
	The concentration of the lens conditioner being used is too high.	Use the correct concentration of lens conditioner.
Why do I have a lens pair in which the right and left lenses are different colors and/or different transmissions?	One of the following may have occurred: • The lenses are from different manufacturers.	Attempt to choose lenses that are better matched before dyeing. Ensure that the dye temperature is hot enough. Low temperatures will cause more differences

*Herrick T: It's up to hue, 20/20 March 2000, p 134.
[†]For what to do to correct color of the lens itself, see Table 11-1 on color balancing.

TABLE 11-2		
Troubleshooting for Tinting—cont'd		
PROBLEM	PROBABLE CAUSE(S)	CORRECTION
	• The lenses are from different batches from the same manufacturer. • One lens is a stock lens, and the other is a surfaced lens.	between lenses in these situations.[‡]
	Lenses may have considerably different thicknesses, such as minus and plus lens combinations.	Match the two lenses by hand using a color-balancing table (see Table 11-1).
Why is the heat transfer fluid popping?	Water or tint solution has gotten into the transfer fluid.	The heat transfer fluid has a higher boiling point than water. If water or anything else with a low boiling point gets into the heat transfer fluid, the foreign fluid will boil and pop, just as when water in hot oil pops. If only a small amount of contaminant is in the fluid, turn the temperature of the unit down to 130° F and allow the spilled liquid to evaporate.
The heat transfer fluid appears dirty. Is something wrong?	It is considered normal for the heat transfer fluid to appear dark. To check and ensure whether the fluid is in fact dirty, use a teaspoon and scoop some out. If the fluid is too dark and the bottom of the spoon is not visible, the fluid needs to be changed.	At the same time the fluid is changed, the heating element should be checked. If it feels crusty, clean the element with a plastic or nylon cleaner. Take care not to scratch the element. Failure to clean the unit will result in early element burnout.
I have dye on my hands that will not wash off. How can I remove it?	Unless you use latex gloves, this can be a problem.	Dye manufacturers generally have one or more soaps or cleansers specially formulated for hand cleaning. If this is a continuous problem, use latex gloves.
I splashed dye on my clothes. Are they ruined?	The best solution is prevention. Wear a laboratory jacket or old clothing on which you do not mind stains.	Try using neutralizer to remove splashed lens dye from clothing. However, there is always the possibility that the original color of the clothing may be affected.
Some of my scratch-resistant coated lenses are having problems with color variations, white spots, and blotchy areas. What should I do?	There may be variations in lens surface charges.	Use a solution made for lenses with hard coatings, such as BPI Spotless. Add the recommended amount to the tint solution.

[‡]DeFranco LM: Eye on equipment, *Eyecare Business* Jan 2000, p 34.

BIBLIOGRAPHY

Seiko Tinting Guide, Mahwah, NJ, Seiko Optical Products (undated publication).

Silor Recommended Tinting Procedures, St Petersburg, Fla, Essilor of America (undated publication).

Wertheim HA et al: *How to tint lenses made from CR-39 monomer for prescription eyewear,* ed 2, Pittsburgh, 1981, PPG Industries.

Proficiency Test Questions

1. Which of the following does not describe one of the three main ways in which ophthalmic lenses may be tinted?

    a. By introducing a coloring substance into the lens material before it becomes a lens
    b. By vacuum coating the color onto the surface of the lens in much the same way that antireflection coatings are applied to lenses
    c. By spray-coating the lens with an aerosol spray
    d. By immersing the lens in a liquid dye so that the dye is absorbed into the lens

2. True or False? All tint base units use a heat transfer fluid to convey the heat to the tint.

3. Tinting a lens with first one color, then with another, results in a green lens. Which two of the following colors are they?

    a. Blue
    b. Red
    c. Yellow

4. Is it advisable to use tap water to dye lenses?

    a. Yes
    b. No

5. To make the tint for lens dyeing, the concentrated dye is best mixed with which of the following?

    a. Lens conditioner
    b. Neutralizer
    c. Tap water
    d. Distilled water
    e. There is no mixing. The dye comes ready to use.

6. When starting a new batch of dye, which of the following choices describes the point at which the concentrate should be added to the tint tank?

    a. Before the water is added to the tint tank
    b. While the water in the tank is still cold
    c. When the water in the tank is 140° F
    d. After the water in the tank is heated to 200° F

7. Which of the following best describes what happens if pigment residue is left in the bottom of a single-use bottle of concentrate?

    a. The lenses may be a slightly different color from what they should normally be.
    b. Not as many lenses may be dyed in this batch.
    c. The lenses will not dye as darkly as they should.

8. To maintain the tint at optimum temperature, which of the following should happen?

    a. Buy a laboratory-grade thermometer to measure dye temperature in the tanks.
    b. Use the temperature dial on the tint unit. It is custom made for the unit. Using another thermometer is both time consuming and a waste of money.

9. Which of the following is true of a lens that has been slowly cured in the manufacturing process as it went from a liquid resin to a solid lens?

    a. It is called a *soft lens*.
    b. It will accept dye more rapidly than one that has been cured rapidly.
    c. It will accept dye more slowly than one that has been cured rapidly.

10. Which of the following happens when one surfaced lens and one stock lens are used together as a pair?

    a. One lens will be thicker than the other and appear different, even when identically tinted.
    b. A difference may occur in the color and/or transmission of the two lenses.
    c. No difference occurs in the color and/or transmission of the two lenses.
    d. Surfaced and stock lenses should never be mixed when tinted under any circumstances.

11. True or False? It is not possible to use too much lens conditioner. It may be a wasteful habit, but it will not affect the lens.

12. Which of the following is true of lens neutralizer?

    a. It works OK when it is hot, but works best when it is room temperature.
    b. It works OK when it is at room temperature, but works best when it is hot.
    c. It works the same at room temperature as it does when it is hot. There is no difference.
    d. It should not be used at room temperature, only hot.
    e. It should not be used hot, only at room temperature.

13. Which of the following choices describes the way in which a lens should be lowered into the tint bath when it is to be tinted?

    a. Quickly to prevent a boil-over of the tint solution
    b. Slowly to prevent a boil-over of the tint solution
    c. The speed at which the lens is lowered is inconsequential.

14. True or False? After the lens is removed from the tint tank, it helps to put the lens in the lens neutralizer, then rinse the lens with water.

15. Which of the following is the instrument used to measure visible and UV light transmission?

    a. Colmascope
    b. Lens analyzer
    c. Colorimeter
    d. Comparator
    e. Photometer

16. Which of the following statements is *false?*

    a. Over a period of time, dyed plastic lenses fade when exposed to sunlight.
    b. Over a period of time, dyed plastic lenses fade when exposed to incandescent or fluorescent lighting.
    c. Over a period of time, dyed plastic lenses fade when placed in a drawer, but not as fast as lenses exposed to sunlight or artificial light.
    d. Dyed plastic lenses do not ever fade.

17. To create a simple gradient tint, which of the following should be done first?

    a. Mount the lenses right side up in the lens holder.
    b. Mount the lenses upside down in the lens holder.

18. Which of the following is one way to smooth out a gradient line that is too harsh?

    a. Hold the lens right side up and dip it part way into lens conditioner.
    b. Hold the lens upside down and dip it part way into lens conditioner.
    c. Hold the lens right side up and dip it part way into lens neutralizer.
    d. Hold the lens upside down and dip it part way into lens neutralizer.

19. True or False? A dyed plastic prescription sunglass lens always contains protection from UV radiation.

20. True or False? A properly coated, clear polycarbonate prescription spectacle lens always contains protection from UV radiation.

21. True or False? Polycarbonate lenses are harder to dye because the lens material is the only thing that takes the dye. The dye must pass completely through the lens coating to get to the lens.

22. A noncitrus dish detergent may be used in all of the following ways *except* which one?

    a. Put a capful of noncitrus dish detergent in water, heat the water to 200° F, and use the solution to lightly bleach polycarbonate lenses.
    b. Use noncitrus dish detergent to wash tint tanks.
    c. Use three drops of noncitrus dish detergent in each tank of tint when tinting polycarbonate lenses.
    d. Use a capful of noncitrus dish detergent in lens conditioner when prepping polycarbonate lenses.
    e. All of the above are appropriate uses for noncitrus dish detergent.

23. Which of the following are true of hard-coated CR-39 plastic lenses?

    a. They dye more quickly than uncoated CR-39 plastic lenses because both the coating and the lens material absorb the dye.
    b. They dye more slowly than uncoated CR-39 plastic lenses because only the coating absorbs the dye.
    c. They dye more slowly than uncoated CR-39 plastic lenses because the coating must first absorb the dye before it can get into the lens itself.

24. An order calls for a light blue fashion tint in a CR-39 plastic lens with an 82% transmission and an AR coating. How should the lens be tinted in preparation for AR coating?

   a. It should be first tinted to a transmission of 57%, then be placed in neutralizer until it has a transmission of 72%. After that it may be AR-coated.
   b. It should be first tinted to a transmission of 68%, then be placed in neutralizer until it has a transmission of 75%. After that it may be AR-coated.
   c. It should be first tinted to a transmission of 75%, then be placed in neutralizer until it has a transmission of 82%. After that it may be AR-coated.
   d. It should be first tinted to a transmission of 82%, then be placed in neutralizer until it has a transmission of 89%. After that it may be AR-coated.
   e. Just tint the lens to 82%, then AR coat it.

25. An order calls for a dark gray sunglass tint in a CR-39 plastic lens with an 18% transmission and an AR coating. How should the lens be tinted in preparation for AR coating?

   a. It should be first tinted to a transmission of 18%, then be placed in neutralizer until it has a transmission of 23%. After that it may be AR-coated.
   b. It should be first tinted to a transmission of 13%, then be placed in neutralizer until it has a transmission of 18%. After that it may be AR-coated.
   c. It should be first tinted to a transmission of 8%, then be placed in neutralizer until it has a transmission of 13%. After that it may be AR-coated.
   d. It should be first tinted to a transmission of 3%, then be placed in neutralizer until it has a transmission of 8%. After that it may be AR-coated.
   e. Just tint the lens to 18%, then AR coat it.

26. True or False? Plastic polarizing lenses may not be dyed because if they are dyed, they will delaminate.

27. After turning the tint unit off, which of the following should be performed next?

   a. Put the lids back on the tint tanks right away. Forgetting this step will cause the dye to evaporate.
   b. Wait until the dyes have reached 180° F before putting the lids back on the tint tanks.
   c. Wait until the dyes have reached 130° F before putting the lids back on the tint tanks.
   d. Wait until the dyes have reached room temperature before putting the lids back on the tint tanks.

28. True or False? The best thing that may be used to clean a tint tank that has burnt-on pigment is steel wool.

29. Which of the following is *not* a possible cause for a streaked lens?

   a. The tank of tint that was used had not been used for a while.
   b. The lens was cured unevenly during manufacture.
   c. The lens holders have dried pigment on them.
   d. The dye was contaminated with heat transfer fluid.
   e. Tap water was used instead of distilled water.
   f. The concentration of lens conditioner being used is too high.

30. Your heat transfer fluid has started to pop. Which of the following describes what this is most likely to indicate?

   a. The heat transfer fluid is too hot.
   b. The heat transfer fluid is too old.
   c. The stainless steel tanks are getting worn.
   d. There is tint solution contaminating the heat transfer fluid.
   e. The lens has been left in the dye too long.

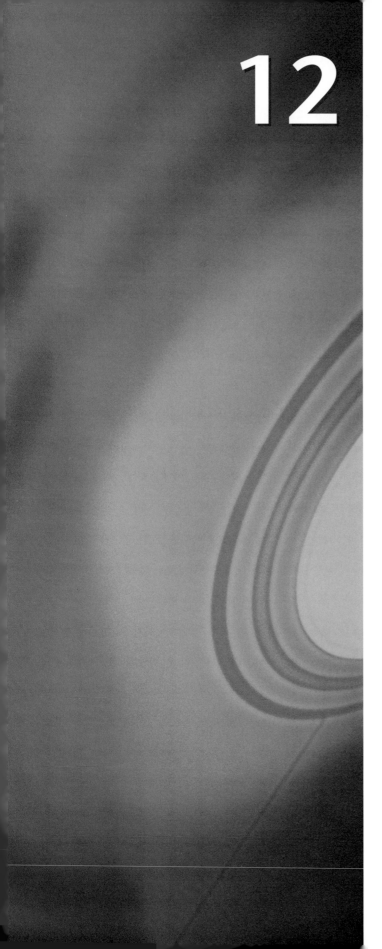

Lens Insertion and Standard Alignment

Seeing the Full Picture

Once the lenses are edged and, if needed, have been hardened or tinted or coated, they are ready to be placed in the frame. Once inserted into the frame, the completed eyeglasses need to be aligned and verified.

This chapter provides an overview of how spectacle lenses should be inserted and the frame aligned. For more detailed information on this process, the reader is referred to the book *System for Ophthalmic Dispensing*[1], in which these processes are addressed in greater detail. The book also contains a complete explanation of the verification process.[2] *System for Ophthalmic Dispensing* is the appropriate companion book to use with *Essentials of Ophthalmic Lens Finishing*.

INSERTING LENSES INTO PLASTIC FRAMES

People insert lenses into the frames in a variety of ways. If the lenses are inserted without damaging the frame and are secure and are not rotated off axis, the task has been accomplished. However, some ways have proven to be efficient and are a good starting point for gaining proficiency in the process.

The procedure explained here is for standard plastic frames made from cellulose acetate material. The following are two methods used for lens insertion. Both

---

[1]Brooks CW, Borish IM: *System for ophthalmic dispensing*, ed 2, Boston, 1996, Butterworth-Heinemann [Chapters 7 and 8].
[2]Brooks CW, Borish IM: *System for ophthalmic dispensing*, ed 2, Boston, 1996, Butterwoth-Heinemann [Chapter 6].

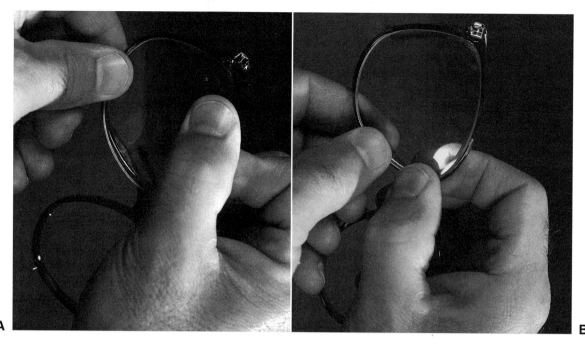

A   B

FIGURE **12-1**   Method 1. **A,** The temporal edge of the lens is placed in the frame groove. (The first moments of lens insertion are crucial in proper alignment of the lens bevel with the frame groove and must be done quickly.) **B,** The lens should snap in place fairly easily. If extreme force must be used in attempting to snap the lens in place, the process is better carried out using Method 2. (From Brooks CW, Borish IM: *System for ophthalmic dispensing,* ed 2, Boston, 1996, Butterworth-Heinemann [Figure 7-3].)

begin by heating the frame, then curving the top and bottom of the frame to match the curved top and bottom of the lens.

Method 1

The eyewire of the frame is heated and the temporal (outer) edge of the lens is inserted into the corresponding portion (outer edge) of the frame (Figure 12-1). With the thumbs on the surface of the lens and the fingers on the nasal (inner) edge of the frame eyewire, the lens is snapped into the frame from the nasal (inner) side by application of pressure with the thumbs and fingers (Figure 12-1, *B*).

Method 2

The eyewire of the frame is heated and the upper outer (temporal) edge of the lens is inserted into the frame groove (Figure 12-2, *A*). The upper inner (nasal) edge is pushed into the eyewire so that the whole upper edge of the lens is in the frame (Figure 12-2, *B*). Next, the lower tempered edge of the lens is pushed into place (Figure 12-2, *C*). The final step is pulling the lower eyewire of the frame around the lower half of the lens and snapping the lower nasal corner of the lens into place (Figure 12-2, *D*). Box 12-1 provides for a review of these methods.

BOX **12-1**
Inserting Lenses into Plastic Frames

Method 1
1. Heat and shape the frame top to match the lens top.
2. Heat the eyewire.
3. Place the outer part of the lens in the outer part of the frame.
4. Push the inner edge of the lens in with the thumbs.

Method 2
1. Heat and shape the frame top to match the lens top.
2. Heat the eyewire.
3. Place the upper outer edge of the lens into the frame.
4. Place the upper inner edge of the lens in the frame. (The whole top of the lens is now in the frame.)
5. Pull the lower eyewire around the lens, beginning temporally and ending nasally.

CHECKING ITEMS AFTER LENS INSERTION

After lenses are inserted, they are checked to ensure the lens is entirely in the groove of the eyewire. The eyewire must be flat or uniformly rounded on the outside. If it

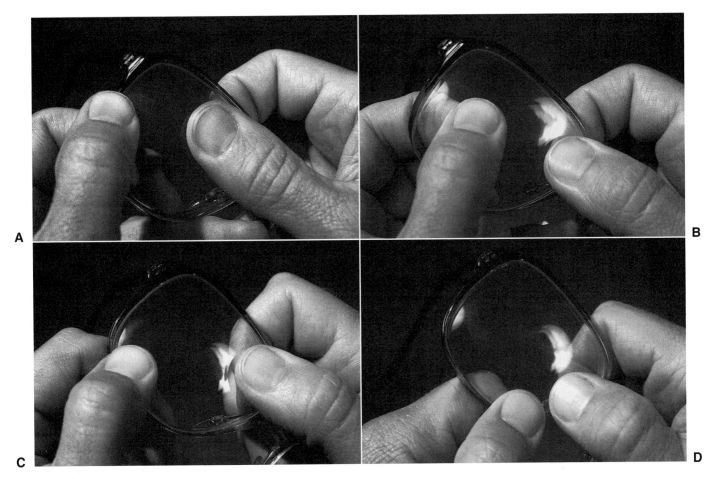

FIGURE **12-2** Method 2. **A,** Method 2 also starts with alignment of the lens bevel and frame groove, beginning in the upper temporal corner. **B,** When the upper and lower rims of the eyewire have been preshaped to the lens configuration, lens insertion into the entire upper half of the frame may be completed well before the frame cools. **C,** When the upper part of the lens is in the frame, the next step is to start temporally and pull the lower eyewire around the lens. **D,** The insertion process is concluded by snapping the bevel of the lower nasal part of the lens into the groove. (From Brooks CW, Borish IM: *System for ophthalmic dispensing,* ed 2, Boston, 1996, Butterworth-Heinemann [Figure 7-4].)

is slanted, the eyewire has been rolled. The practitioner can correct a roll by heating that portion of the eyewire involved and either twisting it with the fingers or pressing the frame against a flat surface with a counter-rolling motion. If uncorrectable by this method, removal of the lens and correction of the eyewire without the lens in it is best. Then the lens is reinserted properly after heating the frame. Antireflection-(AR)coated lenses should not be heated and should be removed from the frame during correction for a rolled eyewire.

Checking the Lens for Rotation

The eyewire containing the lens is compared with the empty eyewire adjacent to it. If the lens is rotated (Figure 12-3), lens-twisting pliers are used to correct the problem. The frame may first need to be heated, and

hot air is the recommended method. However, if hot salt is used to prevent scratching on the lens surface, both the lens and the plier surfaces are inspected to ensure that they are free of salt before the lens is rotated.

The practitioner should check to ensure that the top edges of *flat-top bifocals* are straight by placing a ruler in front of both segments for reference. With *progressive addition lenses,* the marked 180-degree reference marks should be horizontally straight. This is accomplished also by placing a ruler along the 180-degree line.

NONCELLULOSE ACETATE

For most plastic frames, basic lens insertion technique is fairly standard. However, each frame material has its own peculiarities. Table 12-1 shows what those important

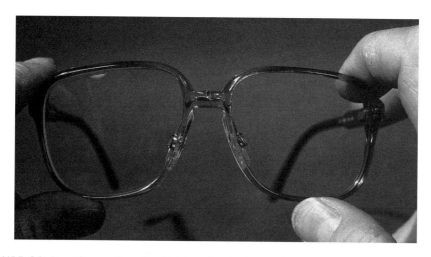

FIGURE **12-3**   After putting the first lens in the frame, lens orientation for the inserted lens should be compared with the empty eyewire. This frame shows too much nasal humping. (From Brooks CW, Borish IM: *System for ophthalmic dispensing,* ed 2, Boston, 1996, Butterworth-Heinemann [Figure 7-8].)

TABLE **12-1**
Plastic Frame Material Differences in Lens Insertion

MATERIAL	AMOUNT OF HEAT	HEATING METHOD(S)	EDGED LENS SIZE	HOW TO SHRINK MATERIAL	NOTES
Cellulose acetate	Minimal heat until pliable	Hot air best; hot salt or beads acceptable	On size or up to 0.5 mm larger than frame size	Plunge in ice water; material will shrink if previously stretched.	Cellulose acetate is the standard material used for most plastic frames.
Nylon	Hot water	Hot water preferable for penetration; hot air used if hot water unavailable	= 0.2 mm larger than frame size	Material does not shrink.	To retain adjusted shape, hold frame in the desired shape until cool. (Running cold water will speed cooling.)
Carbon fiber	None to minimal; preferable insertion method: cold snap	When heat used, hot air at low temperature	On size to just slightly larger in some cases	Material does not shrink.	Types of carbon fiber material vary, as will heat and insertion techniques.
Polyamide	No heat; lenses cold-snapped in place	Hot air for temples only	Exactly on size	Material shrinks slightly when heated.	After insertion, loose lenses may be tightened as the frame is heated slightly.
Polycarbonate	None	Cold snap	On size	Material does not shrink.	Material does not adjust.
Optyl	High heat until material bends under its own weight	Hot air, high temperature	= 0.6 to 1.0 mm larger than frame size	Material will not shrink but instead expands with heat. It gradually returns to size as the temperature cools.	Material returns to original shape when reheated. Quick cooling stops the shrinking process and results in loose lenses.

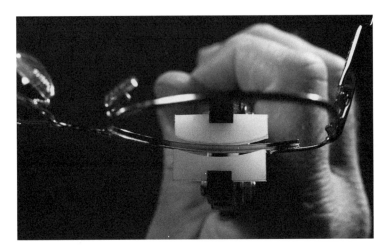

FIGURE **12-4** Eyewire forming pliers are used to cause the frame eyewire to conform to the meniscus curve of the lens bevel. (From Brooks CW, Borish IM: *System for ophthalmic dispensing,* ed 2, Boston, 1996, Butterworth-Heinemann [Figure 7-15].)

differences are for some plastic frame materials. Of particular importance are the following considerations:

- How (or even *if*) the frame material is heated
- What it takes to "shrink" the material down around the lens to achieve a tight fit

Inserting Lenses into Metal Frames

Lenses to be inserted into a metal frame must be edged to the exact size. To put a lens in a metal frame, the curves of the top and bottom of the lens are compared with the corresponding curves of the upper and lower frame eyewires. Using *eyewire-forming pliers* occasionally will be necessary to reshape the frame eyewire. To increase the meniscus curve, the pliers are positioned along the eyewire (Figure 12-4) and squeezed lightly. Then the pliers are repositioned along the upper and possibly lower eyewire until the new curve is evenly formed.

The eyewire screw is removed to place the lens in the eyewire. Use of an *eyewire closure pliers* (Figure 12-5) may be helpful to aid in seating the lens in the eyewire groove. Closure pliers are especially useful during edging to see if the lens will be the correct size (Figure 12-6).

Standard Alignment of Plastic Frames

Before a pair of glasses leaves the laboratory it should be adjusted so that it will sit symmetrically when placed on an individual of average head shape and size.

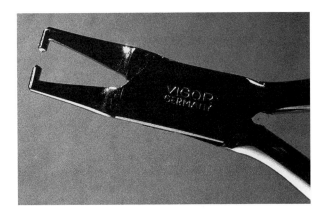

FIGURE **12-5** Eyewire closure pliers are made to fit into the top and bottom of the eyewire barrel. (From Brooks CW, Borish IM: *System for ophthalmic dispensing,* ed 2, Boston, 1996, Butterworth-Heinemann [Figure 7-16].)

For standard alignment, this procedure begins with the bridge and then follows next with the endpieces. The temples are handled last. Obviously, changes made in one part of a frame may influence the alignment in another part. Bending the bridge, for example, may change the relationship of the temples. Handling the bridge first, and the other parts in order, helps to eliminate the need to go back and realign parts.

In general, plastic frames must be heated for most alignments. Box 12-2 summarizes how frames are heated using forced hot air or a salt bath. Hot air is best for frames that can be adjusted with heat. Salt is fast and appropriate if no danger exists of damaging the type of frame or lenses being used.

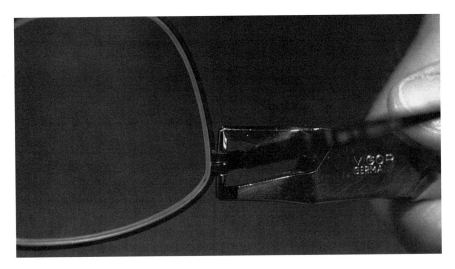

FIGURE **12-6** By using eyewire closure pliers to squeeze the eyewire around the lens, it is possible to see how well the lens will fit without having to replace the screw. Such pliers are especially handy during the edging process. (From Brooks CW, Borish IM: *System for ophthalmic dispensing,* ed 2, Boston, 1996, Butterworth-Heinemann [Figure 7-17].)

With Hot Air
1. Check the type of frame material. Some materials can stand more heat than others.
2. Heat only the portion of the frame on which work is to be performed.
3. Rotate the frame in the heat. (This step is important for warmers with heat from one direction only.)

With Salt or Beads
1. If in doubt as to whether the frame material or the lenses should be subjected to salt or beads, use hot air.
2. Always stir the salt (or glass beads) before use.
3. Keep the area of the frame being heated parallel to the surface of the salt.
4. Keep the frame moving slowly.
5. Heat only the portion of the frame on which work is to be performed.

BRIDGE

Bridge alignment is judged mainly by the effect it has on the plane of the lenses. If alignment is "off," the lenses are readjusted to their proper planes by first heating the bridge area, then grasping the frame by the lens areas.

If the lenses deviate from the horizontal plane (one lens appears to be higher or lower than the other), they are said to be out of *horizontal alignment.* If the lenses deviate from the vertical plane (one lens appears to be farther forward or backward than the other), they are said to be out of *vertical alignment.*

Rotated Lens

Two common causes exist for a frame being out of horizontal alignment: rotated lens and skewed bridge. A lens rotated in the frame causes the top of the eyewire to hump up at the nasal bridge or one endpiece to appear somewhat upswept in shape. An example of a rotated lens was shown in Figure 12-3.

Skewed Bridge

When viewed from the front, a skewed bridge causes one lens to appear higher than the other. This should not occur on a new frame unless the frame has been poorly manufactured or mishandled during processing.

Vertical Alignment (Four-Point Touch)

To check for *vertical alignment,* or *four-point touch,* a ruler or straight edge is placed so that its edge goes across the inside of the entire front of the spectacles below the nosepad area. Theoretically the frame eyewire should touch at four points on the ruler, that is, at each place where the ruler crosses the eyewire (Figure 12-7). This will be the case only if the frame is small compared with the wearer's head size; otherwise face form is required. If the lenses are decentered inward because the frame's A + distance between lenses (DBL) is greater than the wearer's PD, then face form is appropriate.

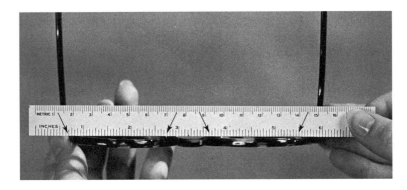

FIGURE **12-7** Checking for four-point touch. The frame eyewire touches at each place where the ruler crosses the eyewire. This indicates correct alignment when the "frame PD" equals the wearer's interpupillary distance. (From Brooks CW, Borish IM: *System for ophthalmic dispensing,* ed 2, Boston, 1996, Butterworth-Heinemann [Figure 8-5].)

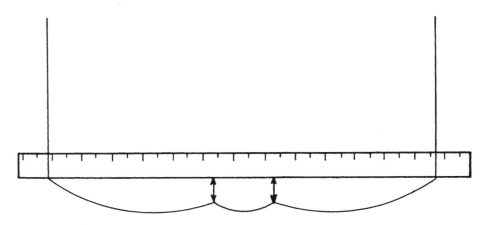

FIGURE **12-8** For those frames that will not or should not conform to a perfect four-point touch, the nasal sides of the eyewire should be equidistant from the ruler. (From Brooks CW, Borish IM: *System for ophthalmic dispensing,* ed 2, Boston, 1996, Butterworth-Heinemann [Figure 8-6].)

Face Form

Face form or *wraparound* is when the frame front is just slightly rounded to the form of the face. Frames with face form will not conform to the four-point touch test. But the temporal sides of the eyewires should touch, and the nasal sides should be equidistant from the ruler (Figure 12-8).

'X-ing'

The frame front may be somewhat twisted. This is called "X-ing" (Figure 12-9). X-ing causes the temples to be out of line with each other.

Variant Planes

Another form of vertical misalignment is when the lens planes are *variant,* or *out of coplanar, alignment.* When the lens planes are parallel, but one lens is farther forward than the other, the frame is out of coplanar

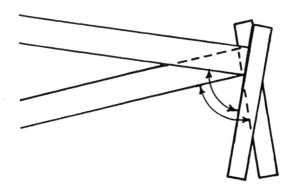

FIGURE **12-9** X-ing may be identified by the characteristic "X" the eyewires make with one another when viewed from the side. (From Brooks CW, Borish IM: *System for ophthalmic dispensing,* ed 2, Boston, 1996, Butterworth-Heinemann [Figure 8-9].)

alignment. This almost never occurs with a new frame unless it has been stressed during lens insertion.

Open Temple Spread

After horizontal and vertical preadjustments have been made to the bridge and eyewires, the next aspect considered is how far the temples are spread.

To allow a good picture of temple spread, temple shafts must be straight. Any curve to the temple shaft should be eliminated by heating the temple and straightening it with the hands. The *open temple spread* is the angle that open temples form in relationship to the front of the frame.

Temples Spread Too Far

Temples flaring more than 95 degrees are spread too far for standard alignment. The endpiece must be heated and bent around so that the temple will not be able to open out as far.

The practitioner begins by heating the endpiece. The temple should already be spread to the wide-open position. Then the endpiece is bent inward with use of one of the following methods:

1. Heat the endpiece and press it back with the thumb.
2. Heat the endpiece and press it against the tabletop.
3. Remove the lens and bend the endpiece and eyewire near the endpiece. Reinsert the lens.
4. When the frame is old or does not respond to the above methods, grasp the temple butt with half-padded pliers and bend the *temple* as close to the pliers as possible.
5. Sink the hidden hinge deeper into the frame front using a soldering iron or Hot Fingers unit.

Temples Not Spread Enough

Occasionally the temples are not spread enough after the lenses have been inserted. This may happen more if lenses with steep front curves are used. If the temples are not spread enough, the following may be attempted:

1. File the temple where it abuts with the front.
2. Bend the endpiece forward.

Temple Parallelism

In standard alignment (but not necessarily after frame fitting) the two temples must be parallel to one another when viewed from the side. If the "pantoscopic angles" the left and right temples make with the frame front are unequal, the temples will not be parallel.

The following steps are used to test whether the temples are parallel:

1. Position the glasses *upside down* on a flat surface with the temples open.
2. Note whether both temples sit flat or whether one temple is not touching the flat surface.
3. Touch first one temple and then the other to see whether the frame wobbles back and forth or sits solidly.

This procedure is known as the *flat surface touch test* (Figure 12-10). If the frame wobbles, it needs correction. If left uncorrected, the frame will likely sit on the face at an angle.

A common mistake is to check for temple parallelism with the glasses placed on the table right side up instead of upside down. If this mistake is made and either the bent-down portion of one temple is bent down the slightest bit more than the other, or if one temple bend is located even the least bit farther forward than the other bend, then the flat surface touch test for temple parallelism will not work.

Several possible sources exist for incorrect temple parallelism, as follows:

- A bent endpiece
- A broken rivet or loose hidden hinge (the temple will be loose and tightening the screw will not help)

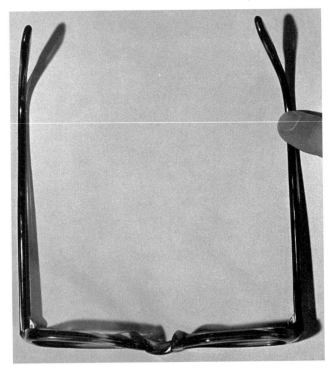

FIGURE **12-10** Testing for parallelism using the flat surface touch test. (From Brooks CW, Borish IM: *System for ophthalmic dispensing*, ed 2, Boston, 1996, Butterworth-Heinemann [Figure 8-21].)

- A bent temple shaft
- A bent hinge
- A twisted bridge

Aligning the Temple Ends

A good standard alignment is one in which the ends of both temples are bent down equally. They also should be bent inward slightly.

Temple-Fold Angle

The final alignment step is to fold the temples to the closed position and observe the angle formed as the temples cross. The temples should fold so that they are parallel to one another or form slight angles from parallel. The temples should cross each other exactly in the center of the frame. A proper temple fold angle permits the spectacle to easily fit into a standard glasses case.

Changing the temple-fold angle on a plastic frame by simply bending the temple with the hands does not work as successfully as using pliers. Using hands alone may cause the temple to split at the hinge. Instead, angling pliers can be used to grasp the top and bottom of the hinge screw. Because the metal hinge is being bent, heating the frame is not necessary.

The second method of angling the temple fold uses *finger-piece pliers*. These pliers, sometimes referred to as *Fits-U pliers*, are made with parallel jaws. With the temple folded, the pliers are held parallel to the endpiece hinge screw so that the hinge is grasped on both sides. While the frame front is held with the other hand, the hinge is angled until it reaches the proper position (Figure 12-11).

Standard Alignment of Metal Frames

Metal frames are aligned using the same standards as were used in evaluating plastic frames. Metal frames require heating only in those places where plastic coats the metal. All other bends are done "cold."

Pliers are used for the majority of adjustments. Because the pressure of the metal jaws may mar or disfigure the finished surface of the frames, to use padded pliers or to cushion one jaw of nonpadded pliers by attaching friction or adhesive tape to it is essential. The order of procedure for aligning metal frames is the same as that used for plastic frames, beginning with the bridge. The frame must be checked for horizontal alignment, a rotated lens, face form, and X-ing.

One of the primary areas in which adjustments are different than those outlined for plastic frames is when the temple angles are adjusted. Adjusting the temple angles encompasses open temple spread, temple parallelism, and temple-fold angles, which are discussed in the following sections.

Metal Temples Spread Too Far

If the temples are spread too far apart, a few selected methods that may be used to correct them, as follows:

1. Use a pair of thin pliers that has a small metal jaw on one side and a nylon-padded jaw on the other as bending pliers. Grip the outside of the endpiece (Figure 12-12) but hold the front firmly near the

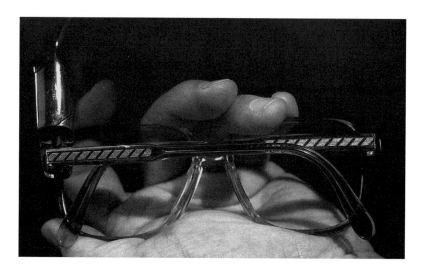

FIGURE **12-11** While the frame is held with the other hand, the hinge is angled until it reaches the proper position, as shown. (From Brooks CW, Borish IM: *System for ophthalmic dispensing,* ed 2, Boston, 1996, Butterworth-Heinemann [Figure 8-32].)

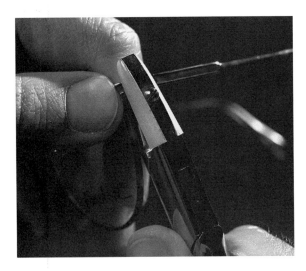

FIGURE **12-12**   If the temples are spread too far apart, a pair of half-padded pliers may serve as bending pliers and grip the outside of the endpiece. (From Brooks CW, Borish IM: *System for ophthalmic dispensing,* ed 2, Boston, 1996, Butterworth-Heinemann [Figure 8-41].)

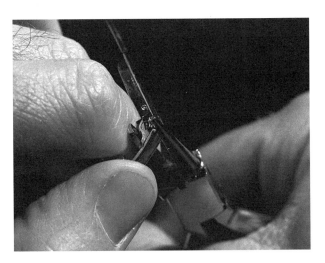

FIGURE **12-13**   The hand is used to grasp the frame front firmly at the endpiece. Temple spread is decreased with the pliers. If risk of chipping the lens is possible, the lens is removed first. (From Brooks CW, Borish IM: *System for ophthalmic dispensing,* ed 2, Boston, 1996, Butterworth-Heinemann [Figure 8-42].)

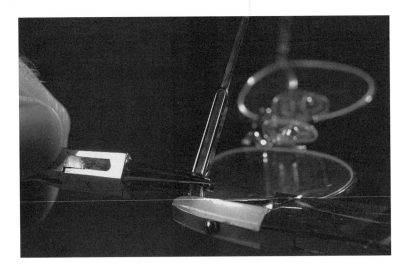

FIGURE **12-14**   The risk of lens chipping can be reduced by using holding pliers while reducing temple spread. (From Brooks CW, Borish IM: *System for ophthalmic dispensing,* ed 2, Boston, 1996, Butterworth-Heinemann [Figure 8-43].)

endpiece with the free hand. (When the endpiece is wide enough, a second pair of thin pliers is used to hold the endpiece where it joins the eyewire.) Rotate the bending pliers until the temple has reached and maintains the desired temple-spread angle.

2. Close the temple and grip the hinge from below with the thin pliers. (Because no visible external frame areas are being gripped, the pliers do not have to be padded.) Rotate the pliers and bend the endpiece area inward (Figure 12-13). Because of the risk of

chipping the lens, whenever there is sufficient space available, a second pair of pliers is used to grip the frame near the lens so that the eyewire area is not stressed (Figure 12-14).

3. Bend the endpiece using a method that does not involve pliers but only a smooth flat surface. With both hands, hold the frame by the lens and eyewire just adjacent to the endpiece. (The closer to the endpiece the frame is held, the less danger there is of breaking a lens.) Hold the frame front perpen-

dicular to the table surface and push the endpiece against the surface.

Temples Not Spread Enough

When the temple spread is too small, it can be increased by several methods. The outside section of the endpiece is grasped with padded pliers in the same manner as for decreasing the temple spread. (This was shown in Figure 12-12.) The endpiece is bent outward to the proper spread, while the front is supported at its junction with the endpiece.

The second method listed in the previous section is used to close the temple and grasp the hinge. (This was shown in Figure 12-13.) As noted previously and seen in Figure 12-14, certain kinds of frames allow enough space at the endpiece to permit a second pair of pliers next to the eyewire as holding pliers. This takes any possible strain off the eyewire, which reduces the possibility of chipping a lens.

Temple Parallelism

The glasses are placed upside down on a flat surface and notice taken as to whether one or both temples touch the surface (flat surface touch test). This is done as first one temple and then the other is touched, as shown for plastic frames in Figure 12-10. If the frame wobbles, the angle the frame front makes with the temple must be adjusted until the two temples are parallel and both touch the surface.

Several ways exist for bending the temple of a metal frame up or down, as follow:

1. Using the simplest way, grasp with one hand the eyewire and lens close to the endpiece on the same side of the frame as the temple that needs to be angled and bend the temple up or down with the other hand.
2. Using a pair of bracing pliers with one metal and one nylon jaw, hold the endpiece on the front of the frame if there is room, or just anterior to the hinge if there is not. (The second pliers, used for bending, should be double-padded nylon jaw pliers to grasp the temple close to or directly on the hinge. It may be prudent to remove the lens if the frame is stiff or there appears to be a possibility of chipping the lens.) Grasp the frame as shown in Figure 12-15 and reangle it upward or downward.
3. It may be possible to do the bend just described in the previous method but without using a pair of bracing pliers. This is shown in Figure 12-16. Take care to prevent chipping the lens.

After the temples have been aligned for parallelism, the bend-down end positions of the temples are aligned for symmetry. Both ends must be bent downward equally

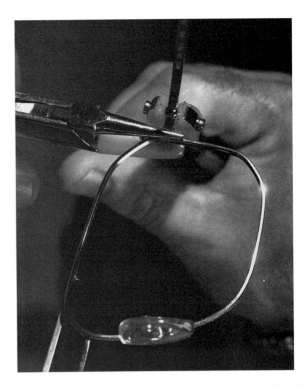

FIGURE **12-15** To change the pantoscopic angle, the endpiece is held, the top and bottom of the hinge area are grasped, and the temple reangled. (From Brooks CW, Borish IM: *System for ophthalmic dispensing,* ed 2, Boston, 1996, Butterworth-Heinemann [Figure 8-46].)

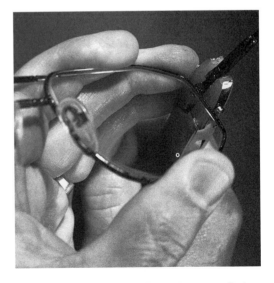

FIGURE **12-16** When the endpiece is too small, the pantoscopic angle can be changed without holding pliers. If the frame does not have enough flexibility, the lens may be removed first. (From Brooks CW, Borish IM: *System for ophthalmic dispensing,* ed 2, Boston, 1996, Butterworth-Heinemann [Figure 8-47].)

and inward slightly so that they are mirror images of each other.

Temple-Fold Angle

To change the fold angle on the commonly used types of metal frames, hold the front in the hand firmly, with the temples closed, and bend the temple upward or downward.

To accomplish this same adjustment using pliers, with the temples closed, the frame front is held firmly in one hand. The top and bottom of the hinge area is gripped with double-padded pliers similar to the manner pictured in Figure 12-15 but with the double-padded pliers pointing toward the center of the frame along the direction of the closed temple. The pliers are rotated in the direction necessary to line up the temples.

Nosepads

Nosepads[3] already should be properly aligned at the factory. From the laboratory standpoint, the most important thing to keep in mind is symmetry. The nosepads should be aligned to be mirror images of one another, as follows:

- Both pads should be at the same height.
- Both pads should be the same distance from the frame front.
- Both pads should be equally angled so that the tops of the pads are closer together than the bottoms.
- Both pads should be equally angled so that the back edges of the pads are slightly farther from each other than the front edges.

[3]For more information on standard alignment of nosepads, see Brooks CW, Borish IM: *System for ophthalmic dispensing,* ed 2, Boston, 1996, Butterworth-Heinemann, pp 171-174.

Proficiency Test Questions

1. True or False? Eyewire forming pliers are used to reshape the upper and sometimes lower rims of a metal frame so that it conforms to the meniscus curve of the edged lens.

2. True or False? Eyewire closure pliers squeeze the top and bottom rims of a *plastic* frame together so that there are no gaps between lens and rim.

3. True or False? In general, metal frames are heated for most adjustments.

4. Which of the following items may be helpful in identifying a lens that is rotated from its correct position in the frame? (*Note:* More than one response may be correct.)

    a. Incorrect cylinder power
    b. A tilted flat-top segment top
    c. Temples that are not parallel with each other
    d. Nasal humping of the eyewire
    e. An off-axis cylinder

5. To check for temple parallelism, the glasses are placed on the table, with the temples open, so that they are in which of the following positions?

    a. Right side up
    b. Upside down
    c. It makes no difference.

6. Vertical alignment or four-point touch is done using which of the following?

    a. Tabletop
    b. Lensmeter
    c. Ruler
    d. Pliers

7. True or False? If the temples are spread to 95 degrees each, they should be re-adjusted so that they are both spread 90 degrees. If this is not done, the frame is not properly standard aligned.

8. True or False? For plastic frames, the temple fold angle should be changed without using heat.

9. Which of the following statements about nosepad alignment is false?

    a. Both pads should be at the same height.
    b. Both pads should be the same distance from the frame front.
    c. Both pads should be equally angled so that the tops of the pads are closer together than the bottoms.
    d. Both pads should be equally angled so that the back edges of the pads are slightly farther from each other than the front edges.
    e. All of the statements about nosepad alignment are true.

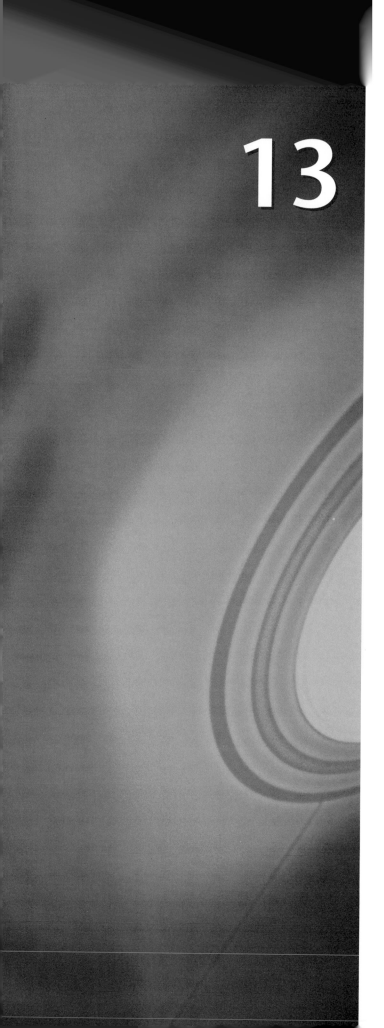

13

Drilled, Slotted, and Notched Mountings

A variety of ways exist to hold lenses in eyeglass frames. The most common method is to bevel the edge of the lens and place it in a frame that has a groove in the rims. One of the most popular methods of mounting lenses that has survived numerous changes in frames and lenses is to drill holes in the lenses and attach the lenses to the frame with screws or other types of posts through the lenses.

Another long-standing method for keeping frames and lenses together is achieved by cutting a groove in the edge of the lens. The lens is held to the frame with a nylon cord.

This chapter explains how to work with drilled, slotted, and notched lenses. The next chapter discusses grooved mountings.

Rimless Defined

Almost any type of frame that does not have a plastic or metal rim around the lens has been called rimless. Many different types of rimless-style frames exist. From a technical standpoint, frames that may be classified as rimless are called *mountings* instead of frames. In this chapter the terms are used interchangeably.

TYPES OF RIMLESS MOUNTINGS

If a frame has no rims at all and no connection between the bridge and endpiece areas, other than the lenses, it is referred to as a *three-piece mounting* (Figure 13-1). Without the lenses, the frame is three separate pieces.

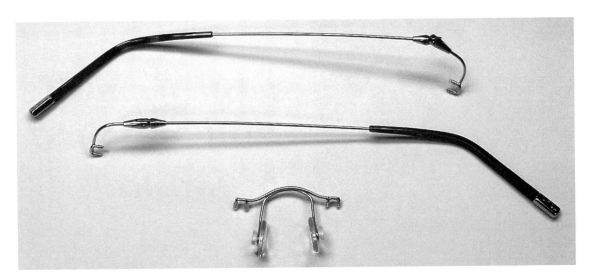

FIGURE **13-1** Without the lenses, a rimless, three-piece mounting consists of three pieces: one centerpiece and two endpieces with temples.

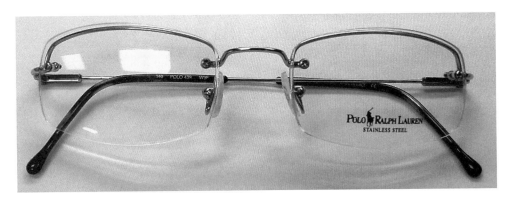

FIGURE **13-2** A semirimless mounting has a top bar that connects the center and endpieces. Without the lenses, the mounting is one unit, not the three pieces characteristic of a true rimless mounting.

Mountings that have the central bridge area attached to the endpieces with a metal bar that runs along the top, back side of the lens are called *semirimless mountings* (Figure 13-2).

Rimless mountings may be further classified by how the lenses are attached. A style of mounting that holds notched lenses in place by spring tension, with clips, is called *Balgrip mountings*. Notching is now seldom used alone. More often it is used in combination with drilling to lend stability to the mounting.

Frames whose lenses are grooved around the edge then held in place with nylon cord are called *nylon cord frames, string mounts,* or *nylon supras*. Nylon cord frames are a category by themselves. However, they still sometimes are referred to as *rimless*. Nylon cord frames are considered in the next chapter and are shown in Figure 14-1.

PARTS OF A RIMLESS MOUNTING

Parts of a rimless frame are unique and have specific terminology. If a rimless mounting attaches the lenses to the frame with screws, the screw passes through a part of a traditionally designed mounting called a *strap*. Technically the strap is an *area* of the mounting. In the original type of rimless mounting, this area consisted of the following parts (Figure 13-3):

- The *shoe* (or *shoulder*) that braces against the edge of the lens
- Between the shoe and the lens edge may or may not be a thin metal *spring*
- An *ear* (or *tongue*) extends behind the lens. Sometimes the lens has two of these—one on the front surface of the lens and one on the back. Together

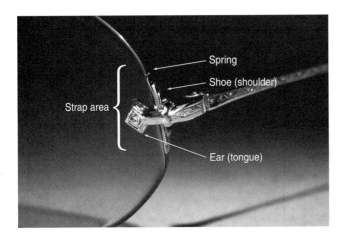

FIGURE **13-3** A close-up of the strap area of an old-fashioned rimless mounting. Newer mountings will not have as many parts. In most cases, only one "ear" or "tongue" is on either the front or back of the lens, but not on both sides. Or, this part of the strap area may not even exist on many new mountings. (From Brooks CW, Borish IM: *System for ophthalmic dispensing,* ed 2, Boston, 1996, Butterworth-Heinemann [Figure 1-22].)

with the screw they clamp the lens in place. Most people call the ear the *strap,* even though technically the strap is the entire area. However, because of common usage, this chapter does the same.

Now, however, mountings are widely different in the specifics of how the frame is constructed at the point of attachment to the lens.

Types of Lens Drills

A number of options are available for drilling lenses. These include the following:

- Nonelectric hand-held drills
- Basic electric stand drills
- In-edger drills
- Computer-assisted drills

The information contained in this chapter begins with principles and builds with explanations of drilling options in the following sections. Procedures explained in sections on the most basics methods are applicable to other methods also and help in an overall understanding of how lenses are mounted.

Wearer Safety Issues

In 1971 the Food and Drug Administration passed a ruling that mandates that lenses must be capable of

withstanding an impact of a $^5/_8$ inch steel ball dropped from a height of 50 inches. All glass lenses had to be hardened to increase their impact resistance. The only available method for hardening glass lenses was heat tempering. Heat tempering creates internal stress in the lens. Drilling a lens and screw mounting it to the frame also sets up stress on the lens. The combination of heat tempering stress and lens mounting stress almost guarantees that the lens will break if struck on the edge. Because glass lenses were still a large segment of the market, this drastically reduced the use of rimless mountings.

Chemical tempering is now the method of choice for hardening glass. Chemical tempering makes it possible to drill-mount a glass lens. This type of lens passes the drop ball test but is still not a good option for rimless eyewear compared with other lens choices available in plastic materials. An Optical Laboratories Association (OLA) technical paper states that drilling (or grooving) a glass lens "produces microscopic surface cracking, which will inevitably propagate and spread. The OLA strongly advises its members against it."[1] For liability reasons most laboratories are not willing to put glass lenses in a rimless mounting, although no specific prohibitions exist against it.

COMPARING LENS MATERIALS FOR RIMLESS USE

Of the available lens materials, glass is the least desirable for rimless eyewear. For a number of years the standard lens material used in rimless eyewear was the standard CR-39 plastic. However, CR-39 is not as good as some other lens materials because it has a tendency to flake and crack at the mounting points.[2]

Polycarbonate material is used regularly for rimless eyewear, but its use is associated with a few downsides. Because polycarbonate lenses are softer than regular plastic lenses, if the lens is not drilled properly and too much heat is produced, the hole may enlarge and cause the mounting assembly to loosen. Because of internal stress when mounted, polycarbonate can still crack at the mounting points, although it is much less likely to do so than conventional plastic materials.

Trivex is emerging as a highly desirable material for rimless eyewear. Like polycarbonate, Trivex is also highly impact resistant, yet it does not crack or distort around the holes of a rimless mounting, even when surfaced thin.[3]

---

[1]Bruneni JL: Ask the labs, *Eyecare Business,* February 1996.
[2]Morgan E: Working with Trivex, *Eyecare Business,* February 2003, p 30.
[3]Bruneni JL: Ask the labs, *Eyecare Business,* January 2003, p 30.

Edge Thickness for Rimless Lenses

No one wants a thick edge on a rimless lens. Everyone sees the edge. This should be a consideration for dispensers. On the other hand, rimless lenses have to have enough thickness for the drill mountings. This raises the question of what types of lens shapes and materials are most appropriate for rimless. Although the question addresses plus and minus lens edges, one type of lens is not well suited for rimless: the Franklin-style (Executive) lens. This lens is unwieldy for drilled lenses and for the type of grooved mountings that are discussed in Chapter 14.

MINIMIZING MINUS EDGES

In making a minus-powered lens for a rimless mounting, thickness can become an issue, especially for higher-powered minus lenses. Edge thickness can be a problem from a cosmetic standpoint because, without frame rims, the lens edges are highly visible. Edge thickness also can make mounting the lenses more difficult. Dispensers should be advised of the possibilities of producing a thinner lens edge if the minus lenses they order are producing thick edges. The following are some ways to make the edges look better:

- Using a higher-index material
- Using a lens material that can be made thinner in the center, which produces thinner edges (e.g., polycarbonate, Trivex, and a number of high-index plastics)
- Using an aspheric design to reduce minus edge thickness
- Polishing the edges to reduce visibility
- Using as small an eyesize as feasible
- Using a lens shape that does not have long corners— in other words, a frame shape in which the effective diameter is not much bigger than the eyesize
- Using an antireflection coating to reduce lens visibility

PLUS LENS EDGE THICKNESS ERRORS

Plus lenses may have edges that are either too thick or too thin. Each situation is discussed individually, beginning with the plus lens with a thick edge.

Overly Thick Plus Edges

Usually two possibilities exist when a plus lens edge thickness is too thick for a rimless mounting. The first is that a plus lens has been taken from stock as an uncut lens and is edged for a small frame. To bring the edges down to a reasonable size, the whole thickness of the lens must be reduced. To do this, a semifinished lens is

surfaced to power for that particular frame. Using a large, higher–plus-powered finished lens blank for a small frame is inappropriate. (This was explained in Chapter 2 and shown in Figure 2-3.)

The other occurs through frame selection error. The following are some ways to equalize and minimize lens thickness around the whole circumference of a plus lens:

1. Choose a frame that does not require much decentration. In other words, the A and distance between lenses (DBL) of the frame should not be much larger than the wearer's PD to prevent a thick nasal edge.
2. Choose a shape that is closer to a round shape than it is to a narrow oval shape. A frame that is narrow vertically causes a plus lens to have thick upper and lower edges.
3. Choose a shape in which the effective diameter of the frame is not much larger than the frame eyesize.
4. Use an aspheric lens design.

Of course high-index materials reduce overall lens thickness. However, a stock high-index lens will not necessarily have a thinner edge compared with a lower-index lens that is custom surfaced for the wearer's frame.[4]

Thin Edges

A plus lens edge can be too thin for a rimless mounting. A low minus lens with a thin center also can have an edge that is too thin to use for rimless mountings. Because no rim exists to protect the edge of the lens, an edge that is too thin may chip. It also must be thick enough to endure the stress of being mounted at only two points on the lens. A lens that is too thin can break or crack at the mounting point.

How thin is too thin? Opinions vary regarding how thin a lens may be. Some say that the minimum edge thickness for a rimless lens should not be less than 1 mm.[5] If the particular lens material being used at this thickness would not be able to withstand the required impact test, 1 mm will be too thin. Others state the "absolute minimum" to be 1.5 mm, whereas still others say to plan for a minimum of 2.0 to 2.2 mm.[6]

Polycarbonate lenses and lenses made from Trivex are strong enough to hold up extremely well in rimless, even with somewhat thinner lens edges. Most other mid- to high-index plastic materials are suitable for

---

[4]For more on correct frame/lens selection, see Brooks CW, Borish IM: *System for ophthalmic dispensing*, ed 2, Boston, 1996, Butterworth-Heinemann [Chapter 4].)

[5]Herrick T: Three-piece mountings, when lenses *are* the frame, *Lenses & Technology*, April 2000, p 20.

[6]DeFranco LM: Eight tips for processing rimless (or semirimless) eyewear, *Eyecare Business*, August 1999, p 36.

rimless, although they do not have as much resistance to fractures at the drilled areas as do polycarbonate and Trivex. The primary weak point with plastic lenses made from another material than polycarbonate and Trivex is that they may not have as much edge strength as desired if edges are thin.

Flatter Base Curves

It is generally easier to mount a rimless lens with a flatter base curve than one with a steeper base curve. If the plus-powered lens prescription is one that calls for a steep base curve, then an aspheric lens, instead of a regular, nonaspheric lens, should be used. Aspheric lenses may be designed with flatter base curves without degrading the optical quality of the lens. Going to an aspheric design is much more preferable than simply flattening the basic curve of a nonaspheric lens.

Marking and Drilling the Lens

Before drilling a lens, the operator must know exactly where the holes are to be located. If the hole is misplaced, the lens will be too high, too low, or tilted in the frame. Or it may be impossible to mount if the holes do not line up with the mounting points on the frame. Therefore the lenses must be marked or the drilling unit programmed for the correct hole locations ahead of time.

If the lens hole locations are to be marked, they may be marked with use of a drilling template or chart if it is available. If a chart is not available, then the actual frame may be used.

LENS-DRILLING CHARTS, GUIDES, AND TEMPLATES

A lens-drilling chart is a series of pictures of pairs of drilled lenses. These pictures are actual size drawings of the lens shape in every available eyesize. A number of different lens shapes may exist for the same mounting, because rimless lenses are not constrained by rims that limit their shape. The same mounting may look totally different when the shape of the lens changes.

Rimless frames should come with a drill-guide, a template, or an actual-size pattern with drill markings on the pattern. If none is with the frame, it should be available upon request. A drill guide is a picture of the lenses and where the holes are supposed to be. A template looks just like the lens and is placed on the lens. Holes are drilled through the template and on through the lens.

Before using a mounting chart, the operator must first think about the finished product. Even a mounting

chart must be considered in perspective. For example, older types of rimless eyewear have straps that end up on the front and back surfaces of the lens. If the lens is a high-minus lens, the holes in the straps will be closer to the edge of the lens than for a plus lens. This is because they have to be bent open farther to accept the thickness of the lens and therefore are closer to the edge of the lens. The operator should bear in mind how lens power and frame construction may affect lateral hole position before marking the lens for drilling. The vertical position of the holes always will be as indicated on the chart.

Steps to Mark a Lens Using a Drilling Chart

1. Find the size and shape that matches the edged lens.
2. Place the edged lens on the corresponding picture.
3. Line up the lens exactly over the drawn shape. To line the lens up exactly, one eye is closed and the open eye positioned exactly above the lens.
4. When ready to mark the lens, shift position so that the sighting eye is exactly over the location of the hole to be marked.
5. Use a fine-point felt-tipped marking pen to dot the location of the center of the hole with a small dot (Figure 13-4).
6. Reposition yourself so that your open eye is exactly above the next hole. Repeat the procedure for each additional hole to be drilled. Both lenses must be marked.
7. When both lenses have been marked, check to ensure that both lenses are identical by holding right and left lenses back-to-back. Their shapes must overlap exactly. Corresponding dots must be lined up over one another.

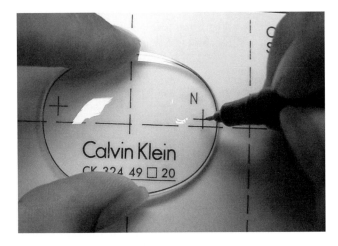

FIGURE **13-4** When using a drilling chart, the operator should be positioned with the sighting eye directly over the place on the lens being marked.

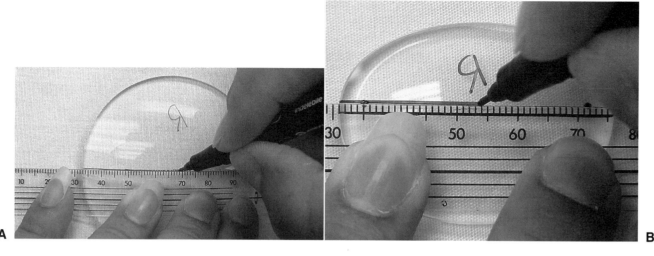

A   **B**

FIGURE **13-5**   Marking a horizontal, 180-degree reference line on a lens before drilling the lens will help keep the lens oriented correctly during drilling and serve as a check after mounting is complete. **A,** A line is being drawn on the uncut. **B,** A line is being drawn through the edged lens. In both cases the three lensmeter dots are used for reference, although this is more visibly evident in **B**.

USING COQUILLES TO MARK THREE-PIECE MOUNTINGS

Three-piece mountings have certain advantages over semirimless mountings regarding lens drilling. The distance between the screws on a semirimless mounting does not have much flexibility. The distance between the nasal and temporal holes in the lens cannot be incorrect.

For a three-piece mounting, the distance between nasal and temporal lens holes is not limited by the top bar. Nothing is connecting the central nosepiece area of the frame to the temporal endpieces.

Before the positions of the drill holes are marked, many recommend drawing a 180-degree reference line across the three lensmeter dots with a permanent felt-tipped overhead transparency pen. The line remains throughout the process. When the lenses are mounted, the lines on both right and left lenses should go straight across the frame. This line may be drawn before or after edging (Figure 13-5). After drawing 180-degree lines on the lenses, edged lenses are held back-to-back to be sure both have identically straight 180-degree lines (Figure 13-6). If they do not, the axis of one lens may be off. If one line is higher than the other, unwanted vertical prism may be present. Finding an error at this point will save wasted time later on.

Many frames come with thin plastic demonstration lenses to make the frame look better on display and to lend stability to the frame. These lenses are called *coquilles,* or *dummy lenses.* If the frame came with attractively

mounted coquilles, the coquilles may be used as guides rather than a chart. To use the coquilles, they are removed from the mounting. Some recommend holding the right edged lens in a back-to-back position with the left dummy lens. (When using this technique the lenses

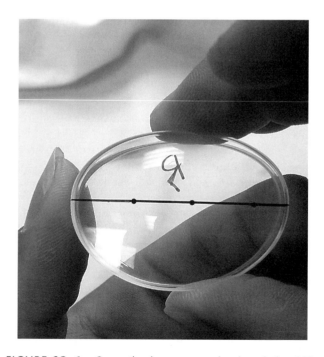

FIGURE **13-6**   Once the lenses are edged and the 180-degree lines drawn on both, hold the lenses back to back. When the shapes are superimposed, the drawn lines should overlap exactly.

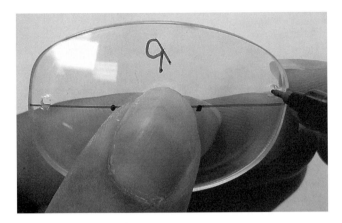

FIGURE **13-7** When using the frame's sample lens or the wearer's old lens as a guide, the eye should be positioned directly over the hole and its location marked.

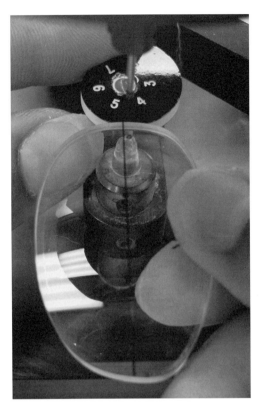

FIGURE **13-8** Some drills have a small-millimeter gauge. The gauge is rotated until the marked drill point is exactly over the proposed location of the hole.

must be right-with-left or left-with-right. This is harder than just holding the edged right lens directly over the dummy right lens, back-to-front. Those who advocate this right-with-left technique, as backward as this seems, maintain that marking right-with-right is more likely to cause the lenses to come out incorrectly.)[7] With experience, each will choose the method that brings them the best results. When the two lenses are aligned, the eye is positioned directly over the place where the hole is to be drilled and the desired location of the hole is marked (Figure 13-7).

DRILLING THE LENS WITH BASIC ELECTRIC STAND DRILLS

The electric stand drill is made like a miniature drill press. The difference between the various types of stand drills is in the way the lens is steadied and held in place so that the drill will create the hole in the intended position on the lens.

A basic stand drill has a base that the back surface of the lens is rested against. The lens is hand held. The marked location for the hole is centered on the base and in some models may be braced against a small millimeter gauge that is rotated to increase or decrease the distance from the edge of the lens to align the location of the hole (Figure 13-8). Once positioned, the gauge is locked in position (Figure 13-9). The gauge is especially useful when the vertical position of the hole is marked on the lens. The horizontal position is set for a certain number of millimeters from the edge of the lens by using the gauge.

The lens should be held so that the angle of the hole will be *perpendicular* to the *front* surface of the lens[8] (Figure 13-10). Without turning the drill on, the drill bit is lowered to a position just above the mark on the lens. If the lens is accurately aligned, the drill is turned on and used to slowly drill through the lens (Figure 13-11). A foot switch is almost a must when drilling because both hands are usually busy with the lens. Pressing too hard causes the lens hole to chip as the drill passes out the back surface of the lens.

The drill bit should go through the lens smoothly. If it does not go through smoothly or goes through more slowly than it should, it is dull and needs to be replaced.

Unless the drill has a lens mounting system that allows the lens to be exactly flipped over, or unless the drill has two drill bits that drill the lens from both sides at once, it is not advisable to turn the lens over and drill from the other side. (Glass lenses are the exception.) Drilling from both sides without the appropriate mechanical assistance makes it too easy to line the hole up wrong and mess up the lens. This is especially true for high minus lenses with thick edges.

[7]Levoy BM: How to work with rimless, *Optometric Weekly*, February 17, 1977, p 34.

[8]Field C: Processing drill-mounted eyewear, *LabTalk*, 28(42):32, 2000.

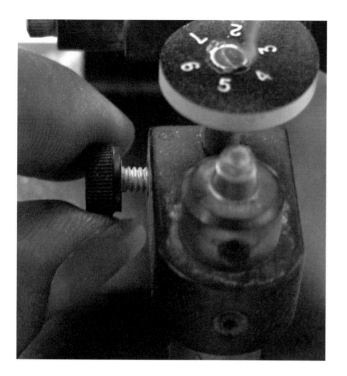

FIGURE **13-9** Once the gauge is correctly positioned, it is locked.

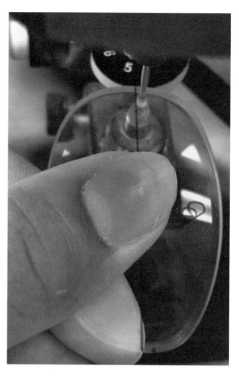

FIGURE **13-11** When pressing the drill bit through the lens, do not press too hard. Drilling through the lens too quickly will cause the back side of the hole to chip.

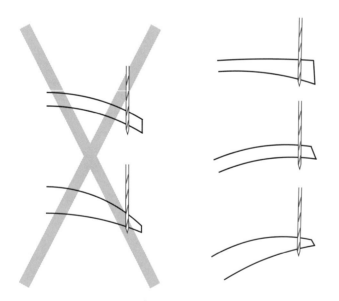

FIGURE **13-10** The left-hand side of the figure shows the angle of a hole incorrectly drilled. The hole is perpendicular to the lens plane, but not perpendicular to the lens surface at the location of the hole. The right-hand side shows the correct angle. The lens must be angled so that the hole is approximately perpendicular to the front surface of the *lens at the location of the hole.*

If the angle of the hole is slanted instead of being perpendicular to the front surface the lens may not mount properly. If this is the case, the hole is straightened by putting the drill back in the hole and, with drill running, the lens is turned to the correct angle. This elongates the hole somewhat and may make it possible to mount the lens.

Chamfering and Smoothing Holes

A drill hole that has not had the sharp edges taken off is just like an edged lens that has not been safety beveled. It is likely to chip. Smoothing off the sharp edges of the hole is called *chamfering.* Chamfering is the equivalent term for safety or pin beveling. To chamfer the edges of the hole either a round diamond burr that is at least twice the diameter of the hole[9], or a small cone tool (Figure 13-12, *A*) is used. The front and back entrances of the hole should be smoothed lightly (Figure 13-12, *B*).

The inside of the hole can be smoothed with a rat-tail file. A rat-tail file is a small-diameter, round file that starts narrow at the tip and increases slightly in diameter

9Yoho A: Keeping the rimless lens tight, *Eyecare Business,* August 2000, p 34.

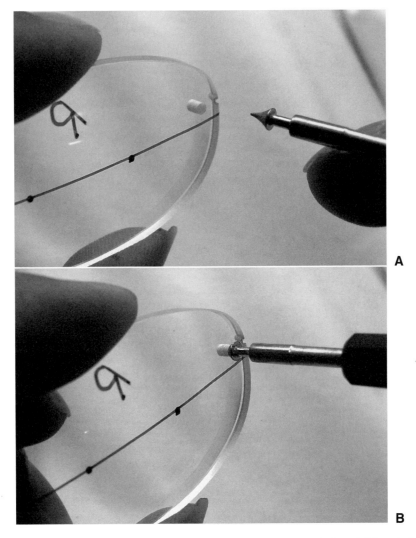

FIGURE **13-12** **A,** A small abrasive cone tool works well to safely bevel (chamfer) the edges of a drilled hole. Leaving the edges of the hole sharp often will cause the hole to chip either during assembly or after the spectacles have been delivered to the wearer. **B,** Chamfering a drilled hole by rotating the tool in the hole.

toward the center of the file (Figure 13-13). The same file may be used to chamfer the edges in the absence of a diamond burr or cone tool (Figure 13-14). However, a rat-tail file cannot be expected to provide the same uniform smoothness.

ATTACHING THE DRILLED LENS TO THE MOUNTING

When assembling the drilled lens and mounting, the operator should use a screwdriver that has a plastic sleeve around the blade to reduce the chance of slipping and gouging the lens surface (Figure 13-15). Lens screws are no different from other screws in that they may

loosen with time. For this reason some people like to use a screw-locking compound on the screw to keep it from loosening. These locking compounds are available from optical suppliers.

Often hex nuts are used to hold the lens in place and are screwed on with a hex wrench (Figure 13-16). To cushion the lens and reduce lens fractures, use of plastic bushings in the drilled holes may be advisable. A plastic bushing looks like a miniature top hat. The plastic bushings are put in from both sides of the hole before the lens is mounted.

Many rimless mountings have only one strap. That strap may be on the front or the back of the lens. If the strap is on the front, the back side of the lens will have

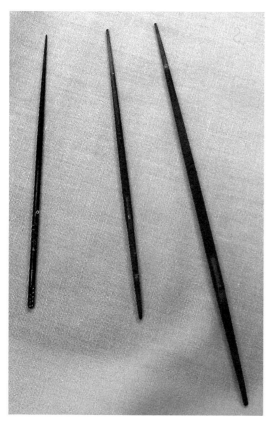

FIGURE **13-13** Rat-tail files are tapered and come in a variety of sizes.

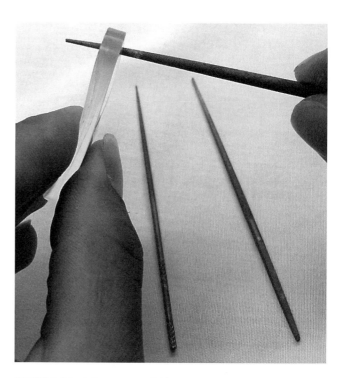

FIGURE **13-14** A rat-tail file may be used to smooth the inside of a drilled hole or to enlarge its diameter.

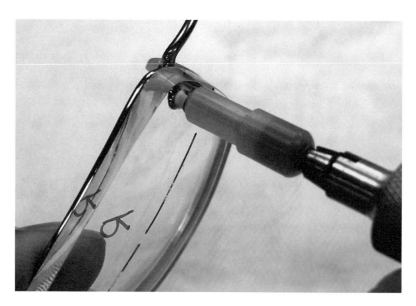

FIGURE **13-15** A screwdriver with a plastic sleeve helps in reducing lens spoilage caused by the blade slipping from the head of the lens screw. This lens is being mounted into a semirimless mounting.

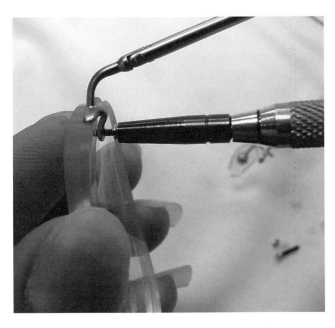

FIGURE **13-16** A hex wrench is used to tighten a nut down. The head of the bolt is held in place with the finger of the other hand to keep it from turning.

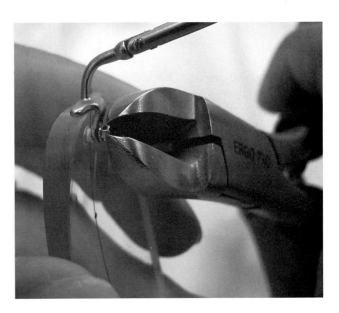

FIGURE **13-17** Once the screw is in place, it needs to be clipped with a cutting pliers to remove excess length.

a nut. A small metal washer is used between the nut and the bushing to keep the nut from crushing the bushing and possibly gouging the lens.[10]

The screw is clipped flush with the nut or strap (Figure 13-17). Next the screw is filed flush. A good file to use is a riffler file (Figure 13-18).

DETECTING MOUNTING FLAWS

One common mounting flaw is to tighten the mounting screws too hard. Screws should be tight. A visible slight amount of pressure distortion on the lens surface is even acceptable. But they should not be so tight that distortion is obvious.[11] This means heavy pressure is in the area and an increased potential exists for the lens breaking at that point. Overtightening a screw also may cause an antireflection (AR) coating on a lens to craze. One suggested method for getting the correct tightness is to tighten the screw as far as it goes, then back it off a half turn.[12]

If two mounting holes are on one side of the lens for style or stability, those two holes must be spaced accurately. If they are too close together or too far apart, they will cause more stress on the lens. Using a high-end manual

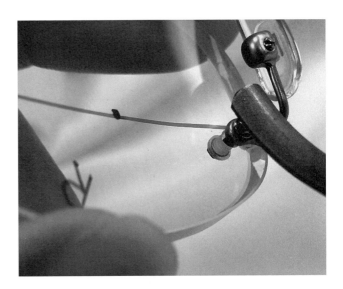

FIGURE **13-18** A clipped screw has a rough end. The end of the screw is smoothed after it has been clipped. The file being used is a spoon-shaped riffler file. Its form helps keep the rough file surface away from the surface of the lens.

lens drill or a computer-assisted drill system will reduce this type of flaw.

Notching Lenses

Lenses may be notched on either side and held in place with clips on the frame that fit into the notches. This type of mounting is called a *Balgrip mounting* or *spring tension semirimless mounting*. The clips are on either side

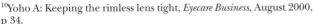

[10]Yoho A: Keeping the rimless lens tight, *Eyecare Business*, August 2000, p 34.
[11]Yoho A: Keeping the rimless lens tight, *Eyecare Business*, August 2000, p 34.
[12]Herrick T: Three-piece mountings, when lenses *are* the frame, *Lenses & Technology*, April 2000, p 22.

of the top bar of the frame. The top bar is curved so that it must be pulled apart slightly so that the clips fit into the lens. The lenses are held in place with spring tension from the top bar. Use of notches alone to hold the lenses in place is rare. Instead notches are used in combination with drilled holes to increase the stability of the mounting.

When mountings with notched lenses were used more commonly, it was not unusual to see small machines called *Balgrip Lens Groovers* in the laboratory. These used a narrow grinding wheel to notch the lenses. When a request for notched lenses occurs, a piece of machinery like this is not necessary. Lenses even may be notched by hand with a rat-tail file. However, to use the drill with a milling bit to make the notch is much easier.

USING A MILLING BIT TO NOTCH A LENS

A milling bit may be used to notch the edge of a lens. It is much easier than trying to notch a lens by hand and does a better job. The milling bit may be lowered onto the edge of the lens as in drilling (Figure 13-19), or the lens may be pressed against the side of the milling bit. After the notch is created, the edges of the notch are smoothed (Figure 13-20).

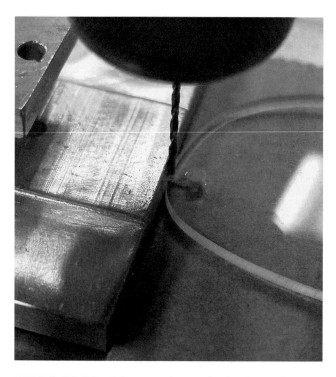

FIGURE **13-19** A lens may be notched with a milling bit. In this photo there is a small piece of cardboard under the temporal half of the lens. This allows the lens to be angled some and also allows extra space under the lens for when the milling bit comes out the other side.

Once drilled or notched lenses have been mounted, the drawn 180-degree lines should be along the 180 of the frame (Figure 13-21).

DRILLING POLYCARBONATE LENSES

For polycarbonate lenses the lens should not be drilled straight through in one pass. Instead about 0.5 mm at a time should be drilled. After each 0.5 mm, the drill is backed out and the drill operator waits for the material to cool. Then the next half-millimeter is done. Pressing through all at once "will push the material through and blow it out in a hump on the back side of the lens."[13] It also will cause the hole to be larger than intended and result in an unstable mounting.[14] Drilling with a dull bit will also create unwanted heat, even when proper drilling techniques are applied. This, too, may result in a hole that is slightly larger than intended.

AN HISTORICAL NOTE ON HAND DRILLS

With plastic lenses, drilling a lens without an electric drill is possible but not necessarily efficient. The correct size drill bit can be mounted in a hand chuck with a swivel handle. To start the drill hole, the lens should be indented with a pointed instrument. The drill bit is placed in the indentation and turned but without a lot of pressure. Too much pressure with a hand *or* electric drill causes hairline cracks around the hole. When using a hand drill, the operator should not drill more than halfway through the lens before turning it over and drilling from the other side. Again, the operator begins by indenting the back surface of the lens with a sharp instrument at the intended point of drilling, then drills from the back. Applying too much pressure will cause plastic to break away next to the hole.

Notes Regarding Glass Lenses

Because plastic, polycarbonate, and Trivex lens materials are so much less likely to break in a rimless mounting than is glass, glass is no longer considered a good option for rimless mountings. If glass lenses are used in a rimless mounting, the lens must be drilled alternately first from one side, then the other, until the two holes meet halfway through the lens. This prevents the hole from chipping and ruining the lens as the drill comes out the other side. Glass lenses almost always chip out around the hole unless this is done. When drilling glass the operator should lubricate the place where the lens

[13]DeFranco LM: Eight tips for processing rimless (or semirimless) eyewear, *Eyecare Business*, August 1999, p 37.
[14]DeFranco LM: Drilling polycarbonate can be hot, *Optical Dispensing News*, No. 1, September 26, 2000.

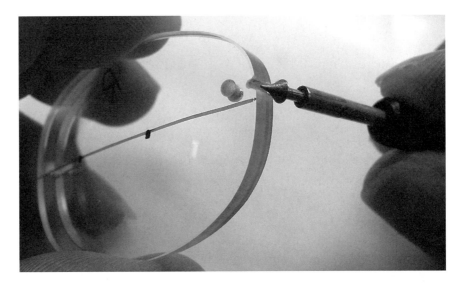

FIGURE **13-20**   Notches need to be safety beveled too. A cone tool works for both holes and notches.

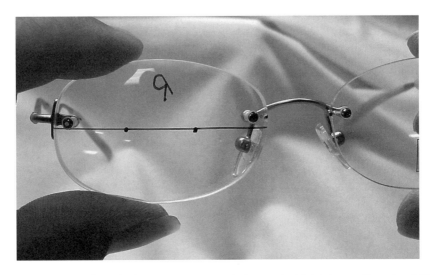

FIGURE **13-21**   When the lenses are mounted, the marked 180-degree lines should both be on the same level. They should both be exactly horizontal as if they were one continuous line.

and drill meet with oil to prevent heat buildup. Without oil, breakage increases and drill bits are ruined quickly.

Once again, glass lenses are not recommended for rimless or grooved mountings. The lens is weaker than a normally beveled and mounted lens and, though not illegal, is not advisable.

USING THE FRAME TO MARK FOR SEMIRIMLESS MOUNTINGS

With semirimless mountings, the shape of the top of the lens matches the curve of the top bar of the mounting. The following is the procedure:

1. With the frame flat on the table, hold the lens in front of the mounting as it should appear after it has been mounted.
   a. The top of the shape should follow the curve of the top bar.
   b. When correctly aligned, the top bar should have about one third of its thickness showing above the edge of the lens.[15]
2. Use a fine-point, felt-tipped marking pen to dot the location of the nasal screw hole.

---

[15]Levoy BM: How to work with rimless, *Optometric Weekly*, February 17, 1977, p 39.

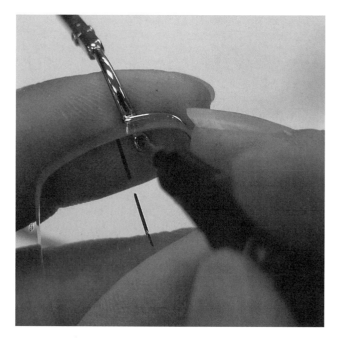

FIGURE **13-22**   This is a semirimless mounting. When no chart is available, the frame may be used as a guide for marking and drilling the lenses. First the nasal hole is marked and drilled. The lens is mounted in the nasal hole. With nasal hole drilled and lens mounted nasally, the lens is swung into position as it should appear when finished. Next the location of the temporal hole is marked as shown here.

3. Repeat the procedure for the other lens.
4. Hold the just-marked lenses back-to-back. The two nasal marks must overlap exactly.
5. Drill the hole for the first lens and smooth it as described in the section on lens drilling.
6. Mount the nasal side of the lens, leaving it loose enough to swing it away from its normal position.
7. Hold the half-mounted lens as it should look when correctly mounted. Mark the location of the temporal screw hole (Figure 13-22). (The biggest pitfall here is the possibility of misaligning the axis of the cylinder.)
8. Either remove the lens from the mounting and then drill it, or swing the lens upward or downward and drill the temporal hole with the lens still in the mounting (Figure 13-23).
9. Repeat the process to mark and drill the temporal hole for the other lens.

DRILLING GUIDES

Some frame manufacturers make drilling guides available to simplify drilling. Silhouette uses a plastic guide for double-hole mountings. To use this system, the 180-degree line is marked on the uncut lens before

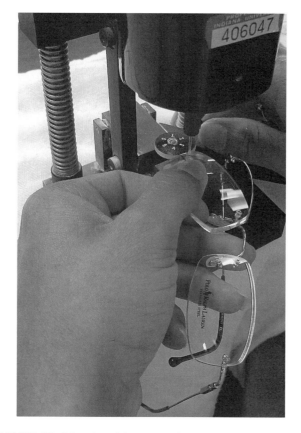

FIGURE **13-23**   On this semirimless mounting the nasal hole has been drilled and mounted. The temporal hole has been marked with the lens mounted nasally. Now the temporal hole may be drilled. As in this photo, it may be possible to drill the lens without removing the lens from the frame.

edging (as discussed earlier in the chapter). After edging, transparent tape is placed on the front of the lens to protect the surface. The nasal and temporal lens drilling positions are marked by using the notches on the edge of the pattern as guides (Figure 13-24). Next a strip of double-sided adhesive tape is placed on the inside of the drilling guide to hold it to the lens (Figure 13-25).

To drill the nasal holes, the drill guide is stuck on the lens so that the center line of the guide is parallel to the 180-degree line marked on the lens. For the temporal holes, the bottom line of the guide is parallel to the lens' 180-degree line (Figure 13-26). The lens is drilled by pressing the drill bit into the holes in the drill guide (Figure 13-27).

Improvements in Electric Drills

A variety of options are available with basic electric drills. These options become increasingly important because

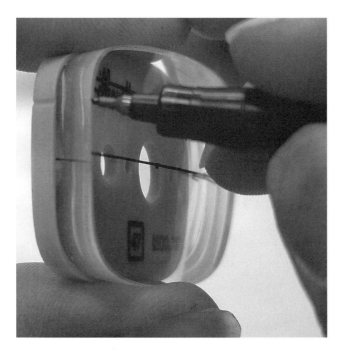

FIGURE **13-24**   Here the pattern has been made to serve as a type of template in the drilling sequence. The edge of the lens is marked at the level of the notch on the pattern. This establishes the height where holes will be drilled.

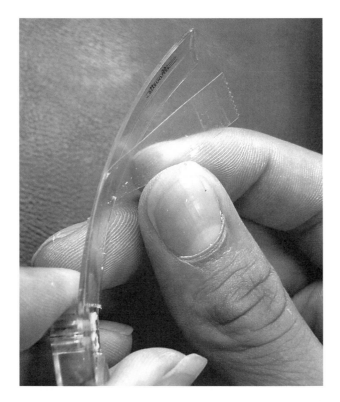

FIGURE **13-25**   Double-sided tape on the drilling guide will hold the guide to the lens during drilling.

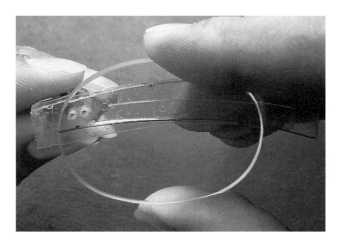

FIGURE **13-26**   Here the lens guide is being applied to the lens.

of (1) the large variety of rimless designs available, (2) the necessity for drilling more than just two holes in one lens, and (3) the increased number of lenses that are slotted or notched. The following list outlines some improvements available with some electric stand drills (with options varying according to drill manufacturer):

- *An edge gauge:* An edge gauge allows the hole to be positioned a known distance inward from the edge of the lens (see Figure 13-8).
- *A clamp-down holding system to hold the lens securely for drilling*
- *The ability to transfer measurements from one lens to the other:* If the drill base guide has horizontal and vertical scales, one lens is marked first. It is then aligned and clamped in the drill base guide. The second lens then is clamped symmetrically in place. Hole location measurements are transferred to the second lens.
- *A lens-holding system that leaves the adhesive-pad blocks on the lenses and uses the blocks to hold the lenses in the drill*[16] (Figure 13-28): This system has several advantages. It assures that the lenses will be on axis. The 180-degree line is exactly as it was for edging. It confirms that both lenses will be drilled the same. It makes replacement of a single lens easier if one lens was incorrect or if one lens has to be replaced later because of damage to the lens or a prescription change.
- *The ability to tilt both lenses at once:* When drilling a lens, the hole should be drilled approximately perpendicular to the first surface. If both lenses are mounted at the same time and one lens is angled for drilling, the second lens will be angled identically. This way both nasal holes will be tilted the same and

---

[16]One such drill is The Smart Drill (Smart Lab Equipment Co, Grants Pass, Ore.).

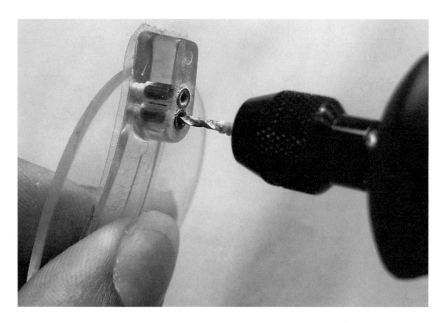

FIGURE **13-27**   When using a drilling guide, the drill can be held "free hand" without having to be mounted on a stand.

drilled. Then after readjusting the tilt, the operator may drill both temporal holes.

- *The ability to transfer the frame manufacturer's hole location specifications to the scale on the drill base guide:* For example, vertical hole location could be specified as distance above or below the boxing center; horizontal location as distance from the edge of the lens. For example, if a lens has two temporal holes their locations could be specified as 5 mm above center and 3 and 6 mm in from the temporal edge of the lens, respectively.
- *Twin drill bits:* Twin drill bits approach the lens from both front and back sides at the same time. Drill bits meet in the middle and produce chip-free guide-holes that will ream out smoothly.[17]
- *Variable-hole diameters:* Hole diameters can be varied without having to change drill bits.
- *The ability to move the drill or table in a controlled manner to allow for slotting and notching of lenses*
- *Reflective screen:* The reflective screen option allows a parallax-free view of the lens and drill.[18]

DRILLING BLOCKED LENSES

Some drills allow the lenses to remain blocked during drilling. Because the lenses are held in place by the

blocks, the cylinder axis cannot be off if the lens was correctly edged. The following is a representative drilling sequence for the type of drill that was shown in Figure 13-28.

Before edging, the base curve of the lens is measured (Figure 13-29). Once the lens is edged, it is mounted on the drill base. The lens is angled by tilting the lens to the corresponding base curve setting (Figures 13-30 and 13-31). This angles the lens so that the drill enters the front surface at the correct angle. (The importance of this was discussed earlier and illustrated in Figure 13-10.)

Drilling charts designed for ease of use with this particular drill show both horizontal and vertical measurements for all the holes and notches in the mounting. These charts also tell which drill bit sizes are needed for each hole (Figure 13-32). The vertical distance from the 180-line to the first hole is dialed. This moves the lens vertically (Figure 13-33).

With the horizontal scale set to zero, the edge of the lens is "zero-ed in" by sliding the base of the stand until the edge touches the drill (Figure 13-34). Now the stand is moved to the notch or hole location indicated on the chart using a screw-mechanism to set the horizontal distance on the scale (Figure 13-35). At this point the lens may be notched or drilled as needed (Figure 13-36). In this example a notch and a hole are on the nasal side. After notching the lens, the measurements are reset. When necessary, a different size bit is used to drill the second hole (Figure 13-37).

---

[17]The LAB-Tech DM-3 Drilling System (LAB-Tech, Inc., Miami) has this feature.
[18]The Drillrite Automatic Lens Drill (Nu-Tec Optical Equipment, Richardson, Texas) has this feature.

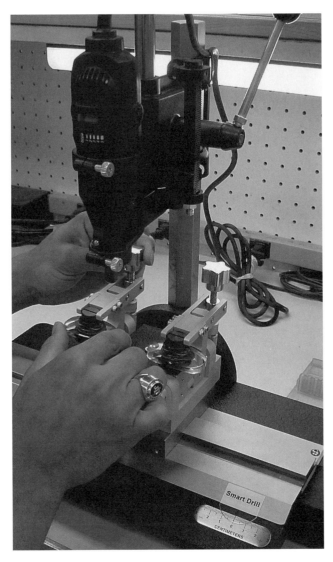

FIGURE **13-28** This lens drilling system holds the lenses in place by the lens blocks. Because lenses are still blocked, it is not necessary to draw a 180-degree line on the lens. The clamping system ensures an accurate 180-degree alignment.

Slotted Lenses

Some lenses are held in place with a *clip* (Figure 13-38). The clip is slipped into a slot in the lens and stays in place by a tensile spring effect. This happens because the slot is slightly smaller than the distance between the two sections of the wire that makes up the clip. Clips may come in different lengths, depending upon lens thickness at the location of the slot. To provide enough lens substance for the clip, the lens must be no less than 2.7 mm thick at the position of the slot.[19]

---

[19]Air Titanium Optician's Video (Lindberg Optic Design, Frichsparken, Denmark).

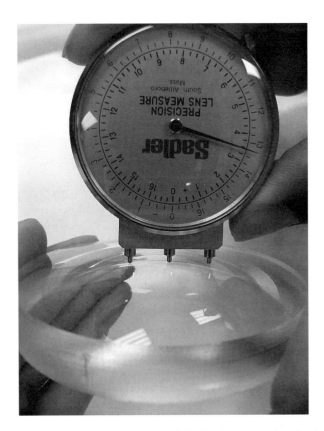

FIGURE **13-29** With certain drills the lens may be tilted for drilling according to base curve. This lens has a +3.50 D base curve.

The lens is marked with a 180-degree line, *R* or *L*, and an *N* for the nasal side and placed on the drilling chart. In preparation for slotting, the center of the slot is dotted (Figure 13-39). Then the lens is marked with a line drawn perpendicular to the center of the slot (Figure 13-40). Unless the nasal and temporal slots are at exactly the same height, two lines will be on the lens, one for each slot.

If the slot is vertical, the line(s) will be parallel to the 180. The lens is secured in place on the table and the desired position of the slot centered (Figure 13-41). The table is placed on the base of the stand[20] and locked into position (Figure 13-42).

A drill cuts into a plastic lens by being pressed into the lens from above. However, with use of a "milling drill bit," the "drill" can now cut sideways. To cut a slot in a lens, the milling bit must have the ability to move laterally.[21] The milling drill bit is now set to move left

---

[20]A space bar is used between the back edge of the table and the stand. The thickness of the bar causes the location of the slot to come out as needed.
[21]It would be possible to construct a table for the drill stand that moved the lens laterally.

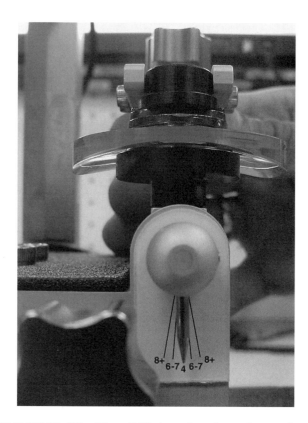

FIGURE **13-30** The +3.50 base lens from the previous figure has been edged. It is still blocked and has been mounted on the drill. For this drill, lenses with a base curve of +4.00 D and below are considered flat enough not to require any tilt when drilled.

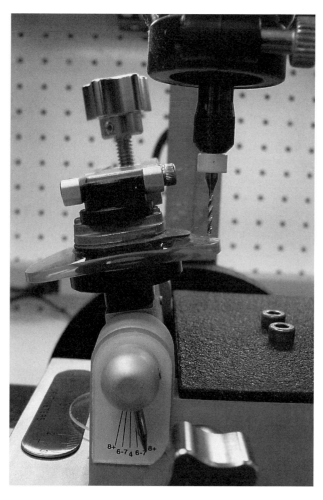

FIGURE **13-31** For comparison we see how much tilt is required to drill this +8.00 D base curve lens. The drill is basically perpendicular to the front surface of the lens.

and right from the center point of the slot by equal amounts. The total length of the move corresponds to the length of the slot.

The milling bit is lowered onto the lens and drilled through the center of where the slot will be (Figure 13-43). A locking mechanism is loosened (Figure 13-44), the milling bit pressed slightly into the lens surface, and then moved laterally. This removes plastic along the whole length of the slot (Figure 13-45). The bit is lowered into the lens a little at a time, each time moving the bit back and forth. This process is repeated about 15 to 20 times until the slot goes all the way through the lens. (The number of times varies, depending upon lens thickness.)

Once the slot is through the lens, the bit is raised. It is moved to one end of the slot and the end of the slot "drilled." This process is repeated for the other end. This smoothes the inside ends of the slot.

Next the slot needs to be chamfered (safety beveled). This may be done with the drill, a cone-shaped tool, or by hand with the same type of tool. When done with the drill, the cone-shaped tool is mounted like a drill bit. The lens is held in the hands and moved back and forth

across the spinning cone in the drill. Both the front and the back of the slot must be beveled. When safety beveled with the hand tool, the cone-shaped hand tool is rotated in the slot (Figure 13-46).

The clip is cleaned with alcohol (Figure 13-47) and the clip/slot fit is checked (Figure 13-48). The clips should slide into the lens easily. If force is used, stress will be introduced into the lens and the possibility of breakage increases. Clips from looped wire may be expanded or compressed (Figure 13-49). However, the top and bottom wire must remain parallel with each other so that they contact the ends of the slots evenly.

When all is prepared, glue is added to the inside slot of the lens or to the clip (Figure 13-50) and the clip secured in the lens (Figure 13-51). When glue is applied to the inside of the slot, excess glue should be wiped off the lens surface with alcohol before the clips are pressed into the slots.

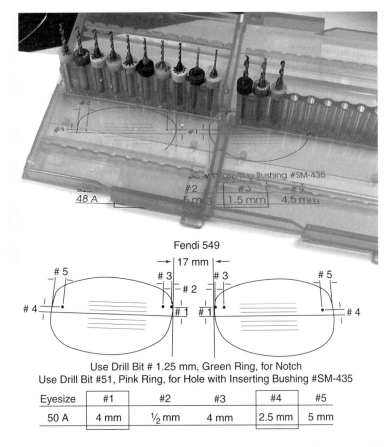

Fendi 549

Use Drill Bit # 1.25 mm, Green Ring, for Notch
Use Drill Bit #51, Pink Ring, for Hole with Inserting Bushing #SM-435

Eyesize	#1	#2	#3	#4	#5
50 A	4 mm	½ mm	4 mm	2.5 mm	5 mm

FIGURE **13-32** This chart indicates that the nasal hole is 4 mm above the 180-degree line (measure #1), the temporal hole is 2.5 mm above the 180-degree line (measure #4), the nasal notch is 0.5 mm in from the nasal edge (measure #2), the nasal hole is 4 mm in from the nasal edge (measure #3), and the temporal hole is 5 mm in from the temporal edge (measure #5). It also tells exactly which diameter drill to use for each hole or notch.

COMPUTER-ASSISTED DRILLS

The reason for going to a computer-assisted drill is not necessarily to achieve a higher quality drill-mounting job than would otherwise be possible with other drills. Using a good quality manual drill that has some of the better available options will produce a drilled lens mounting of outstanding quality. The reason many elect to use a computer-assisted drill is to "maintain the quality of workmanship while increasing productivity."[22] In other words, a computer-assisted drill should decrease the amount of time required for each job.

Another reason for going to a computer-assisted drill is to increase the number of people who are able to participate in the drilling process. Computerizing many of the steps in the process makes it easier to train others to do drill-mounts. However, the comparatively high

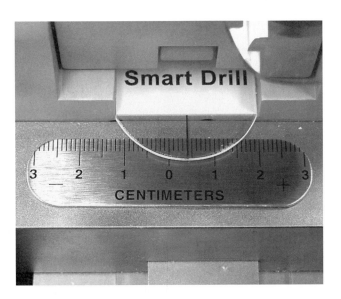

FIGURE **13-33** To set up the nasal side for drilling for the mounting in the previous figure, the hole is set for 4 mm above the midline.

---

[22]Freeburg S et al: L & T review, OptiDrill CNC Drilling System, *Lenses & Technology*, April 2001, p 20.

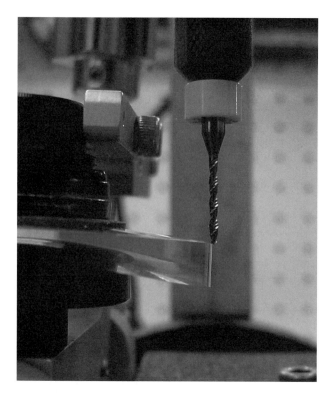

FIGURE **13-34** With the horizontal scale set for zero, the stand table is moved until the edge of the lens is pressed tight against the tip of the drill bit. This establishes the horizontal zero point for the nasal holes of the right lens.

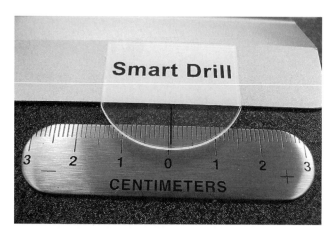

FIGURE **13-35** In preparation for cutting the notch, the table is moved 0.5 mm using a crank handle.

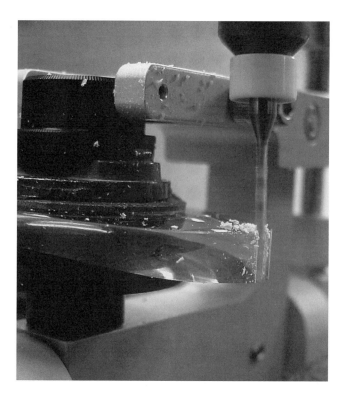

FIGURE **13-36** The drill accurately "notches" the lens 0.5 mm.

Other features available for computer-assisted drills will be similar to those features listed for manual drills. In evaluating computer-assisted drills, the same features that are attractive for manual drills should be searched for in a computer-assisted drill.

Computer-assisted drills generally interface with a personal computer (Figure 13-52).

THE IN-EDGER DRILL

WECO has an edger that drills the lens while it is still in the edger (Figure 13-53). To use this option, the WECO blocker also must be used. An image of the drilled demo lens or the wearer's old drilled lens is projected on a screen in the blocker during layout. Then a cursor is moved to the location of the hole and an X is placed over the future position of the holes. The edger edges the lenses then drills them as indicated in the blocking process.

Working with Older-Style, Double-Strap Mountings

Older style rimless mountings have a double-strap assembly and were used extensively in years past.

cost of computer-assisted drills is justifiable only for laboratories that have a high volume of drill mountings.

Computer-assisted drills have, or should have, a capacity to store and recall a database of drill, slot, and notch positions for a large number of mountings in their full range of available sizes and shapes.

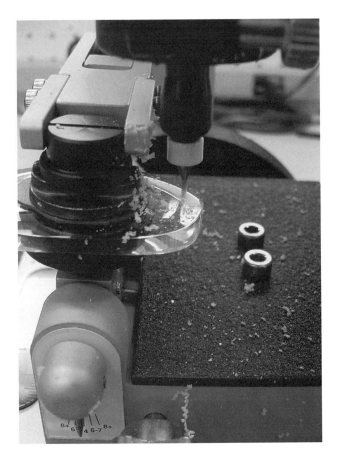

FIGURE **13-37** After notching the lens, the lens table is horizontally repositioned to 4 mm. The hole is drilled using a different sized drill bit.

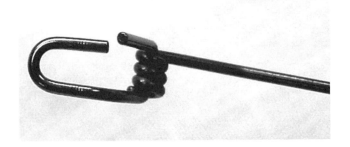

FIGURE **13-38** One type of Air Titanium frame design uses a clip that slips into a slot in the lens. The clip stays in the lens slot primarily because of the spring-tension effect of the clip.

Fortunately, laboratories seldom have to deal with these types of mountings now. When these mountings appear, the following discussion provides guidance on how to work with them.

Double-strap mountings have a strap on the front and on the back of the lens. This helps stabilize the

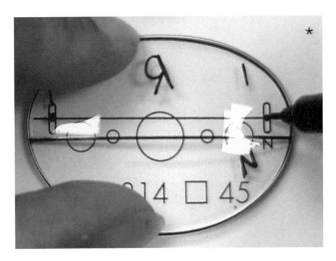

FIGURE **13-39** This drilling chart is on a translucent sheet of plastic that is used first for one lens, then is turned over for the second lens. The centers of the slots are dotted.

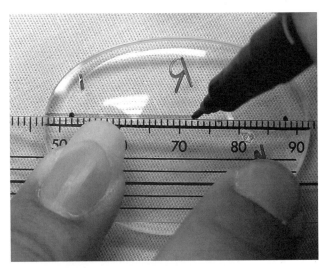

FIGURE **13-40** After the slot centers are dotted, each gets a horizontal line drawn through it. On this lens both slots are at the same height, so the same line goes through both slot centers.

lens/frame assembly. The problem is that each lens has a slightly different edge thickness. Therefore the straps have to be realigned for the width of the lens edge. If the edge is wider, the straps go farther out before they bend around the lens edge. This positions the hole closer to the edge. For normal-thickness lenses, the procedure for marking and drilling the lens is basically the same as for any other rimless mounting. A lens-mounting chart or a dummy lens is used to mark the lenses. Next the lens is drilled.

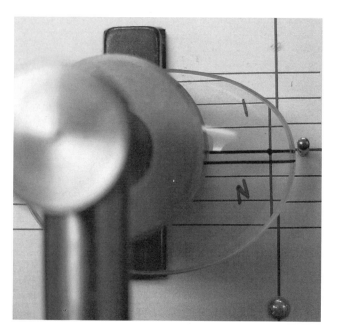

FIGURE **13-41**   The lens is placed in the lens holder on the mounting table so that the slot center is on the intersection of vertical and horizontal lines. The horizontal line running through the slot center overlaps the horizontal line on the table. This way the finished slot will be precisely vertical.

ADJUSTING THE DOUBLE-STRAP AREA

The way the straps are adjusted before mounting the lenses strongly influences the alignment of the assembled spectacles. For example, if the straps are bent forward, even though they are still parallel to one another, the temple will be spread too widely.

The nasal and temporal lens straps are bent to the correct angles, beginning with the nasal straps. Next the centerpiece on the lens is held so that the lens edge is between the two straps. This way it is possible to see if the "front" of the spectacles will align properly. When satisfied, the lens hole is aligned with the holes in the straps and a "tap" used to rethread the straps (Figure 13-54). (A tap is a lens threader mounted in a chuck handle.) Rethreading allows the screw to go through the straps at the proper angle. Next the temporal straps are done.

The shoe and spring section of the strap area contribute to the stability of the lens mounting. The shoe and spring should be touching the edge of the lens above and below the strap with moderate pressure. (To view this area of the frame, see Figure 13-3.) If necessary, the shoe is bent to establish proper tension against the lens edge.

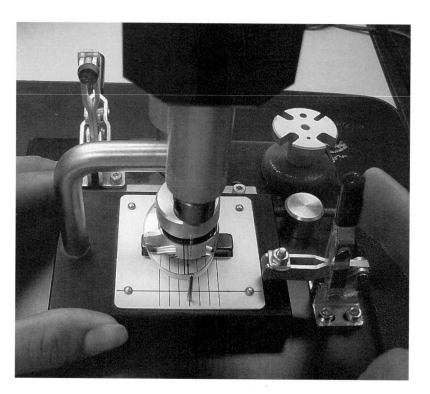

FIGURE **13-42**   The table is placed on the base of the stand and locked into position.

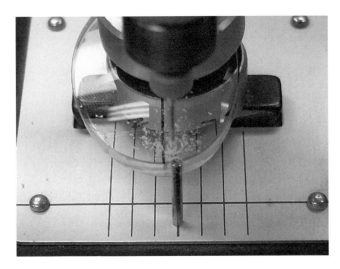

FIGURE **13-43** A hole is drilled through the center of where the slot will be.

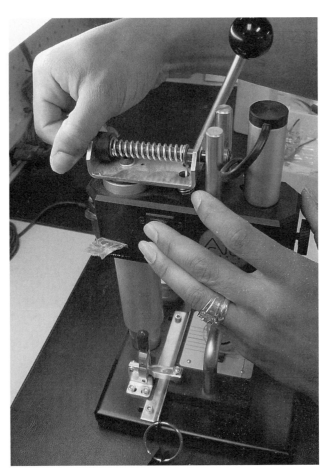

FIGURE **13-44** To make a slot, the locking mechanism is loosened to allow the drill to swing back and forth as it cuts the slot.

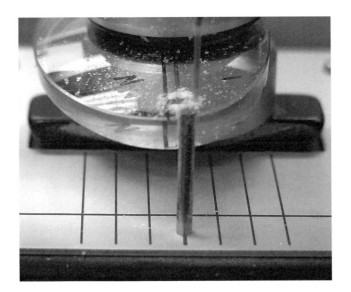

FIGURE **13-45** The drilling bit is pressed lightly into the surface and moved back and forth to remove plastic along the length of the slot. The process is repeated 15 or 20 times until the slot goes all the way through the lens.

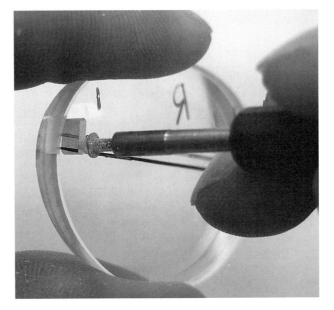

FIGURE **13-46** A cone-shaped tool will safety bevel (chamfer) the lens slot and will keep the slot from chipping.

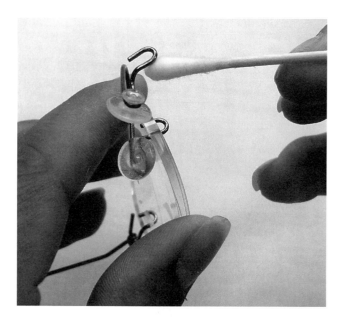

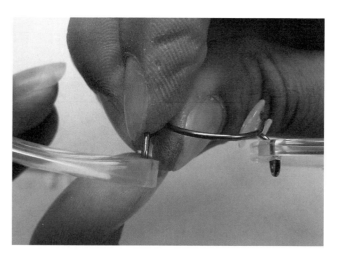

FIGURE **13-48**   Before applying lock glue, the fit of the clip in the slot is checked. If the tension is not correct, the clip needs to be widened or narrowed.

FIGURE **13-47**   The clip needs to be free of any dirt or oils before being put into the slot. Cleaning it with alcohol helps the lock-glue to adhere better as well.

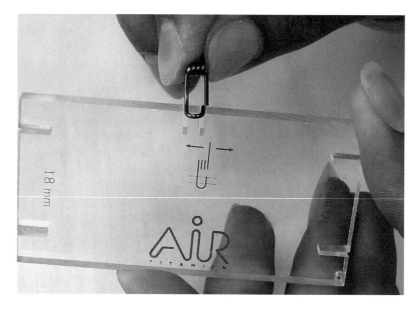

FIGURE **13-49**   Clip width may be adjusted so that it has the correct amount of tension in the slot. Both sides of the clip must be parallel after adjustment.

The shoe should contact the lens all along the edge. To have this happen, the face of the straps must parallel the up and down plane of the spring/shoe portion of the assembly (Figure 13-55).

MODERATELY THICK LENS EDGES

If the lens edge is moderately thick, the location of the holes is marked, but the holes are not drilled yet. Instead the straps are adjusted to fit the edge of the lens at the location of the proposed hole. If the straps need to be narrowed or widened, an old-fashioned strapping pliers is used (Figure 13-56). This widens or narrows the distance between the straps as shown in Figure 13-57. The straps also should be shaped to conform to the curve of the lens, lying flat against it.

When in doubt as to how close to the edge the holes should be, the operator should remember that it may be better to have the hole too far in from the edge than too close to the edge. If the hole is too close to the edge,

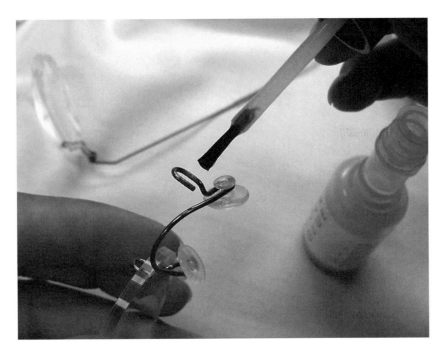

FIGURE **13-50** Applying "lock glue" to the inside of the slot and/or the clip before inserting the clip helps retain the clip in the lens.

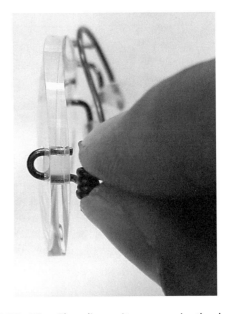

FIGURE **13-51** The clip as it appears in the lens. Clips come in different lengths, depending upon the edge thickness of the prescription.

the lens will be loose. But if the hole is too far in from the edge of the lens, the front or back surface of the lens under the strap can be filed. (See the next section.)

Once the straps are adjusted, the new location for the hole is marked. That location will be closer to the lens edge than it would have been. Yet it will be at the same vertical height as it was before.

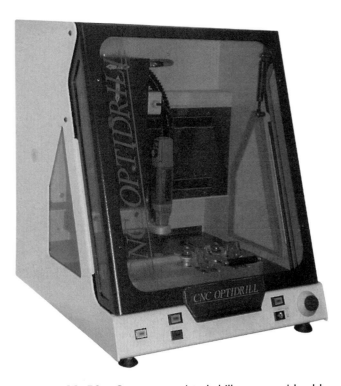

FIGURE **13-52** Computer-assisted drills are considerably more expensive but are faster and require less training.

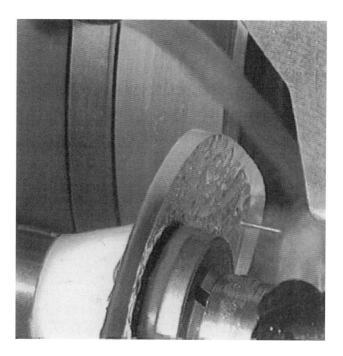

FIGURE **13-53**   One type of WECO edger drills the lenses immediately after they have been edged. For this feature to work, the locations of the drill holes, slots or notches are set up in the blocking process with the corresponding WECO blocker.

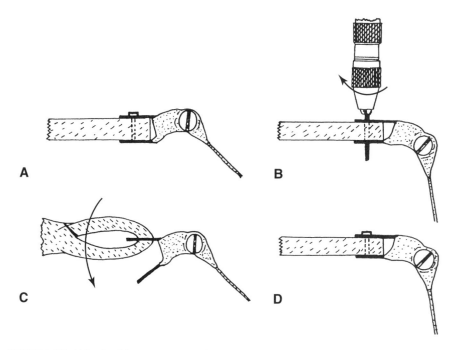

FIGURE **13-54**   In this sequence, **A** shows straps that are improperly angled, causing the temple to open out too far. In **B** the straps are being reangled, and in **C** rethreaded, using a tap. When corrected as shown in **D**, the temple once more shows proper positioning. (From Brooks CW, Borish IM: *System for ophthalmic dispensing,* ed 2, Boston, 1996, Butterworth-Heinemann [Figure 8-67].)

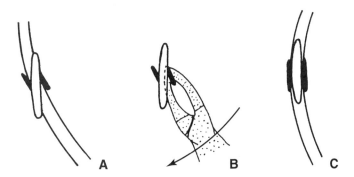

FIGURE **13-55**   **A,** The straps are misrotated, causing the lens to be angled. **B,** The straps are re-angled using hollow snipe-nosed pliers. **C,** The straps are shown correctly positioned. (From Brooks CW, Borish IM: *System for ophthalmic dispensing,* ed 2, Boston, 1996, Butterworth-Heinemann [Figure 8-75].)

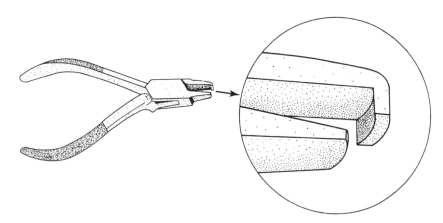

FIGURE **13-56**   Strapping pliers are made to help in spreading or narrowing the distance between the double straps of an old-fashioned rimless mounting. (From Brooks CW, Borish IM: *System for ophthalmic dispensing,* ed 2, Boston, 1996, Butterworth-Heinemann [Figure 8-73].)

LENS TOO THICK FOR THE STRAPS

If the lens edge is too thick for the size of the straps, again, the location of the holes is marked. Their marked location is for vertical reference only.

Next the back surface of the lens is filed to thin the edge where the strap will grip the lens. On extremely thick lenses, it may be necessary to file some off the front surface, too. A rat-tail file is used to file the lens surface. When the lens edge is thin enough to accommodate the strap, the strap is adjusted to fit. The location of the new hole is marked and the lens is drilled.

BIBLIOGRAPHY

Air Titanium Optician's Video, Frichsparken, Denmark, Lindberg Optic Design (undated).

DeFranco LM: Eight tips for processing rimless (or semirimless) eyewear, *Eyecare Business,* August 1999, pp 36-37.

Field C: Processing drill-mounted eyewear, *LabTalk* 28(42):32-34, 2000.

Geeren H: *Werkstatt buch,* Pforzheim, Germany, 1981, Verlag Neues Optikerjournal.

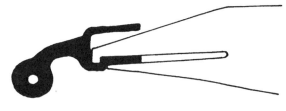

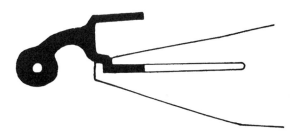

FIGURE **13-57**   A strapping pliers can be used to either widen or narrow the distance between straps to accommodate varying lens thickness. (From Brooks CW, Borish IM: *System for ophthalmic dispensing,* ed 2, Boston, 1996, Butterworth-Heinemann [Figure 8-74].)

Herrick T: Three-piece mountings: when lenses *are* the frame, *Lenses & Technology,* April, 2000, pp 18-22.

How to assemble 1776 and other Balgrip mountings, Rochester, NY, Bausch & Lomb, (publication A-1907), undated.

Levoy BM: How to work with rimless, *Optometric Weekly,* February 17, 1977, pp 33-40.

Yoho A: Keeping the rimless lens tight, *Eyecare Business,* August 2000, p 34.

Proficiency Test Questions

1. True or False? Polycarbonate is not well suited for any type of rimless eyewear because the material is so soft.

2. True or False? Using glass lenses in a rimless mounting, even when they are chemically hardened, is against FDA regulations.

3. Which of the following is not a good option for minimizing minus lens edges for rimless eyewear?

   a. Use a lens with an ED at least 5 mm larger than the A dimension of the lens.
   b. Use high-index material.
   c. Polish the edges.
   d. Use a small eyesize.
   e. Use an AR coating.
   f. All of the above are good options for minimizing minus lens edges for rimless eyewear.

4. To minimize and equalize plus lens edges for rimless eyewear, all but one of the following may help. Which one of the following will not help?

   a. Choose a frame size such that A+DBL is close to the wearer's PD.
   b. Choose a shape with a narrow B dimension.
   c. Choose a shape with an ED not much bigger than the A dimension.
   d. All of the above will help minimize and equalize plus lens edge thickness.
   e. None of the above will help minimize and equalize plus lens edge thickness.

5. For lenses of the same power, which of the following may be more difficult to mount in a rimless mounting?

   a. One with a flat base curve
   b. One with a steep base curve
   c. One with an aspheric base curve
   d. No difference exists in how easy or hard these lenses are to mount in a rimless frame

6. A drilling template describes which of the following?

   a. A picture of the lens, including where the holes are to be drilled on the lens
   b. Something that is shaped just like the lens. It is placed on the lens. Holes are drilled through the "holes" in the template and on through the lens.

7. A coquille describes which of the following?

   a. The mounting assembly of a double-drilled mounting
   b. A tool used to guide the drill through the lens, reducing chipping and spoiled lenses
   c. A type of French monocle that is drill-mounted
   d. The plastic display lens that comes in a frame
   e. A flowerlike decorative piece that is drill-mounted to a spectacle lens

8. You must drill a lens for a semirimless mounting without the help of drill guides. Using only the frame, with which of the following would you begin?

   a. The right lens
   b. The left lens
   c. The nasal hole
   d. The temporal hole
   e. Any lens or any hole; it will all end up the same anyway

9. Of the possibilities listed below, which is considered to be the most proper sequence of steps for drilling and mounting of plastic lenses for semirimless eyewear when a drilling chart is not available?

1. Drill the nasal hole.
2. Hold the lens in the proper position and mark the location for the temporal hole.
3. Hold the lens in the proper position and mark the location for the nasal hole.
4. Mount the lens temporally.
5. Mount the lens nasally.
6. Drill the temporal hole.

   a. 3, 1, 2, 6, 5, 4
   b. 2, 6, 4, 3, 1, 5
   c. 3, 1, 2, 6, 4, 5
   d. 2, 6, 3, 1, 5, 4
   e. 3, 1, 5, 2, 6, 4

10. To drill a lens, the drill should be positioned as which of the following?

    a. The lens lies flat and the drill is positioned perpendicular to the flat surface.
    b. The lens is angled so that the drill goes through the lens perpendicular to the front surface.
    c. The lens is angled so that the drill goes through the lens and exits perpendicular to the back surface.

11. Which of the following describes the proper procedure for drilling polycarbonate material?

    a. Drill straight through in a slow steady motion.
    b. Drill straight through, exerting moderate to heavy pressure on the lens.
    c. Drill halfway through, then turn the lens over and drill from the other side until the two holes meet.
    d. Drill 0.5 mm at a time, backing the drill out each time to wait for the material to cool.

12. To drill a glass lens, which of the following is correct?

    a. Drill straight through in a slow steady motion.
    b. Drill straight through, exerting moderate to heavy pressure on the lens.
    c. Drill halfway through, then turn the lens over and drill from the other side until the two holes meet.
    d. Drill 0.5 mm at a time, backing the drill out each time to wait for the material to cool.
    e. Glass lenses are never drilled.

13. Smoothing off the sharp edges of a drilled hole is called which of the following?

    a. Chamfering
    b. Counter-rolling
    c. Sacheting
    d. Stoning
    e. Blending

14. True or False? One option available on some lens drills will allow the diameter of the hole to be varied without changing bits.

15. True or False? The number one reason to get a computer-assisted drill is to increase the quality of drill mountings. It is not possible to obtain the same high-quality drill jobs with a manual drill.

16. True or False? Balgrip mountings use notches alone to hold the lenses in place. However, notches are also sometimes used with a drilled mounting to further stabilize the mounting.

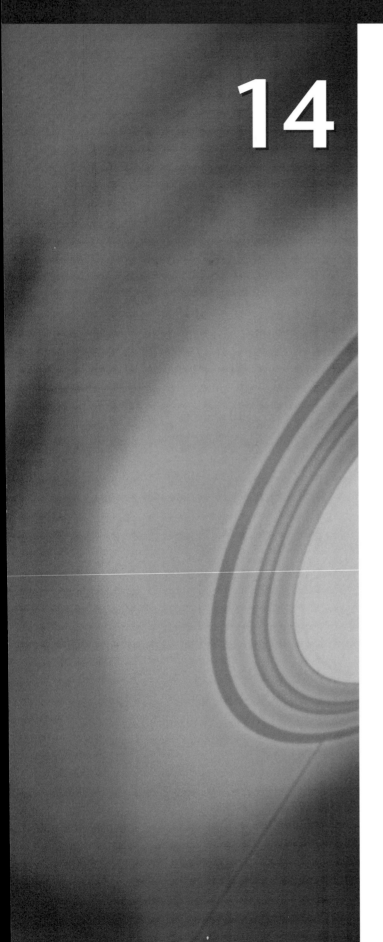

14

Nylon Cord and Other Groove Mountings

One method to keep frames and lenses together holds the lens in place with a nylon cord that resides in a groove cut in the edge of the lens (Figure 14-1). Alternatively some frames have a rim that slips into the groove (Figure 14-2). When the frame rim slips into the groove, the groove must be wider than for nylon cords.

A nylon cord frame is also referred to by a number of names, including *nylon supra,* a *string mount, Rimlon, Nylor,* and *suspension mounting.*

Wearer Safety Issues

Wearer safety issues[1] for grooved lenses are essentially the same as for rimless mountings and were discussed in Chapter 13. Reviewing these issues is recommended.

The issue of whether to use glass lenses in nylon cord frames is not as clear-cut as it is with drilled lenses. Most laboratories either do not put glass lenses in nylon cord frames, or if they do, they do so with reservations. The Optical Laboratories Association (OLA) addressed the issue in a 1993 technical paper. Even though a hardened glass lens will pass the required impact resistance test for a new lens in a nylon cord mounting, the edge of the lens is left unprotected. Putting the lenses on a rough surface or dropping them on a hard surface can

For more information, refer to *Instruction for the automatic groove master,* Los Angeles, Novamatic Systems (undated).
[1]The information in this section was taken from Bruneni JL: Ask the labs, glass lenses/nylon suspension mountings, (response by Dan Torgersen, technical director, Optical Laboratories Association), *Eyecare Business,* November 2000, p 36.

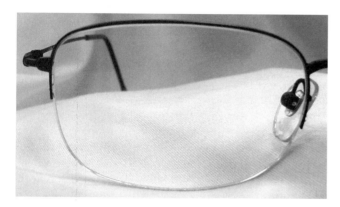

FIGURE **14-1** A nylon cord frame holds the lenses in place with a nylon cord that slips into a groove on the edge of the lens.

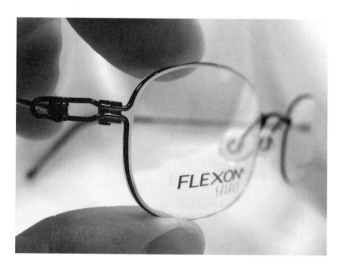

FIGURE **14-2** Some frames have thin metal rims. The lens edges are grooved and the rim slips into the groove on the lens and is tightened.

cause small edge chips or microcracks. These may reduce the impact resistance of the lens by a significant amount. A previous OLA technical director, George Chase, suggested that if the laboratory decides to make a grooved glass lens at the insistence of the prescriber or dispenser, a warning label should accompany the eyewear. The suggested wording is as follows:

To Prescriber/Dispenser: The glass lenses in this rimless mounting were made according to your work order. Instruct your patient to take care to avoid damaging the edge. Should the exposed edge of the lens become damaged, have it replaced immediately. Edge damage

reduces the original impact resistance of the lenses. Plastic lenses[2] are strongly recommended for such mountings.

Edge Thickness for Grooving

The edges of a rimless lens will be visible and should be as thin as possible for best cosmetic effect. However, lens edges need to be thick enough to allow them to be grooved but still have enough lens material left on either side of the groove so that it will not chip off.

Chapter 13, on rimless eyewear, includes a section titled "Edge Thickness for Rimless Lenses." If the reader has not yet read or does not recall the section, that section should be reviewed now, including the subsections on plus and minus lens edge thickness. These sections include cosmetic, safety, and functional considerations for edge thickness and apply equally to grooved mountings.

Another factor is important to remember when grooving a lens. The groove for the nylon cord is 0.5 mm wide. After the lens is grooved, enough thickness must remain on either side of the groove to keep the edge from chipping. Apart from safety factors, ideas on just how much extra thickness is required vary. Most practitioners recommend a minimum edge thickness of 2.3 mm.

Many polycarbonate and high-index minus lenses have thin centers. When these are edged for small frames, the lens edge can be less than 2.3 mm in places. These lenses may not be thick enough to be grooved. To keep the same frame, either a different finished lens will have to be selected, or lenses will have to be surfaced to ensure enough edge thickness for grooving.

Grooving Methods

The groove can be cut into the edge of the lens by using either a specially equipped *lens edger*, or a separate piece of equipment called a *lens groover*. The groover is currently the most common method.

The first type of edger to incorporate a grooving option was a dry-cut router-blade-type edger. By replacing the normal V-bevel blade with a flat blade having a small cutting nib, the lens may be edged flat and grooved at the same time (Figure 14-3). Several types of edgers have

---

[2]Polycarbonate and Trivex lenses are included in this broad plastic lens material classification.

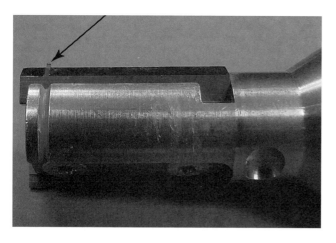

FIGURE **14-3** The cutting blade that can edge and groove a lens simultaneously. The *arrow* shows where the blade cuts the groove.

a grooving option as part of the edging cycle (Figure 14-4). This topic is discussed again later in the chapter.

Lens Grooving Method

Although several different types of manually operated groovers are available, the explanation that follows is primarily for one commonly occurring type of groover. Each groover operates somewhat differently. However, the basic principles are the same.

PREPARING THE LENS FOR GROOVING

A lens groover requires a lens that has been edged flat, as if it were to be drill-mounted. Lenses to be grooved should have a safety bevel—but only a moderate one. Excessive safety beveling of a thin-edged lens that is to be grooved causes the lens edge to be weak after grooving.[3]

Setting Up the Groover

The cutter wheel in a lens groover is a water-cooled diamond abrasive wheel. Because the wheel is thin and so narrow, only a wet sponge is needed to keep it cooled and cleaned. The sponge is placed against the wheel from underneath and should be wet thoroughly before each use if it is not already sitting in a reservoir of water (Figure 14-5).

The cutter wheel protrudes through a wheel dome. The edge of the lens rests on the wheel dome and the lens turns on the groover. The wheel cuts into the lens at the same depth that the wheel protrudes from the dome.

The groover has a groove depth adjustment. To calibrate groove depth, the depth dial is turned until the cutter wheel is flush with the wheel dome. The depth dial should register zero (Figure 14-6). If it does not, the zero-adjuster knob is used to reset the dial to zero.

---

[3]Rimlon mounting instructions, Hoya Corporation, 1983, p 4.

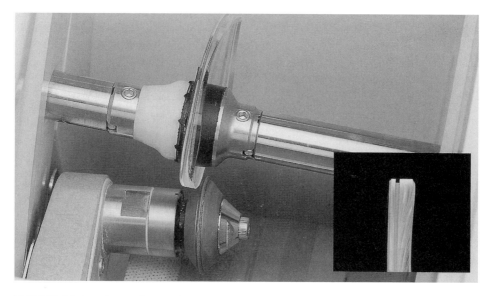

FIGURE **14-4** Some diamond-wheel edgers have the capability of grooving the lens immediately after it has been edged. (Courtesy Nidek, Fremont, Calif.)

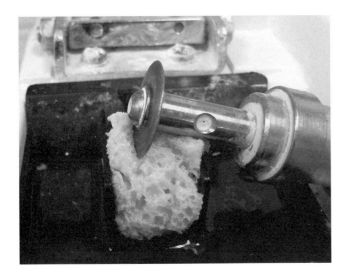

FIGURE **14-5**   A wet sponge keeps the cutting wheel of a lens groover clean and cool.

Before the grooving process begins, the depth for the desired cut is set. The groove depth required for nylon cord frames is normally between 0.4 and 0.5 mm.

POSITIONING THE GROOVE ON THE LENS EDGE

The position on the lens edge on which the groove is placed depends on the power of the lens and sometimes on the type of lens. When a lens has a fairly thin edge that is uniform in thickness all the way around the circumference of the lens, the only logical position for a groove is halfway between the front and the back surfaces. When the lens edge thickens or varies in thickness around the lens, the possibilities for groove location increase. The groove can be placed in one of the following positions:

- In the middle of the edge
- At a constant distance from the front edge and usually closer to the front
- At a constant distance from the back edge and usually closer to the back

Grooving the Lens in the Middle of the Lens Edge

When the lens is thin, the groove is placed in the middle of the edge (Figure 14-7, *A*). This occurs with low minus and low–plus-powered lenses and keeps the groove from getting too close to either surface.

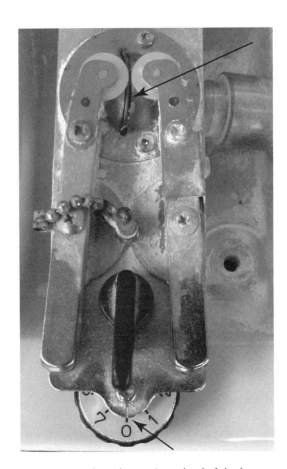

FIGURE **14-6**   When the cutting wheel of the lens groover is flush with the wheel dome, the cutting depth dial should register zero. The *top arrow* shows the cutting wheel.

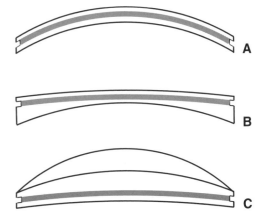

FIGURE **14-7**   **A,** For the thin-edged, low-powered lens shown in **A,** the groove is placed exactly in the middle of the lens edge. **B,** For thick-edged high minus lenses, the groove position is the same distance from the front edge of the lens, all the way around the lens. This is especially the case for high minus lenses with high cylinder. **C,** High plus lenses often base the groove location on the back surface of the lens. These lenses are viewed from the top. Lenses, particularly lenses **B** and **C,** vary in edge thickness around the perimeter of the lens.

To center-groove a lens, the operator begins by correctly setting the guide arms. The groover has two spring-controlled *guide arms* with rollers. The rollers follow along the front and back surfaces of the lens as the lens rotates to hold it on center. To keep the lens centered for center grooving, these arms must be locked together in such a way that they may spread apart evenly as the lens passes between them. The two guide arms are locked together from underneath when two coupling pins connected with a spring are set for centering (Figure 14-8, *A*). In addition, a centering pin (Figure 14-8, *B*) locks the unit into a centered position.

The lens is placed between the two lens groover chucks (Figure 14-9). The lens should be positioned in the groover so that the front surface is always facing in one direction. For the groover shown, the correct direction is toward the right. The lens must face this way because the cutting wheel is angled slightly so that the groove angle conforms to the normal meniscus curve of the lens (see Figure 14-5). Once the pins are set, the guide arms are spread and the lens is lowered onto the wheel between the arms (Figure 14-10).

The groover has two switches. One switch causes the lens to rotate; the other turns the small grinding wheel on and off. The switch to rotate the lens is turned on and the lens begins to rotate. After the lens rotates about one quarter turn, the cutting wheel is turned on and begins to groove the lens.

After the lens has been grooved all the way around, the sound of the cutter wheel changes. When this happens, the cutter wheel is turned off. Afterward the lens rotation switch is turned off.

The lens is taken out of the groover and rinsed to remove ground up lens material. To remove ground lens material from the groove, either a toothbrush or an ultrasonic cleaner, or both, are used (Figure 14-11). When using an ultrasonic cleaner and leaving the lens in the unit for cleaning, the operator should be sure the lens is placed face up to prevent surface scratching. The operator should not reach into the water in the ultrasonic unit before turning the unit off. Continued exposure of the joints of the fingers to ultrasonic vibration causes arthritis. The unit is turned off or a metal basket used to lower objects into and remove objects from the ultrasonic cleaner.

Grooving the Lens toward the Front of the Lens Edge

The groover may be reset so that the groove will be based on a specific distance from the *front* of the lens edge rather than positioned in the center of the lens edge. The groove position normally is based on the front edge of the lens for higher minus lenses, especially when the lens has more than a small amount

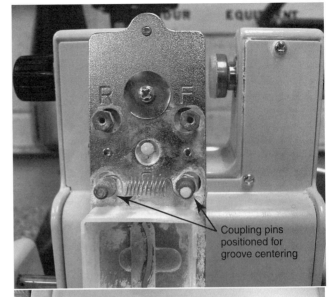

Coupling pins positioned for groove centering

A

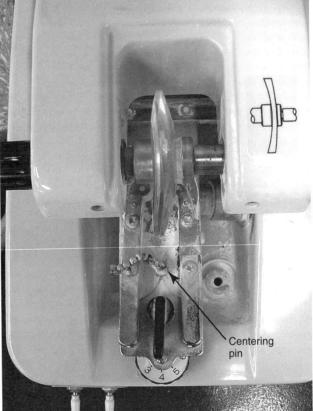

Centering pin

B

FIGURE **14-8** **A**, To cut a lens groove in the middle of the lens edge, first the two spring-connected coupling pins need to be positioned for centering. **B**, A centering pin locks the groover so that the lens groove will center.

of cylinder power. (The cylinder normally is created on the back surface of the lens.) This is not to say that the groove needs to be *close to* the front of the lens. The distance the groove may be offset from the front

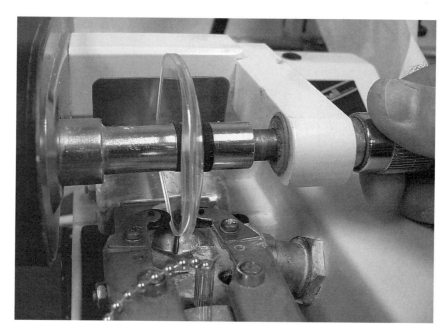

FIGURE **14-9** To begin the grooving process, the lens is held in place between the two chucks of the lens groover.

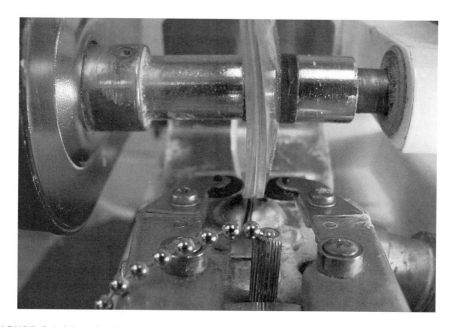

FIGURE **14-10** The lens is positioned between the guide arms for grooving.

surface may be varied. The distance from the front of the lens is based on how the groove will be positioned when it reaches the thinnest edge of the lens. Therefore groove location should be set at the location of the thinnest portion of the edge. Once set, the groove maintains that same distance from the front surface (see Figure 14-7, *B*).

To change the settings of the groover so that the groove location is based on the front of the edge, one of the spring-coupled pins is moved to the "F" or front position (Figure 14-12, *A*). The centering pin is removed. (The centering pin was shown in Figure 14-8, *B*.)

The lens is chucked and lowered between the guide arms. Next the operator looks to see where the cutting

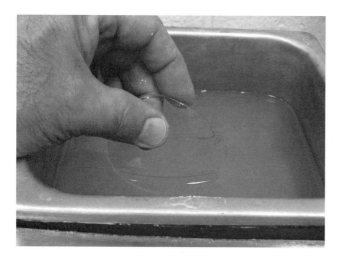

FIGURE **14-11** When the groove is cleaned with an ultrasonic cleaner, the fingers must not dip into the solution with the unit running.

wheel will meet the lens edge and decides how far the groove should be from the front surface of the lens. The groove position control lever is turned (Figure 14-12, *B*). This will move the front surface guide arm, shifting the lens left or right, until the groove location is at the desired position.

To help in deciding exactly where the groove should be located, the operator rotates the lens and observes where the groove will fall. Noting where the groove will be as it comes around to the thinnest part of the lens edge is especially important. Opinions vary regarding what distance from the front surface to put the groove. One suggestion is to position the groove just far enough back from the front surface so that when it reaches the thinnest part of the minus lens edge it bisects the edge.[4]

---

[4]Lisa J: Answers to challenges that arise when grooving and drilling lenses, (contributed by Chris Farley, Gerber/Coburn), *Eyecare Business*, October 1998, p 20.

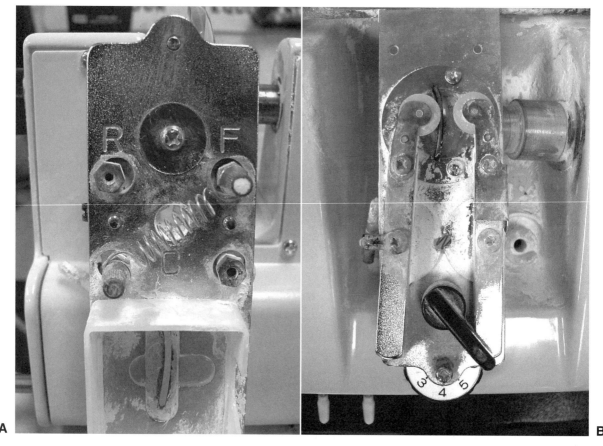

FIGURE **14-12** **A**, If the groove is to take its location based on a uniform distance from the front surface of the lens, one of the spring-coupled pins is moved to the front position. **B**, To set the distance from the front surface to the groove, the lever is turned to the right by varying degrees. Here the lever is turned to the extreme right. This would result in a large distance from the front of the lens to the groove.

Grooving the Lens toward the Back of the Lens Edge

Occasionally it is helpful to position the groove a certain distance from the back surface of the lens. Some people like to use this positioning for higher plus lenses (see Figure 14-7, *C*). This positioning is especially appropriate for Franklin-style (Executive) lenses. Franklin-style lenses have a shelf between the distance and near portions that goes all the way across the lens. If the groove is based on either the center or the front edge of the lens, the groove will track well on the upper part of the lens then "drop off" the lens edge at the shelf. Steps to prevent this problem include ensuring that the thinner, lower portion of the lens edge is sufficiently thick and basing the groove position on the back surface (Figure 14-13). In reality, the best solution is not to use a Franklin-style lens at all for grooved or drill-mounted lenses. If so desired, switching to a flat-top 35 will provide a wide near viewing area.

To change the settings of the groover so that the groove location is based on the back of the edge, one of the spring-coupled pins is moved to the "R" or rear position (Figure 14-14, *A*). Because the groove will not be centered, the centering pin must be removed.

The lens is chucked and lowered between the guide arms. The operator should notice where the cutting wheel will meet the lens edge and then decide how far the groove should be from the back surface of the lens.

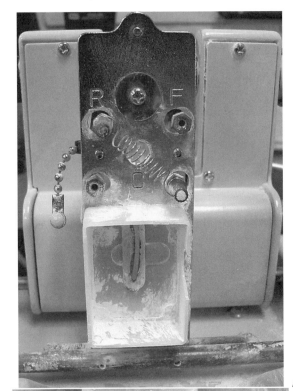

A

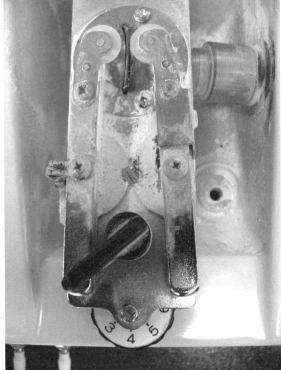

B

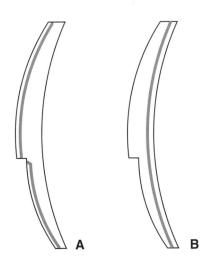

A   B

FIGURE **14-13** Grooved Executive lenses must have the groove based on the back surface of the lens. Otherwise the groove can go off the lens edge at the ledge. The lens shown in **A** was grooved based on the front surface. The groove drops off the ledge from the top and then must reposition itself on the lower half of the lens. This type of groove is unusable. The lens shown in **B** was based on the back surface of the lens and does not encounter the ledge.

FIGURE **14-14** **A**, The setting for basing the groove position on the rear surface of the lens. **B**, Turning the groove position control lever to the left moves the groove farther from the back surface of the lens. Here the lever is to the extreme left. This is farther than normally would be used.

The groove position control lever is turned until the groove location is at the desired position (Figure 14-14, *B*).

For Franklin-style lenses, the lens is rotated to the places where the lens shelf separates distance and near portions and the position of the groove is noted. (For any style lens, the operator should look to see where the groove will be located when it tracks along the thinnest part of the lens edge.) When it is certain that the groove will be placed properly along the entire circumference of the lens edge, the operator starts the lens rotating and turns on the cutting wheel.

For a summary of groove placements, see Table 14-1. See Figure 14-15 for another type of groover.

TOUCHING UP THE GROOVE

If one part of the lens groove is not exactly as wanted, the groove may be touched up by hand. The plate supporting the guide arms is lifted, which exposes the cutting wheel. The operator holds the lens in the hand and smoothes out the groove where needed.

TABLE **14-1** *Groove Position by Lens Type*	
TYPE OF LENS	GROOVE LOCATION
Low-powered plus or minus lenses	In the center of the edge
High minus lenses	A uniform distance from the front surface of the lens
High plus lenses	A uniform distance from the back surface of the lens
Franklin-style (Executive) lenses	A uniform distance from the back surface of the lens

SAFETY BEVELING THE GROOVE

Grooves on the edge of lenses chip if they are too sharp. This is true especially for lenses with wider grooves. Two ways exist to safety bevel the inner groove edges[5]:

[5]DeFranco LM: Rimless and faceted eyewear, (contributed by Matt Vulich, AIT Industries), *Eyecare Business*, December 2000, p 24.

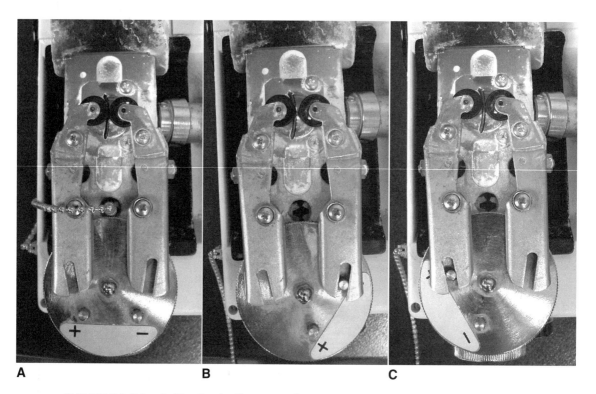

A   **B**   **C**

FIGURE **14-15**   **A,** The Santinelli groover also uses a centering pin to keep the groove in the middle of the lens edge. **B,** To base the groove location on the front surface of the lens, the centering pin is removed and the plus/minus dial is turned toward the minus. The farther the dial is turned, the farther the groove moves away from the front surface of the lens. **C,** For high plus lenses, the dial is turned toward the plus direction, basing groove location on the back surface.

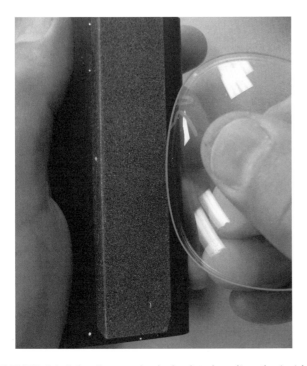

FIGURE **14-16** One method of safety-beveling the inside edges of the lens groove is to hand-smooth it with the corner edge of a ceramic block.

1. A ceramic wheel with a 90-degree angle is used. The groove is touched lightly to the corner of the wheel. The lens is turned evenly without pressure.
2. A ceramic block is used to rub a corner of the block along the inner edge of the groove by hand (Figure 14-16).

GROOVING POLYCARBONATE

Polycarbonate material softens with heat. Therefore, making multiple passes around the lens when grooving is advisable. The first pass is done at one half the groove depth. The second pass is done at or close to the final groove depth.[6]

The following steps can help ensure a nice-looking polycarbonate lens:

1. Groove the lens dry.
2. Leave only a little depth ungrooved.
3. For the last pass, groove the lens wet. This eliminates the frosted look and gives a more polished appearance to the groove.

If the edge of the lens is to be polished, it should be polished before it is grooved, instead of afterward. Polishing over a groove will wallow out the groove,

affecting appearance and possibly security of the lens in the frame.

GROOVING FOR A RECESSED METAL RIM

Some frames are made with a metal eyewire rim that slips into a groove in the lens edge (see Figure 14-2). The rims of these types of frames are thin but not as thin as a nylon cord. This means that the groove in the edge of the lens must be wider than the normal 0.5 mm width.

Because the groove must be wider, the minimum edge thickness for these lenses also will be greater than for regular nylon cord frames. Minimum edge thickness recommendations may vary. A recommendation of 2.4 edge is minimum.[7] A 2.4 edge thickness works best with high-index or polycarbonate lenses. For CR-39 lenses, a 2.8 minimum edge thickness is less likely to chip in the course of normal handling.

To create a wider groove, either a wider cutting wheel must be used, or the lens must be grooved more than once. Using a wider wheel is certainly easier and is more likely to give a better-looking end result.

Grooving for Recessed Metal Rims with a Wide Cutting Wheel

The groove-cutting wheel for recessed-rim mountings is 0.3 mm thicker than the standard cutting wheel.[8] The cutting wheel protrudes through a slot in a small dome (see Figure 14-6). The slot is wide enough for the standard-width wheel but might be too small for the new, wider-width wheel. If the slot is not wide enough, the dome will need to be replaced with one that has a wider slot.

Grooving for Recessed Metal Rims with a Standard-Width Cutting Wheel

To groove the lens more than once, the groover is set to trace off either the front surface or the back surface of the lens. (It should not be set for centering, otherwise the additional groove simply will overlap the original groove.) The groove is set at a certain distance from the front (or back) surface of the lens. The lens is grooved as usual. Next the lens is reset slightly farther away from the front (or back) surface than it was before. If the groove is 0.3 mm larger than the standard groove, then the groove is moved back an additional 0.3 mm and regrooved for this distance. This widens the groove by an amount equal to the difference between the first setting and the second setting.

---

[6]DeFranco LM: Eight tips for processing rimless (or semi-rimless) eyewear, *Eyecare Business,* August 1999, p 37.

[7]Air Titanium Rim, *Optician's video.* Section C. Frichsparken, Denmark, Lindberg Optic Design (undated).
[8]Air Titanium Rim, *Optician's video.* Section C. Frichsparken, Denmark, Lindberg Optic Design (undated).

Grooving a lens twice with a narrow wheel and achieving the desired result is more difficult than grooving the lens once with the correct wheel width.

The process for mounting a lens-recessed rim is similar to that for lenses for nylon cord mountings. A ribbon is used to pull the rim around the lens. This procedure is described later in the chapter.

Grooving in the Edger

Many newer patternless edgers offer the option of grooving the lens in the edger. The increased precision of these edgers allows control that includes variable groove depth, groove width, and groove location. Figure 14-17 shows how the screen appears for lens grooving on one such edger.

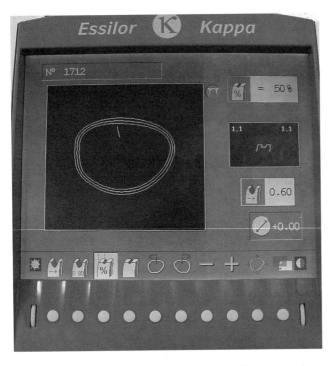

FIGURE **14-17** This grooving screen shows the lens shape. The highlighted groove % icon shows that 50% of the edge of the lens is in front of the groove center (leaving 50% behind the groove center). In other words the groove is centered on the edge. The almost vertical line in the lens shape shows where the second box down on the right is measuring finished lens thickness. The distance measures 1.1 mm from the center of the groove to the front and 1.1 mm from the center of the groove to the back. The third box down on the right side shows that the groove depth is 0.60 mm. The third icon from the left shows a groove width of 0.8 mm.

Mounting a Grooved Lens

The procedures for mounting a new grooved lens in a nylon cord frame or replacing a broken cord and remounting the lens are similar. Restringing requires a few extra steps but includes everything required for mounting a new lens in a new frame. The following is the procedure for restringing:

1. *Remove the old cord.* Sometimes it is difficult to remove the end of the cord from the frame groove because it is wedged in the groove. If this is the case, a dental pick can be useful for pulling the end of the cord out of the groove (Figure 14-18).

2. *Cut the end of the new cord at an angle.* The end of the cord should be cut at an angle to make threading easier. A razor blade works best (Figure 14-19). If the old cord is unbroken, a new length of cord can be cut to match the old. Many choose to purchase monofilament fishing line as replacement line for nylon cord frames. The line is 0.4 mm (0.016 inch) in diameter. The old cord is used as a guide and the new cord length is cut to match.

3. *Thread the cord into one side of the frame.* The cord must be attached to the mounting at two locations. Each point of attachment consists of two small holes. Some people prefer to start with the nasal point of attachment; others the temporal. For illustration purposes, this example begins temporally.

   Starting with the temporal point of attachment, one end of the nylon line is threaded into the *lower* hole from the *lens* side. Then the same end is

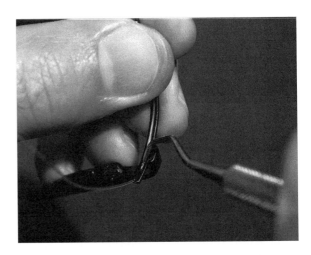

FIGURE **14-18** When it is difficult to remove a nylon cord from the lens groove of a nylon cord frame, a dental pick makes the job easier. (From Brooks CW, Borish IM: *System for ophthalmic dispensing,* ed 2, Boston, 1996, Butterworth-Heinemann [Figure 7-18].)

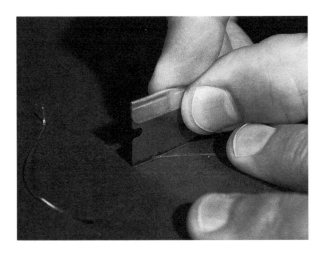

FIGURE **14-19** Cutting the nylon cord at an angle makes it easier to thread it through the holes in the frame and allows it to seat smoothly in the groove under the lens. (From Brooks CW, Borish IM: *System for ophthalmic dispensing,* ed 2, Boston, 1996, Butterworth-Heinemann [Figure 7-19].)

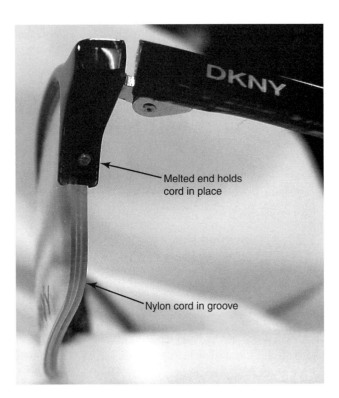

FIGURE **14-21** With certain types of nylon cord frames an alternative method used to secure the lens in place is to melt the end of the string. This hard melted ball will not pull through the hole.

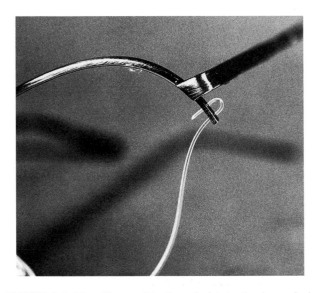

FIGURE **14-20** The cord is threaded into the lower hole from the inside and back into the upper hole. (From Brooks CW, Borish IM: *System for ophthalmic dispensing,* ed 2, Boston, 1996, Butterworth-Heinemann [Figure 7-20].)

threaded into the upper hole, and a length of 1.5 to 2 mm is left (Figure 14-20). For frames that will allow, an alternative method of securing the cord is to melt the end. The nylon balls up and will not slip through the hole (Figure 14-21).

4. *Size the lens.* The other end of the cord is slipped through the lower hole from the lens side at the nasal point of attachment. It is not threaded

through the upper hole. With the end of the nylon cord still loose, the lens is slipped into the upper part of the frame. It is not shoved tight into the frame eyewire. The cord is threaded around the lens and the cord is pulled snug (Figure 14-22). The cord is not pulled so tight that it stretches.

5. *Remove the lens.* The excess end of the cord is held with the thumb so that it does not slide out, and the lens is removed. (Because the lens was not pressed up tight into the eyewire it should be able to be removed without loosening the cord and losing the point of reference for cord length.)

6. *Take up the slack in the cord.* Because the cord was not pulled tight around the lens, it must be pulled 1.5 to 2 mm *farther* through the lower hole so that the lens will be tight enough.

7. *Thread the excess cord through the remaining hole.* The excess cord is threaded through the upper nasal hole while the new position of the cord is maintained in the lower hole.

8. *Clip the excess cord.* The excess cord is clipped, which leaves 1.5 to 2 mm inside the eyewire. It should be clipped at an angle so that it lays down in the groove smoothly (Figure 14-23; nail clippers work as well as regular cutting nippers.)

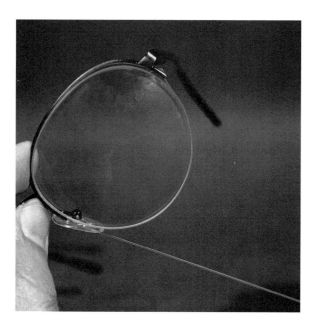

FIGURE **14-22**   When a nylon cord of unknown length is replaced, the cord is pulled snug around the lens but should not stretch. (From Brooks CW, Borish IM: *System for ophthalmic dispensing,* ed 2, Boston, 1996, Butterworth-Heinemann [Figure 7-21].)

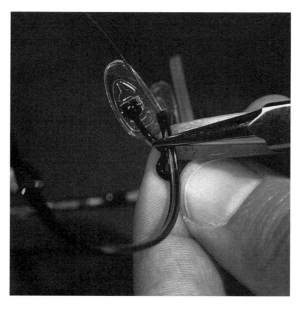

FIGURE **14-24**   Using a half-padded pliers, the free end of the cord at each point of attachment is pressed into the groove. (From Brooks CW, Borish IM: *System for ophthalmic dispensing,* ed 2, Boston, 1996, Butterworth-Heinemann [Figure 7-23].)

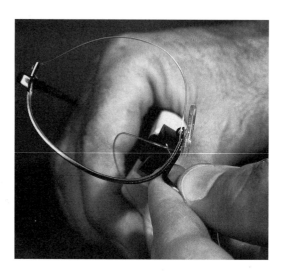

FIGURE **14-23**   Once the cord has been sized, extra cord is cut off. (From Brooks CW, Borish IM: *System for ophthalmic dispensing,* ed 2, Boston, 1996, Butterworth-Heinemann, [Figure 7-22].)

9. *Press the end of the cord into the frame groove.* A pair of half-padded nylon jaw pliers is used to push the loose end of the cord down into the groove in the eyewire (Figure 14-24). (Failure to tuck the cord into the groove causes the lens to chip or flake because of the pressure of the cord between the

edge of the lens and the edge of the eyewire.) This is done nasally and temporally.

10. *Secure the lens in the upper half of the frame.* The lens is inserted into the upper half of the frame beginning in the upper nasal area (Figure 14-25), followed by the upper temporal area (Figure 14-26). The lens should come in behind the nylon cord so that the cord rests on the front surface of the lens.

11. *Stretch the cord into the groove around the lens.* To secure the lens in the frame, the cord must be stretched to fit into the lens groove. This is done with a plastic strip. Many people use a fabric ribbon. However, a ribbon often frays, which leaves threads wedged between the lens and the cord. These threads are extremely difficult to remove.

    Some metal hooks are made specifically for stringing lenses. The main hazard of these hooks is the possibility of causing a small flake of the lens to chip out at the groove area. When this occurs the lens must be replaced.

    The plastic strip is slipped between the nylon cord and the lens. The strip then is folded back, and both ends are grasped together. Beginning at the thinnest portion of the lens edge and using the strip to pull the cord around the edge of the lens, the lens is seated into the groove on the way around (Figure 14-27).

12. *Check the cord tension.* Cord tension can be checked as the plastic strip slides toward the bottom of the

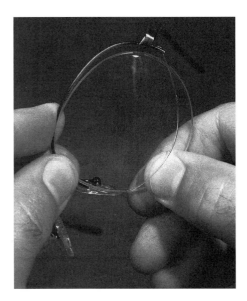

FIGURE **14-25** The lens is inserted in the frame beginning with the upper nasal corner. (From Brooks CW, Borish IM: *System for ophthalmic dispensing,* ed 2, Boston, 1996, Butterworth-Heinemann [Figure 7-24].)

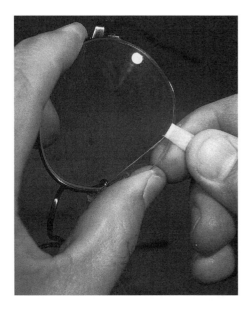

FIGURE **14-27** To thread a nylon cord into the lens groove, the cord is pulled around the lens, beginning temporally and continuing in a nasal direction. The cord must be on the front side of the lens. (From Brooks CW, Borish IM: *System for ophthalmic dispensing,* ed 2, Boston, 1996, Butterworth-Heinemann [Figure 7-26].)

and the length of the cord altered. (Using the dental pick may be necessary to free the end of the cord from the frame groove.) Usually the cord will be loose and have to be shortened. If this is the case, the earlier steps are repeated, beginning with step 8.

Once the lens is securely seated, one end of the plastic strip is released and pulled from between the lens and cord.

RETIGHTENING A LOOSE LENS

If a lens in an old nylon cord frame is loose or has fallen out, it is better to replace the cord, rather than to retighten the existing cord. An old cord may have lost some of its elasticity. The new cord has more elasticity and is less likely to break later.

Some have resorted to removing the lens and heating the old cord. The heat will cause the cord to shrink. When the lens is reinserted it will be tighter but only temporarily. Tightening a lens in this manner is not a good practice. The cord will not remain tightened long and the lens may fall out unexpectedly, breaking or scratching the lens.

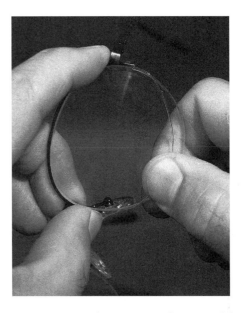

FIGURE **14-26** Once the upper nasal corner of the lens is in place, the upper edge of the lens is seated in the rim. This is done through temporal movement across the upper rim while the rim is slipped into the groove. (From Brooks CW, Borish IM: *System for ophthalmic dispensing,* ed 2, Boston, 1996, Butterworth-Heinemann [Figure 7-25].)

NYLON CORD FRAMES WITH LINERS

Some nylon cord frames have liners that fit into the top eyewire channel of the frame. These liners are called

lens until it is close to the midpoint of the lens cord. The strip should be pulled fairly hard. The strip should pull the cord about 0.5 to 1.0 mm away from the edge of the lens (Figure 14-28). If the tension is incorrect, the lens should be removed

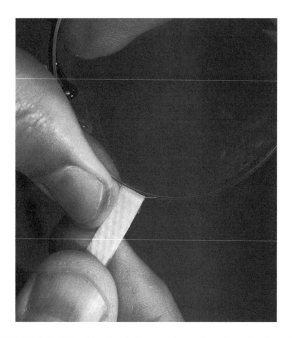

FIGURE **14-28**   To check for cord tension, the plastic strip is slid toward the bottom central part of the cord and pulled fairly hard. As shown, the cord should stretch some; no more than a 1.0-mm gap should show between the cord and the lens. A gap between 0.5 and 1.0 mm indicates the correct amount of tension. (From Brooks CW, Borish IM: *System for ophthalmic dispensing,* ed 2, Boston, 1996, Butterworth-Heinemann, [Figure 7-27].)

figure-8 liners because, when viewed from the end (in cross-section) the liner looks like the number 8. One part of the 8 is smaller than the other.

If it is necessary to replace the figure-8 liner in the top eyewire, a knife blade, file, or dental pick is used to dig into the liner and slide it out either end. The old length of liner is measured and a new piece of the same length is cut. To aid in insertion of the figure-8 liner back into the top eyewire, the new piece should be cut at an angle.

Using the smallest side of the figure 8 first and beginning either nasally or temporally, the operator slides the liner into the top eyewire channel. The entire piece of liner is fed in and centered in the channel. If the liner seems loose, it is turned around and the larger side is used. Care should be taken not to block any of the four holes used to hold the nylon cord in place.

Some frames use a thin, raised *metal ridge* in the top rim of the nylon cord frame to lend stability to the mounting instead of a figure-8 liner. Regrooving that section of the lens with a wider groove may be advisable. Then when the frame flexes, the lens is less likely to chip along the groove.

1. Which of the following is *not* a synonym for a nylon cord frame?

   a. Nebulon
   b. String mount
   c. Nylor
   d. Suspension mounting
   e. Nylon supra

2. True or False? FDA regulations prohibit the use of glass lenses in nylon cord frames.

3. Which of the following is the minimum edge thickness that is recommended for grooved high-index and polycarbonate lenses?

   a. 1.5 mm
   b. 2.4 mm
   c. 2.8 mm
   d. 3.2 mm
   e. No recommended minimum edge

4. True or False? Edging and grooving lenses on some lens edgers is possible.

5. True or False? A heavy safety bevel on a grooved lens may cause the edge to be weak.

6. If a lens is ordered with polished edges, the edges should be polished at which of the following times?

   a. Before the lens is grooved
   b. After the lens is grooved
   c. Either before or after the lens is grooved—it makes no difference

7. Normally the required groove depth for a lens to be mounted in a nylon cord frame is which of the following?

   a. 0.4-0.5 mm
   b. 0.9-1.0 mm
   c. 1.4-1.5 mm
   d. 1.9-2.0 mm

8. Match the lens with the most likely groove placement.

   1. In the middle of the edge
   2. Closer to the front edge
   3. Close to the back edge

   a. High-powered minu powered lens
   b. Low-powered plus or minus lens
   c. Franklin-style lens

9. True or False? If the lens grooving process progresses in the normal manner, a change in the sound of the cutting-wheel means that the lens groove has been cut all the way around the edge.

10. On a lens groover that has two switches—one for lens rotation and the other for cutting wheel rotation—which of the following is turned on first?

   a. The cutting wheel rotation switch
   b. The lens rotation switch
   c. Both must be turned on at the same time.
   d. It makes absolutely no difference.

11. On a lens groover that has two switches—one for lens rotation and the other for cutting wheel rotation—after the lens has been grooved all the way around, which of the following switches is turned *off* first?

   a. The cutting wheel rotation switch
   b. The lens rotation switch
   c. Both must be turned off at the same time.
   d. It makes absolutely no difference.

12. Reaching into an ultrasonic cleaning unit repeatedly with the unit still on may cause which of the following?

   a. Fingernail damage
   b. Skin cancer
   c. Arthritis
   d. Dry skin
   e. All of the above

13. During grooving of a polycarbonate lens, because polycarbonate is soft, which of the following is correct?

   a. The lens should be grooved slightly deeper than normal.
   b. The lens should be grooved slightly less deep than normal.
   c. The lens should be grooved in two or more passes, with the first pass being half the depth and the second, the full depth.
   d. Both *a* and *c* are correct.
   e. Both *b* and *c* are correct.

14. When threading the nylon cord into one side of a nylon cord frame, the operator should start with which of the following?

   a. The upper hole and thread it in from the outside of the frame
   b. The upper hole and thread it in from the lens side
   c. The lower hole and thread it in from the outside of the frame
   d. The lower hole and thread it in from the lens side

15. For a nylon cord frame, how much extra cord length should there be on each end of the cord?

   a. 0.5-1.0 mm
   b. 1.5-2.0 mm
   c. 2.5-3.0 mm
   d. 3.0-3.5 mm
   e. 4.0-4.5 mm

16. To check for the correct amount of cord tension on a nylon cord frame, using a plastic strip, pull the cord away from the lens edge fairly hard. The strip should pull the cord how far from the lens edge?

   a. The cord should not pull away from the lens edge at all.
   b. The cord should pull away less than 0.5 mm.
   c. The cord should pull away between 0.5 mm and 1.0 mm.
   d. The cord should pull away between 1.5 mm and 2.0 mm.

17. True or False? A rapid and acceptable method for retightening a loose lens in a nylon cord frame is to remove the lens, heat the cord in the frame heater to shrink it, and remount the lens.

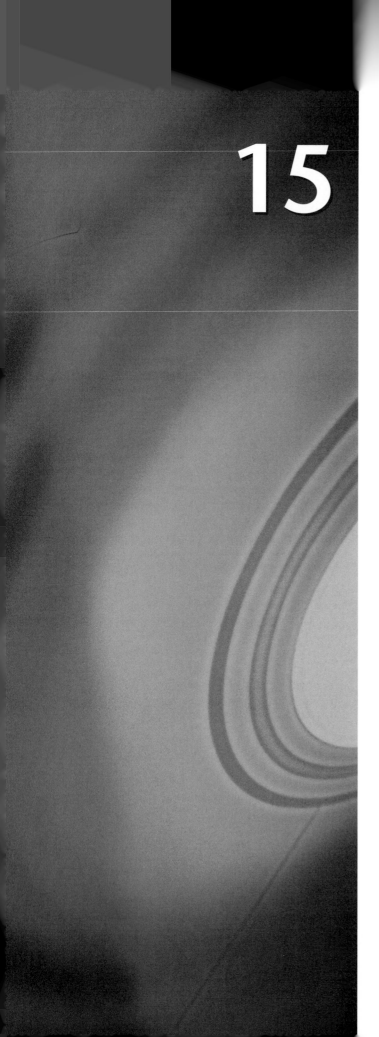

15

Lens Impact Resistance and Testing

The optical finishing laboratory is the last step before lenses and frame become finished eyewear. When the product is assembled, it must be suitable for wear. The product's suitability involves legal, optical, and aesthetic aspects. To be suitable for wear, the spectacles must be safe enough to pass certain preestablished standards. This section investigates impact resistance and how impact resistance is determined to be sufficient.

General Eyewear Categories

Eyewear is divided into the following three broad categories:

1. *Dress eyewear:* designed for everyday use
2. *Safety eyewear:* designed to meet higher standards of impact resistance because it will be worn in situations that could be potentially hazardous to the eyes
3. *Sports eyewear:* designed to protect the eyes and/or enhance vision in specific sports situations; the design varies by sport

Requirements for Dress Eyewear

There did not used to be any impact-resistance requirements for dress ophthalmic lenses in the United States. The United States is currently the only country with an impact-resistance requirement for dress eyewear.[1]

---

[1]*Impact resistance compliance guide: street/dress eyewear (not industrial eyewear),* Falls Church, Va, 1998, Optical Laboratory Association, p 3.

In many countries it is possible to surface glass lenses as thin as 0.3 mm and still dispense the lenses for regular spectacle lens wear. Such lenses appear thin and are still considered optically excellent. However, they afford little protection for the eyes, and in many situations end up becoming a hazard to the wearer.

FOOD AND DRUG ADMINISTRATION

The U.S. Food and Drug Administration (FDA) began mandating impact resistance for dress ophthalmic lenses in 1971. Since then all eyeglass and sunglass lenses must be impact resistant, except when the optometrist or physician finds that they will not otherwise fulfill the patient's visual requirements. If the lens cannot be rendered impact resistant, this must be recorded in the patient's record and the patient also must be notified in writing.

Situations for Dispensing Non–Impact-Resistant Lenses

Some dispensers may assume that a written agreement having the patient assume responsibility makes it possible to dispense non–impact-resistant lenses. This does not ensure freedom from liability. The following are the FDA's responses to three frequently asked questions regarding dispensing non–impact-resistant lenses[2]:

Q: Under what circumstances may retailers dispense lenses that are not impact resistant?
A: Lenses that are not impact resistant may be dispensed when a physician or optometrist determines that impact-resistant lenses will not fulfill the visual requirements of a particular patient. The physician or optometrist directs this in writing and gives written notification to the patient.
Q: Can a retailer supply a non–impact-resistant lens if a patient requests it or if the patient/customer agrees to assume all responsibility?
A: No. Non–impact-resistant lenses may be provided only when the physician or optometrist determines that impact-resistant lenses will not fulfill the visual requirements of the patient.... In such cases the physician or optometrist must give notice in writing

to the patient, explaining that the patient is receiving a lens that is not impact resistant.
Q: May a physician or optometrist prescribe non–impact-resistant lenses for a patient for purely cosmetic reasons?
A: No. If medical problems are related to cosmetic considerations, however, the physician or optometrist may invoke special exemption provisions of the regulation based on professional judgment. For example, if the patient's prescription cannot be filled by impact-resistant lenses because the physician or optometrist knows from previous experience that the weight of the heavy lenses may cause headaches, undue pressure on the bridge of the nose or ears, pressure sores, etc., the physician or optometrist may find that the visual requirements of the patient cannot be met by use of impact-resistant lenses.

For lenses to qualify for impact resistance, they must meet certain qualifications.

MINIMUM THICKNESS FOR DRESS OPHTHALMIC LENSES

Formerly the American National Standards Institute (ANSI) Z80.1 prescription lens standards had a minimum thickness recommendation of 2.0 mm. Now no thickness recommendation exists. FDA impact-resistance requirements are—and have always been—performance-based; the lens must be capable of withstanding a predetermined amount of impact. If that requirement can be met with lenses that are thinner than 2.0 mm, the lens is acceptable. Today many lenses can meet current impact-resistance requirements and still be below 2.0 mm, including some types of glass lenses.

IMPACT-RESISTANCE TEST REQUIREMENTS

The standard "referee test" for determination of impact-resistance suitability for dress ophthalmic lenses is the drop-ball test. This test has specific administration guidelines. However, the FDA states that this does not inhibit the lens manufacturer from using equal or superior test methods to test for impact resistance.

THE DROP-BALL TEST

To be judged acceptable, first a lens is placed front-side-up on a neoprene gasket. It must be capable of

---

[2]Snesko WN, Stigi JF: *Impact resistant lenses: questions and answers,* HHS Publication FDA 87-4002, Rockville, Md, Revised September 1987, US Department of Health and Human Services, Public Health Service, Food and Drug Administration, Center for Devices and Radiological Health, pp 11-12.

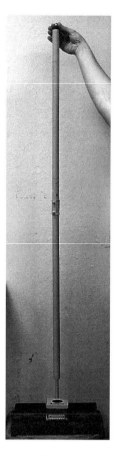

FIGURE 15-1 A drop-ball tester drops a steel ball on the front surface of a lens from 50 inches.

withstanding the impact of a $^5/_8$-inch steel ball weighing 0.56 ounce, dropped from a height of 50 inches (Figure 15-1). (The exact specifications for the drop-ball test are given in Appendix C.)

The area of contact that the dropped steel ball makes with the surface of the lens influences the outcome of the test. Because with use these steel balls deform over time they should be replaced periodically. Similarly, the neoprene gasket compresses and loses some elasticity over time. If a worn gasket is not replaced, the percentage of glass lenses that pass the drop-ball test will decrease by 25%.[3]

Timing of Drop-Ball Test

Glass lenses must be tested after the lens has been edged and hardened and before it is placed in the frame. Plastic lenses may be tested in the "uncut-finished" stage before they have been edged.

Drop-Ball Testing of Glass Lenses

With few exceptions, all glass lenses must be hardened *and* individually subjected to the drop-ball test. Only lenses that could be damaged by the test are exempt. These lenses must still be hardened but do not need to be tested. Glass lenses that are exempt from testing are the following:

- Raised multifocal lenses (lenses that have a ledge area on the lens, such as an Executive lens)
- Prism segment multifocals
- Slab-off lenses
- Lenticular cataract lenses
- Iseikonic (size) lenses
- Depressed-segment one-piece multifocals
- Biconcave, myodisc, and minus lenticular lenses
- Custom laminate lenses (such as polarizing lenses)
- Cement assembly lenses

INDIVIDUAL VERSUS BATCH TESTING

Batch testing is the practice of selectively testing a statistically significant number of lenses in a manufactured group. This prevents having to test individually lenses that could sustain damage by the test. The practice of batch testing is permitted for plastic lenses and nonprescription lenses such as mass-produced sunglass lenses. Glass, plano-powered sunglass lenses that are produced individually in a finishing laboratory must still be individually drop-ball tested.

Performing Batch Testing

Most—but not all—lens manufacturers normally batch-test for finished lens product impact resistance. This allows finished plastic lenses edged in a finishing laboratory to avoid individual testing or batch testing. Currently, nearly every lens manufacturer states that laboratories must perform testing to ensure impact resistance for lenses that have been surfaced from semifinished product.

If the lens is altered after having been received, as when it is sent out for antireflection (AR) coating, its impact resistance is altered. A great many types of coatings could be applied to the lens. Each of these coatings affects the impact resistance of the lens differently.

The envelope or box that the lens comes in should state whether the lens has been batch tested. If the package has nothing on it about impact testing, even if it is polycarbonate, it must be tested for FDA compliance.[4]

Typically the AR-coating laboratory batch tests lenses being coated. Laboratory personnel use lenses of the

[3]Torgersen D: Impact resistance questions and answers, *OLA Tech Topic* (Optical Laboratories Association), February 1998, pp 3-4.

[4]Young J: Technical Information for Labs, *Lab Talk*, 25(11):25, 1997.

same material and minimum thickness as those sent to them for coating. Finishing laboratory personnel are responsible to communicate with the company that applies the coating to determine that testing requirements have been fulfilled.

DEFINING 'MANUFACTURER'

A large number of participants are involved in the process of making a pair of glasses. One company makes the lenses, another may surface the lenses, a third may edge the lenses, and someone else could coat the lenses. Who then is the manufacturer of the finished eyeglasses? Although in a lawsuit, each participating party is likely to be named, final responsibility lies heavily with the unit that performed the final process on that lens. The following is the FDA's response to the question:

> **Q:** In terms of the regulation, who is the manufacturer?
>
> **A:** The manufacturer is the person who puts the lens in the form ready for its intended use or who alters the physical or chemical characteristics of the lens by such acts as grinding, heat treating, beveling, or cutting. For the purpose of this regulation the term "manufacturer" includes a company that imports eyeglasses for resale.[5]

In this chain of manufacturing events, the question of record-keeping may arise. The following is how the FDA poses and answers this question:

> **Q:** What are the record keeping requirements on partially finished lenses furnished by one manufacturer for completion by another?
>
> **A:** Records must be kept to show how lenses were rendered impact-resistant, when and how they were tested for impact resistance, and by whom in the processing chain these actions were accomplished.[6]

This means that if the retailer is the manufacturer, then the record-keeping requirements of the manufacturer apply. Retailers also have a 3-year requirement of keeping the names and addresses of persons buying prescription eyewear.

EFFECT OF LENS PROCESSING ON IMPACT RESISTANCE

A number of processes can be performed on a lens that affect the way the lens is able to resist the impact of an object. One of the most obvious is lens thickness: the thinner the lens, the less the impact resistance will be. Other factors may reduce impact resistance. Some of the more significant ones are listed below.

Effect of Lens Coatings on Impact Resistance

When a plastic lens is either scratch-resistant–coated or antireflection-(AR-)coated, the impact resistance of the lens normally decreases. This seems opposite to what would be expected.

Both scratch-resistance and AR coatings are harder than the plastic lens material to which they adhere. When a lens breaks, the break starts at the weakest point. If a plastic lens is hit by an object, the lens may flex but may not break. However, if the coating is harder than the lens, as the lens flexes, the harder (more brittle) coating cracks before the uncoated lens would. When the coating is bonded strongly to the lens, the energy that is concentrated at the first crack is released. The released energy travels through the lens and may cause it to break.

Corzine and colleagues[7] used a static load form of testing[8] and compared uncoated CR-39 lenses to the following:

- Scratch-resistance–coated lenses
- Five-layer AR-coated lenses
- Lenses that had been prepped for AR coating but were not yet AR-coated

The mean fracture load required to break the lenses in each category were as follows:

> Uncoated CR-39: 587
> Scratch-resistance coated CR-39: 505
> AR-coated CR-39: 465
> AR-prepped, but not AR-coated CR-39: 609

As can be seen from the results, the weakening of the lens is as a result of the coating itself, not by the process the lens is subjected to in preparation for coating.

This tendency of the coating to reduce impact resistance can be countered to some extent by using cushion coatings or primers applied to the surface of the lens before the application of a hard coating.[9]

[5]Snesko WN, Stigi JF: *Impact resistant lenses: questions and answers,* HHS Publication FDA 87-4002, p 7, Rockville, Md, Revised September 1987, US Department of Health and Human Services, Public Health Service, Food and Drug Administration, Center for Devices and Radiological Health.

[6]Snesko WN, Stigi JF: *Impact resistant lenses: questions and answers,* HHS Publication FDA 87-4002, p 10, Rockville, Md, Revised September 1987, US Department of Health and Human Services, Public Health Service, Food and Drug Administration, Center for Devices and Radiological Health.

[7]Corzine JC, Greer RB, Bruess RD, et al: The effects of coatings on the fracture resistance of ophthalmic lenses, *Optometry and Vision Science* 73:8, 1996.

[8]Static load testing is where an increasing amount of pressure is applied to the lens until the lens finally breaks.

[9]Torgersen D: Impact resistance questions and answers, *OLA Tech Topic* (Optical Laboratories Association), February 1998, p 5.

Newer methods of coating probably will be engineered with impact resistance in mind.

In consideration of the effect a coating may have, a point worth remembering is that highly impact-resistant lenses such as polycarbonate still have plenty of impact resistance, regardless of the coating. The main concern is for plastic lenses, especially some high-index plastic lenses. These lenses might be surfaced very thin and then have a coating applied without the benefit of cushion or primer coatings. As the number of finished stock lenses that have been AR-coated at the factory increases, there may be a resulting increase in impact-resistance quality. This result is because cushion or primer coatings can be engineered for the specific plastic substrate/lens coating combination being delivered in a factory-finished, already-coated, uncut lens blank.

Lenses sent out for coating have the chemical characteristics of the lens altered by the coating process. It then becomes the responsibility of the coating laboratory to comply with testing requirements for impact resistance. The edging laboratory personnel should be certain that the coating laboratory personnel fulfill these responsibilities. Otherwise the edging laboratory becomes responsible.[10]

Effect of Re-edging on Impact Resistance

Re-edging a plastic lens to another shape after it has been edged once does not significantly affect impact resistance. However, edging or re-edging a glass lens that already has been hardened will affect impact resistance. So may a hardened glass lens be re-edged to a new shape and then worn? The following is the FDA's response to the question:

> **Q:** May a glass lens, after it has been chemically or thermally treated for impact resistance, be processed further in any way?
> **A:** Lenses that are treated for impact resistance by induced surface compression may be re-edged or modified for power. However, the beneficial effects of surface compression may be reduced substantially. Such lenses must be retreated and tested before they are dispensed to the patient.[11]

Effect of Drilling and Grooving on Impact Resistance

Drilled glass lenses that are heat treated are not safe to wear. They may pass the drop-ball test in their unmounted state, but the compounded stress brought about by the mounting causes the mounted lenses to fail too easily.

Drilled lenses that are tempered chemically will pass the drop-ball test and are not as affected by drill mounting as are heat-treated lenses. Nevertheless, glass lenses are seldom used in a drill mounting even when chemically tempered.

In fact, glass lenses are seldom used with grooved lenses either. In 1993, Optical Laboratories Association Technical Director George Chase addressed the glass lens grooving/drilling issue in an OLA Tech Topics paper. He indicated that even though drilled and grooved glass lenses normally would pass the drop-ball test, the unprotected, exposed lens edges were likely to chip or microcrack with normal use and reduce impact strength. If drilled or grooved glass lenses are to be made, the OLA encourages optical laboratories to first obtain a waiver from the person ordering the lenses.[12]

Effect of Surface Scratches on Impact Resistance

A scratched lens surface reduces impact resistance. The scratch introduces a weak spot on the lens and creates a sort of "fault line." The scratch provides an easy area for stress to build during impact, which makes breakage more likely. To better imagine how this works, the reader may think about how panes of glass are "scored" with a diamond so that they may be broken along the scored line.

Contrary to intuition, scratches on the back surface of a lens reduce lens impact resistance *more* than front surface scratches. Glass or CR-39 lenses with front surface scratches were reduced in impact resistance by 20%, whereas CR-39 lenses with back surface scratches were reduced in impact resistance by 80%.[13]

'Duty To Inform'

Eyeglasses come in a large variety of lens materials. Each of these materials varies in impact resistance. Lenses that have a lower impact resistance may be acceptable for a person with a sedentary lifestyle but would not be appropriate for children who run and play. Laboratory personnel have no way of knowing the lifestyle of the person whose name appears at the top of

[10]Torgensen D: The effect of coatings on impact resistance, *Clearvisions* (Optical Laboratories Association), 3(7):8, 2000.
[11]Snesko WN, Stigi JF: *Impact resistant lenses: questions and answers,* HHS Publication FDA 87-4002, p 9, Rockville, Md, Revised September 1987, US Department of Health and Human Services, Public Health Service, Food and Drug Administration, Center for Devices and Radiological Health.

[12]Chase G (as quoted by Torgerson D): Impact resistance questions and answers (May 26, 1993), *OLA Tech Topic* (Optical Laboratories Association), February 1998, p 4.
[13]Torgersen D: Impact resistance questions and answers, *OLA Tech Topic* (Optical Laboratories Association), February 1998, p 4.

the prescription form. Yet the laboratory usually is named in a lawsuit.

The optical laboratory personnel must lower their potential liability and ensure the wearer of the eyeglasses knows of variability in protection given by different options in spectacles. The Optical Laboratories Association and others recommend a program of ensuring that wearers are informed of the availability of highly impact-resistant lens material. This type of program is called "Duty to Inform."

A similar phrase, "duty to warn," was used originally in a 1980s court case. In that case it was maintained that the eye injury was a result of negligence by the dispenser. Lawyers argued that "the dispenser, owner, laboratory, manufacturer, and all other parties down the line had a duty to inform the patient about all products and options, including the ones purchased."[14] In other words, laboratories and optical dispensers may not have a legal responsibility but do have a professional responsibility to warn prospective wearers of the dangers that may be associated with wearing spectacles that are not suited for certain potentially hazardous situations.

HOW THE PROGRAM WORKS

The "duty to inform" program that the Optical Laboratories Association recommends starts with the eye examination and includes the optical dispensary and the laboratory. The following is an overview of the OLA Program, which is currently under revision.

At the time of the visual examination the patient would receive a "Lens Menu." This pamphlet describes the variety of options available in lenses. It includes an explanation of lens materials, lens designs (e.g., aspherics, bifocals, progressives), specialty glasses such as sports or computer, and lens treatments such as ultraviolet (UV) protection. The pamphlet is used as a basis for the prescriber and dispenser to explain available lens options. A clear "Vision Safety Notice," is being revised to inform the patient of lens materials capable of withstanding high impact. At present, these materials are polycarbonate and Trivex (PPG Industries, Pittsburgh, Pa.), but new materials with high-impact capabilities are sure to emerge.

When the laboratory personnel complete the spectacles, a printed warning is enclosed with each. These warnings vary, depending upon whether the finished spectacles are dress eyewear, glass safety spectacles, hard resin safety spectacles, polycarbonate safety spectacles, or unfinished eyewear components. Except in the case of unfinished components, the warning

is meant for the wearer and is not to be removed by the dispenser.

This particular OLA program is only one method of ensuring that the wearer is informed fully regarding the choices available in lens material and is able to make an informed decision. The mechanics of such a program and the methods of passing along the information may be varied, depending upon the eyecare practice. The most important aspect is getting that information conveyed in a clear, documented, and regular manner that reflects a consistent practice policy.

FDA LABORATORY LABELING REQUIREMENTS

When an optical laboratory sends a finished spectacle prescription to an account, the FDA requires certain labeling, as follows:

Under 21 C.F.R. § 801.1, the label on prescription spectacle lenses, or finished spectacles containing those lenses, must conspicuously contain the name and address of the optical laboratory (city, state, Zip code, and street address, if not in current telephone directory) and such name and address should be prefaced with the phrase, "Distributed by _____ ." The name of the corporation must be the actual corporate name, which *may* be preceded or followed by the name of a particular division of the corporation.

In addition, the label on prescription spectacle lenses, or finished spectacle lenses containing those lenses, must contain the Rx legend, which is simply the text, "Rx Only."

The label must be "open the immediate container" (not including package liners) of each set of lenses or finished spectacles.[15]

These requirements must be fulfilled by use of the laboratory invoice as a "label." The invoice is printed with the name and address of the laboratory, along with the words "Rx Only." It is then folded to expose this printing and secured to the eyeglasses or slipped into the plastic bag holding the eyeglasses so that it may be seen through the bag. Alternatively, the label address and the words "Rx Only" can be printed on the outside of the bag or packing material that encloses the eyeglasses.

The FDA also requires that "...copies of invoices, shipping documents and records of sale for distribution of all impact resistant lenses be kept and maintained for a period of *three years*."[16]

[14]Duty to Warn: how to set up a program, *Eyecare Business*, June 1998, p 53.

[15]Hart HA, Smith R: *Checklist of federal statutes and regulations of particular interest to the optical lab*, Falls Church, Va, 2002, Optical Laboratories Association, p 7.
[16]Hart HA, Smith R: *Checklist of federal statutes and regulations of particular interest to the optical lab*, Falls Church, Va, 2002, Optical Laboratories Association, p 9.

Safety Eyewear

Safety eyewear has been an extremely important factor in reducing eye injuries. Although safety eyewear is a must in industry, 60% of eye injuries occur because of a failure to wear eye protection at the time of the accident. According to the U.S. Department of Labor, of the remaining 40%, "these workers were most likely to be wearing protective eyeglasses with no side shields... ."[17]

REGULATION OF SAFETY EYEWEAR

The standards used for safety lenses and frames are put forth by the American National Standards Institute (ANSI). The requirements for use of safety eyewear are regulated by the Occupational Safety and Health Administration (OSHA).

ANSI

The American National Standards Institute (ANSI) is an industry-based standards-setting association. ANSI is not just an agency for ophthalmic matters, but it addresses standards throughout all of industry, of which the ophthalmic industry is only a small part.

ANSI's Relation to OSHA

ANSI standards for dress eyewear are unrelated to OSHA requirements. However, for safety eyewear, the situation changes. For safety eyewear the American National Standard Practice for Occupational and Educational Eye and Face Protection (ANSI Standard Z87.1) has the power of a regulatory instrument. This is because OSHA has incorporated the Z87.1 standard into their requirements. The Z87.1 standard defines what constitutes a pair of safety glasses. The standard goes beyond safety glasses, however, to include the whole area of nonprescription eye and face protective devices.

Impact Requirements for Safety Eyewear

At the time of this writing the Z87.1 requirements for safety eyewear are those that were passed in 1989 and reaffirmed in 1998. However, new standards for safety eyewear are out for review. It appears likely that these

standards will be affirmed. The older standard has one set of requirements for all safety eyewear. The new standards may have two levels of standards. One is called *basic impact*; the other, *high impact*. The 1998-affirmed Z87.1 standard is the same as the basic-impact level for what the new standard is expected to be. In the next sections of the chapter, the two levels of impact resistance requirements that may become the new standard are explained.

Basic-Impact Requirements for Safety Eyewear

Because two levels of safety eyewear may be set forth by ANSI, the logical question is, why would anyone want to wear a basic-impact lens when high-impact lenses are available? Glass lenses are in the basic-impact category. In a number of work situations workers are cleaning their glasses constantly; for example, places with a lot of dust and places in which liquids or mists are present. In these situations, plastic and polycarbonate lenses may scratch. Glass lenses withstand scratching better and will not have to be replaced constantly. Badly scratched lenses are irritating to wear and, if vision is impaired, may create a safety hazard.

BASIC-IMPACT THICKNESS REQUIREMENTS

Historically thickness requirements for prescription safety lenses are a minimum thickness of 3.0 mm, with the exception being for plus lenses that have a power of +3.00 D or higher in the most plus meridian of the distance portion of the lens. Because high plus lenses are so much thicker in the center, these lenses may be thinned to a 2.5 mm minimum edge thickness. These standards continue on in the basic-impact category.

BASIC-IMPACT TESTING REQUIREMENTS

The testing requirements for basic-impact safety lenses are similar to those for dress ophthalmic lenses. Dress lenses are required to withstand the impact of a $^5/_8$-inch steel ball dropped from 50 inches. Basic-impact safety lenses must withstand the impact of a 1-inch steel ball dropped from 50 inches.

BASIC-IMPACT MARKING REQUIREMENTS

Basic-impact safety lenses must be marked with the manufacturer's logo or identifying marking. The markings are applied after edging. In-house laboratories

---

[17]*Eye protection in the workplace,* US Department of Labor Program Highlight, Fact Sheet No. OSHA 93-03, GPO: 1993 0-353-374, Washington, DC, 1993, US Department of Labor.

TABLE **15-1**
Current and Anticipated ANSI Z87.1 Lens Marking Requirements

LENS TYPE	REQUIREMENT*	BASIC-IMPACT[†] EXAMPLE	HIGH-IMPACT EXAMPLE
Clear lenses	Manufacturer's monogram and sometimes +	JO	JO+
Tinted (absorptive) lenses, except for special-purpose lenses	Manufacturer's monogram, shade number, and sometimes +	JO-2.5	JO-2.5+
Photochromic lenses	Manufacturer's monogram, letter V for "variable shade," and sometimes +	JO-V	JO-V+
Special-purpose lenses[‡] (These lenses provide eye protection during the performance of visual tasks that require unusual filtering of light. Examples include didymium-containing lenses, cobalt-containing lenses, uniformly tinted lenses, and lenses prescribed by an eye specialist for particular vision problems.)	Manufacturer's monogram, letter S for "special purpose," and sometimes +	JO-S	JO-S+

JO, James Optical (fictitious optical company).
*All markings must be legible and permanent and placed so that interference with the vision of the wearer is minimal.
[†]Basic-impact requirements are historically the same as the Z87.1-1989 standard and are part of the projected new standard that would include both basic and high-impact lenses.
[‡]"Many such (special purpose) lenses offer inadequate ultraviolet and/or infrared protection; caution shall be exercised in their use. For each application, the responsible individual shall ensure that the proper ultraviolet, infrared, and visible protection is provided. Spectral transmittance data shall be available to buyers upon request." *(ANSI Z87.1-1989 American National Standard Practice for Occupational and Educational Eye and Face Protection,* New York, 1989, American National Standards Institute, Inc, p 14.)

that do their own edging of safety lenses must mark the lenses. Marks on the surface of the lens should not interfere with straight-ahead viewing; they must, however, be visible. They usually appear at the center of the top of the lens or in the upper, outer corner. If the lens is other than a clear lens, it may require an additional marking. A summary of these marking requirements is found in Table 15-1. A lens that is thick enough to be classed as a safety lens and strong enough to pass safety lens impact testing is not acceptable as a safety lens until it is marked with the required manufacturer identification.

Methods Used to Mark Safety Lenses

Several methods may be used to mark safety lenses. These include sandblasting, indenting, and laser engraving.

Sandblasting is the only method that works for glass lenses. The same sandblasting unit (Figure 15-2) works equally well for plastic lenses. To mark the lens, a thin rubber "mask" is used. This mask has a cutout of the manufacturer's mark. Before each use the rubber mask is brushed clean (Figure 15-3). The lens is placed on the mask at the desired location of the mark (Figure 15-4).

Then the mask is sandblasted. The cutout area exposes the lens to the sand and etches the exposed lens surface, which creates the desired symbol (Figure 15-5).

Plastic lenses may be marked by indentation of the surface. To do this, a small branding-iron–like tool is mounted on a specifically designed pair of pliers. The tool has the shape of the manufacturer's symbol. When it is squeezed against the lens surface, the surface indents.

A third option is to "tattoo" the lens using a discreet method of laser engraving.

WARNING LABELS FOR BASIC-IMPACT LENSES

Basic-impact safety glasses are not as impact resistant as high-impact safety glasses. The person wearing the lenses needs to know this. Therefore, if the standards pass as anticipated, a warning must accompany basic-impact eyewear. That warning will be in the form of a hang tag or label to be removed only by the wearer. The label must say that the lenses meet the basic-impact requirements but should not be relied upon for protection from high-impact exposure.

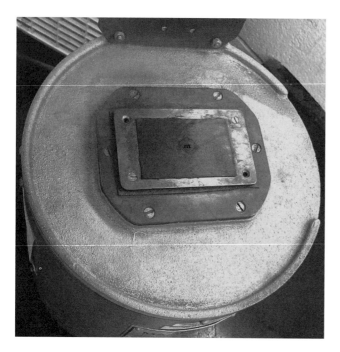

FIGURE **15-2** A sandblasting unit may be used to mark safety lenses.

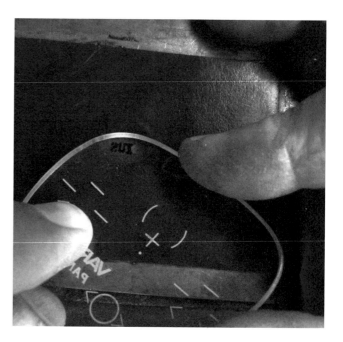

FIGURE **15-4** The lens is placed on the rubber mask where the safety marking is to be etched. The mask is sandblasted from underneath, leaving an imprint of the logo on the lens.

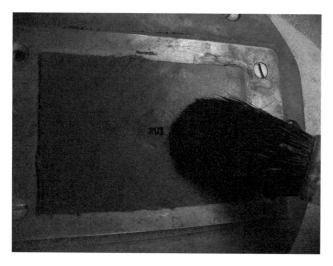

FIGURE **15-3** A rubber mask stenciled with the identifying lens and laboratory marking is positioned in the sandblasting unit. Before each use it should be brushed clean. Loose sand particles can scratch the lens.

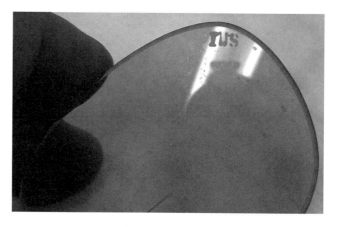

FIGURE **15-5** An identifying marking on a safety lens.

High-Impact Requirements for Safety Eyewear

High-impact requirements allow the lenses to be thinner than basic-impact lenses. However, the tests that high-impact lenses must withstand are more stringent.

HIGH-IMPACT THICKNESS REQUIREMENTS

The thickness requirement for high-impact safety lenses is that they be 2.0 mm thick or more. This includes both prescription and nonprescription (plano) safety lenses.

HIGH-IMPACT TESTING REQUIREMENTS

High-impact safety lenses must pass the high-velocity impact test. In this test the lens must be capable of withstanding the force of a $1/4$-inch steel ball traveling at 150 feet/sec when mounted on a special holder.

TABLE **15-2** *Safety Lens Requirements*			
TYPE OF REQUIREMENT	THICKNESS	MARKING*	IMPACT TESTING
Basic impact[†]	3.0 mm 2.5 mm if power in most plus meridian is +3.00 D or more	Manufacturer's logo	1-inch steel ball dropped from 50 inches
High impact	2.0 mm	Manufacturer's logo +	1-inch steel ball dropped from 50 inches *and* $^1/_4$-inch steel ball traveling at 150 feet/sec

*See also Table 15-1.
[†]Basic-impact requirements are historically the same as the Z87.1-1989 standard and are part of the projected new standard that would include both basic- and high-impact lenses.

HIGH-IMPACT MARKING REQUIREMENTS

High-impact safety lenses are marked in the same manner as basic-impact lenses, except that they are to be additionally marked with a plus (+) symbol—not just the manufacturer's logo (Table 15-2).

Safety Frames

In 1989 the ANSI standards for safety frames dropped specific design requirements, including groove design. Instead, requirements are performance based. Safety frames must withstand certain specific impact tests that are not required of normal dress frames. Frames are placed on a head model. When impact occurs, the frame cannot break. Nor can the frame or lens come into contact with the eye.

One test is the *high-velocity impact test*. This test simulates a high-velocity, low-mass object. In the high-velocity impact test a series of $^1/_4$-inch steel balls traveling at 150 feet per second are directed at 20 different parts of the glazed frame[18] (Figure 15-6). A new frame is used for each impact. Neither the frame nor the lens can break, nor can the lens come out of the frame.

The second test simulates the impact of a large, pointed, slow-moving object. In this *high-mass impact test* a pointed, conical-tipped projectile, 1 inch in diameter, weighing 17.6 ounces, is dropped 51.2 inches through a tube and onto the eyeglasses (Figure 15-7). The lens must not break, nor come out of the frame.

[18]A glazed frame is a frame with lenses. In this case the lenses are plano in power.

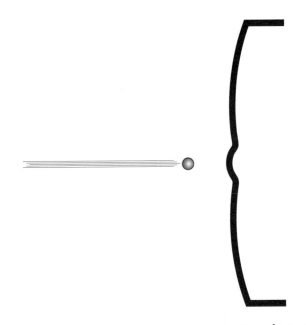

FIGURE **15-6**   The high-velocity impact test fires a $^1/_4$-inch steel ball at 150 feet/sec at a frame or lens.

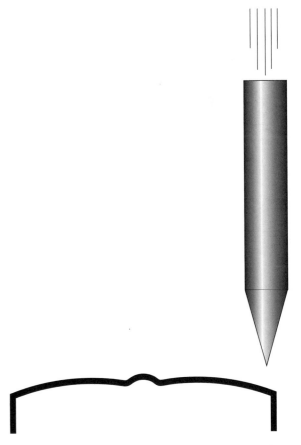

FIGURE **15-7**   The high-mass impact test drops a pointed, 1-inch diameter projectile onto the eyeglasses from 51.2 inches.

MARKING SAFETY FRAMES

With safety requirements, a clear distinction between "dress" frames and safety frames must be kept in mind. *Dress* frames are those worn for everyday purposes. No matter how sturdy the construction of a dress frame, it is still not a safety frame unless it meets certain requirements and is marked as a safety frame.

The first requirement is that it be capable of withstanding a series of stress tests. If the frames are capable of passing these tests and have been so certified, they may be marked as safety frames. Without these markings, the frames are not safety frames. Markings consist of size, the manufacturer's trademark, and the all-important Z87 marking on temples and front, indicating compliance with ANSI Z87 standards.

With the anticipated passage of new requirements in the form of a high-impact category of safety lenses, safety frames intended for use with 2.0-millimeter thick lenses must be tested for 2.0-mm thick lenses. When successfully designed and tested, these frames are to be marked Z87-2 instead of just Z87. The "2" signifies that the frame is suitable for lenses with a minimum thickness of 2 or 3 mm (Box 15-1). The new requirements will be for all safety frames, meaning that all frames will need to be marked "Z87-2."

DEFINING SAFETY GLASSES

Safety frames should be used only with safety lenses. *Regular lenses must not be put into a safety frame,* even to save the wearer money. A pair of regular "dress" lenses placed in a safety frame may give the wearer the impression that they are wearing safety glasses. A safety frame with dress-thickness lenses is no more safety eyewear than a dress frame with safety lenses. Eyeglasses are not safety glasses until both the frame and lenses are in compliance.

Intentionally thick lenses should not be placed in a pair of regular frames for increased safety. If safety is important enough to warrant thick lenses, it is important enough to warrant safety or sports-type frames. "Safety" lenses in regular frames can give the wearer a false sense of security and the mistaken impression than this is a "safe" prescription. *Under no circumstances should a pair of lenses be marked as safety and placed in a nonsafety frame.*

SIDE SHIELDS

Now that eye protection is required and used in many more settings, eye injuries that happen to people wearing safety glasses usually occur from the side. Therefore "use of protectors providing side protection should be encouraged whenever practical."[19]

Side shields may be removable or permanent (Figure 15-8). Most people would rather not wear side shields if given the choice. If side shields are constantly required, then permanent side shields are logical. Removable side shields have the advantage of being able to be taken off when working in a nonhazardous situation. The drawback is that removable side shields often end up not being worn when they should.

Side shields are not universally interchangeable. A removable side shield designed for one particular type

---

[19]*American National Standard practice for occupational and educational eye and face protection,* Z87.1-1989, New York, 1989, American National Standards Institute, Inc, p 15.

BOX 15-1
Safety Frame Marking Requirements

Fronts
- A-dimension (eyesize)
- DBL (distance between lenses)
- "Z87-2"*
- Manufacturer's identifying trademark

Temples
- Overall length
- "Z87-2"*
- Manufacturer's identifying trademark
- "Z87-2" markings also required for side shields

*The marking "Z87" indicates frame compliance with Z87.1-1989 standards. After new standards take effect, the "Z87-2" marking will indicate frame compliance with high-impact standards. Thereafter, frames with removable lenses will only be marked "Z87" if the lenses in the frames are non-Rx (plano).

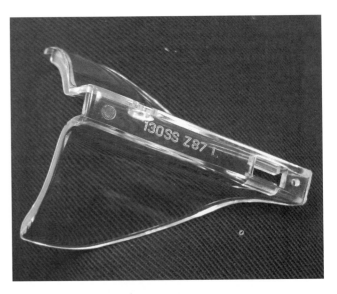

FIGURE 15-8   Some side shields are removable.

of frame will not necessarily provide the ANSI-standard-approved protection required if used on a different type of frame.

Hardening Glass Lenses

Glass lenses are not impact resistant enough to pass the FDA-mandated impact test unless they are hardened. Currently two methods are used to harden glass lenses. One uses a heat-treating process and the second a chemical-tempering process. Not all types of glass are capable of being tempered. These types may be used only in the United States if no other type of lens material is acceptable for the visual needs of the wearer.

Scratched lenses are more likely to break than unscratched lenses regardless of the method used to harden a lens. Scratches introduce weak points on the lens. A scratched heat-tempered lens loses more of its impact resistance than a scratched chemically tempered (or *chemtempered*) lens. For maximum safety, scratched lenses should be replaced.

HEAT-TREATING PROCESS

Heat treating is done by placement of the edged glass lens into a small kiln, where the temperature is high enough to almost bring the glass to the softening point. The lens is left in the kiln for about 2 or 3 minutes. The exact amount of time depends upon (1) lens thickness, (2) type of glass, and (3) lens tint. (For more exactness, lens weight may also be considered.)

The lens is removed from the heat and cooled rapidly by blowing forced air against both front and back surfaces (Figure 15-9).

To understand how this process could cause an increase in impact resistance, the reader should

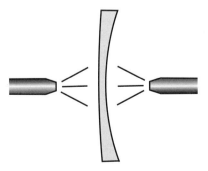

FIGURE **15-9** When air strikes front and back surfaces of a lens that has been heated just below the softening point, it "freezes" the outside, setting up a controlled internal stress that makes the lens more impact resistant.

remember that as glass heats, it expands and becomes more like a liquid. When the hot lens is struck by cool air against its outer surfaces, the outer surfaces "freeze." The inner part of the lens cools more slowly. As it is cooling it is trying to contract. But the outer part of the lens is already "frozen" and refuses to shrink farther. This creates an inner pull on the lens, which induces stress. Part of the stress is surface compaction or squeezing called *maximum compressive stress*. Another part of the stress is called *maximum tensile stress*. This stress creates strength in the same way that the tightened spokes on a bicycle wheel add strength to the rim. These forces result in a compression of the lens surface. The depth from the outside surface of the lens where compressive stress and tensile stress meet is called the *depth of compression*.

The advantage to heat treating is that it is fast. The disadvantage is that the heat-tempered lens is not as impact resistant as lenses that are chemically tempered.

CHEMICAL TEMPERING

Glass lenses are hardened chemically by immersing them in molten salt. The salt used for clear crown glass and tinted crown glass lenses is potassium nitrate (KNO_3). During the process of chemical tempering, smaller Sodium (Na) or Lithium (Li) ions from the glass are drawn out of the lens surface and replaced by larger potassium (K) ions from the salt. This crowds the surface, setting up a surface tension that "squeezes" the lens. This surface tension increases impact resistance by creating compressive stresses. The actual amount of compressive stress is 28 to 50 kg/mm^2, compared with 6 to 14 kg/mm^2 for heat-tempered glass[20] (Figure 15-10).

The salt used to temper photochromic lenses is different from the salt used for crown glass lenses. Salt used for photochromic lenses is a mixture of 40% sodium nitrate ($NaNO_3$) and 60% potassium nitrate (KNO_3). Both of these salts are hazardous in dry or molten states. Salts are available in both commercial and reagent grades. Reagent grade is more expensive, but being purer, does not require conditioning and prevents salt-related problems.

If the proportion between salts is incorrect, or if the salt is contaminated or has been used too long, the lenses will have problems. Lenses may break in the bath, come out hazy, or show hairline cracks. Processing a crown glass lens in a salt bath intended for photo-chromics will cause the lens to craze, showing a meshwork of hairline surface cracks (Figure 15-11).

[20]Krauser RP: *Chemtempering today*, Corning, NY, 1974, Corning Glass Works, p 4.

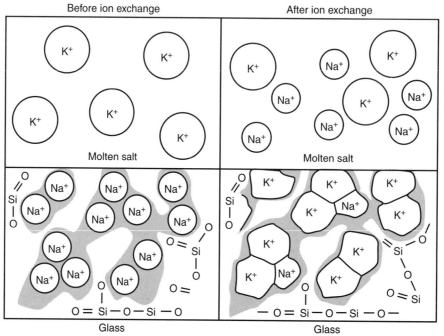

FIGURE **15-10**　In chemical tempering, smaller sodium (Na) or lithium (Li) ions from the glass are replaced by larger potassium (K) ions from the molten salt.

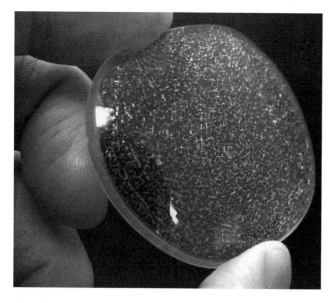

FIGURE **15-11**　A crown glass lens mistakenly placed in a photochromic salt bath will craze.

Salt needs to be replaced on a regular basis. As salt pH rises above neutral, some salt should be removed and replaced with new salt to lower the pH. When sediment builds up in the bottom of the tank, all of the salt should be replaced.

To chemically temper crown and tinted glass lenses together, the temperature of the salt is 450°± 5° C (842°

±9° F). To temper photochromic glass lenses the salt is heated to 400° ± 5°C (752° ± 9° F).[21]

This temperature is especially critical for photochromic lenses and should be verified with use of a calibrated stainless steel thermometer with a long stem. The stem should be long enough so that the thermometer may be read without having to hold it with the hands near the salt. Thermometers are important even though the chemical tempering unit has a temperature control that reads in degrees.

If the temperature of the bath is not exact, problems will occur with photochromic lenses being off-color, splotching, or not lightening or darkening properly.

Chemical Tempering Process

Lenses are cleaned and placed in a lens holder. That holder is held above the bath for 15±2 minutes for crown glass lenses. For photochromics these times may vary from 0 to 15 minutes. This allows the lenses to preheat, which prevents breakage resulting from extreme temperature changes. The lenses are then immersed in the molten salt bath for 16 hours. (It is possible to leave the lenses over the weekend for 64 hours. Impact resistance drops slightly, but the amount of drop is normally insignificant.) At the end of the cycle the lenses are again held above the bath. The postbath-cool times are the same as the preheat times. Lenses are then removed from the unit, allowed to cool at room temperature, then rinsed in hot water to remove the salt.

(A special process makes it possible to chemically harden standard photochromic lenses in 2 hours.[22])

Chemically hardened crown glass lenses are more impact resistant than thermally hardened crown glass lenses and maintain their strength better, even when scratched. They will not warp during the chemical tempering process, as do some lenses during the heat tempering process. Because their internal tensile stress is less than that of a heat-tempered lens, chemically tempered lenses may be re-edged or resurfaced without breaking.

If a pair of chemically tempered glass lenses has been removed from a broken frame and reshaped for a new frame, the lenses should be rehardened. (Heat tempered lenses should never be re-edged on an edger or hand edger unless they have been dehardened[23] first.)

Compared with heat tempering, chemical tempering of crown glass lenses is clearly the method of choice.

Determining whether a Lens Has Been Hardened

Determining whether a lens has been heat treated is possible by viewing it between two crossed polarizing filters. An instrument with a light source and two crossed polarizing filters made for this purpose is called a *colmascope* or *polariscope*. Viewed through a colmascope, a heat-treated lens shows a maltese cross pattern (Figure 15-12). A perfectly shaped maltese cross pattern does not mean that the lens is any more impact resistant than a lens showing a misshapen maltese cross. Rotating the lens while viewing it though the colmascope will cause the maltese cross to change in appearance. This pattern shows up because surface compression in a heat-treated lens is nonuniform.[24]

Chemically tempered lenses have an even surface compression and therefore show no stress patterns when viewed through crossed polarizing filters. A chemically tempered lens can be identified only by taking the lens out of the frame and immersing it in a glycerin solution while viewing it between crossed polarizing filters. A chemically hardened lens shows a halolike, bright band around the edge of the lens. Because of the time-consuming inconvenience of this process, almost everyone depends upon notification enclosed with the

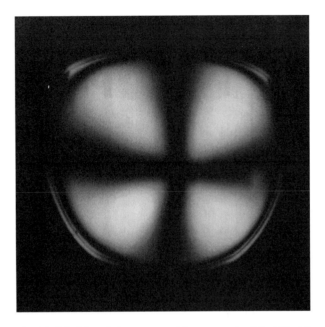

FIGURE **15-12** A heat-treated lens may be identified by the characteristic maltese cross pattern seen when the lens is viewed through the crossed polarizing filter of a colmascope. (From Brooks CW, Borish IM: *System for ophthalmic dispensing*, ed 2, Boston, 1996, Butterworth-Heinemann [Figure 21-1].)

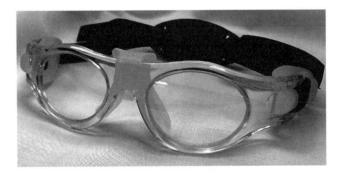

FIGURE **15-13** Sports eyewear is not just safety glasses for sports. Each sport has particular visual and eye protective needs.

finished spectacle lenses as assurance that the lens has been chemically hardened.

Sports Eyewear

Standards for sports eyewear vary. Most of that variation takes place in the frame. Generally the same lenses that are appropriate for high-impact safety eyewear also are appropriate for sports. However, standard Z87–type safety frames are not necessarily appropriate. Specialized sports require specialized frames (Figure 15-13). None of the lenses placed in sports frames are marked with a manufacturer's logo as safety lenses.

---

[22]The 2-hour photochromic process is used for PhotoGray Extra, PhotoBrown Extra, PhotoGray II, and PhotoSun II. It may not be used for PhotoGray, PhotoBrown, PhotoSun, PhotoGray Extra 16, or PhotoBrown Extra 16.

[23]A heat-tempered lens is "dehardened" by heating it as if it were to be heat tempered again. When the lens comes out of the furnace, the cold air is turned off and the lens allowed to cool slowly.

[24]Wilson-Powers B: Chemtempering photochromic lenses, *Optical Management*, 8(5):39, 1979.

Proficiency Test Questions

1. Which of the following is the term for eyewear used for everyday and not for sports or safety?

   a. Casual eyewear
   b. Everyday eyewear
   c. Formal eyewear
   d. Dress eyewear
   e. Standard eyewear

2. Which of the following is the minimum thickness requirements mandated by the FDA for dress eyewear?

   a. 1.0 mm
   b. 1.5 mm
   c. 2.0 mm
   d. 2.2 mm
   e. No minimum thickness requirements exist.

3. When may retailers dispense prescription lenses that are not impact resistant?

   a. When the wearer signs a waiver accepting responsibility
   b. When no other types of impact-resistant lenses will fulfill the visual requirements of the wearer
   c. When the lenses are high-index glass and are unable to be either heat treated or chemically tempered
   d. In any of the above circumstances
   e. In none of the above circumstances

4. Which of the following is the standard "referee test" for determining impact resistance suitable for dress ophthalmic lenses?

   a. A 1-inch steel ball dropped on the front surface of the lens from a height of 50 inches
   b. A 1-inch steel ball dropped on the front surface of the lens from a height of 52 inches
   c. A $5/8$-inch steel ball dropped on the front surface of the lens from a height of 50 inches
   d. A $5/8$-inch steel ball dropped on the front surface of the lens from a height of 52 inches
   e. A $1/4$-inch steel ball shot at the front of lens at a speed of 150 feet per second

5. Which of the following lenses must be individually drop-ball tested and not just batch tested or exempted from testing?

   a. A stock high-index plastic AR-coated lens
   b. A crown glass executive bifocal lens
   c. A fused flat-top 25 photochromic glass bifocal lens
   d. A glass slab-off lens
   e. All of the above must be individually drop-ball tested.
   f. None of the above must be individually drop-ball tested.

6. True or False? Plano sunglasses manufactured in quantity do not have to be impact resistant.

7. An edging laboratory orders a single vision photochromic glass lens from a surfacing laboratory because it is a high cylinder and is not available as a stock lens. Which of the following parties is responsible for drop-ball testing the lens?

   a. The surfacing laboratory
   b. The edging laboratory before it has been edged
   c. The edging laboratory after it has been edged
   d. Neither, because the lenses are batch tested
   e. Neither, because glass photochromics are exempt

8. Arrange the following lenses in order, estimating what you think the relative impact resistance might be, from the most impact resistant to the least impact resistant. (Variations may occur.)

   1. An uncoated plastic lens
   2. A lens coated with scratch-resistant and AR coatings
   3. A lens coated with scratch-resistant and AR coatings, with cushion coatings and/or primers

   a. 1, 2, 3
   b. 3, 2, 1
   c. 2, 1, 3
   d. 1, 3, 2
   e. 2, 3, 1

9. A wearer breaks his frames. You find a new frame, but the old glass lenses are too large. Which of the following is true?

   a. New lenses must be used in the new frame. Chemically tempered lenses cannot be re-edged.
   b. The lenses can be re-edged and put back in the frame as is. The chemical tempering is unaffected because the chemical change occurs on the surfaces of the lens.
   c. The lenses can be re-edged but must be chemically tempered all over again before being put into the new frame.
   d. The lenses can be re-edged but must be chemically tempered again and drop-ball tested again before being put into the new frame.

10. True or False? It is illegal to use a glass lens in a nylon cord frame.

11. Which of the following lenses is most likely to break?

    a. An unscratched lens
    b. A lens that has been scratched on the front surface
    c. A lens that has been scratched on the back surface
    d. All lenses are equally likely to break

12. The "duty to inform" is which of the following?

    a. A legal responsibility
    b. A professional responsibility
    c. Both

13. Which of the following is the basic-impact* safety eyewear minimum thickness?

    a. 2.0 mm
    b. 2.2 mm
    c. 3.0 mm (except +3.00 D in the most plus meridian and above, which have a minimum thickness of 2.5 mm)
    d. 3.2 mm (except +3.00 D in the most plus meridian and above, which have a minimum thickness of 2.8 mm)

14. Which of the following is the anticipated high-impact safety eyewear minimum thicknesses?

    a. 2.0 mm
    b. 2.2 mm
    c. 3.0 mm (except +3.00 D in the most plus meridian and above, which have a minimum thickness of 2.5 mm)
    d. 3.2 mm (except +3.00 D in the most plus meridian and above, which have a minimum thickness of 2.8 mm)

15. Which of the following is the standard "referee test" for determining impact resistance suitable for basic-impact prescription safety lenses?

    a. A 1-inch steel ball dropped on the front surface of the lens from a height of 50 inches
    b. A 1-inch steel ball dropped on the front surface of the lens from a height of 54 inches
    c. A $5/8$-inch steel ball dropped on the front surface of the lens from a height of 50 inches
    d. A $5/8$-inch steel ball dropped on the front surface of the lens from a height of 54 inches
    e. A $1/4$-inch steel ball shot at the front of lens at a speed of 150 feet per second

16. How must a safety *frame* suitable for high-impact safety lenses be marked on the front and temples, assuming that the projected standards become actual standards?

    a. Size and manufacturer
    b. Size, manufacturer, and Z87
    c. Size, manufacturer, and Z87+
    d. Size, manufacturer, and Z87-2

17. True or False? Putting 2.0-mm thick CR-39 lenses in a safety frame but not marking the lenses for safety is acceptable if the person just wants the glasses for regular wear.

18. True or False? Putting 2.0-mm thick polycarbonate lenses in a safety frame but not marking the lenses for safety is acceptable if the person just wants the glasses for regular wear.

---

*Basic-impact requirements are historically the same as the Z87.1-1989 standard and are part of the projected new standard that would include both basic- and high-impact lenses.

19. Which of the following lenses is the most impact resistant?

    a A 2.2-mm thick crown glass lens that has not been heat treated or chemically tempered
    b. A 2.2-mm thick crown glass lens that has been heat treated
    c. A 2.2-mm thick crown glass lens that has been chemically tempered

20. Chemically tempered photochromic lenses are treated in a bath of molten salt that consists of which of the following?

    a. Sodium nitrate
    b. Potassium nitrate
    c. A combination of sodium nitrate and potassium nitrate
    d. Sodium chloride
    e. Potassium chloride
    f. A combination of sodium chloride and potassium chloride

21. True or False? A lens may be identified has having been chemically tempered by placing it in a colmascope. (A colmascope consists of two crossed polarizing filters that are backlighted.)

16 Maintenance and Calibration

Having the best and newest equipment does not ensure prescription accuracy and quality craftsmanship if that equipment is not properly maintained and correctly calibrated. Many fine apprenticeship programs in optical craftsmanship begin, not with an explanation of optics, but with instruction on cleaning and care of the equipment vital to the functioning of the laboratory. The material presented in this chapter is more than reference material to consult only in an emergency situation—the maintenance of equipment is important to the successful operation of an optical laboratory.

Maintenance Schedules

A master maintenance schedule that outlines how often each piece of equipment should be lubricated, greased, cleaned, or calibrated is helpful. This master list should detail how often each of these tasks must be done and leave enough space to enter the date when the service was performed and the signature or initials of the individual who performed it. In this way deficiencies may be noted at a glance.

As much as is possible, maintenance services should be done on a regularly scheduled basis so that each workday concludes with cleaning and wiping of equipment. A section of time at the end of the week could, for example, be devoted to more thorough maintenance, including lubrication, coolant changes, and calibration checks.

Care of the Lensmeter

Prescription accuracy begins and ends with the lensmeter. A laboratory lensmeter must be highly accurate. Those who use the lensmeter regularly must know how to adjust it for exact measurements so that they are confident that the power being read is the power the lens actually has. Many a disagreement between laboratory and account would never have occurred if both instruments had been used correctly and rightly calibrated.

CALIBRATION OF POWER

Before any instrument is calibrated, the individual must be certain that it is adjusted properly for his or her eye. The eye's accommodative (focusing) mechanism and refractive error can directly influence lens power readings. The eyepiece is turned out (counter-clockwise) and slowly turned inward until the black reticle lines *first* come into focus. (For better illumination holding a sheet of white paper in the lensmeter where the lens would be normally to reflect light back and provide a white background may be helpful.) Looking at the 1.0Δ ring is helpful for best reference. Once the eyepiece is in focus, then power accuracy may be checked.

Those wearing bifocals and progressive addition lenses should look through the lensmeter through the *distance* part of the prescription. The instrument is set for distance vision. They should not look through the segment or the progressive zone, even though the instrument target appears to be close. It is easy to make a mistake with progressive addition lenses, looking through a slightly different part of the progressive lens each time. Those who wear bifocals and progressive addition lenses should ensure they are well into the upper, distance portion of the progressive addition lens correction when using the lensmeter.

With no lens in the instrument, the power wheel is turned from a minus direction[1] until the target clears. The wheel is not rocked back and forth to obtain a focus; instead, the operator simply stops when the target first clears. (This rule applies equally for reading lens power. For more on how to use a lensmeter, see Brooks CW, Borish IM: *System for ophthalmic dispensing*, ed 2, Boston, 1996, Butterworth-Heinemann.) The power should read zero. If the instrument does not read zero, the process is repeated several times to be certain of obtaining a clear target. If the target still does not focus at zero, the instrument must be recalibrated.

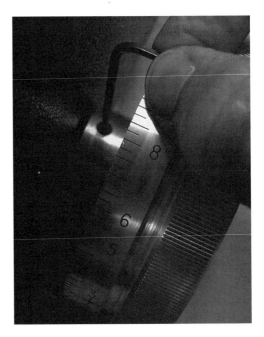

FIGURE **16-1** If the lensmeter does not read zero without a lens in place, a manual model may often be readjusted by loosening the power wheel set screw and turning the wheel to zero.

Once the target is accurately sharp and zeroed, the power is recalibrated by loosening the power wheel with the appropriate tool, such as a screwdriver or Allen wrench (Figure 16-1). This allows the wheel to turn freely. The zero setting on the power wheel is turned to the index mark and the wheel retightened. (Some instruments allow for correction of small errors by an adjustment of the index mark.)

PRISM

With both reticle and target in focus, the instrument is checked for prism accuracy. With no lens in the instrument, the target should cross exactly at the center of the reticle. *Note:* If the lensmeter has an auxiliary rotary prism system, it must be set on zero. Otherwise the instrument will show prism when no prism exists.

If prism is evident without lenses present, as is seen in Figure 16-2, the instrument manual should be consulted for corrective measures. It may require factory realignment.

OPTICS

The optics of a lensmeter or other optical instrument may be blown free of dust using a syringe or canned compressed air (such as is employed for photography lenses). Alternatively, a camel's hair brush may be used

---

[1]*ANSI Z80.1-1999 American National Standard for ophthalmics— prescription ophthalmic lenses—recommendations*, Merrifield, Va, 2000, Optical Laboratories Association, p 12.

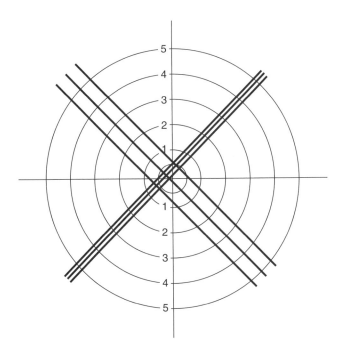

FIGURE **16-2** An off-center target is difficult to compensate for and should be fixed as soon as possible. (Instruments with prism compensation devices should be checked to ensure that the device registers zero.)

to wipe dust from the lenses. Any solution that would not damage a fine, vacuum-coated camera lens may be used to clean away oily film or smudges.

EXTERIOR

Smooth-finish exteriors may be cleaned with a damp cloth. To restore polish to enamel exteriors on lensmeters, edgers, or other instruments having a shiny enameled look, a high-quality automotive paste wax is used.

Black crackle-finish exteriors are wiped clean with a damp cloth then polished with mineral oil to return their original luster.

INKING

If the spotting mechanism is giving splotchy and incomplete dots, or is depositing too much ink on the lens, the pad and reservoir are cleaned; then the pad is reinked. Ordinary stamp pad ink works well.

The marking pins should move freely, be clear of debris, and be smooth-tipped so as not to scratch the lens. If the pins do not move freely, the assembly is cleaned and lubricated with a light oil.

Centration Blockers

The centration blocker places the block on the lens. The traditional centration blocker always puts the block exactly at the same place in the instrument. However, because the lens is decentered, the block is not at the same place on the lens every time. The centration blocker places the block at the center of the background grid of the instrument. The lens is moved to create the correct amount of decentration. The center of the block should always correspond to the zero point on the background grid both horizontally and vertically. Centration blockers have a movable vertical line and a background grid. The background grid does not move.

The 180-degree line of the block must overlap with the 180-degree line of the background grid.

- If the block is displaced horizontally, the PD will be off.
- If the block is displaced vertically, major reference point (MRP) heights, fitting cross heights, and bifocal heights will be wrong.
- If the block is tilted relative to the background 180, the cylinder axis will be incorrect and bifocal lines will not be straight.

To check the accuracy of a centration blocker, a lens with the flattest front curve available is chosen. First this lens is hand-marked with a long horizontal and short vertical line through the center. A flexible ruler should be used to ensure that the line is straight.[2] The hand-drawn mark is aligned on the grid as if no decentration existed. The mark must be exactly on the origin of the background grid. The lens is blocked in the customary manner.

After blocking, the mark on the lens should be exactly in the center of the block. Figure 16-3 illustrates how the 180-degree line marked on the lens should overlap the 180-degree reference line(s) on the block.

Some adhesive pad blocks have a small central hole used in some blocking alignment systems. This hole should be at the center of the hand-drawn mark. Other blocks have vertical and horizontal lines at the center of the front of the block. This also can be seen in Figure 16-3.

If the marker/blocker is off horizontally or vertically, the problem is corrected by readjusting the background grid. Readjustment of the background grid varies according to the type of instrument. Figure 16-4, *A*, shows one example of how a centration blocker is recalibrated. A cap is on each side of the screen. The cap is removed and an Allen screw is loosened as shown in the figure. This allows the tabletop to be pushed left or right as shown in Figure 16-4, *B*.

---

[2]Using a higher base curve lens causes the ruler to curve when pressed against the lens. Therefore the use of a flat base curve lens for these purposes is important.

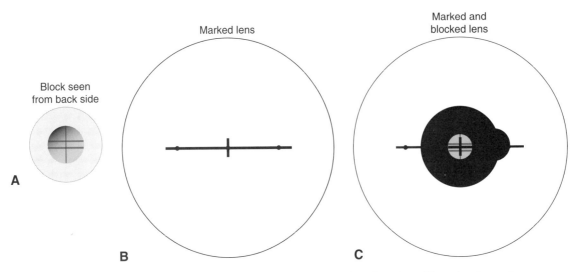

FIGURE **16**-3   Lens blockers may be checked by first hand-marking the lens, then placing the center of the mark on the grid origin and blocking the lens. **A,** The back of the lens block. Most blocks have horizontal markings and a central reference point or line. **B,** The marked lens before blocking. **C,** The lens after it is blocked. If the block conforms to the marked 180-degree line both horizontally and vertically, the blocker is in adjustment. If the marked cross is not in the middle of the block both horizontally and vertically, or is tilted, the blocker is not aligned properly and should be readjusted.

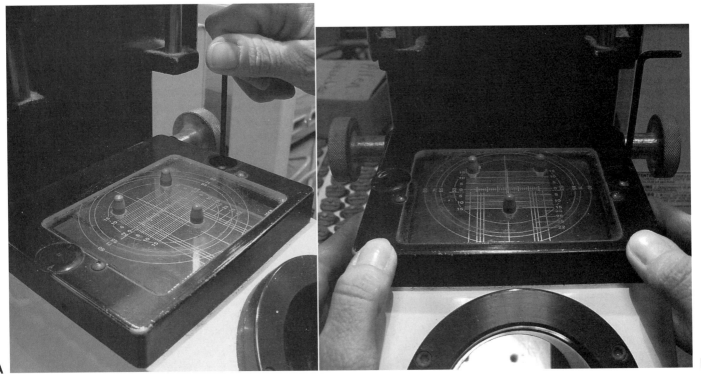

FIGURE **16-4**   **A,** Translucent background grids may be readjusted by Allen screws (setscrews), or other similar means. Here set screws are being loosened to allow for horizontal alignment. **B,** Once the tabletop containing the background grid is loosened, it may be moved left or right until it is properly realigned.

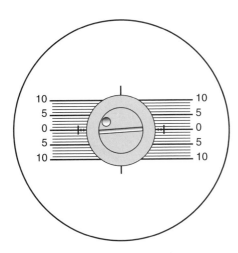

FIGURE **16-5** A centration device that blocks at an angle will result in cylinder axis errors and tilted bifocal segments.

If the block is tilted relative to the 180-degree line on the lens, the axis is out of adjustment (Figure 16-5). This means that every cylinder lens will be off axis and every bifocal top tilted. If the block is tilted, the blocking mechanism that lowers the block onto the lens may be at fault.

Calibration of Edgers

When considering calibration and maintenance of edgers, the reader must keep in mind that the information included here is not an adequate substitute for material provided with each individual edger. This discussion should be regarded as an overview of general maintenance and calibration requirements.

No attempt is made to cover calibration of patternless edgers. These requirements vary considerably. Calibration is unique and usually built into the program that runs the edger.

CHECKING AXIS ACCURACY FOR PATTERNED EDGERS

In edging lenses, it is essential that the 180-degree line on the pattern is always parallel to the 180-degree line on the lens. However, because the pattern and lens are some distance apart and each is held in place by a separate mechanism, the possibility of misalignment is understandable. For this reason patterned edgers are made so that axis alignment may be fine-tuned for reliability.

To check for accuracy of the axis, a pattern is chosen whose shape comes close to being a square or octagon.

It is helpful if pattern corners are squared-off and distinct, with sides, tops, and bottoms as straight as possible.

A pair of lenses is marked carefully along the 180-degree line. The lenses are blocked on this line. The mark must be either non–water-soluble or protected with tape or spray to withstand the washing effect of the coolant. (Test lenses do not need to be cylindrical because the point of reference is the marked cutting line and not the cylinder axis.)

Next, the lenses are edged. As the two lenses must be held back-to-back exactly over one another when cut, it is helpful to have a flat edge on the lenses. Therefore the lenses should be either cut on the rimless program or stopped after they have been roughed. (*Reminder:* Lenses are being edged as if they were a pair; therefore the pattern must be turned after edging the first lens.)

When edging is completed, the lenses are held back to back. Their shapes must match exactly. If the marked lines exactly overlap each other, the edger axis is properly set. (The sequence for checking the edger axis is reviewed in Box 16-1.) If, however, these marked lines are *not* coincident (Figure 16-6), then the axis of the edger must be readjusted. This is further clarified in Figure 16-7, *A*. Figure 16-7 and Table 16-1 help clarify the possible sources of error.

BOX **16-1**
Edger Axis Checking Sequence

1. Clearly mark one lens pair with non–water-soluble ink.
2. Accurately block both lenses with no decentration.
3. Choose a squared pattern.
4. Flat-edge or rough only.
5. Hold the edged lenses back to back.
6. Check to ensure that the marks on the lenses overlap.

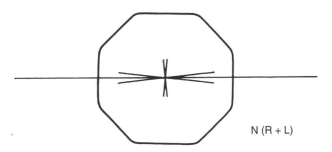

N (R + L)

FIGURE **16-6** When edged lenses are held back to back and their reference marks do not overlap, the origin of the problem could stem from a variety of possible sources. This particular error is shown in a different manner in Figure 16-7, *A*, where it is also discussed in more detail.

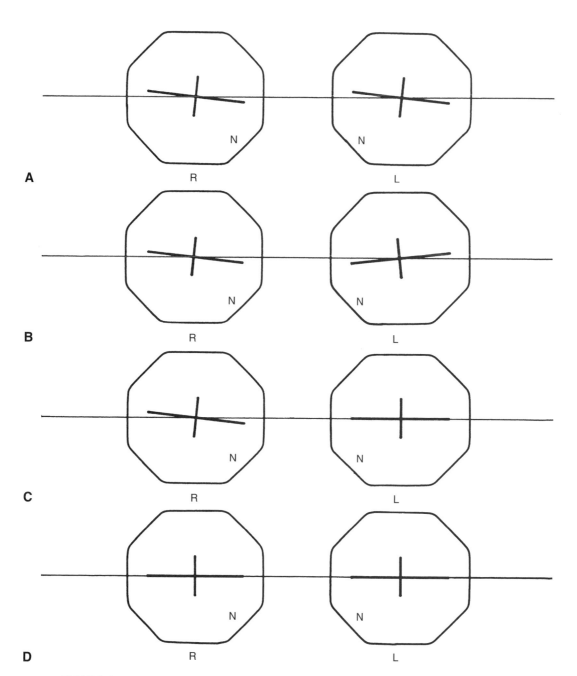

FIGURE **16-7**   **A,** The lenses are placed face up and correctly turned; the marks are off axis. (These lenses are the same as those shown in the previous figure.) When the error manifests itself in this manner, the problem could stem from an axis error in either the edger or the blocker. **B,** If these lenses were placed back to back, the two marks would overlap exactly, masking the problem. The possible source of this error is a pattern that has been cut off axis. (It could be that the lenses are actually correct, but the frame shape has been misinterpreted and the lenses are twisted wrong.) **C,** Two sources of error are possible here: human error or the block slipped during edging. **D,** If the marks are correct after edging, but the cylinder axis is off for both lenses when checked in the lensmeter, then the problem lies with the centration device.

TABLE **16-1**
Possible Sources of Axis Errors

CHECKPOINT	SOURCE OF ERROR
An axis error shows up when a second lensmeter is used.	The two lensmeters should be compared. One of the lensmeters may be out of adjustment.
An axis error shows up when the same lensmeter is used as was used for spotting.	Lensmeter error is ruled out. The error may be caused by the edger or the centration instrument.
Formally check the edger with marked lenses. Afterward, hold the lenses back to back.	If the marks on the lenses are not coincident, consult Figure 16-7 for the source of the error.
Formally check the centration device by premarking the lens with a horizontal line. Block the lens on the line to determine whether the line is parallel to the 180-degree line of the block.	If the drawn line is not parallel to the 180-degree line on the lens block, the centration device is at fault.

Methods for readjusting the edger axis vary. The edger manual will detail exactly how to do this for the edger being used.

CHECKING WHEEL DIFFERENTIAL (GRINDING ALLOWANCE)

Wheel differential is the difference in size of a lens after it has been rough edged compared with its final size. Because the finishing wheel uses fine-grit diamond particles, it cuts slowly and has the potential of wearing down quickly if used excessively. For maximum speed and best wheel life, the lens should be cut as small as possible on the coarse-grit roughing wheel first. Computer-assisted patternless edgers also must be checked for wheel differential.

Roughing wheels cut rapidly but coarsely and leave a rough edge along the lens periphery. This rough edge should be removed on the finishing wheel. Generally the roughed lens must be reduced in size by about 2 mm.

Wheel differential increases as a metal bonded roughing wheel wears down and should be monitored. Normally this is not an issue with electroplated wheels because little wear occurs with this type of wheel from plastic lenses. (For more on edger wheel types, see Chapter 17.) Failure to check wheel differential with bonded roughing wheels causes an unnecessary increase in edging time with a corresponding decrease in edge quality and finishing wheel life.

MEASURING WHEEL DIFFERENTIAL

To measure wheel differential, a blocked lens blank is placed in the edger and the edging cycle starts. After the roughing cycle is completed, but before the finishing cycle starts, the cycle is stopped. The roughed lens is removed and its A dimension measured. Afterwards the lens is returned to the edger and the cycle is allowed to continue until the lens is fully beveled. Upon completion of the cycle, the lens is measured a second time. The difference in size between the first and second measurements is the wheel differential. This is summarized in Box 16-2. Use a round lens and a vernier caliper-like the one that was shown in Figure 3-12.

Example 16-1

A lens is to be edged to a 50-mm eyesize. If the pattern is a "set −10" pattern, the edger is set for 40.0. To check for wheel differential, the edging cycle is started but stopped after roughing. The lens is removed from the edger, measured with a caliper, and found to have an eyesize of 52.8 mm. The lens is put back in the edger and edged to completion. It is taken out and measured with the caliper. Now the lens has an eyesize of 50 mm. What is the wheel differential for this edger?

Solution

The difference between the two measurements is taken to find wheel differential:

$$\text{Wheel differential} = 52.8\,\text{mm} - 50\,\text{mm}$$
$$= 2.8\,\text{mm}$$

Because this measured wheel differential is larger than recommended, it should be reduced to about 2.0 mm.

BOX **16-2**
Wheel Differential Checking Sequence

1. Begin to edge a lens.
2. Stop the cycle after roughing the lens.
3. Measure the eyesize of the roughed lens.
4. Replace the lens and complete the cycle.
5. Measured the finished lens eyesize.
6. Wheel differential = Roughed eyesize − Finished eyesize

ADJUSTING FOR WHEEL DIFFERENTIAL

Methods for wheel differential adjustment vary considerably from edger to edger. Sometimes the position of the clapper plate upon which the pattern turns during roughing must be readjusted. These plates also must be reset after installation of new or retrued wheels. (Exact procedures are found in the manual that accompanies each edger.) Make no attempt to recalibrate eyesize until the correct wheel differential has been properly set.

EYESIZE ADJUSTMENTS FOR MANUAL, PATTERNED EDGERS

In simplest terms, lens edger eyesize accuracy is checked by first edging a lens and then measuring to see whether its size corresponds to what was intended. There are two methods for checking eyesize accuracy—one that uses the A dimension of the lens and another that uses lens circumference.

Adjusting Edger Setting Accuracy Using the A Dimension

When checking eyesize accuracy it is best to use a round pattern, or a pattern whose A dimension is easily measured. If the pattern is not round, the pattern chosen must be widest at the midline. With this shape less error in measurement is likely. If the pattern size is not exactly known, the pattern is measured with vernier calipers and its set number determined.

The set number is calculated by subtracting the pattern A dimension from the standard size of 36.5 mm. If the pattern measures 46.5 mm, the set number would be −10, as follows:

$$36.5 - 46.5 = -10$$

The pattern is placed on the edger. The eyesize is set. (For a 50-mm eyesize, a 40-mm setting would be chosen.) With a test lens in place, the edger is run through its complete cycle. The edged lens is removed and measured with the vernier caliper in the same manner as was done for the pattern. The edged lens size should come out right. In this example, the lens would be exactly 50 mm. If it does not have the expected eyesize, the edger size needs to be recalibrated.

For many edgers, recalibration is as easy as loosening the setscrew on the eyesize dial. This allows the dial to turn freely. The dial is turned to the *setting that corresponds to the eyesize actually produced* by the edger and the setscrew is tightened up again.

In summary, the following steps are involved in checking eyesize setting accuracy:

1. Choose a round or easily measured pattern.
2. Measure the pattern.
3. Set the edger to an average value eyesize setting for the pattern.
4. Edge a test lens.
5. Measure the test lens.

Example 16-2

The edger seems to be edging large; a set-10, round pattern is chosen. The edger is set at 40 to provide a 50-mm eyesize lens. The lens is edged and measured with a vernier caliper. Instead of 50-mm, it edges out as 50.5 mm. How would the edger be recalibrated for this error?

Solution

The setting that *should* produce a 50.5-mm lens using a set −10 pattern is the following:

$$\text{Edger setting} = \text{Eyesize} + \text{Set number}$$

or

$$\text{Edger setting} = 50.5 - 10$$
$$= 40.5$$

Therefore the dial is loosened, turned to 40.5, and retightened.

Adjusting Edger Setting Accuracy Using Circumference

Recalibration of the edger size setting is possible with use of a round pattern and a circumference gauge. The following is the procedure.

The circumference of a round pattern is measured. The edger is set for slightly more than 36.5 mm. That pattern is used to edge a lens. The edged lens is measured with the circumference gauge. The circumference of the lens should come out larger than the circumference of the pattern. The edger setting is reduced step-wise; each time the operator checks the circumference of the lens. When the lens reaches the circumference of the pattern, the edger should be reading 36.5 mm. If it is not, loosen the edger setting dial until it moves freely. The loosened dial is turned until it reads 36.5 mm and is retightened.

Cleaning and Lubricating Edgers

Glass and plastic sludge should not be allowed to build up hard deposits anywhere within or upon the edger because they can be removed only through mechanical action that is damaging to machine surfaces.

To clean the edger, the grinding chamber is flushed with water so that excess glass or plastic sludge is flushed down into the coolant tank for removal. A small hose run from a faucet or other source is most effective.

The coolant tank must not run over while the chamber is flushed. An alternative to a hose is to use a water-filled spray bottle. The bottle is kept next to the edger and used to clean out the inside of the grinding chamber several times during the course of the day.

If it has been a while since any of this has been done, the sludge will have hardened and will have to be brushed or scraped off. Therefore it is best to clean the edger lightly at the end of each day by rinsing off excess sludge and wiping the exterior with a damp cloth. The machine should be cleaned thoroughly at least once a week, or as often as the coolant is changed, whichever occurs more frequently. To clean the edger thoroughly, the following steps are performed:

1. Remove all glass or plastic sludge from the chamber by rinsing and wiping.
2. Clean the exterior thoroughly.
3. If the edger requires greasing, wipe grease from the gears or moving parts and regrease. If thorough greasing is not carried out when indicated, glass or plastic sludge can creep into moving parts, which causes excessive wear and possible freeze-up.
4. Oil those areas indicated in the manual, such as hinges and springs, using a light machine oil like those suitable for sewing machines. (Some areas require oiling only once every few months. These maintenance requirements are recorded on a master maintenance sheet.)

Edger Coolants

Some system of cooling the lens and flushing the abraded lens material off of the wheel is absolutely essential during the conventional edging operation with use of diamond wheels. The most basic coolant is water and water often is used by itself. If a coolant is added to water, it should help to keep particles of ground material in suspension. This prevents sludge build-up on the wheel and in the grinding chamber. Commercial coolant also serves as a rust inhibitor.

With a water-only coolant system, with some edgers the use of a defoamer may be helpful to prevent the coolant tank from foaming up and overflowing.

CHANGING THE COOLANT

The coolant tank may be designed for the edger or simply be a 5-gallon bucket. The tank can be pulled out from under the edger and the liquid drained off, which leaves sludge in the plastic bag liner. The sludge-filled liner is removed and tied at the top for disposal. (See Chapter 18 on Safety and Environmental Concerns regarding disposal of coolant liquids and solids.)

Before new coolant is added, the coolant pump is cleansed and any residue is rinsed from drains and electrical cords. If this is done regularly, it is easy to do. If not, residues become increasingly difficult to remove.

Coolants come in varying concentrations that are added to fresh water. Coolant replacement is the *last* in a series of maintenance procedures. Some procedures that may precede coolant changes are the following:

1. Stoning (dressing) the diamond wheel
2. Cleaning the coolant chamber
3. Lubricating the edger

Because the coolant pump is located inside and toward the top of the coolant tank, coolant level should be checked to ensure that the pump remains covered. Water may be added to raise the coolant back up to the required level to compensate for evaporation.

Proficiency Test Questions

1. True or False? Focusing the lensmeter eyepiece allows the instrument to compensate for either the lack of accommodation or for a refractive error on the part of the operator. This means two individuals may well require two different eyepiece settings. Failure to refocus the eyepiece before using the instrument may cause discomfort to the operator, but it in no way affects the accuracy of the reading.

2. Which of the following is not normally recommended for cleaning lenses in an optical instrument?

   a. AR lens cleaners
   b. Camel's hair brush
   c. Ammonia
   d. Canned compressed air

3. True or False? It is possible to use ordinary stamp pad ink in the lensmeter marking device when plastic lenses are being marked.

4. Which of the following lens shapes is best used to check edger axis accuracy?

   a. Round
   b. Square
   c. Oval

5. In which of the following instances is it most helpful to have a flat edge on test lenses?

   a. When checking edger eyesize
   b. When checking lensmeter accuracy
   c. When checking edger axis

6. When verifying completed work in the finishing laboratory and using the same lensmeter as was used in marking up the lenses, errors in axis are discovered as follows:

LENS ORDERED	CURRENT REALITY
R: +2.00 –1.00 X 180	+2.00 –1.00 X 8
L: +2.25 –1.25 X 5	+2.25 –1.25 X 13
R: –3.75 –2.00 X 48	–3.75 –2.00 X 56
L: –4.00 –1.75 X 136	–4.00 –1.75 X 144

   All lenses are edged for metal frames. The lenses are straight in the frame. Which of the following piece(s) of equipment may be responsible for the errors?

   1. Lensmeter
   2. Centration device
   3. Edger

   a. 1, 2, 3
   b. 1, 2
   c. 2, 3
   d. 1

7. Both left and right lenses are correctly inserted into a metal frame with their blocks still intact. Assuming the frame is properly manufactured, if the blocks on the right and left lenses are both at a 10-degree angle instead of at 180 degrees, which of the following might describe the problem?

   a. The edger axis may be out of adjustment.
   b. The centration device may be off.
   c. The pattern may have been cut off axis.
   d. Any of the above could have caused the problem.

8. Both left and right lenses are correctly inserted into a metal frame with their blocks still intact. Assuming the frame is properly manufactured, if the block on the right lens marking cross is turned to a 10-degree axis and the block on the left marking cross is turned to a 170-degree axis, which of the following might describe the problem?

   a. The edger axis may be out of adjustment.
   b. The lens marker stamp may be rotated.
   c. The pattern may have been cut off axis.
   d. Any of the above could have caused the problem.

9. While checking the edger for eyesize accuracy, it is discovered that the wheel differential is also in need of adjustment. Which of the following should normally be corrected first?

   a. Eyesize
   b. Wheel differential

10. Which of the following describes the wheel differential?

    a. Difference in the width of the wheel edge between roughing and finishing wheels
    b. The ratio between the speed of rotation of the lens drive motor and the speed of rotation of the edger wheel itself
    c. The wheel speed of the edger in question as compared to a standard wheel speed
    d. The size difference a lens has after being rough edged on the roughing wheel in comparison to the size it has after being edged on the finishing wheel
    e. The difference between the wheel speed as measured at the edge of the roughing wheel in comparison to the speed as measured at the edge of the finishing wheel

11. An edger is checked for accuracy of eyesize. An accurate pattern with a "set –12" size is used. The edger dial is set for 45. Which of the following identifies the lens A dimension measure when it is cut?

    a. 45
    b. 33
    c. 57
    d. 36.5
    e. None of the above is correct.

12. A sizing pattern that has an A dimension of 46.5 is used to check the edger for correctness in cutting eyesize. The edger is set on 45 and a trial lens is edged. When removed and measured, the lens is found to be 54.5 mm. To reset the edger, the thumb screw is loosened and the sizing dial knob turned. The thumb screw is then retightened. The edger should now cut a lens correctly. Which of the following identifies the new, correct edger setting?

   a. 45
   b. 54
   c. 54.5
   d. 44.5
   e. 55.5

13. To check for edger eyesize accuracy, a "set −15" pattern is used. When edged, the lens measures 49.2 instead of the 49.0 mm that was called for by the dial setting. To correctly calibrate the edger, its eyesize dial is loosened. To which of the following measures should it be turned to be recalibrated correctly?

   a. 49.2
   b. 48.8
   c. 33.8
   d. 34.2
   e. None of the above is correct.

14. Place the following edger maintenance jobs in their optimum order, from first job to be carried out, to last.

   1. Cleaning the grinding chamber
   2. Changing the coolant
   3. Stoning the wheel
   4. Lubricating the edger

   a. 1, 3, 4, 2
   b. 4, 3, 2, 1
   c. 2, 1, 3, 4
   d. 3, 1, 4, 2
   e. 1, 4, 2, 3

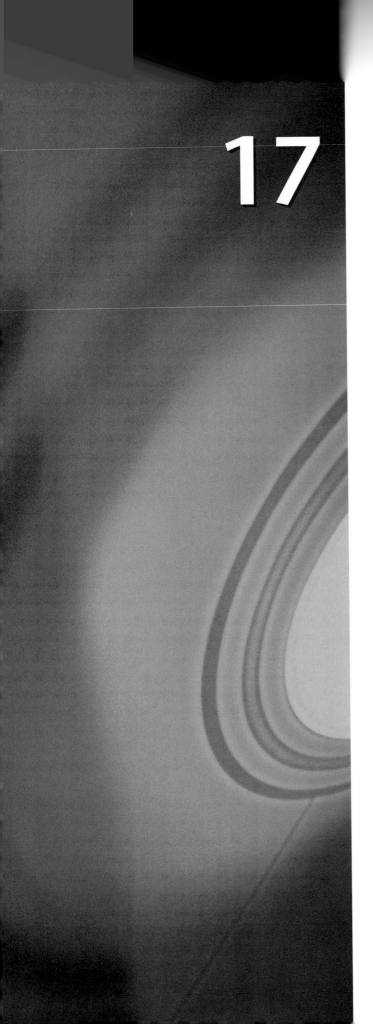

17 Edger Wheels and Cutters

A number of diamond wheels are marketed through a variety of sources. Knowledge of wheel construction and variable factors is important for comparison of wheels. In addition, diamond wheel care varies according to type. Even if a wheel is chosen with care, if it is not properly maintained, it will not give optimum service.

Four Construction Factors

Four main variable factors exist in the construction of diamond wheel surfaces and include grit size, diamond concentration, depth of the diamond layer, and type of bond used to hold the diamond to the wheel.

GRIT SIZE

A diamond abrasive works in much the same manner as does ordinary sandpaper. Coarse grade sandpaper contains large chunks of abrasive and removes surface material rapidly. A surface coarsely sanded shows visible grooves and feels rough to the touch. On the other hand, fine grade sandpaper gives a smooth, clean finish. However, because it can abrade away only small amounts of material, it is inappropriate for anything but a fine finish. The same is true for diamond wheels. If the main task of the wheel is to grind away large quantities of material, large, chunky diamond particles are appropriate.

Wheels having a coarse grit grind rapidly but leave ragged edges. Large grit diamond particles are used for making roughing wheels. Finer particle sizes are used for finishing wheels and, although slower, produce smooth edges. Diamond polishing wheels have diamond particles that are finer still.

Because they are used as industrial abrasives, diamond particles are sorted by size. If a screening process were used for this, progressively finer mesh would be used to trap larger particles. If a diamond particle is small enough to fall through one screen but is stopped by the next, then its size is between the two screen sizes. Because screens are measured by the number of wires or fibers per unit area, diamond grit numbers are based on this system. Therefore the *higher* the diamond code number, the *smaller* the diamond particle size.

When grit size is extremely small, the diamond material takes on a flourlike consistency and is referred to as *diamond powder*.

Two or more different grit sizes may be used in combination on the same wheel. In this manner a better cutting speed can be achieved while producing a more acceptable edge finish.

Grit size also becomes a factor in how well a wheel holds its form. The finer the grit used in a wheel, the faster it will be worn away during the edging process. As would be expected, V-bevels and hidden bevels lose their configuration as the wheel wears. Therefore a compromise results between how smooth and flake-free the bevel will be, in contrast to how long the wheel will cut distinct edges before retruing is needed.

CONCENTRATION

The second factor in diamond wheel evaluation is the amount of diamond per cubic unit. A wheel having only a small amount of diamond in comparison with the bonding material that holds it is of low concentration.

The highest concentration wheel normally used in the optical industry contains 25% diamond and 75% bonding material. This concentration is designated by volume and is given a code number of 100, as is Table 17-1. A high concentration wheel is not necessarily the best wheel for all situations.

Roughing wheels having a high concentration of diamond are excellent for edgers with a heavy head pressure, but a high concentration wheel on a low-pressure edger cuts poorly.

As would be expected, high concentration wheels wear slower. Therefore they are the correct choice for finishing wheels made to cut distinct edge shapes. If a medium or low concentration of diamond were to be used, sharp bevel angles would soon begin to round.

TABLE 17-1 *Diamond Concentrations*			
CONCENTRATION NUMBER	CARATS*/ CUBIC INCHES	CARATS/ CUBIC CENTIMETERS	% DIAMOND BY VOLUME
100	72	4.4	25
75	54	3.3	18.75
50	36	2.2	12.5
25	18	1.1	6.25

*One carat of diamond is 0.2 g.

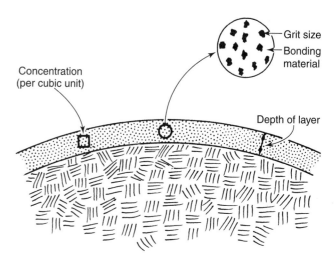

FIGURE **17-1** Important factors in specifying wheel type include concentration (particles per cubic unit of area), grit size (how big the abrasive particles are), bonding material (what is used to hold the abrasive particles in place), and depth of layer (how thick the abrasive particle layer is).

DEPTH OF LAYER

Were a wheel to have a good concentration of the proper grit diamond material, it would still have no lasting value if the depth of layer were too thin (Figure 17-1). A wheel is only useful while abrasive material remains on the core. Once this layer has worn thin, the wheel must be replaced.

TYPE OF BONDING

Diamond material must be bound solidly to the core of the wheel and simultaneously allow exposure of sharp diamond edges. Bonding usually is accomplished in one of two ways:

1. *Metal-bonded or impregnated* wheels are made by mixing diamond material with powdered metal. This mixture is placed in a mold containing the core of the wheel. The filled mold is heated in a furnace until the metal begins to melt. When cooling takes place, the diamond grit is bound to the core of the wheel with solidified metal.
2. *Electroplated or electrometallic* wheels are made by electrolytically depositing metal onto the wheel. During this process diamond particles are encompassed by a thickening layer of metal that is transferred electrolytically from the ion-laden plating solution.

Generally, metal-bonded wheels are used to grind glass lenses, although they also may be used for plastic lenses. Electroplated wheels, though, are used almost exclusively for plastic lenses. Some wheel types are shown in Figure 17-2. Edging a hard glass lens on an electroplated wheel causes an extreme reduction in wheel life because diamond particles are torn easily from the electroplated metal.

Although the edging of plastic lenses on metal-bonded *roughing* wheels that are intended primarily for glass is acceptable, results are satisfactory only up to a point because the wheel clogs with plastic between the diamonds. In other words, the wheel glazes.

During the *finishing* cycle, excellent results may be obtained for plastic lenses using either an electroplated or a metal-bonded wheel. Figure 17-3 summarizes the process.

Dressing Diamond Wheels

From time to time a diamond wheel begins to lose some of the sharp cutting ability that it had when new. This is generally a result of (1) a "glazed" wheel or (2) diamonds that have become dull.

GLAZED WHEEL

When the empty spaces between exposed diamond particles begin to fill up with ground lens material, the diamonds are unable to dig or bite into the lens as deeply. This condition is known as *glazing*. A glazed wheel looks smooth and feels relatively smooth to the touch. When a wheel becomes glazed, it must be cleaned by dressing.

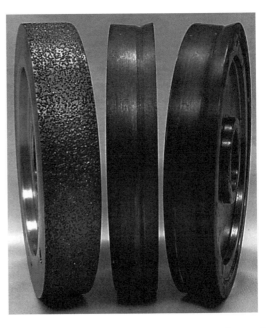

FIGURE **17-2**   The wheel on the left is an electroplated roughing wheel. The center wheel is a metal-bonded finishing wheel, and the wheel on the right is an extremely fine grit metal-bonded wheel for polishing.

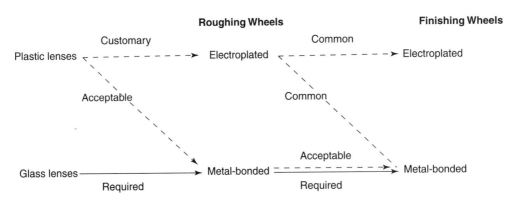

FIGURE **17-3**   Types of wheels and sequence used in the edging of glass and plastic lenses. This figure represents possible paths plastic *(dashed lines)* and glass lenses *(solid lines)* may take in the edging process.

DRESSING THE WHEEL

Wheels may lose their cutting ability because their exposed diamonds have dulled through use.

If the outermost diamonds can be removed to allow exposure of ones slightly deeper in the bond, cutting integrity can be restored. The outer surface of the metal bond that holds the diamond in place is attacked. This is referred to as *dressing* or *stoning*. The procedure involves holding an abrasive stick against the spinning wheel. Figure 17-4 shows the abrasive stick, most often made up of aluminum oxide or silicone carbide grit formed into a squared stick and held together with a soft bonding material. When the abrasive stick is held against the wheel, exposed diamonds easily furrow through the loosely bonded stick surface. This allows the stick to rub against the bonding material surrounding the diamond particles. The bonding is ground down far enough that old, dull diamonds no longer are embedded in enough bonding material to hold them and so they drop off. As in Figure 17-5, other diamonds embedded more deeply in the bonding are exposed, which gives a fresh, sharp cutting surface.

Dressing of an edger wheel should be done before changing coolant. In this manner, the spent abrasive material from stick and wheel is not left to recirculate in the coolant, which increases the risk of scratching lens surfaces during edging. The proper sequence is as follows:

1. Dress the wheel.
2. Cycle the machine empty to flush abrasive material from the wheel.
3. Rinse or clean the grinding chamber.
4. Change the coolant.

Dressing Metal-Bonded Roughing Wheels

Only metal-bonded wheels are to be dressed because attempts to dress an electroplated wheel only causes the soft bonding material to glaze over the diamonds, which decreases wheel effectiveness.

The procedure for dressing a metal-bonded roughing wheel begins by soaking a correctly chosen abrasive stick in coolant. A coarse grit is the appropriate choice and most sticks are recognizable by color. If the stick is not soaked, no lubricating effect occurs.

Then the edger coolant pump is disconnected and the wheel turned on. Because roughing wheels should *not* be dressed at full speed the power is turned off and the abrasive stick pressed firmly against the wheel until rotation is halted. This is repeated until the stick is rapidly and easily consumed by the wheel, indicating exposure of fresh cutting surfaces. The stick should not be dragged laterally across the wheel even if the stick is

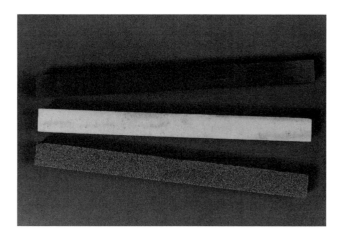

FIGURE **17-4** Dressing sticks for diamond wheels are themselves abrasive. Coarse sticks are used for roughing wheels and fine sticks for finishing wheels.

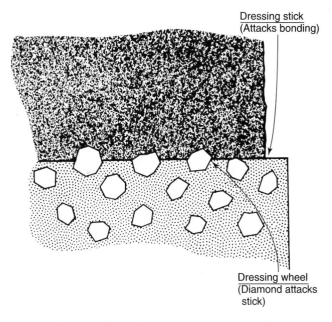

FIGURE **17-5** The dressing stick attacks the softer bonding material, which allows worn diamonds to drop out and expose fresh, new diamond particles.

In summary, to dress metal-bonded roughing wheels, perform the following:

1. Soak a coarse-grit abrasive stick in coolant.
2. Disconnect the edger pump.
3. Turn the wheel on full speed.
4. Turn the wheel off.
5. Stop the wheel quickly with the stick.
6. Repeat this process until the stick is consumed quickly.

narrower than the width of the wheel. The stick is lifted off the wheel each time and one section of the wheel is done at a time.

Dressing Metal-Bonded Finishing Wheels

Finishing wheels require dressing when their cutting speed slows. (Dressing is also needed if the edger uses an older free-float method and no longer properly situates the bevel even when the machine is level.) Finishing wheels should not be dressed unless clearly needed. Just because one wheel needs dressing does not mean that all wheels in the laboratory should be done as a preventive measure. A wheel should not be dressed until it needs it.

To dress a finishing wheel, the operator begins with a pumice or fine grit stick that has been soaked in coolant. (Extreme caution is exercised in dressing finishing wheels because bevel configuration can be ruined if improper procedures are followed.) A round pattern is placed on the edger and the size setting increased to a maximum so that the edger head is out of the way. For finishing wheels the coolant is left *on* and the wheel runs at *full power*. Power is not turned off during dressing. In this way the rapidly spinning exposed diamonds tend to protect the bonding from excessive erosion and loss of bevel form.

With both coolant and power on, the stick is pressed *lightly* against the wheel for a few seconds. All portions of both flat and V portions should be touched, one after the other (Figure 17-6). When dressing is complete, no shiny portions should be left on the wheel. The entire surface should have an even, matte appearance.

Changing the Lens Bevel Location

For manual edgers with a free-float beveling system, selectively dressing a finishing wheel is possible to change the way the bevel is positioned on the lens edge. Because dressing an edger wheel causes it to cut faster, if only one side of a finishing wheel groove were dressed, it seems the dressed side would cut faster. If this is the side corresponding to the front bevel, more

In summary, to dress metal-bonded finishing wheels, perform the following:

1. Soak a fine-grit abrasive stick in coolant.
2. Place a round pattern on the edger.
3. Set the edger to a large eyesize.
4. Turn the wheel and coolant on. (Do not turn them off!)
5. Lightly press the stick against the wheel for a few seconds.

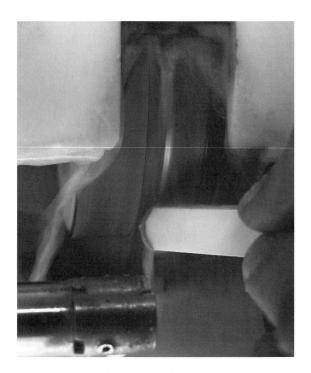

FIGURE **17-6** In dressing the finishing wheel, the power and coolant flow are turned on and the stick pressed lightly against each surface of the wheel. In this photo the right side of the bevel groove is being dressed.

lens material will be ground from the front than the rear. This places the bevel apex toward the back of the lens, which, of course, is undesirable. However, by selectively dressing only portions of the edger wheel, the bevel apex can be moved either forward or backward.

For example, an edger consistently is edging lenses with the bevel either exactly in the middle or somewhat farther back. It is desirable to place the bevel apex more at the one-third/two-thirds location. (That is, one third of the lens edge is ahead and two thirds are behind the apex of the bend.) This may be done by selectively dressing the rear (minus) surface of the groove. Thus the minus side of the lens is cut away faster; the lens shifts *back* toward the dressed half of the groove; and the bevel apex moves forward. See Figure 17-7 for a summary of the procedure.

Bevel apex location also can be shifted by selectively *dulling* one section of the finishing wheel. *D*ulling serves to *d*raw the bevel apex toward the dulled side, just as *s*harpening *s*hoves the apex sharp side. The location of the bevel apex is controlled as listed in Table 17-2.

Selectively dulling one portion of the edger wheel may be accomplished using a tungsten carbide tool, a carbide chip, or even an Allen wrench. Without coolant and with the wheel at full power, the tool is lightly touched to the side of the groove. To make certain that

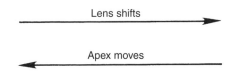

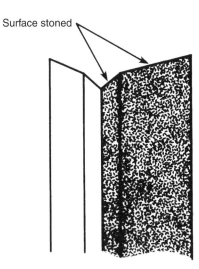

FIGURE 17-7 Dressing the right-hand side of the wheel causes it to cut more aggressively. Therefore the rear surface of the lens bevel is ground away more rapidly. This moves the bevel apex forward.

In summary, to position the bevel apex, perform the following:

1. Dress the metal-bonded finishing wheel.
2. Run the test lens.
3. If the bevel is still positioned improperly, dull the side toward which the bevel apex is to be drawn, as follows:
   a. Turn off the coolant.
   b. Turn on the power to the wheel.
   c. Lightly hold the dulling tool against the predetermined side of the groove.
4. Run the test lens, again turning the coolant back on.
5. If the bevel apex has moved too far in the desired direction, dress both groove sides simultaneously.

---

the desired result has been obtained, a test lens may be run. If the bevel apex has moved too far, the surface may be resharpened a bit by holding the proper abrasive stick against both sides of the groove simultaneously.

Cleaning Electroplated Wheels

If electroplated wheels show a tendency to become glazed, they must be cleaned rather than dressed. Cleaning may be accomplished by using a stiff bristle brush in combination with a scrubbing kitchen cleanser. Any attempt to dress an electroplated wheel will result in further glazing because the soft bonding material will be forced over the diamond cutting surfaces.

Truing Diamond Wheels

When edger wheels no longer cut to the proper configuration despite careful attention to proper machine maintenance and correct dressing of wheels, then the wheel must be trued.

The truing process itself consists of recutting a new surface on the wheel that duplicates the shape of the original surface. This is done at the factory rather than in the laboratory. After truing, the wheel surface is shaped like new, but the diamond layer is thinner and the wheel radius is slightly smaller than it was originally.

RETRUING ROUGHING WHEELS

Retruing of roughing wheels is of questionable value and should be done only after all other options have been tried. Most edgers have a system of setting the lens down on the roughing wheel in slightly different areas each time. This gives a more even wear to the wheel.

Because the roughing wheel does not give the lens edge its final configuration, the fact that the wheel has become grooved is not a major consideration. Truing would be considered only if it were felt that the uneven edge shape produced on the lens after roughing was creating too much wear in one location on the finishing wheel. Usually, however, excessive finishing wheel wear is a result of failure to compensate for a worn down roughing wheel by resetting the wheel differential.

When a roughing wheel is factory retrued, all of the diamond surface that extends above the lowest level of the worn part of the wheel will be removed.

TABLE **17-2** *Controlling Bevel Apex Location*	
DESIRED OUTCOME	ACTION
To move the bevel apex forward	Dull the front (plus) side of the groove *OR* Sharpen (dress) the rear (minus) side of the groove
To move the bevel apex back on the lens	Sharpen the front (plus) side of the groove *OR* Dull the rear (minus) side of the groove

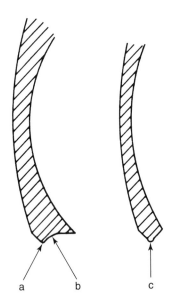

FIGURE **17-8** Failure to retrue finishing wheels often enough results in loss of sharp, distinct edges (*a* and *b*) or a rutting out of the groove apex of the V-bevel (*c*).

FINISHING WHEEL RETRUING

Finishing wheels should be retrued when it is noted that bevels are formed poorly. This could manifest itself as rounded bevel apices or loss of a sharp demarcation between bevel and hidden-bevel ledge, as shown in Figure 17-8. Failure of lenses to fit well in metal frame eyewires also can be an indication for a needed retrue.

Finishing wheels should not be allowed to deteriorate excessively between retrues. Excessive deterioration necessitates removing a great deal of diamond material to bring the wheel back to its correct shape, thus reducing the number of times a wheel may be trued. The alternative results in consistent high-quality workmanship and more retrues from each wheel.

When feasible, having an extra finishing wheel is best. If two finishing wheels can be interchanged, a freshly trued wheel always will be available when wear begins to manifest itself as a reduction in quality. With a spare wheel on hand, the temptation to forestall the process "just a while longer" is reduced.

Cutter Blades

Dry cut edgers use rotating blades to edge plastic and polycarbonate lenses (see Figure 8-23). These blades have a long, flat area on the blade where the lens is cut down to the correct shape. This corresponds to the roughing cycle for edgers with diamond wheels. At one end of the blade is a notched-out V shape. This is where the lens is taken down the last few millimeters in size while the bevel is being applied.

Cutter blades are fast and versatile. They can be shaped to produce a variety of edges and include beveling, modified Hide-a-Bevel, grooving, faceting, and shelving. Each option uses a different cutter blade.

Cutter blades dull over time but can be returned for retruing. Carbide steel blades give excellent results for both plastic and polycarbonate lenses. Although diamond-edged cutter blades increase the number of lenses that can be edged before changing the blade, the quality and smoothness of the edge is not considered to be as high as with use of carbide blades.

Proficiency Test Questions

1. How does a diamond wheel having a coarse grit cut in comparison to one with a fine grit?

   a. At a faster speed
   b. At a slower speed
   c. At the same speed

2. The numbers used in classifying diamond grit size for optical grinding wheels become which of the following?

   a. Larger as the particle size becomes smaller.
   b. Larger as the particle size becomes larger.

3. A diamond wheel described as having a concentration of 50 contains which of the following percentages of diamond by volume?

   a. 75%
   b. 50%
   c. 25%
   d. 12.5%
   e. None of the above because percent always is specified by weight.

4. Metal-bonded diamond wheels are made by which of the following processes?

   a. Bonding diamonds to the wheel through an electrolytic process
   b. Fusing a powdered metal and diamond particle mixture together at a high temperature

5. Glass is edged using which of the following?

   a. A metal-bonded wheel
   b. An electroplated wheel
   c. A milling cutter
   d. A router blade
   e. Any of the above is acceptable, although some methods are better than others.

6. In ophthalmic use, for which of the following lens types are electroplated wheels used more often?

   a. Photochromic glass lenses
   b. Crown glass lenses
   c. High-index glass lenses
   d. CR-39 plastic lenses

7. In reference to ophthalmic lens grinding wheels, which of the following best defines the term *glazing*?

   a. Dressing of the wheel with an abrasive stick
   b. Accumulation of lens material between abrasive particles on the edger wheel surface
   c. Turning of the wheel so that it spins in the opposite direction
   d. Dulling of a portion of the groove with a hard, blunt instrument, for purposes of controlling bevel placement

8. True or False? A small number of crown glass lenses may be regularly edged on electroplated wheels designed for plastic lenses, as long as the wheel is properly dressed afterwards.

9. Which of the following lists the proper sequence for the performance of each job listed?

   1. Rinse or clean the grinding chamber.
   2. Change the coolant.
   3. Dress the wheel.
   4. Cycle the machine empty.

   a. 3, 1, 2, 4
   b. 2, 4, 1, 3
   c. 2, 3, 1, 4
   d. 3, 4, 1, 2

10. True or False? When dressing an edger wheel, the stick is dragged across the wheel laterally until the stick is consumed rapidly and easily by the wheel.

11. Which of the following types of dressing stick should be used to dress an electroplated finishing wheel?

    a. White (fine grit) used wet
    b. White (fine grit) used dry
    c. Brown (80 grit) used wet
    d. Brown (80 grit) used dry
    e. Electroplated finishing wheels should not be dressed.

12. True or False? Wheels should be dressed only when they show signs of needing it and not as part of a regular maintenance schedule.

Matching

For Questions 13 through 17, an answer may be used more than one time.

13. Which type of wheel is dressed when it is running under full power?

14. Which type of wheel is dressed after turning power off?

15. Which type of wheel is dressed with coolant running?

16. Which type of wheel is dressed with coolant off?

17. Which type of wheel is not dressed?

    a. Metal-bonded (impregnated) roughing wheel
    b. Metal-bonded (impregnated) finishing wheel
    c. Electroplated roughing wheel
    d. None of the other responses is appropriate.

18. Dressing only the front side of a finishing wheel groove causes the bevel apex to do which of the following?

    a. Move forward toward the front surface of the lens
    b. Move backward toward the back surface of the lens
    c. Become somewhat more pointed
    d. Move forward for plus lenses and backward for minus lenses

19. If the effect of dulling one side of the finishing wheel groove has caused the bevel position to move *too* far in the desired direction, the best correction procedure is to do which of the following?

    a. Resharpen just the dulled side with an abrasive stick.
    b. Dull the opposite side of the groove slightly.
    c. Resharpen *both* sides of the groove with an abrasive stick simultaneously.

20. In the event that an electroplated diamond wheel shows a tendency to become glazed, it may be corrected by which of the following?

    a. Using a pumice abrasive stick
    b. Using a coarse grit abrasive stick
    c. Using a stiff bristle brush and scrubbing cleanser

21. Which type of wheel requires the most frequent retruing?

    a. A metal-bonded roughing wheel
    b. A metal-bonded finishing wheel
    c. Electroplated roughing wheel
    d. Electroplated finishing wheel

22. Which of the following is the best statement about the truing of metal-bonded diamond

    a. Metal-bonded roughing wheels should be trued regularly to prevent grooving of the surface.
    b. Roughing wheels should be trued when grooving first appears.
    c. Retruing of metal-bonded roughing wheels is of questionable value.
    d. Metal-bonded roughing wheels cannot be retrued.

23. True or False? The roughing wheel on a diamond edger is dressed with the wheel running at full RPM.

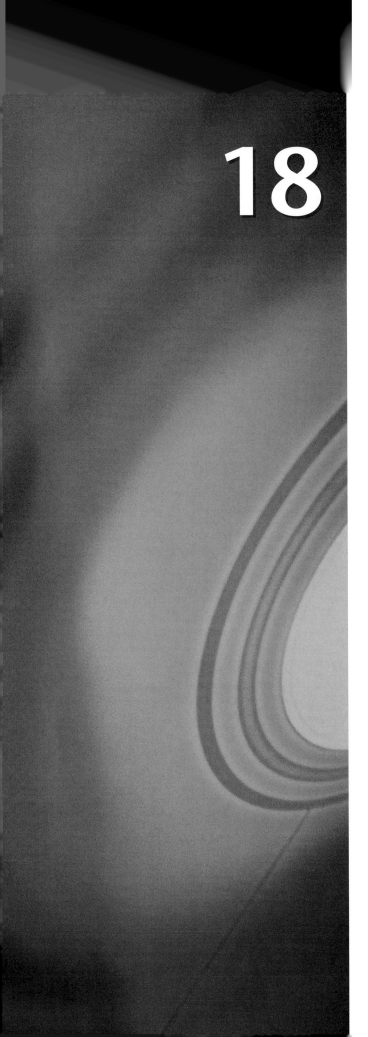

18 Safety and Environmental Concerns

Like any place of business that employs people, including eye care practices and optical dispensaries, the optical laboratory also is subject to federal, state, and local regulations. Some of those regulations involve worker safety.

Worker safety includes physical safety from injury, such as the necessity for eye protection in situations that involve dangers of eye injury. Worker safety also includes safety from chemicals or substances that may not cause immediate injury but that are hazardous to a person's health, even if the effects may not be evident for several years. A well-known example is the danger that asbestos poses to the long-term health of individuals exposed to it. The federal agency that oversees worker safety issues is the Occupational Safety and Health Administration (OSHA).

Some of the substances that might or might not be harmful to workers may be harmful to the environment. The federal agency responsible for regulations that protect the environment is the EPA or Environmental Protection Agency. State and local regulations determine what is or is not permissible regarding worker safety and the environment.

Disclaimer: The information presented in this chapter should not be considered all-inclusive. It is meant as an aid for the optical laboratory in establishment of a safe and healthy work environment and as a beginning for complying with appropriate federal, state, and local requirements. It is not a laboratory action plan. Regulations change. Even if this writing were all-inclusive, it could be superceded at the time of publication. In short, this chapter is meant as help in establishing policy but should not be taken as policy.

Occupational Safety and Health Administration

The Occupational Safety and Health Administration (OSHA) was created in 1971. Since its creation, occupational deaths have been cut in half and injuries have declined by 40%.[1]

OSHA regulations are sometimes called "Employee Right To Know" laws. In addition to having specific rules on workplace safety, OSHA requires employers to "make their employees aware of potential hazards in the workplace and to provide their employees with appropriate training in how to handle hazardous material and what to do in case of an emergency."[2] An employer must provide documented training on subjects relating to hazardous materials.

Environmental Protection Agency

The Environmental Protection Agency (EPA) makes regulations that govern how a company that generates materials classified as "hazardous" must store, transport, and dispose of such materials. "A business or organization that generates waste is responsible for that waste until it has been disposed of at a licensed facility and notification has been received that it has been properly disposed of."[3]

In other words, just paying someone to haul off hazardous waste does not absolve the "waste generator" of responsibility should that waste be improperly disposed of and create an environmental hazard later on. Hazardous wastes must be disposed of by a licensed contractor in a regulated site.

Agencies Overseeing OSHA Requirements

A total of 23 states operate their own job safety and health programs in place of the federal OSHA program. This practice is encouraged as long as the state plans provide standards and enforcement programs that are either identical to or "at least as effective as" the federal OSHA program. Most state plans are similar to federal standards, but states with approved plans may have different and independent standards.[4]

An Employer's Responsibility under OSHA

The OSH Act that established OSHA makes employers responsible for a safe workplace. A multitude of possible work situations exist, each with different workplace hazards. OSHA requirements therefore have general and specific aspects. In certain industries hazards are common and protection from them is standardized. These industries have specific OSHA standards.

Other industries are smaller and more individualized. It is not possible to make detailed standards for every industry. Therefore the requirements are more general for these industries.

OSHA STANDARDS AND THE 'GENERAL DUTY CLAUSE'

In general, standards require that employers do the following[5]:

- Maintain conditions or adopt practices reasonably necessary and appropriate to protect workers on the job
- Be familiar with and comply with standards applicable to their establishments
- Ensure that employees have and use personal protective equipment when required for safety and health
- Comply with the OSH Act's "general duty clause" in situations for which no specific standards exist

Where no specific standards exist, the guiding factor is OSHA's "general duty clause." The general duty clause, or Section 5(a)(1) of the OSH Act, requires that each employer "furnish...a place of employment which is free from recognized hazards that are causing or are likely to cause death or serious physical harm to employees."[6]

Overall responsibilities under OSHA are listed in Appendix 18-1, *What Are My Responsibilities under the OSH Act?*, found in the back of the chapter.

[1]About OSHA: frequently asked questions (webpage), Washington, DC, accessed June 2001, US Department of Labor, Occupational Safety and Health Administration (http://www.osha.gov/as/opa/osha-faq.html).

[2]Moody DP: What to do when they come for you, *Vision Monday*, 1995, p 7.

[3]Moody DP: What to do when they come for you, *Vision Monday*, 1995, p 7.

[4]*All about OSHA*, OSHA publication 2056, Washington, DC, 2000 (revised), US Department of Labor, Occupational Safety and Health Administration, p 9.

[5]*All about OSHA*, OSHA publication 2056, Washington, DC, 2000 (revised), US Department of Labor, Occupational Safety and Health Administration, p 15.

[6]*All about OSHA*, OSHA publication 2056, Washington, DC, 2000 (revised), US Department of Labor, Occupational Safety and Health Administration, p 15.

HAZARDS ADDRESSED BY OSHA

OSHA issues standards covering a wide variety of workplace hazards, including the following[7]:

- Toxic substances
- Harmful physical agents
- Electrical hazards
- Fall hazards
- Hazardous waste
- Infectious diseases
- Fire and explosion hazards
- Dangerous atmospheres
- Machine hazards

Many of these are only secondarily applicable to the optical laboratory. Certain hazards, such as electrical hazards, are common to many work situations.

OSHA INSPECTIONS

OSHA enforces workplace standards by conducting inspections. Inspections are unannounced. The four stages of a typical OSHA inspection are the following[8]:

- Presentation of inspector credentials
- Opening conference
- Inspection walkaround
- Closing conference

Ordinarily OSHA chooses the most hazardous workplaces to inspect. They inspect under the following conditions[9]:

- Imminent danger
- Catastrophes and fatal accidents resulting in the death of an employee or the hospitalization of three or more employees
- Employee complaints
- Referrals from other agencies
- Planned or programmed inspections in high-hazard industries
- Follow-ups to previous inspections

DIFFERENT TREATMENT FOR SMALL AND LARGE BUSINESSES

Small businesses are exempt from certain OSHA requirements. For example, most firms with less than 11 employees do not have to keep a Log and Summary of Occupational Injuries and Illnesses nor a Supplementary Record of Occupational Injuries and Illnesses.

OSHA is expected to be responsive to questions by small businesses and have a penalty reduction for small businesses. For information specific to small businesses, the OSHA *Handbook for Small Businesses* (OSHA publication 2209) is helpful.

DEVELOPING A SAFETY PROGRAM

OSHA recommends that every safety program should have the following five elements[10]:

1. *Management leadership and employee participation:* Employers and employees work together to make safety and health a priority. Employer and employee involvement and communication on workplace safety and communication on workplace safety and health issues are essential.
2. *Workplace analysis:* A worksite analysis means that you and your employees analyze all worksite conditions to identify and eliminate existing or potential hazards. This should be done on a regular and timely basis. A current hazard analysis should be performed for all jobs and processes that all employees know and understand.
3. *Hazard prevention and control:* The next part of a good safety and health program means that you continually review your work environment and work practices to control or prevent workplace hazards.
4. *Safety and health training and education:* It is important that everyone in the workplace be properly trained, from the floor worker to the supervisors, managers, contractors, and part-time and temporary employees.
5. *Program evaluation:* Program evaluation is done by either requesting an OSHA program evaluation through the OSHA Consultation Service or having a knowledgeable third party to evaluate the program developed.

The Chemical Hazard Communication Standard

One of the important standards that applies to the workplace, including the optical laboratory, is the Chemical Hazard Communication Standard (HAZCOM). This standard has specific requirements that must be

---

[7]*All about OSHA,* OSHA publication 2056, Washington, DC, 2000 (revised), US Department of Labor, Occupational Safety and Health Administration, p 15.
[8]*All about OSHA,* OSHA publication 2056, Washington, DC, 2000 (revised), US Department of Labor, Occupational Safety and Health Administration, p 27.
[9]*All about OSHA,* OSHA publication 2056, Washington, DC, 2000 (revised), US Department of Labor, Occupational Safety and Health Administration, p 26.

[10]*Q's and A's for small business employers* [website], OSHA 3163, Washington, DC, US Department of Labor, Occupational Safety and Health Administration, accessed March 2003 (http://www.osha.gov/Publications/osha3163.pdf).

individually tailored for the firm. It includes the following:

- A written portion
- A list of all hazardous chemicals in the workplace
- Material Safety Data Sheets
- Labels on all containers of hazardous materials
- Employee training.

This is an important section of every safety program and has specific, verifiable elements:

> OSHA's Hazard Communication Standard (HCS) is based on a simple concept—that employees have both a need and a right to know the hazards and identities of the chemicals they are exposed to when working. They also need to know what protective measures are available to prevent adverse effects from occurring. OSHA designed the HCS to provide employees with the information they need to know.[11]

A WRITTEN HAZARD COMMUNICATION PROGRAM

The Occupational Safety and Health Administration's *Hazard Communications Standard* requires all employers to provide their employees with information and training about any possible exposure to hazardous chemicals in the workplace.[12] Information is to be in written form and should explain workplace policy on protection from hazards.

The written program is not necessarily a compendium of safety procedures but rather a set of guidelines on what an employee can expect the organization to do in providing information and training. It is written for the employee.

At a minimum, the following should be included in the written program:

- A current file of Material Safety Data Sheets
- A list of the hazardous chemicals in each work area
- A description of the means the employer will use to inform employees of those issues required by OSHA to comply with the Hazardous Communications Standard
- Information regarding labels on hazardous chemicals

The written hazard communication program, consisting of all of the parts described in this section, including a list of hazardous chemicals and the MSDS sheets about those chemicals, must be readily accessible to employees.

A sample of a written Hazard Communication Program is included as Appendix 18-2 in the back of the chapter. It is a template published by OSHA as part of their Hazard Communication Compliance Kit but is not meant as a fill-in-the-blanks form. It is a good starting point in the process of creating a written Hazard Communication Program.

LIST OF HAZARDOUS CHEMICALS

Preparation of an effective employee training program relies on knowledge of those chemicals that would be hazardous in the form of liquids, solids, gases, fumes, or mists.[13] Not all chemicals are hazardous. Only those that are hazardous need to go on a *Hazardous Chemicals List* (see Appendix 18-3). This includes materials such as those that are flammable or poisonous, cause skin irritation, and are carcinogenic. A list of some types of potentially hazardous chemicals is shown in Box 18-1.

[13]Neary J: Can you pass an OSHA inspection? *Optometric Management,* December 1997, p 41.

BOX 18-1
Potentially Hazardous Chemicals

The following list identifies some types of potentially hazardous chemicals that may be present in the workplace:

Acids	Insecticides
Adhesives	Herbicides
Aerosols	Janitorial supplies
Battery fluids	Kerosene
Benzene	Lacquers
Catalysts	Lead
Caustics	Lye
Cleaning agents	Oxalic acid
Coal tar pitch	Paints
Coatings	Pesticides
Degreasing agents	Plastics
Detergents	Process chemicals
Dusts	Resins
Etching agents	Sealers
Fiberglass	Shellacs
Flammables	Solders
Foaming resins	Solvents
Fuels	Strippers
Fungicides	Surfactants
Gasoline	Thinners
Glues	Varnishes
Greases	Water treatments
Industrial oils	Wood preservatives
Inks	Xylene

From *Hazard communication: a compliance kit,* OSHA Publication 3104, Washington, DC, 1988, US Department of Labor, Occupational Safety and Health Administration, p D-2.

---

[11]*Hazard communication guidelines for compliance,* OSHA publication 3111, Washington, DC, 2000 (reprinted), US Department of Labor, Occupational Safety and Health Administration, p 1.
[12]*OSHA office guidelines,* Indianapolis, Indiana Optometric Association, accessed March 2003, (http://www.ioa.org/members/osha.htm).

Information must be available to employees about each substance that is considered hazardous. This information is made available to employees in the form of a Material Safety and Data Sheet (MSDS).

Materials are listed on the Hazardous Chemical List by the name of the chemical as it appears on the MSDS and on the label on the container and by other names as well. The entire workplace may have one master list, or separate lists may be generated for each work area. Everything on this list must have a corresponding MSDS for employee reference.

Material Safety Data Sheets

OSHA requires certain information about materials. That information is collected on what is called a *Material Safety Data Sheet* (MSDS). Although OSHA does not mandate a standard format for an MSDS, most use the standardized form as shown in Appendix 18-4. The following are some important points about MSDSs:

- An MSDS should be maintained and available in the laboratory for every potentially hazardous material or chemical.
- All employers are required to set up and maintain MSDSs for their employees to reference. Most keep these posted in the form of a loose-leaf notebook or on a bulletin board in a readily accessible place.
- MSDSs may become outdated if new information about the effects of the material becomes known. Employers are expected to replace outdated sheets with the most recent ones available.
- MSDSs should include physical and chemical characteristics, known acute and chronic health effects, exposure limits, precautionary measures, and emergency and first aid procedures.
- Possible materials that would have MSDSs in the optical laboratory include alcohol, acetone, heat transfer fluid for tint units, lens neutralizer, and dyes.
- Management must request MSDSs from the manufacturer of the substance, whose responsibility it is to supply it. It is advisable to document when these were requested and any follow-up required to obtain them. That way if a delay occurs, documentation exists that a good-faith effort is being made to comply.[14]
- One of the responsibilities of an employer is to make sure that employees have a basic understanding of how to find information on a Material Safety Data Sheet, and how to use that information.

LABELS ON ALL CONTAINERS

All containers must be properly labeled. Hazardous chemicals must be labeled with the following:

1. The name of the hazardous chemical
2. A hazard warning

A hazard warning can be any type of message, words, pictures, or symbols that convey the hazards of the chemical in the container.[15] The label can be directly on the container, or on a tag attached to the container.

According to OSHA's website:

> If the hazardous chemicals are transferred into unmarked containers, these containers must be labeled with the required information, unless the container into which the chemical is transferred is intended for the immediate use of the employee who performed the transfer.[16]

EMPLOYEE TRAINING

Employee safety training is a necessity. However, no established training standards exist[17] because each work situation is unique. However, OSHA does provide information on safety training and periodically conducts regional "Training Institutes" appropriate for general industry. One piece of useful information on training is found in OSHA publication 3104, *Hazard Communication: a Compliance Kit*, in the "Training Guidelines" section. Following are some areas to include in an employee personal safety training program[18]:

- How the hazard communication program will be implemented in the workplace
- How to read and interpret information on labels and on MSDS forms
- How an employee can obtain and use the available hazard information.
- What the hazards of the chemical in the work area are
- How an employee may protect themselves from workplace hazards
- How to follow specific procedures put into effect by the employer to provide protection, such as work practices and the use of and care for personal protective equipment

---

[14]Neary J: Can you pass an OSHA inspection? *Optometric Management*, December 1997, p 41.

[15]*OSHA office guidelines*, Indianapolis, Indiana Optometric Association, March 2003, (http://www.ioa.org/members/osha.htm).
[16]*What are the container labeling requirements under HAZCOM?: frequently asked questions: hazard communication (HAZCOM)* [website], Washington, DC, Occupational Safety and Health Administration, accessed March 2003 (http://www.osha-slc.gov/html/faq-hazcom.html).
[17]Hill RS, Lamperelli K: Safety first, *Eyewear*, July1998, p 52.
[18]*OSHA office guidelines*, Indianapolis, Indiana Optometric Association, accessed March 2003 (http://www.ioa.org/members/osha.htm).

- Methods and observations, such as visual appearance or smell, that workers can use to detect the presence of a hazardous chemical

Training in the above areas should include how exposure to specific chemicals may aggravate certain medical conditions. Training also should include information on the proper way to work with each type of hazardous chemical or substance present in the work environment.

Box 18-2 shows a checklist to use to ensure all elements of the Chemical Hazard Communication Standard have been addressed.

An Effective Safety Program

A safety program includes more than just compliance with regulations on hazardous chemicals. The following are some elements that should be included in an effective safety program. These elements are explained further in the next few sections of the chapter. (Some of the items [5 through 7] have been covered already in the Chemical Hazardous Communications section of the chapter.)

1. Having clear management support for the program by the following:
   a. Appointing someone to implement and oversee the program
   b. Asking employees for help in finding problems
   c. Correcting identified problems quickly
2. Cleaning up your place of business
3. Identifying and implementing OSHA requirements for safety by posting signs and properly labeling containers of hazardous materials
4. Providing employees with personal protective equipment
5. Correcting identified hazards
6. Having written safety policies
7. Training employees in safety issues
8. Keeping documentation on the following:
   a. Training of employees
   b. Accidents and injuries
   c. Communication with government officials and others relating to environmental and safety issues.
9. Reviewing appropriate OSHA checklists. (An extensive set of checklists may be found in OSHA Publication 2209, OSHA *Handbook for Small Business*.)

CLEAR MANAGEMENT SUPPORT

Success of a safety plan relies on management support. By appropriate delegation, staff involvement, a plan of

---

BOX 18-2
Hazardous Communication Checklist

1. Is there a list of hazardous substances used in your workplace?
2. Is there a written hazard communication program dealing with Material Safety Data Sheets (MSDS), labeling, and employee training?
3. Is each container for a hazardous substance (i.e., vats, bottles, storage tanks) labeled with product identity and a hazard warning (communication of the specific health hazards and physical hazards)?
4. Is there a Material Safety Data Sheet readily available for each hazardous substance used?
5. Is there an employee training program for hazardous substances?
6. Does this program include the following:
   a. An explanation of what an MSDS is and how to use and obtain one?
   b. MSDS contents for each hazardous substance or class of substances?
   c. Explanation of "Right to Know"?
   d. Identification of where an employee can see the employers written hazard communication program and where hazardous substances are present in their work areas?
   e. The physical and health hazards of substances in the work area and specific protective measures to be used?
   f. Details of the hazard communication program, including how to use the labeling system and MSDSs?
7. Are employees trained in the following:
   a. How to recognize tasks that might result in occupational exposure?
   b. How to use work practice and engineering controls and personal protective equipment and to know their limitations?
   c. How to obtain information on the types selection, proper use, location, removal handling, decontamination, and disposal of personal protective equipment?
   d. Whom to contact and what to do in an emergency?

From *Self-Inspection Checklists Hazard Communication* [website], Washington, DC, US Department of Labor, Occupational Safety and Health Administration, March 2003, (http://www.osha.gov/SLTC/smallbusiness/chklist.html#HAZCOM).

---

enforcement, and a willingness to correct problems, a safety plan can become an effective program.

Implementation and Oversight
Even with the best plan on paper, a safety program may not happen if no strategy is in place for putting it into effect. Specific steps must be mapped out ahead of time

to ensure agreement upon action and a follow-up is necessary to enforce action.

One of the best ways to implement a safety program is to appoint someone capable of effectively implementing the program and work toward active, ongoing employee involvement.

Employee Involvement

Interested employee involvement is best. Otherwise a safety plan can be an aggravation to employees and difficult to carry out. If employees recognize that their input is taken seriously, implementation is much easier.

A positive way to help ensure ongoing employee involvement is to form a safety committee. If a safety committee is formed, minutes of the meetings should be kept. The best safety plans are ones that ensure an open line of communication with employees about safety issues and that document everything.[19]

Correcting Employee-Identified Problems Quickly

If a safety problem is identified, it should be corrected quickly for several reasons, as follow:

- If employees identify a problem that they consider hazardous and the problem is ignored, they will feel that management does not value their input and is not concerned for their safety.
- Once a problem is identified, failure to correct the problem before a mishap occurs would lead to greater liability.
- Uncorrected problems that are reported, yet left uncorrected, provide reason for a disgruntled employee to contact OSHA with a complaint, which is likely to trigger an inspection.

An Enforcement Plan

Without some type of enforcement, a safety plan is not likely to succeed. For example, just as many people still do not wear seat belts while driving, not everyone wears safety glasses voluntarily. If something takes extra time or is an inconvenience, even in safety matters, not everyone will comply unless required to do so.

CLEANING UP THE WORKPLACE

OSHA's *Handbook for Small Business* recommends beginning a safety program by cleaning up the place of business. A neat, clean establishment makes a better impression in the event of an inspection than a sloppy one. The *Handbook* provides the following direction:

Poor housekeeping is a major contributor to low morale and sloppy work in general, even if it is not usually the cause of major accidents. Most safety action programs start with an intensive clean-up campaign in all areas of business.

Get rid of rubbish that has collected; make sure proper containers are provided; see that flammables are properly stored; make sure that exits are not blocked; if necessary, mark aisles and passageways; provide adequate lighting, etc.[20]

REQUIREMENTS FOR POSTING AND LABELING

For labeling of hazardous chemicals, see the "HAZCOM" section on labeling.

The following sections describe a few types of signs and pieces of information required in almost all work settings. The list should not be considered all-inclusive.

OSHA Poster

OSHA issues a poster that informs employees of what OSHA expects and therefore what employees should expect from their employers. (The poster is available for viewing or download at http://www.osha.gov/Publications/osha3165.pdf and may also be requested from OSHA.) It should be put up on a bulletin board or posting area where required information is visible to all. Display of this poster will be verified if an OSHA inspection occurs. Poster requirements can be expected to change, and new requirements should be checked periodically.

Safety Signs

Safety signs should be posted in the areas of the laboratory where personal safety equipment is required. For example, a sign stating "Safety Eyewear Required" should be in those areas where machinery is operated. An area with loud equipment should post a "Hearing Protection Required" sign (Figure 18-1).

Exit Signs

Exit signs should be posted on all exits. Exit signs should be either glow-in-the-dark or lighted with backup power in case of power failure.

'No Smoking' Signs

Many buildings are completely no-smoking facilities. However, if smoking is not generally banned, then "No Smoking" signs should be posted in the laboratory because of any flammable chemicals.

---

[19]Brauner A: OSHA—the good, the bad, and the ugly, *Frames,* July 1994.

[20]*OSHA handbook for small business,* Safety Management Series, OSHA 2209, Washington, DC, 1996 (revised), US Department of Labor, Occupational Safety and Health Administration, p 9.

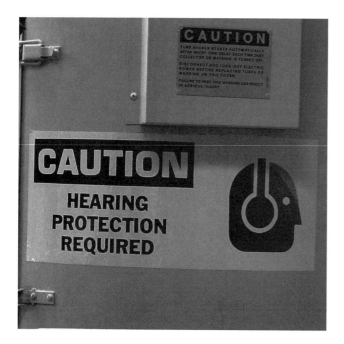

FIGURE **18-1** Safety signs are to be displayed where appropriate.

Emergency Telephone Numbers

Emergency telephone numbers should be posted. Numbers should be posted on an appropriate bulletin board and near the phone. These would include fire, police, and medical emergency numbers.

Fire Evacuation Route

One of the requirements for OSHA is an evacuation route in case of fire. This should be done even if the exit is obvious. For example, it may be possible to go out the laboratory door, turn left or right, and end up outside. It seems unnecessary to have an evacuation route in such a case, but it is required. If other possible disasters such as tornado or hurricane could occur, disaster plans should be posted for these, too.

Posting Requirements for Businesses with 11 or More Employees

If the business has 11 or more employees, a written *Emergency Action Plan* must be in place in case of a disaster like a fire, tornado, or personal injury. Also required is a written *record of work-related illness or injury.*[21] Even if no injuries or illnesses have occurred, that record must be kept up-to-date.[22] This is summarized on OSHA Form 300, *Log of Work-Related Injuries and Illnesses,* and must be

posted each year from February 1 through April 30. (This does not include minor injuries requiring only first aid.)

PERSONAL PROTECTIVE EQUIPMENT

The employer is usually responsible for providing most personal protective equipment. However, what is or is not the employer's responsibility may vary, depending on what the equipment is and negotiated agreements between management and employees. Personal protective equipment would include such things as safety glasses, hearing protection, and latex gloves, as follow:

- *Safety glasses* should be worn in the optical laboratory.
- If a noise hazard is present, *hearing protection* should be worn. Continuous noise levels that exceed 85 dBA are problematic.[23]
- *Latex gloves* should be worn if the hands are to come into contact with dyes or similar product.
- A *mask* that filters air should be used if there is plastic dust in the air when edging polycarbonate lenses.[24]

Safety Equipment for Chemical Tempering

Chemical hardening of glass lenses involves heating salt to the molten state, also known as *chemtempering*. If employees are exposed to this hazard, they require heat-resistant protective equipment such as gloves, aprons, or other body protection.

MAINTAINING DOCUMENTATION

From an internal standpoint, accurate, complete documentation is essential. Good documentation decreases misunderstanding and discord.

From an external standpoint, documentation is the only thing that gives evidence of an ongoing, compliant program. Inspecting agencies consider anything not documented as not done.[25]

Documenting Training

Documentation is important when attempting to comply with governmental regulations. With this in mind, each employee must sign a form or a roster stating that he or she has been advised about possible hazards in the laboratory and how to prevent harm. An outline summary of the material covered is an appropriate method of documenting training.

[21]This is reported on Forms 300, *Log of Work-Related Injuries and Illnesses,* and 301, *Injury and Illness Incident Report.*
[22]Bruneni J: In-office labs must face up to legal problems too, *Eye Quest Magazine,* 3(5):18, 1993.

[23]*OSHA handbook for small business,* Safety Management Series, OSHA 2209, Washington, DC, 1996 (revised), US Department of Labor, Occupational Safety and Health Administration, p 33.
[24]DeFranco LM: Environmental concerns in the lab, *Eyecare Business,* July 2000, p 40.
[25]Hill RS, Lamperelli K: Safety first, *Eyewear,* July 1998, p 52.

All training may not be done at one time. In this case appropriate documentation is necessary for each section of training that has occurred. Documentation should state specifically what was included in that training. The employee should sign a roster or individual form for each section completed.

Documenting Accidents and Injuries

As mentioned earlier, documentation of accidents and injuries must be kept for firms with 11 or more employees. This documentation is as follows[26]:

1. A report on every injury requiring medical treatment (other than first aid)
2. A record of each injury on OSHA Form No. 200. The annual Form No. 200 summary must be posted for the month of February
3. A supplementary record of occupational injuries and illnesses for recordable cases either on OSHA Form No. 101 or on worker's compensation reports giving the same information
4. These records must be kept for at least 5 years

Documenting Conversations

Another aspect of documentation is important but is not a legal requirement. This optional but prudent documentation is of conversations with federal, state, and local officials regarding safety issues. In addition, records should be kept of all conversations with regulatory agencies and with any private contractors that might be assisting in the setting up or ongoing oversight of safety and environmental program concerns. These are important in showing an ongoing effort and are helpful if disagreements arise.

REVIEWING APPROPRIATE CHECKLISTS

There are any number of possible workplace hazards. Therefore how is it possible to know which hazards exist in the laboratory? One quick way of screening for possible hazards or OSHA requirements is to use checklists. Following are some applicable checklists that range from general to specific:

- Responsibilities of management under the OSH Act. Appendix 18-1 is a list of employer and employee responsibilities set forth by the OSHA. (This was referenced previously.)
- General areas in which possible problems may exist. A general "Self-Inspection Scope" checklist is shown in Box 18-3.

- 21 Pages of checklists for specific areas starting with "Employer Posting" and ending with "Tire Inflation" are found in OSHA's publication 2209, *Handbook for Small Business.*[27] Though most of the items listed have little to do with the optical laboratory, some will. A checklist is a quick way to be certain nothing is overlooked.

INSURANCE

The laboratory is a manufacturer and must have product liability insurance. Professional liability insurance for either a doctor's office or an optical dispensary that includes an optical laboratory will probably not cover product liability. Anyone doing any laboratory work is considered a manufacturer—even if it is only tinting.[28]

A FEW SPECIFICS

It is beyond the scope of this chapter to list every potential hazard or every necessary hazard prevention. Such a list becomes quickly outdated. Only a few specifics that are common to most laboratories are mentioned.

Fire Extinguishers

Fire extinguishers should be placed appropriately. In most cases the dry chemical extinguisher (red in color) is most appropriate for the optical laboratory.[29]

First-Aid Kit

A first-aid kit should be available. If an eyewash station is not available, then sterile solution should be on hand for splash injuries (Figure 18-2).

Wet and Slippery Hazards

Other potential hazards exist to employees that may not be readily apparent. One such example would be areas that are or could be wet, slippery, and hazardous. For example, the area near the tint unit in a laboratory could fit this description. In this case, nonslip mats are advisable, which make the floor slip-safe and, in some cases, easier to stand on for extended periods of time (Figure 18-3).

Electrical Hazards

Common sense rules about electricity apply in the workplace. Safety requirements are what would be expected. Some examples follow:

[26]*OSHA handbook for small business*, Safety Management Series, OSHA 2209, Washington, DC, 1996 (revised), US Department of Labor, Occupational Safety and Health Administration, p 6.

[27]*OSHA handbook for small business*, Safety Management Series, OSHA 2209, Washington, DC, 1996 (revised), US Department of Labor, Occupational Safety and Health Administration, pp 15-36.
[28]Bruneni J: In-office labs must face up to legal problems too, *Eye Quest Magazine*, 3(5):18, 1993.
[29]Hill RS, Lamperelli K: Safety first, *Eyewear*, July 1998, p 54.

BOX **18-3**
Self-Inspection Scope

The scope of your self-inspections should include the following:

- *Processing, receiving, shipping and storage:* equipment, job planning, layout, heights, floor loads, projection of materials, materials-handling and storage methods, and training for material handling equipment
- *Building and grounds conditions:* floors, walls, ceilings, exits, stairs, walkways, ramps, platforms, driveways, and aisles
- *Housekeeping program:* waste disposal, tools, objects, materials, leakage and spillage, cleaning methods, schedules, work areas, remote areas, and storage areas
- *Electricity:* equipment, switches, breakers, fuses, switch-boxes, junctions, special fixtures, circuits, insulation, extensions, tools, motors, grounding, and national electric code compliance
- *Lighting:* type, intensity, controls, conditions, diffusion, location, and glare and shadow control
- *Heating and ventilation:* type, effectiveness, temperature, humidity, controls, and natural and artificial ventilation and exhaust
- *Machinery:* points of operation, flywheels, gears, shafts, pulleys, key ways, belts, couplings, sprockets, chains, frames, controls, lighting for tools and equipment, brakes, exhausting, feeding, oiling, adjusting, maintenance, lockout/tagout, grounding, work space, location, and purchasing standards
- *Personnel:* experience training, including hazard identification training; methods of checking machines before use; type of clothing; personal protective equipment; use of guards; tool storage; work practices; and methods of cleaning, oiling, or adjusting machinery
- *Hand and power tools:* purchasing standards, inspection, storage, repair, types, maintenance, grounding, use, and handling
- *Chemicals:* storage, handling, transportation, spills, disposals, amounts used, labeling, toxicity or other harmful effects, warning signs, supervision, training, protective clothing and equipment, and hazard communication requirements
- *Fire prevention:* extinguishers, alarms, sprinklers, smoking rules, exits, personnel assigned, separation of flammable materials and dangerous operations, explosive-proof fixtures in hazardous locations, and waste disposal
- *Maintenance, including tracking and abatement of preventative and regular maintenance:* regularity, effectiveness, training of personnel, materials and equipment used, records maintained, method of locking out machinery, and general methods
- *Personal protective equipment:* type, size, maintenance, repair, storage, assignment of responsibility, purchasing methods, standards observed, training in care and use, rules of use, and method of assignment
- *Transportation:* motor vehicle safety, seat belts, vehicle maintenance, and safe driver programs
- *Review:* evacuation routes, equipment, and personal protective equipment

From *OSHA handbook for small business,* Safety Management Series, OSHA publication 2209, Washington, DC, 1996 (revised), US Department of Labor, Occupational Safety and Health Administration.

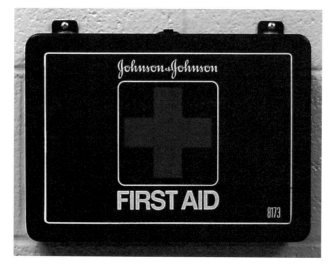

FIGURE **18-2**   A first-aid kit should be available in case of minor injuries.

- Overloading electric circuits with equipment that pulls more power than the circuit is designed to handle is inappropriate.
- Frayed cords should be replaced, not just wrapped with electrical tape.
- Use of multiple adapters and overloading a plug-in are unsafe.
- Outlets that are not grounded with a third prong ground wire need to be changed.
- Ground fault interrupters are required if an electrical outlet is within 6 feet of a sink. These are the same type of outlet as routinely found in bathrooms.
- Emergency lights in case of power failure are needed so that easy exiting is possible (Figure 18-4).

The Need for Proper Ventilation

If ventilation for tint units is inadequate, or if state regulations require, it may be necessary to vent the unit outside. Dry cut edgers are normally not a problem

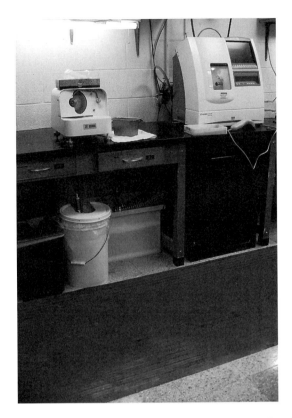

FIGURE **18-3** Where surfaces are often wet or continually wet and could cause falls, a nonslip mat increases safety. It also makes standing for long periods of time easier.

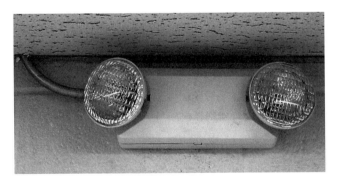

FIGURE **18-4** An example of emergency lights that come on when the power goes off.

unless the vacuum is blowing plastic dust back into the room.

Environmental Concerns

Employee safety concerns and environmental concerns are linked closely. When considering an overall safety plan, it is logical to tie in a plan for addressing environmental concerns at the same time. The primary envi-

ronmental issue is how to dispose properly of generated waste without harming individuals or the environment.

POTENTIAL PROBLEMS WITH WASTE MANAGEMENT IN THE LABORATORY

Optical laboratories should be sure that the waste materials they are generating are being disposed of properly. First of all, waste management regulations vary across the country. States differ in what is considered hazardous waste, and so do cities. For example, one sewage treatment facility may be capable of handling certain types of liquid waste, whereas another in a nearby town may not. Therefore what is permissible depends on the individual geographic location of the optical laboratory.

According to Moody in *Vision Monday:*

> *"A business or organization that generates waste is responsible for that waste until it has been disposed of at a licensed facility and notification has been received that it has been properly disposed of."*[30]

This means that a business cannot hire a shoddy or dishonest waste handler and be absolved of all responsibility for hazardous wastes generated just because those wastes have been picked up and are off the premises. Responsibility extends to the point at which the business can be assured that hazardous waste has been fully taken care of.

Ignorance of waste disposal requirements will not prevent a citation for violations.

Three Rules
The following are three rules to consider to make waste disposal easier[31]:

1. No chemical is brought into the laboratory without figuring out how to dispose of it.
2. Only as much of a chemical is kept on hand as needed.
3. Products that do not generate hazardous wastes should be used.

All liquid wastes that cannot be filtered and then disposed of in the sewer system must be removed by an approved waste contractor.

Fortunately only a limited number of waste management problems exist in a finishing laboratory. Existing problems are manageable with a bit of foresight. The

[30]Moody, DP: What to do when they come for you, *Vision Monday,* 1995, p 7.
[31]Hill RS: Hazardous-waste management in the optical laboratory, *Lab Talk,* May 1994, pp 12, 14; Hill RA: How to OSHA-proof your lab, part 1 of 2, *Lab Talk,* 26(24):16, 1998.

following are a few areas within the finishing laboratory that should be watched.

Edger and Hand Edger Coolant

Filters may be a part of the edger system and catch lens debris as it leaves the edging chamber. Some systems do not use coolant at all but rather plain water, which is filtered but not recycled. It becomes waste water after filtering. If the edger coolant and defoaming agents being used are water based and biodegradable, the solids may be filtered out and put in the trash, and the filtered liquid poured down the drain.

Even though it may be appropriate to pour edger coolant down the drain with some types of coolant in some areas, it cannot be assumed that this is universally permissible for all coolants in all areas. Some coolants, especially oil-based coolants, are in violation if disposed of in the sewer. A licensed waste hauler must remove these.

Lens Tinting Fluids

A number of fluids are used in the tinting process. These include dyes, heat transfer fluid, lens conditioner, and neutralizers. The MSDS for tint unit dyes and heat transfer fluids commonly state, "Dispose of waste in accordance with all local, state and federal regulations."[32] Dyes and ultraviolet (UV) liquid should not be considered suitable for sewer disposal unless all regulations are checked, even though many dyes are biodegradable and may be poured down the drain. However, because of their color, even biodegradable dyes may interfere with some types of monitoring equipment used in local sewage treatment facilities. If unsure of whether dyes may be disposed of down the drain, laboratory management personnel should check with local authorities.

Neutralizers generally are not suitable for sewer disposal.

Heat transfer fluids contain their original chemical make-up, in addition to lens dye and UV liquids from boilovers. Heat transfer fluid may be a hazardous waste, depending upon the brand of transfer fluid and the products with which it is contaminated.

Lens Cleaning and Other Cleaning Products

The best strategy for disposal of cleaning products is to only buy products as they are needed, buy products that are nontoxic whenever feasible, and then use the product completely. Even so, there may be an issue with some of the empty containers or the rags or tissues used in the process.[33]

Sometimes containers may be disposed of in a household hazardous waste facility in the community. Rags or tissues used with certain compounds may be flammable and could present a fire hazard if not handled properly.

Chemical Tempering Products

Chemical tempering salts are corrosive oxidizers and thus classified as hazardous. Used chemtempering salts may or may not be accepted by trash handlers in an individual area. If not, it may be possible to see if the supplier will take back the used product. Otherwise a licensed hazardous waste hauler must remove it.

Alloy Finish Blocking Wastes

The only justifiable reason for using metal alloy blocking in the finishing laboratory is if the finishing laboratory is connected to a surfacing laboratory that also uses alloy blocking. In that case a system would have to be already in place for appropriate waste disposal. This would include filtering the mop water used in the area of the alloy blocking system. The best solution is to not use an alloy blocking system in lens finishing. Instead a different system entirely should be used.

Spill Cleanups

Certain procedures are to be followed if a hazardous chemical is spilled. Chemical spills are to be cleaned up by trained personnel. If hazardous chemicals are present in the finishing laboratory, someone needs to be trained in spill cleanup. A suitable emergency spill kit should be on hand.

OVERALL RECOMMENDATIONS

The following are some overall recommendations to consider.

'Good Faith Effort'

It is difficult to know and implement every rule for every potential hazard. When a laboratory is chosen for inspection it is possible that not everything will have been done that should have been. One of the things that inspectors will be looking for is whether or not they think that management is making an effort to comply with safety and environmental regulations. If evidence exists that the organization is making a "good faith effort," then any violations are less likely to be penalized to the same degree than if inspectors feel that management has a negative attitude toward safety and environmental concerns.

'Engineering Out the Hazard'

It is easier to "engineer out the hazard" than it is to try

---

[32] *BPI Material Safety Data Sheet Book*, BPI, Inc., Miami.
[33] *SG₂, Processing Manual*, Bellingham, Wash, 1996, Seagreen, p 53.

to protect employees from a hazard.[34] If some chemicals are not hazardous, use those instead of hazardous ones. If a piece of equipment is dangerous, it should be replaced. In the long run it may be far better to replace equipment that requires protective work-arounds with something that does not even present the hazard.

If a process requires a chemical or hazardous substance, the process may be replaced with one that does not even use the same material. For example, if a finishing laboratory were still using a metal alloy finish blocking system, it would cost considerably more to protect against a heavy metal hazard than it would cost to replace that system with an adhesive pad blocking system.

Additional Information

Some businesses cater specifically to the area of OSHA and EPA compliance. How extensive this help needs to be and how much it costs varies.

Interested laboratory personnel may go directly to the government agency responsible for oversight for advice about how to comply with regulations. The advice is free. OSHA posts phone numbers and addresses for state branch consulting services on its OSHA website.[35] This service is run as a separate agency from OSHA and, unless there is a direct refusal to comply, information obtained by the consulting agency of OSHA is said to be kept confidential.[36] Keep in mind, however, that if you ask, you should certainly be prepared to implement any recommendations made.[37]

The following is the introduction to the OSHA-funded consultation service, as explained on the OSHA website[38]:

Using a free consultation service largely funded by the U.S. Occupational Safety and Health Administration (OSHA), employers can find out about potential hazards at their worksites, improve their occupational safety and health management systems, and even qualify for a one-year exemption from routine OSHA inspections.

The service is delivered by state governments using well-trained professional staff. Most consultations take place on-site, though limited services away from the worksite are available.

Primarily targeted for smaller businesses, this safety and health consultation program is completely separate from the OSHA inspection effort. In addition, no citations are issued or penalties proposed.

It's confidential, too. Your name, your firm's name, and any information you provide about your workplace, plus any unsafe or unhealthful working conditions that the consultant uncovers, will not be reported routinely to the OSHA inspection staff.

Your only obligation will be to commit yourself to correcting serious job safety and health hazards — a commitment which you are expected to make prior to the actual visit and carry out in a timely manner.

Before the decision is made to hire a consultant or help is requested from OSHA, laboratory personnel should simply start out and try to get as far with a program as possible with what is already known. Many steps will become obvious in the process and will have to be done sooner or later anyway. Doing as much as possible with what is already known may end up making the job easier in the end. Going as far as possible to bring about a safe, environmentally responsible policy will simplify matters, making the task more understandable and easier to maintain in the long run.

---

[34]Hill RA: How to OSHA-proof your lab, part 1 of 2, *Lab Talk*, 26(24):16, 1998.

[35]The web address at the time of this publication is http://www.osha.gov/oshdir/consult.html. Although it is possible that the specific web address may change, the website should still be possible to locate with an appropriate search.

[36]Jacob JA: Even small doctor offices can face OSHA inspections, *American Medical News*, July 31, 2000, p 2.

[37]Hill RA: How to OSHA-proof your lab, part 1 of 2, *Lab Talk*, 26(24):16, 1998.

[38]*OSHA's consultation service: consultation office directory* [website], Washington, DC, accessed March 2003, US Department of Labor, Occupational Safety and Health Administration (http://www.osha.gov/oshprogs/consult.html).

Proficiency Test Questions

1. True or False? Some states operate their own job safety and health programs in place of the federal OSHA program.

2. The OSH Act makes which of the following responsible for a safe workplace?

   a. OSHA
   b. Employers
   c. Workers
   d. All of the above
   e. The OSH Act does not make anyone responsible. It simply was an act of Congress that established OSHA.

3. True or False? Both small and large businesses are treated alike under OSHA. Worker safety and company size are unrelated.

4. OSHA recommends five elements for every safety program. Which of the following is not specifically listed as one of those five recommendations?

   a. Management leadership and employee involvement
   b. Workplace analysis
   c. Employee safety committees
   d. Hazard prevention and control
   e. Safety and health training and education
   f. Program evaluation

5. True or False? OSHA's Hazard Communication Standard is based on the premise that employees need to know what chemicals they are working with, what the hazards of those chemicals are, and how to protect themselves from those hazards.

6. True or False? One of the requirements of HAZCOM is that employers have a written workplace policy on protection from hazards.

7. True or False? A written safety program is simply a collection of safety procedures.

8. True or False? A safety program requires a "Hazardous Chemicals List." Such a list must include all chemicals found in the workplace.

9. Which of the following statements is true?

   a. Employers must have either a Hazardous Chemicals List or a Material Safety Data Sheet for each hazardous chemical.
   b. A Material Safety Data Sheet must exist for every chemical listed on the Hazardous Chemicals List.
   c. A Material Safety Data Sheet must exist for every chemical found in the laboratory.
   d. Material Safety Data Sheets are not required if the container label includes all information that would otherwise be found on the MSDS.

10. True or False? Never, under any circumstances, may a hazardous chemical be transferred to an unlabeled container.

11. With which of the following steps does OSHA's *Handbook for Small Business* recommend beginning a safety program?

    a. Forming an employer/employee safety committee
    b. Contacting OSHA's independent advisory agency
    c. Devising an enforcement policy
    d. Hiring a consultant
    e. Cleaning up your place of business

12. True or False? Every place of employment must have a written "Emergency Action Plan" in case of a disaster such as a fire, tornado, or personal injury.

13. In which business situation must there be a written record of work-related illness or injury using appropriate OSHA forms?

    a. In every business, but the record does not ever have to be posted
    b. In every business with 11 or more employees, but the record does not ever have to be posted
    c. In every business, and the record must be posted from February 1 through April 30
    d. In every business with 11 or more employees, and the record must be posted from February 1 through April 30
    e. No requirements exist for keeping a written record of work-related illness or injury.

14. True or False? Personal protective equipment for workers is always the employer's responsibility. Employees never have to pay for their own personal protective equipment.

15. True or False? Professional liability insurance carried by an optometrist, optician, or ophthalmologist also, by definition, covers them for product liability if they have an edging laboratory on the premises.

16. True or False? Waste management standards are uniform across the United States and are under the jurisdiction of the Environmental Protection Agency.

17. True or False? A business or organization that generates waste is responsible for that waste only until it has been picked up by a licensed hazardous waste handler.

18. True or False? If the edger coolant and defoaming agents being used are water based and biodegradable, the solids may be filtered out and put in the trash and the filtered liquid poured down the drain.

19. True or False? It may safely be assumed that biodegradable lens dyes may be poured down the drain.

20. True or False? Chemical tempering salts are similar to ordinary table salt and may be disposed of by placing those salts in the normal trash pickup.

Appendix 18-1

What Are My Responsibilities under the OSHA Act?

If you are an *employer* under the OSHA Act, you must do the following:

- Meet your general duty responsibility to provide a workplace free from recognized hazards.
- Keep workers informed about OSHA and safety and health matters with which they are involved.
- Comply in a responsible manner with standards, rules, and regulations issued under the OSHA Act.
- Be familiar with mandatory OSHA standards.
- Make copies of standards available to employees for review upon request.
- Evaluate workplace conditions.
- Minimize or eliminate potential hazards.
- Make sure employees have and use safe, properly maintained tools and equipment (including appropriate personal protective equipment).
- Warn employees of potential hazards.
- Establish or update operating procedures and communicate them to employees.
- Provide medical examinations when required.
- Provide training required by OSHA standards.
- Report within 8 hours any accident that results in a fatality or the hospitalization of three or more employees.
- Keep OSHA-required records of work-related injuries and illnesses (on Forms 300, *Log of Work-Related Injuries and Illnesses,* and 301, *Injury and Illness Incident Report*),* unless otherwise specified (see page 19).
- Post a copy of the OSHA Form 300A, *Summary of Work-Related Injuries and Illnesses,* for the prior year each year from February 1 through April 30 unless otherwise specified (see page 20).*
- Post, at a prominent location within the workplace, the OSHA poster (OSHA 3165) informing employees of their rights and responsibilities.†

- Provide employees, former employees, and their representatives access to the OSHA Form 300 at a reasonable time and in a reasonable manner.*
- Provide access to employee medical records and exposure records.
- Cooperate with OSHA compliance officers.
- Not discriminate against employees who properly exercise their rights under the OSHA Act.
- Post OSHA citations and abatement verification notices at or near the worksite involved.
- Abate cited violations within the prescribed period.

If you are an *employee* under the OSHA Act, you should:

- Read the OSHA poster at the job site.
- Comply with all applicable OSHA Standards.
- Follow all employer safety and health rules and regulations, and wear or use prescribed protective equipment while engaged in work.
- Report hazardous conditions to the supervisor.
- Report any job-related injury or illness to the employer, and seek treatment promptly.
- Cooperate with the OSHA compliance officer conducting an inspection.
- Exercise your rights under the OSHA Act in a responsible manner.

Although OSHA does not cite employees for violations of their responsibilities, each employee must follow all applicable standards, rules, regulations, and orders issued under the OSHA Act. OSHA, however, does not expect employees to pay for guardrails, floor cleaning, equipment maintenance, respirators, training, or other safety and health measures.

Modified from *All about OSHA,* OSHA publication 2056, Washington, DC, 2000 (revised), US Department of Labor, Occupational Safety and Health Administration, p 10.
*These sections are updated to reflect a change in forms required, effective January 1, 2002.
†The poster number has been changed to reflect a change in OSHA's numbering.

Appendix 18-2

Sample Hazard Communication Program

In 1983 OSHA established a standard for protecting workers from harmful exposure to hazardous chemicals. The rule, called "Hazard Communication," now applies to both manufacturing and nonmanufacturing sectors of industry. To comply with that standard, employers must communicate the dangers of hazardous substances to their employees. One form of required communication is a written document. This appendix contains an example of a Hazard Communication Program document and is taken from the following source:

> U.S. Department of Labor, Occupational Safety and Health Administration
> Directive CPL 2-2.38D
> Inspection Procedures for the Hazard Communication Standard
> Standard Number 1910.1200
> Information date: March 20, 1998
> Appendix E: *Sample Hazard Communication Programs*

Sample Hazard Communication Program (B)

INTRODUCTION

The Hazard Communication Standard requires you to develop a written hazard communication program.

The following is a *sample* hazard communication program that you may use as a guide in developing your program.

Our Hazard Communication Program

GENERAL COMPANY POLICY

The purpose of this notice is to inform you that our company is complying with the OSHA Hazard Communication Standard, Title 29 Code of Federal Regulations 1910.1200, by compiling a hazardous chemicals list, by using MSDSS, by ensuring that containers are labeled, and by providing you with training.

This program applies to all work operations in our company where you may be exposed to hazardous chemicals under normal working conditions or during an emergency situation.

The safety and health (S&H) manager, Robert Jones, is the program coordinator, acting as the representative of the plant manager, who has overall responsibility for the program. Mr. Jones will review and update the program, as necessary. Copies of the written program may be obtained from Mr. Jones in Room SD-10.

Under this program, you will be informed of the contents of the Hazard Communication Standard, the hazardous properties of chemicals with which you work, safe handling procedures, and measures to take to protect yourselves from these chemicals. You will also be informed of the hazards associated with nonroutine tasks, such as the cleaning of reactor vessels, and the hazards associated with chemicals in unlabeled pipes.

LIST OF HAZARDOUS CHEMICALS

The safety and health manager will make a list of all hazardous chemicals and related work practices used in the facility, and will update the list as necessary. Our list of chemicals identifies all of the chemicals used in our 10 work process areas. A separate list is available for each work area and is posted there. Each list also identifies the corresponding MSDS for each chemical. A master list of these chemicals will be maintained by and is available from Mr. Jones' office, Room SD-10.

MATERIAL SAFETY DATA SHEETS (MSDSs)

MSDSs provide you with specific information on the chemicals you use. The safety and health manager, Mr. Jones, will maintain a binder in his office with an MSDS on every substance on the list of hazardous chemicals. The plant manager, Jeff O'Brien, will ensure that each work site maintains MSDSs for the hazardous chemicals in each work area. MSDSs will be made readily available to you at your work stations during your shifts.

The safety and health manager, Mr. Jones, is responsible for acquiring and updating MSDSs. He will contact the chemical manufacturer or vendor if additional research is necessary or if an MSDS has not been supplied with an initial shipment. All new procurements for the company must be cleared by the safety and health manager. A master list of MSDSs is available from Mr. Jones in Room SD-10.

LABELS AND OTHER FORMS OF WARNING

The safety and health manager will ensure that all hazardous chemicals in the plant are properly labeled and updated, as necessary. Labels should list at least the chemical identity, appropriate hazard warnings, and the name and address of the manufacturer, importer or other responsible party. Mr. Jones will refer to the corresponding MSDS to assist you in verifying label information. Containers that are shipped from the plant will be checked by the supervisor of shipping and receiving to make sure all containers are property labeled.

If there are a number of stationary containers within a work area that have similar contents and hazards, signs will be posted on them to convey hazard information. On stationary process equipment, regular process sheets, batch tickets, blend tickets, and similar written materials will be substituted for container labels when these documents contain the same information as labels. These written materials will be made readily available to you during your work shift.

If you transfer chemicals from a labeled container to a portable container that is intended only for your immediate use, no labels are required on the portable container. Pipes or piping systems will not be labeled but their contents will be described in training sessions.

NONROUTINE TASKS

When you are required to perform hazardous nonroutine tasks (e.g., cleaning tanks, entering confined spaces, etc.), a special training session will be conducted to inform you of the hazardous chemicals to which you might be exposed and the precautions you must take to reduce or avoid exposure.

TRAINING

Everyone who works with or is potentially exposed to hazardous chemicals will receive initial training on the Hazard Communication Standard and the safe use of those hazardous chemicals. The safety and health manager will conduct these training sessions. A program that uses both audiovisual materials and classroom-type training has been prepared for this purpose. Whenever a new hazard is introduced, additional training will be provided. Regular safety meetings will also be used to review the information presented in the initial training. Foremen and other supervisors will be extensively trained regarding hazards and appropriate protective measures so they will be available to answer questions from employees and provide daily monitoring of safe work practices.

The training program will emphasize these items:

- A summary of the standard and this company's written program.
- The chemical and physical properties of hazardous materials (e.g., flash point, vapor pressure, reactivity) and methods that can be used to detect the presence or release of chemicals (including chemicals in unlabeled pipes).
- The physical hazards of the chemicals in your work area (e.g., potential for fire, explosion, etc.).
- The health hazards, including signs and symptoms of exposure, of the chemicals in work area and any medical condition known to be aggravated by exposure to these chemicals.
- Procedures to protect against chemicals hazards (e.g., required personal protective equipment, and its proper use and maintenance; work practices or methods to ensure appropriate use and handling of chemicals; and procedures for emergency response).
- Work procedures to follow to assure protection when cleaning hazardous-chemical spills and leaks.
- The location of the MSDSs, how to read and interpret the information on labels and MSDSs, and how employees may obtain additional hazard information.

The safety and health manager or his/her designee will review the employee training program and advise the plant manager on training or retraining needs. Retraining is required when the hazard changes or when a new hazard is introduced into the workplace. It will be company policy to provide training regularly in safety meetings to ensure the effectiveness of the program. As part of the assessment of the training program, the safety and health manager will obtain input from employees regarding the training they have received, and their suggestions for improvement.

CONTRACTOR EMPLOYERS

The safety and health manager, Robert Jones, upon notification by the responsible supervisor, will advise outside contractors, in person, of any chemical hazards that may be encountered in the normal course of their work on the premises, the labeling system in use, the protective measures to be taken, and the safe handling procedures to be used. In addition, Mr. Jones will notify these individuals of the location and availability of MSDSs. Each contractor bringing chemicals on-site must provide Mr. Jones with the appropriate hazard information for these substances, including MSDSs, labels, and precautionary measures to be taken when working with or around these chemicals.

ADDITIONAL INFORMATION

All employees, or their designated representatives, can obtain further information on this written program, the hazard communication standard, applicable MSDSs, and chemical information lists at the safety and health office, Room SD-10.

Appendix 18-3

List of Hazardous Chemicals and Index of MSDSs

HAZARDOUS CHEMICALS	OPERATION/AREA USED (OPTIONAL)	MSDSs ON FILE

From *Hazard communication: a compliance kit,* OSHA publication 3104, Washington, DC, 1988, US Department of Labor, Occupational Safety and Health Administration, p D-2.

Appendix 18-4

Material Safety Data Sheet

Material Safety Data Sheet May be used to comply with OSHA's Hazard Communication Standard, 29 CFR 1910.1200. Standard must be consulted for specific requirements.	**U.S. Department of Labor** Occupational Safety and Health Administration (Non-Mandatory Form) Form Approved OMB No. 1218-0072	◈
IDENTITY *(As Used on Label and List)*	*Note: Blank spaces are not permitted. If any item is not applicable, or no information is available, the space must be marked to indicate that.*	

SECTION I

Manufacturer's Name	Emergency Telephone Number
Address *(Number, Street, City, State, and ZIP Code)*	Telephone Number for Information
	Date Prepared
	Signature of Preparer *(optional)*

SECTION II — Hazardous Ingredients/Identity Information

Hazardous Components (Specific Chemical Identity, Common Name[s])	OSHA PEL	ACGIH TLV	Other Limits Recommended	% *(optional)*

SECTION III — Physical/Chemical Characteristics

Boiling Point		Specific Gravity ($H_2O - 1$)	
Vapor Pressure (mm Hg)		Melting Point	
Vapor Density (AIR –1)		Evaporation Rate (Butyl Acetate – 1)	

Solubility in Water

Appearance and Odor

SECTION IV — Fire and Explosion Hazard Data

Flash Point (Method Used)	Flammable Limits	LEL	UEL

Extinguishing Media

Special Fire Fighting Procedures

Unusual Fire and Explosion Hazards

(Reproduce locally)

OSHA 174, Sept. 1985

Continued

SECTION V — Reactivity Data

Stability	Unstable		Conditions to Avoid
	Stable		

Incompatibility *(Materials to Avoid)*

Hazardous Decomposition or Byproducts

Hazardous Polymerization	May Occur		Conditions to Avoid
	Will Not Occur		

SECTION VI — Health Hazard Data

Route(s) of Entry:	Inhalation?	Skin?	Ingestion?

Health Hazards *(Acute and Chronic)*

Cardnogenicity:	NTP?	IARC Monographs?	OSHA Regulations?

Signs and Symptoms of Exposure

Medical Conditions
Generally Aggravated by Exposure

Emergency and First-Aid Procedures

SECTION VII — Percautions for Safe Handling and Use

Steps to Be Taken in Case Material is Released or Spilled

Waste Disposal Method

Precautions to Be Taken in Handling and Storing

Other Precautions

SECTION VIII — Control Measures

Respiratory Protection *(Specify Type)*

Ventilation	Local Exhaust		Special
	Mechanical *(General)*		Other

Protection Gloves		Eye Protection

Other Protection Clothing or Equipment

Work/Hygienic Practices

Standards of Lens and Frame Measurement

Standardization for measuring frames and lenses is essential. The method used in most of the English-speaking world is based upon "boxed" lens size measurements and is called the *boxing system*. The once-popular *datum system* seldom is used.

In the boxing system the *eyesize* or *lens size* is determined by the horizontal distance between two vertical tangents that enclose the lens on the left and right (Figure A-1). The point halfway between these vertical tangents and also halfway between horizontal tangents that enclose the lens in a box is the primary reference point. This is known as the *boxing center* because it is the center of the box enclosing the lens. It is referred to alternately as the *geometrical center* because *after* the lens is edged, it is the geometrical center point. (The term *geometrical center* usually must be qualified because the geometrical center of an uncut lens blank will not be at the geometrical center of the lens once it has been edged.)

The *datum system* (Figure A-2) defines the lens or eyesize as being the width of the lens along the datum line. The *datum line* is a horizontal line halfway between the two horizontal tangents that border the top and bottom of the lens. This measure corresponds to the so-called *C dimension* of the boxing system and is known as the *datum length*, or simply the *eyesize*. The datum eyesize is not necessarily the same size as the boxing eyesize. The central reference point in the datum system is halfway across the lens as measured along the datum line and is called the *datum center*.

The distance between lenses (DBL) is measured differently between the two standards as well. The *datum system* measures this along the datum line. As can be seen from Figure A-2, this distance between lenses may not necessarily be the *smallest* distance between lenses.

Therefore in the datum system the smallest measurable distance between the two lenses (regardless of the level at which this minimum occurs) is called the *minimum between lenses* (MBL). The datum MBL is the same as the boxing system's DBL.

When patterns are being manufactured, the center of rotation is positioned to correspond to the central reference point of the lens shape. Because the boxing center is not located at the same point for a given shape as the datum center, a pattern drilled for the boxing system will not work if the datum system is used to calculate lens decentration, and vice versa.

Decentration calculations are made in exactly the same manner, regardless of the system being used. However, the results are not interchangeable.

For example, a frame has the following dimensions when measuring using the boxing system:

Boxing eyesize (A) = 52
Boxing DBL = 15

When the same frame is measured in the datum system, the dimensions are as follows:

Datum length = 49
Datum DBL = 19
Wearer's PD = 63 mm

Decentration when using the boxing system is as follows:

$$\frac{(\text{Eyesize} + \text{DBL}) - \text{PD}}{2} = \frac{(52 + 15) - 63}{2}$$

Decentration = 2 mm per lens

Decentration when using the datum system is as follows:

$$\frac{(\text{Eyesize} + \text{DBL}) - \text{PD}}{2} = \frac{(49 + 19) - 63}{2}$$

Decentration = 2.5 mm per lens

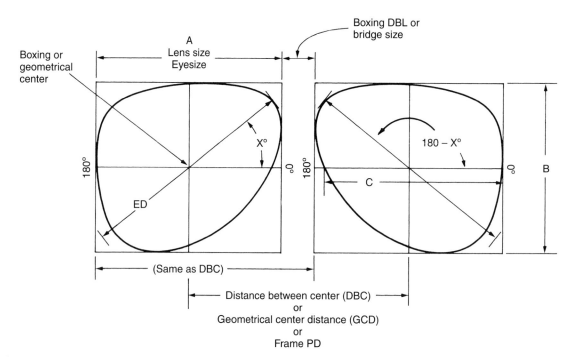

FIGURE **A-1**   In the boxing system, *ED* is the abbreviation for effective diameter, which is twice the longest radius of the shape as measured from the boxing (geometrical) center. The angle from the 0-degree side of the 180-degree line to the effective diameter axis is X for the right lens. Effective diameter is used to determine the minimum lens blank size and to calculate how thin lenses may be ground when surfacing the lens. *DBL,* Distance between lenses; *PD,* interpupillary distance.

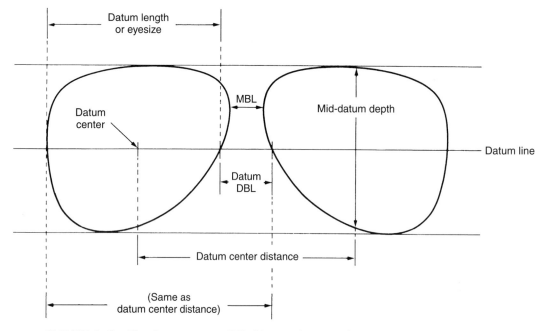

FIGURE **A-2**   The datum system. *DBL,* Distance between lenses; *MBL,* minimum between lenses.

This underscores the importance of correct measurement of the eye and bridge sizes. Measuring the frame using the datum system but using a pattern made for the boxing system results in an incorrect decentration. The finished distance between the lens optical centers does not correspond to the wearer's PD. In the example given, the distance between the two lens optical centers is 1 mm larger than ordered.

Differences and similarities in boxing and datum systems are summarized in Figure A-3. Corresponding boxing and datum system terms are listed in Table A-1. Similarities and differences between boxing and datum multifocal placement terminology are summarized in Figures A-4 and A-5.

TABLE A-1
Comparison of Standard Terms

BOXING SYSTEM	DATUM OR BRITISH STANDARD
A	—
B	—
C	Datum length
Boxing DBL	MBL
—	Datum DBL
—	Datum center distance (DCD)
Distance between centers (DBC) (Geometrical center distance [GCD]) ("Frame PD") (Boxing center distance)	—
—	Mid-datum depth
Horizontal midline	Datum line
Major reference point (MRP) Prism reference point (PRP)	Distance centration point (DCP) or simply *centration point*

DBL, Distance between lenses; *MBL,* minimum between lenses; *PD,* interpupillary distance.

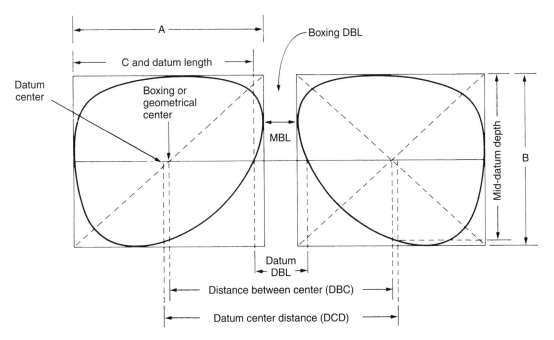

FIGURE **A-3** Diagrammatical comparison of boxing and datum systems. The datum center will not always be outset with respect to the boxing center. For example, for an upswept harlequin shape the datum center will be inset in comparison to the location of the boxing center. *DBL,* Distance between lenses; *MBL,* minimum between lenses.

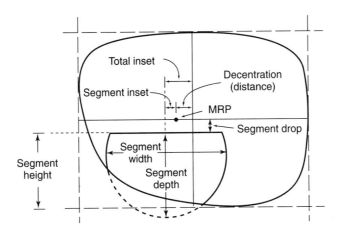

FIGURE **A-4** Accepted boxing system multifocal placement terminology. Decentration is sometimes referred to as *inset*. This must not be confused with segment inset or total inset. *MRP,* Major reference point.

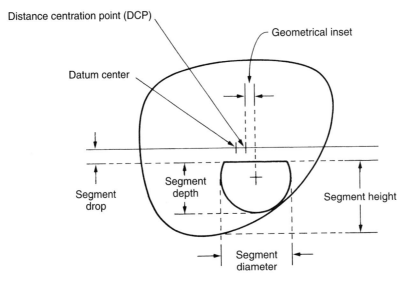

FIGURE **A-5** Accepted datum system multifocal placement terminology. (A right lens is shown in this diagram, whereas a left lens was shown in Figure A-4.)

ANSI Z80.1 Prescription Ophthalmic Lenses— Recommendations

Before the standards are outlined in this section, one point should be clarified. Unlike ANSI standards for safety eyewear, standards for dress prescription eyewear are not requirements, but recommendations. "The standard remains a recommendation. Therefore, it is the intent of the Z80 Committee that this standard not be used as a regulatory instrument."*

The information summarized here in Tables B-1 through B-10 is not meant to be all-inclusive. For complete information the original document should be consulted: *Z80.1-1999 American National Standard for Ophthalmics—Prescription Ophthalmic Lenses—Recommendations*. This standard may be obtained from the following address:

---

*Z80.1-1999 American National Standard for ophthalmics–prescription ophthalmic lenses–recommendations, Merrifield, Va, 2000, Optical Laboratories Association, p ii.

Optical Laboratories Association
P.O. Box 2000
Merrifield, VA 22116-2000

Meridian of Highest Absolute Power

To be able to understand the "meridian of highest absolute power" as referenced in Table B-1, the following must be considered:

- The power of one major meridian is the sphere power.
- The power of the other major meridian equals the sphere power plus the cylinder power.
- Of these two meridians, the meridian having the highest numerical value (plus or minus) is the *meridian of highest absolute power.*

TABLE B-1
ANSI Z80.1-1999: Distance Refractive Power Tolerances

ABSOLUTE POWER OF MERIDIAN OF HIGHEST POWER	TOLERANCE ON MERIDIAN OF HIGHEST POWER	CYLINDER ≥0.00 D ≤2.00 D	CYLINDER >2.00 D ≤4.50 D	CYLINDER >4.50 D
From 0.00 to 6.50 D	±0.13 D	±0.13 D	±0.15 D	±4%
Above 6.50 D	±2%	±0.13 D	±0.15 D	±4%

From *ANSI Z80.1-1999 American National Standard for ophthalmics–prescription ophthalmic lenses–recommendations*, Merrifield, Va, 2000, Optical Laboratories Association, p ii.

TABLE B-2
ANSI Z80.1-1999: Tolerances for Cylinder Axis

CYLINDER POWER STATED EXACTLY	CYLINDER POWER STATED IN QUARTER DIOPTER STEPS	AXIS TOLERANCE IN DEGREES FOR THE STATED CYLINDER POWER
Up to and including 0.37	0.25	±7
>0.37 up to and including 0.75	0.50 and 0.75	±5
>0.75 up to and including 1.50	1.00, 1.25 and 1.50	±3
>1.50	1.75 and above	±2

Note: When measuring for cylinder axis, the lens should be checked at the distance reference point. The distance reference point is that point on a lens at which, according to the manufacturer, the distance power is to be measured. The distance reference point may not correspond to the prism reference point, as in the case of progressive addition lenses.

TABLE B-3
ANSI Z80.1-1999: Tolerances for Addition Power

ADD POWER	TOLERANCE
Up to and including 4.00	±0.12
>4.00	±0.18

TABLE B-4
ANSI Z80.1-1999: Determining Tolerances for Unwanted Vertical and Horizontal Prism Using "Method 1;" Single Vision and Segmented Multifocal Lenses Mounted in the Frame

PRISM AND PRP* PLACEMENT	TOLERANCE
Vertical prism or PRP placement	$1/3$ prism diopter *or* 1.0-mm difference between left and right PRP (prism reference point) heights in high-powered prescriptions with no prism ordered *Note*: The prescription must fail both of the above tolerance limits to be considered out of tolerance for unwanted vertical prism.
Horizontal prism or PRP placement	$2/3$ prism diopter (total from both lenses combined) *or* ±2.5-mm variation from the specified distance PD for high-powered prescriptions *Note*: The prescription must fail both of the above tolerance limits to be considered out of tolerance for unwanted horizontal prism.

PRP, Prism reference point.
*The PRP is that point on a lens where prism power is to be verified. It also has been referred to as the *major reference point* (MRP).

TABLE B-5
ANSI Z80.1-1999: Determining Tolerances for Unwanted Vertical and Horizontal Prism Using 'Method 2;'* Single Vision and Segmented Multifocal Lenses Mounted in the Frame

PRISM	TOLERANCE
Vertical Prism	
For lenses of ±3.375 D or below in the vertical meridian	Unwanted vertical imbalance shall not exceed 0.33Δ
For lenses stronger than ±3.375 D in the vertical meridian	The vertical differences between prism reference points may not be greater than 1.0 mm
Horizontal Prism	
For lenses of ±2.75 D or below in the horizontal meridian	Unwanted horizontal prism for both eyes combined shall not exceed 0.67Δ
For lenses stronger than ± 2.75 D in the horizontal meridian	The horizontal difference from the ordered PD and the actual measured distance between the prism reference points shall not be greater than 2.5 mm

*Both methods 1 and 2 yield exactly the same tolerance results.

TABLE B-6
ANSI Z80.1-1999 Tolerances for Unwanted Vertical and Horizontal Prism; Edged But Unmounted Single Vision and Segmented Multifocals and Uncut Multifocals

Both Horizontal and Vertical Prism

- The tolerance must be within $1/3$ Δ the ordered prism power.
  or
- The PRP placement must be within ±1.0 mm of the ordered position.

Note: The prescription must fail both of the above tolerance limits to be considered out of tolerance.

PRP, Prism reference point.

TABLE B-7
ANSI Z80.1-1999: Tolerances for Progressive Addition Lens Fitting Cross Location

CROSS LOCATION	TOLERANCE
Vertical Fitting Cross Heights	
A single unmounted lens	Actual fitting cross height must be within ±1.0 mm of the ordered fitting cross height
A pair of unmounted lenses	
A pair of mounted lenses	Also, both fitting cross heights should be within 1 mm of each other relative to their ordered heights
Horizontal Fitting Cross Location	
A single unmounted lens	Actual monocular interpupillary distance must be within ±1.0 mm from the monocular interpupillary distance specified
A pair of unmounted lenses	
A pair of mounted lenses	
Horizontal Tilt*	
Mounted lens	2 degrees

*As measured using the hidden reference "circles."

TABLE B-8
ANSI Z80.1-1999: Unwanted Vertical and Horizontal Prism Tolerances for Progressive Addition Lenses

Vertical Prism

When prism thinning is used to reduce lens thickness, the vertical thinning prism is considered as if it were prescribed prism.
- For lenses of ±3.375 D or below in the vertical meridian, vertical prismatic imbalance shall not exceed 0.33Δ.*
- For lenses stronger than ±0.33Δ in the vertical meridian, the combined vertical variation from each PRP must not exceed 1 mm.

Horizontal Prism

- For lenses of ±3.375 D or below in the horizontal meridian, the combined unwanted horizontal prismatic effects must not exceed 0.67Δ at the PRPs.
- For lenses stronger than ±3.375 D in the horizontal meridian, the horizontal variation from the ordered prism reference point location† must not be greater than ±1.0 mm for either lens.

PRP, Prism reference point.
*For lens pairs with different cross heights, finding unwanted vertical prism is not as simple as dotting the stronger lens and sliding the spectacles across to read the other lens vertical prismatic effect. If the two lenses have differing cross heights, the second PRP will be at a different ordered height.
†The horizontal PRP location is the same as the monocular PD.

TABLE B-9
ANSI Z80.1-1999: Tolerances for Multifocal Segment Location and Tilt

SEGMENT LOCATION AND TILT	TOLERANCE
Vertical (Segment and Fitting Cross Heights)	
One unmounted lens	Actual height should be within ±1.0 mm from the ordered segment height
A lens pair (mounted or unmounted)	Actual height should be within ±1.0 mm from the ordered segment height *and* both lens segments in the pair should be within 1 mm of each other
Horizontal Segment Location* (Near PD)	
Mounted lens pair	Near PD should be within ±2.5 mm of the ordered near PD Inset should appear symmetrical and balanced unless specified monocularly
Segment Tilt†	
Mounted lens	2 degrees

PD, Interpupillary distance.
*For an E-line (Franklin style) bifocal, the center of the segment is located at the thinnest point on the segment ledge.
†The amount that the flat top of a segment line deviates from the horizontal.

TABLE B-10
ANSI Z80.1-1999: Miscellaneous Tolerances

CHARACTERISTIC	TOLERANCE
Thickness (measured at the prism reference point)	±0.3 mm (when thickness is specified on the order)
Warpage	1.00 D (not applicable for points within 6 mm of the eyewire)
Base curve	±0.75 D (when specified on the order)
Impact resistance	Capable of withstanding the impact of a 5/8-inch steel ball dropped from 50 inches*

*For more information, see Appendix C.

Determining whether Refractive Power is within Tolerance

The following text outlines a cookbook method that may be used to see if the refractive power of a prescription is within ANSI standards.

EXAMPLE B-1

Following is an example of a prescription in which the meridian of highest absolute power is also the sphere power. Determine whether or not the prescription passes ANSI refractive power tolerances.

EXAMPLE B-2

Following is an example of a prescription where the meridian of highest absolute power is not the sphere power. Determine whether or not the prescription passes ANSI refractive power tolerances.

Example B-1

METHODOLOGY	EXAMPLE
1. Note the refractive power of the ordered prescription.	$+4.25 - 1.75 \times 180$
2. Measure the refractive power of the ordered prescription.	$+4.37 - 1.62 \times 178$
3. Find the power in the meridian of highest absolute power for	
a. the ordered prescription and	a. $+4.25$
b. the measured prescription	b. $+4.37$
4. Using Table B-1, determine the following:	
a. What is the tolerance for the meridian of highest absolute power?	a. Tolerance for a 4.25 D power is ± 0.13 D, giving a possible range of from +4.12 D to + 4.38 D.
b. Is the meridian of highest absolute power within tolerance?	b. The + 4.37 D measured power is within the tolerance range.
5. Using Table B-1 determine the following:	
a. What is the tolerance for the cylinder power?	a. Tolerance for a 1.75 D cylinder is ± 0.13 D, giving a possible range of from −1.62 to −1.88 D.
b. Is the cylinder power within tolerance?	b. The −1.62 measured cylinder power is within the tolerance range.
6. Using Table B-2 determine the following:	
a. What is the tolerance for the cylinder axis?	a. Axis tolerance for a 1.75 D cylinder is ± 2 degrees. This gives a possible range of between 178 and 2 degrees.
b. Is the cylinder axis within tolerance?	b. The measured axis is 178 degrees and thus within the tolerance range.

Conclusion: The prescription passes.

Example B-2

METHODOLOGY	EXAMPLE
1. Ordered power	$-5.00 - 2.00 \times 174$
2. Measured power	$-5.12 - 2.12 \times 174$
3. Power of meridian of highest absolute power for	
a. The ordered prescription	a. $\left| -5.00 - 2.00 \right| = 7.00$
b. The measured prescription	b. $\left| -5.12 - 2.12 \right| = 7.24$
4. a. Tolerance for the meridian of highest absolute power	a. 2% of 7.00 is $0.02 \times 7 = 0.14$ D. This gives a possible range of from − 6.86 D to − 7.14 D.
b. Is the meridian within tolerance?	b. The measured power in this meridian is − 7.24. This is well outside of ANSI standards.

Conclusion: The prescription does not pass.

FDA Policy

The material in this appendix has been reproduced from the following federal publication:

Code of Federal Regulations
Title 21, Volume 8, Parts 800 to 1299
Revised as of April 1, 2000
From the U.S. Government Printing Office via GPO Access
Cite: 21CFR801.410
Pages 24-26

Title 21—Food and Drugs Services—(Continued)

PART 801—LABELING—TABLE OF CONTENTS

Subpart H—Special Requirements for Specific Devices

Sec. 801.410: Use of impact-resistant lenses in eyeglasses and sunglasses.

(a) Examination of data available on the frequency of eye injuries resulting from the shattering of ordinary crown glass lenses indicates that the use of such lenses constitutes an avoidable hazard to the eye of the wearer.

(b) The consensus of the ophthalmic community is that the number of eye injuries would be substantially reduced by the use in eyeglasses and sunglasses of impact-resistant lenses.

(c)(1) To protect the public more adequately from potential eye injury, eyeglasses and sunglasses must be fitted with impact-resistant lenses, except in those cases where the physician or optometrist finds that such lenses will not fulfill the visual requirements of the particular patient, directs in writing the use of other lenses, and gives written notification thereof to the patient.

(2) The physician or optometrist shall have the option of ordering glass lenses, plastic lenses, or laminated glass lenses made impact resistant by any method; however, all such lenses shall be capable of withstanding the impact test described in paragraph (d)(2) of this section.

(3) Each finished impact-resistant glass lens for prescription use shall be individually tested for impact resistance and shall be capable of withstanding the impact test described in paragraph (d)(2) of this section. Raised multifocal lenses shall be impact resistant but need not be tested beyond initial design testing. Prism segment multifocal, slab-off prism, lenticular cataract, iseikonic, depressed segment one-piece multifocal, bi-concave, myodisc and minus lenticular, custom laminate, and cemented assembly lenses shall be impact resistant but need not be subjected to impact testing. To demonstrate that all other types of impact-resistant lenses, including impact-resistant laminated glass lenses (i.e., lenses other than those described in the three preceding sentences of this paragraph [c][3]), are capable of withstanding the impact test described in this regulation, the manufacturer of these lenses shall subject to an impact test a statistically significant sampling of lenses from each production batch, and the lenses so tested shall be representative of the finished forms as worn by the wearer, including finished forms that are of minimal lens thickness and have been subjected to any treatment used to impart impact resistance. All nonprescription lenses and plastic prescription lenses tested on the basis of statistical significance shall be tested in uncut-finished or finished form.

(d)(1) For the purpose of this regulation, the impact test described in paragraph (d)(2) of this section shall be the "referee test," defined as "one which will be utilized to determine compliance with a regulation." The referee test provides the Food and Drug Administration with the means of examining a medical device for performance and does not inhibit the manufacturer from using equal or superior test methods. A lens manufacturer shall conduct tests of lenses using the impact test described in paragraph (d)(2) of this section or any equal or superior test. Whatever test is used, the lenses shall be capable of withstanding the impact test described in paragraph (d)(2) of this section if the Food and Drug Administration examines them for performance.

(2) In the impact test, a $\frac{5}{8}$-inch steel ball weighing approximately 0.56 ounce is dropped from a height of 50 inches upon the horizontal upper surface of the lens. The ball shall strike within a $\frac{5}{8}$-inch diameter circle located at the geometric center of the lens. The ball may be guided but not restricted in its fall by being dropped through a tube extending to within approximately 4 inches of the lens. To pass the test, the lens must not fracture; for the purpose of this section, a lens will be considered to have fractured if it cracks through its entire thickness, including a laminar layer, if any, and across a complete diameter into two or more separate pieces, or if any lens material visible to the naked eyes becomes detached from the ocular surface. The test shall be conducted with the lens supported by a tube (1-inch inside diameter, $1\frac{1}{4}$-inch outside diameter, and approximately 1-inch high) affixed to a rigid iron or steel base plate. The total weight of the base plate and its rigidly attached fixtures shall be not less than 27 pounds. For lenses of small minimum diameter, a support tube having an outside diameter of less than $1\frac{1}{4}$ inches may be used. The support tube shall be made of rigid acrylic plastic, steel, or other suitable substance and shall have securely bonded on the top edge a $1\frac{1}{8}$- by $1\frac{1}{8}$-inch neoprene gasket having a hardness of 40 ± 5 as determined by ASTM Method D 1415-88, "Standard Test Method for Rubber Property—International Hardness" a minimum tensile strength of 1200 pounds, as determined by ASTM Method D 412-97, Standard Test Methods for Vulcanized Rubber and Thermoplastic Rubbers and Thermoplastic Elastomers—Tension and a minimum ultimate elongation of 400 percent, as determined by ASTM Method D 412-68. (Both methods are incorporated by reference and are available from the American Society for Testing Materials, 100 Barr Harbor Dr., West Conshohocken, Philadelphia, PA 19428, or available for inspection at the Center for Devices and Radiological Health's Library, 9200 Corporate Blvd., Rockville, MD 10850, or

at the Office of the Federal Register, 800 North Capitol St., NW, Suite 700, Washington, DC.) The diameter or contour of the lens support may be modified as necessary so that the $1\frac{1}{8}$- by $1\frac{1}{8}$-inch neoprene gasket supports the lens at its periphery.

(e) Copies of invoice(s), shipping document(s), and records of sale or distribution of all impact resistant lenses, including finished eyeglasses and sunglasses, shall be kept and maintained for a period of 3 years; however, the names and addresses of individuals purchasing nonprescription eyeglasses and sunglasses at the retail level need not be kept and maintained by the retailer. The records kept in compliance with this paragraph shall be made available upon request at all reasonable hours by any officer or employee of the Food and Drug Administration or by any other officer or employee acting on behalf of the Secretary of Health and Human Services and such officer or employee shall be permitted to inspect and copy such records, to make such inventories of stock as he [or she] deems necessary, and otherwise to check the correctness of such inventories.

(f) In addition, those persons conducting tests in accordance with paragraph (d) of this section shall maintain the results thereof and a description of the test method and of the test apparatus for a period of 3 years. These records shall be made available upon request at any reasonable hour by any officer or employee acting on behalf of the Secretary of Health and Human Services. The persons conducting tests shall permit the officer or employee to inspect and copy the records, to make such inventories of stock as the officer or employee deems necessary, and otherwise to check the correctness of the inventories.

(g) For the purpose of this section, the term "manufacturer" includes an importer for resale. Such importer may have the tests required by paragraph (d) of this section conducted in the country of origin but must make the results thereof available, upon request, to the Food and Drug Administration, as soon as practicable.

(h) All lenses must be impact-resistant except when the physician or optometrist finds that impact-resistant lenses will not fulfill the visual requirements for a particular patient.

(i) This statement of policy does not apply to contact lenses.

[41 FR 6896, Feb. 13, 1976, as amended at 44 FR 20678, Apr. 6, 1979; 47 FR 9397, Mar. 5, 1982; 65 FR 3586, Jan. 24, 2000]

Effective Date Note: At 65 FR 3586, Jan. 24, 2000, Secs. 801.410 was amended in paragraph (d)(2) by removing "ASTM Method D 1415-68 Test for International Hardness of Vulcanized Rubber," and adding in its place "ASTM

Method D 1415-88, Standard Test Method for Rubber Property— International Hardness"; by removing "ASTM Method D 412-68 Tension Test of Vulcanized Rubber," and adding in its place "ASTM Method D 412-97, Standard Test Methods for Vulcanized Rubber and Thermoplastic Rubbers and Thermoplastic Elastomers—Tension"; and by removing "1916 Race St., Philadelphia, PA 19103, or available for inspection at the Office of the Federal Register, 800 North Capitol Street, NW, Suite 700, Washington, DC 20408" and adding in its place "100 Barr Harbor Dr., West Conshohocken, Philadelphia, PA 19428, or available for inspection at the Center for Devices and Radiological Health's Library, 9200 Corporate Blvd., Rockville, MD 10850, or at the Office of the Federal Register, 800 North Capitol St., NW, Suite 700, Washington, DC," effective June 7, 2000.

Chapter 1

1. False
2. a
3. c
4. True
5. True
6. c
7. b
8. d

Chapter 2

1. True
2. a
3. b
4. b
5. e
6. a and c
7. False
8. d
9. a
10. c
11. False
12. c
13. True
14. True
15. c
16. d
17. d
18. c and d
19. True
20. True
21. d
22. True
23. b
24. False
25. True
26. True
27. e
28. b
29. d
30. a
31. c
32. a and b (unless the lens is polarized, in which case the only answer is B)
33. b
34. c

Chapter 3

1. c
2. d
3. d
4. c
5. e
6. b
7. False
8. a
9. c
10. c
11. e
12. True
13. True
14. 45 mm
15. a
16. b
17. 2.5 mm
18. 5.5 mm
19. d
20. a
21. c
22. 2 mm in, 1.5 mm down
23. e
24. b
25. b
26. a
27. d
28. d
29. f
30. e
31. True
32. d

Chapter 4

1. 67 mm
2. a. 4 total in
   b. 8 total in
   c. 1 total in
3. b
4. R: 3 mm in
   L: 1.5 mm in
5. R: 1.5 mm in
   L: 2 mm in
6. e
7. e (The answer to this problem is the same as the previous problem because the major reference point that included Rx prism already has been found during the spotting.)
8. +3 mm
9. 2 mm in and 2 mm up
10. 1.5 mm in and 4.5 mm up
11. d
12. b
13. d
14. a
15. a
16. a
17. a. 0.6D base out
    b. 1.5D base in
    c. 1.725D base out
18. d
19. b
20. c
21. 1 mm out
22. 4 mm to the left of and 2 mm above the cross

Chapter 5

1. d
2. False
3. a
4. True
5. R: 3 mm inset
   6 mm raise
   L: 1 mm inset
   5 mm raise
6. R: 4 mm inset
   4.5 mm raise
   L: 2.5 mm inset
   4.5 mm raise
7. R: 2 mm inset
   1 mm hidden circle drop
   L: 1.5 mm inset
   0 mm hidden circle raise or drop
8. R: 2.5 mm inset
   1 mm hidden circle drop
   L: 3.5 mm inset
   2 mm hidden circle raise or drop
9. False
10. False
11. For the lower portion of the lens, the powers will be:
    R: $+2.00 -0.50 \times 170$
    L: $+2.25 -0.75 \times 5$
    For the upper portion of the lens, the powers will be:
    R: $pl -0.050 \times 170$
    L: $+0.25 -0.75 \times 5$
12. For the lower portion of the lens:
    R: $+2.00 -0.50 \times 170$
    L: $+2.25 -0.75 \times 5$
    For the upper portion of the lens:
    R: $+0.75 -0.50 \times 170$
    L: $+1.00 -0.75 \times 5$
13. b

Chapter 6

1. c
2. a
3. 3 mm in and 3 mm down
4. 2.5 mm above, 1.5 mm out
5. c
6. b
7. b
8. a
9. a
10. b
11. b
12. b
13. a
14. b
15. b
16. a
17. b
18. c
19. d
20. d
21. b and c
22. b
23. b
24. a
25. a
26. b
27. e
28. a
29. a
30. False
31. a
32. d
33. b, d, and e
34. a
35. c
36. c and d
37. b and d
38. d

Chapter 7

1. a
2. c
3. c
4. c
5. c
6. True
7. e
8. f
9. b

Chapter 8

1. a. 0
   b. 50
   c. 46.5
   d. 38
   e. 44.5
   f. −8
   g. 52
   h. −8
   i. 0
   j. 50
   k. 62
   l. 41.5
   m. −15
   n. 35
   o. −13.5
   p. 38.5
2. d
3. b
4. a
5. c
6. d
7. b
8. c
9. a
10. True
11. a
12. False
13. d
14. c
15. e
16. c and d
17. b
18. d
19. c, e, b, g
20. d
21. False
22. d
23. True
24. False
25. True
26. True
27. False

Chapter 9

1. c
2. False
3. False
4. c
5. False
6. False

Chapter 10

1. b
2. a
3. e
4. True
5. e
6. b
7. a
8. b
9. True
10. True
11. c
12. c
13. a
14. a
15. d
16. a and b
17. True
18. b
19. False

Chapter 11

1. c
2. False
3. a and c
4. b
5. d
6. c
7. a
8. a
9. c
10. b
11. False
12. d
13. b
14. True
15. e
16. d
17. b
18. c
19. False
20. True
21. False
22. d
23. c
24. b
25. c
26. False
27. c
28. False
29. e
30. d

Chapter 12

1. True
2. False
3. False
4. b, d, and e
5. b
6. c
7. False
8. True
9. e

Chapter 13

1. False
2. False
3. a
4. b
5. b
6. b
7. d
8. c
9. e
10. b
11. d
12. c
13. a
14. True
15. False
16. True

Chapter 14

1. a
2. False
3. b
4. True
5. True
6. a
7. a
8. a:2, b:1, c:3
9. True
10. b
11. a
12. c
13. c
14. d
15. b
16. c
17. False

Chapter 15	Chapter 16	Chapter 17	Chapter 18
1. d	1. False	1. a	1. True
2. e	2. c	2. a	2. b
3. b	3. True	3. d	3. False
4. c	4. b	4. b	4. c
5. c	5. c	5. a	5. True
6. False	6. c	6. d	6. True
7. c	7. a	7. b	7. False
8. d	8. c	8. False	8. False
9. d	9. b	9. d	9. b
10. False	10. d	10. False	10. False
11. c	11. c	11. e	11. e
12. b	12. d	12. True	12. False
13. c	13. d	13. b	13. d
14. a	14. d	14. a	14. False
15. a		15. b	15. False
16. d		16. a	16. False
17. False		17. c	17. False
18. False		18. b	18. True
19. c		19. c	19. False
20. c		20. c	20. False
21. False		21. b	
		22. c	
		23. False	

@ Symbol for *at*, or *in the same meridian as*.

Δ Symbol for *prism*. When following a number, it denotes the units known as prism diopters.

⌣ Symbol for *in combination with*.

180-degree line   A synonym for *horizontal midline*.

A

A   The horizontal dimension of the boxing system rectangle that encloses a lens or lens opening.

Abbé value   See *value, Abbé*.

aberration   The resulting degradation of an image that occurs when a point source of light does not result in a single-point image after going through the lens or lens system.

aberration, chromatic   The type of aberration that causes light of different wavelengths (colors) to be refracted differently through the same optical system.

aberration, lateral chromatic   An aberration that produces images of slightly different sizes at the focal length of the lens, depending upon the color of the light. (Synonym: *chromatic power*.)

aberration, longitudinal chromatic   Occurs when a point light source that is composed of several wavelengths (like white light) forms a series of point images along the optical axis. Each of these images is a different color and each has a slightly different focal length.

aberration, monochromatic   An aberration that is present even when light is made up of only one wavelength (one color).

aberration, spherical   An aberration that occurs when parallel light from an object enters a large area of a spherical lens surface and peripheral rays focus at different points on the optic axis than do paraxial rays.

absolute refractive index   See *index, absolute refractive*.

accurate sag formula   See *formula, accurate sag*.

actual power   See *power, actual*.

add   See *addition, near*.

add, nasal   The modification of an existing lens shape by allowing more lens material to remain in the inferior, nasal position than would be indicated otherwise for the purpose of creating a better frame fit.

addition, near   The power that a lens segment has in addition to that power already present in the main portion of the lens.

alignment, horizontal   A lack of deviation of the two datum lines in a pair of spectacles from a single horizontal plane (neither lens higher than the other when viewed from the front).

alignment, standard   An impersonal standard, independent of facial shape, for the alignment of spectacle frames.

alignment, vertical   Lack of deviation of the two spectacle lenses from the vertical plane (one being neither further forward nor backward than the other).

allowance, grinding   Synonym for wheel differential.

allowance, vertex power   The amount by which the front surface curvature of a lens must be flattened to compensate for a thickness-related gain in power.

American endpiece   See *endpiece, American*.

American National Standards Institute   An industry-based, nongovernmental standards-setting association. The American National Standards Institute is an agency that addresses standards throughout all of industry, of which the ophthalmic industry is only a small part. ANSI sets standards for aspects of the ophthalmic industry that includes lenses, frames, and contact lenses.

Amethyst Contrast Enhancer (ACE)   A selectively absorbing glass developed by Schott that is said to enhance contrast and be advantageous for target and trap shooting, hunting, computer terminal viewing, skiing, and bird watching. The lens allows highest transmission around the blue, green, and red regions of the spectrum.

analyzer, lens   A trade name for an automated lensmeter.

angle of deviation   The difference between the angle of incidence and the angle of refraction.

angle, apical   The angle formed by the junction of two nonparallel prism surfaces.

angle, crest   The angle from the tip to the top of the nose (between the eyes) compared with a vertical plane roughly parallel to the brows and cheeks.

angle, effective diameter   The angle from the 0-degree side of the 180-degree line to the axis of the effective diameter. The angle is referred to by the letter X and is measured using the right lens.

angle, frontal   1. The angle with which each side of the nose deviates from the vertical. 2. The angular amount the nosepad face deviates from the vertical when the frame is viewed from the front.

angle, pantoscopic   1. In standard alignment that angle by which the frame front deviates from the vertical (lower rims farther inward than upper rims) when the spectacles are held with the temples horizontal. 2. In fitting, that angle that the frame front makes with the frontal plane of the wearer's face when the lower rims are closer to the face than the upper rims (opposite-retroscopic angle). (Synonym: *pantoscopic tilt*.)

angle, retroscopic   That angle that the frame front makes with the frontal plane of the wearer's face when the lower rims are farther from the face than the upper rims (opposite-pantoscopic angle). (Synonym: *retroscopic tilt*.)

angle, splay 1. That angle formed by the side of the nose with a straight anterior-posterior surface that would bisect it vertically (also called *transverse angle*). 2. The angle the face of a nosepad makes with a plane perpendicular to that of the frame front when viewed from above.

angle, temple fold The angle formed when a temple is folded to a closed position.

angle, vertical When viewed from the side, that angle formed between the plane of the lenses and the long axis of the adjustable nosepads.

anisometropia A condition in which one eye differs significantly in refractive power from the other.

ANSI Abbreviation for American National Standards Institute.

antireflection coating See *coating, antireflection.*

antiscratch coating See *coating, antiscratch.*

aperture 1. An opening or hole that admits only a portion of light from a given source or sources. 2. The central, optically correct portion of a lenticular lens.

aperture, lens The portion of the spectacle frame that accepts the lens. (Synonym: *lens opening.*)

apex The junction point at which the two non-parallel surfaces of a prism meet.

aphake A person whose crystalline lens has been removed.

apical angle See *angle, apical.*

AR An abbreviation for antireflection coating.

arm Also called *bar, browbar,* in a semirimless mounting, the metal reinforcement that follows the upper posterior surface of a spectacle lens and joins the centerpiece to the endpiece.

arms, guard A synonym for pad arms.

arms, pad Metal pieces that connect adjustable nosepads to the front of a frame. (Synonym: *guard arms.*)

aspheric A nonspherical surface.

aspheric lenticular See *lenticular, aspheric.*

aspheric, full-field An aspheric lens that continues in its asphericity in an optically usable manner all the way to the edge of the lens blank.

astigmatic difference See *difference, astigmatic.*

astigmatic error See *error, astigmatic.*

astigmatism The presence of two different curves on a single refracting surface on or within the eye. This causes light to focus as two line images instead of as a single point.

astigmatism, marginal See *astigmatism, oblique.*

astigmatism, oblique 1. An astigmatic eye condition whereby the major meridians of the correcting lens are at an oblique angle, between 30 and 60 degrees or 120 and 150 degrees. 2. The lens aberration that occurs when rays from an off-axis point pass through a spherical lens and light focuses as two line images

instead of a single point. (Synonyms: *radial astigmatism, marginal astigmatism.*)

astigmatism, radial See *astigmatism, oblique.*

ASTM American Society for Testing and Materials.

autolensmeter A lensmeter that measures the power and prismatic effect of the lens in an automated fashion.

axis meridian See *meridian, axis.*

axis of a cylinder An imaginary reference line used to specify cylinder or spherocylinder lens orientation and corresponding to the meridian perpendicular to that of maximum cylinder power.

axis, optical That line which passes through the center of a lens on which the radii of curvature of the front and back surfaces fall.

axis, prism The base direction of an ophthalmic prism, expressed in degrees.

B

B The vertical dimension of the boxing system rectangle that encloses a lens or lens opening.

back base curve See *curve, back base.*

back vertex power See *power, back vertex.*

Balgrip mounting See *mounting, Balgrip.*

bar See *arm.*

barrel The housing for a screw on a pair of glasses.

barrel distortion See *distortion, barrel.*

base In a prism, the edge of maximum surface separation opposite the apex.

base curve See *curve, base.*

base down Vertical placement of prism such that the base is at 270 degrees on a degree scale.

base in Horizontal placement of prism such that the base is toward the nose.

base out Horizontal placement of prism such that the base is toward the side of the head.

base up Vertical placement of prism such that the base is at 90 degrees on a degree scale.

basic impact See *impact, basic.*

BCD Boxing center distance. See *distance, boxing center.*

bent-down portion See *earpiece.*

best form lens See *lens, corrected curve.*

bevel The angled edge of the spectacle lens.

bevel, hidden An edged lens configuration that attempts to reduce the appearance of thickness by creating a small bevel with the rest of the lens edge remaining flat.

bevel, mini A lens edge configuration that has a bevel and an angled ledge.

bevel, pin Synonym for safety bevel.

bevel, safety 1. To remove the sharp interface between lens surface and bevel surface and the sharp point at the bevel apex. 2. The smoothed interface between lens surface and bevel surface and the smoothed lens bevel apex.

bevel, V A lens edge configuration having the form of a V across the whole breadth of the lens edge.

bicentric grinding See *grinding, bicentric.*

bifocal A lens having two areas for viewing, each with its own focal power. Usually the upper portion of the lens is for distance vision, the lower for near vision.

bifocal, blended A bifocal lens constructed from one piece of lens material and having the demarcation line smoothed out so as not to be visible to an observer.

bifocal, curved-top A bifocal lens having a segment that is round in the lower portion and gently curved on the top of the segment.

bifocal, Executive American Optical's trade name for the Franklin-style bifocal.

bifocal, flat-top A bifocal with a segment that is round in the lower half but flat on the top.

bifocal, Franklin A bifocal having a segment that extends the entire width of the lens blank.

bifocal, minus add A bifocal with a large, round segment at the top of the lens. The segment is powered for distance viewing and the rest of the lens for near viewing. (Synonym: *minus add bifocal.*)

bifocal, Panoptik A bifocal lens resembling a flat-top bifocal, but having a segment that has a slightly curved upper edge with rounded corners.

bifocal, Rede-Rite See *bifocal, minus add.*

bifocal, ribbon A bifocal with a segment that resembles a circle with the top and bottom removed.

bifocal, round seg A bifocal with a segment that is perfectly round. The width of the segment is usually 22 mm, but may be larger (usually 38 mm).

bifocal, upcurve See *bifocal, minus add.*

binocular PD See *PD, binocular.*

blank geometric center See *center, blank geometrical.*

blank seg drop See *drop, blank seg.*

blank seg inset See *inset, blank seg.*

blank, finished lens A lens that has front and back surfaces ground to the desired powers but not yet edged to the shape of the frame.

blank, pattern A predrilled, flat piece of plastic from which a pattern may be cut.

blank, rough A lens-shaped piece of glass with neither side having the finished curvature. Both sides must yet be surfaced to bring the lens to its desired power and thickness.

blank, semifinished lens A lens with only one side having the desired curvature. The second side must yet be surfaced to bring the lens to its desired power and thickness.

blended bifocals See *lens, blended bifocal.*

blended myodisc See *lens, blended myodisc.*

block That which is attached to the surface of a lens to hold it in place during the surfacing or edging process.

blocker The device used to place a block on the lens to hold the lens in place during the surfacing or edging process.

blocker, layout A centering device with the capability of also blocking the lens. The layout blocker does not mark the lens first, nor does it have a conversion capacity to allow marking of the lens

blocking, finish The application of a holding block to an ophthalmic lens so that it may be edged to fit a frame.

blocking, surface The application of a holding block to an ophthalmic lens so that one side may be ground to the correct curvature and polished.

Boley gauge See *gauge, Boley.*

box, light A box with a white, translucent piece of plastic on top and a full spectrum bulb inside. When used in the optical laboratory, the white, illuminated background serves as a backdrop for comparison of two lens colors.

boxing center See *center, boxing.*

boxing center distance See *distance, boxing center.*

Boxing system See *system, boxing.*

Box-o-Graph A flat device containing grids and slides, used in the measurement of pattern and edged lens size.

bridge The area of the frame front between the lenses.

bridge, comfort A clear plastic saddle-type bridge that is used on a metal frame.

bridge, keyhole The top, inside area of a keyhole bridge is shaped like an old-fashioned keyhole. From the top, it flares out slightly, resting on the sides of the nose but not on the crest of the nose.

bridge, metal saddle A metal bridge that arches across in a thin band, sitting directly on the crest of the nose. (Synonym: *W bridge.*)

bridge, saddle A frame bridge that is shaped like a saddle in a smooth curve and follows the bridge of the nose smoothly.

bridge, semisaddle A bridge that looks much the same as a saddle from the front but has permanent, nonadjustable nose pads attached to the back of the bridge. (Synonym: *modified saddle bridge.*)

bridge, skewed That misalignment that occurs when one lens in a pair of spectacles is higher than the other yet neither lens is rotated.

bridge-narrowing pliers See *pliers, bridge-narrowing.*

bridge-widening pliers See *pliers, bridge-widening.*

browbar See *arm.*

build-up pads See *pads, build-up.*

C

C size   The circumference of an edged lens.

C   The horizontal width of a lens or lens opening as measured at the level of its geometrical center. (Synonym: *datum length*.)

cable temple   See *temple, cable*.

caliper, vernier   A hand-held width measuring device with a short graduated scale that slides along a longer graduated scale allowing a measure of fractional parts or decimals.

carrier   The outer, nonoptical portion of a lenticular lens.

cataract   A loss in clarity of the crystalline lens of the eye, which results in reduced vision or loss of vision.

cellulose acetate   A material extracted from cotton or wood pulp and used extensively for making spectacle frames.

center, blank geometrical   The physical center of a semifinished lens blank or an uncut finished lens blank. The blank geometrical center is the center of the smallest square or rectangle that completely encloses the lens blank.

center, boxing   The midpoint of the rectangle that encloses a lens in the boxing system.

center, cutting   Synonym for mechanical center.

center, datum   The midpoint of the datum length (C dimension) of a lens along the datum line.

center, edging   Synonym for mechanical center.

center, geometrical   1. The boxing center. 2. The middle point on an uncut lens blank.

center, mechanical   The rotational center of a pattern found at the midpoint of the central hole. (Synonyms: *cutting center, edging center*)

center, optical   That point on an ophthalmic prescription lens through which no prismatic effect is manifested.

center, reading   That point on a lens at the reading level that corresponds to the near PD.

center, rotational   The point on a pattern around which it rotates during edging.

center, seg optical   That location on the segment of a bifocal lens that shows zero prismatic effect when no refractive power is in the distance portion of the lens.

centerpiece   The portion of a rimless mounting consisting of bridge, pad arms, pads, and strap area.

centrad (∇)   A unit of measurement of the displacement of light by a prism. One centrad is the prism power required to displace a ray of light 1 cm from the position it would otherwise strike on the arc of a circle having a 1-m radius.

centration   The act of positioning a lens for edging such that it will conform optically to prescription specifications.

chamfering   The word *chamfer* means to bevel. In lens finishing, chamfering is taken to mean the act of smoothing off or safety beveling the sharp edges of a hole, slot, or notch drilled in a spectacle lens to prevent the chipping of the hole, slot, or notch when the spectacles are worn. *Note:* In British terminology, *chamfering* and *safety beveling* are synonymous.

chemical tempering   See *tempering, chemical*.

chemtempering   See *tempering, chemical*.

chord   A straight line that intersects two points of an arc.

chromatic aberration   See *aberration, chromatic*.

chromatic power   See *aberration, lateral chromatic*.

circumference gauge   See *gauge, circumference*.

C-Lite lens   See *lens, Corlon*.

clock, seg   Designed like a conventional lens measure except that the three points of contact are closely spaced.

coating, antireflection   A thin layer or series of layers of material applied to the surface of a lens for the purpose of reducing unwanted reflections from the lens surface and thus increasing the amount of light that passes through to the eye.

coating, antiscratch   A thin, hard coating applied to plastic lens surfaces to make them more resistant to scratching.

coating, color   A coating applied to the surface of a lens for the purpose of reducing light transmission.

coating, edge   Application of color to the edge of a lens for the purpose of decreasing edge visibility.

coating, mirror   A coating applied to a lens causing it to have the same properties as a two-way mirror.

coating, scratch resistant   A synonym for antiscratch coating.

collar   See *shoe*.

colmascope   An instrument that utilizes polarized light to show strain patterns in glass or plastic. (Synonym: *polariscope*.)

color coating   See *coating, color*.

color, reflex   The residual color of an antireflection coated lens.

coma   The lens aberration that occurs when the object point is off the axis of the lens causing a difference in magnification for rays passing through different zones of the lens. Instead of forming a single, point image off the optic axis, the image appears shaped like a comet or ice cream cone.

combination frame   See *frame, combination*.

comfort bridge   See *bridge, comfort*.

comfort cable temple   See *temple, cable*.

compensated power   See *power, compensated*.

compensated segs   See *segs, R-compensated*.

compounding (of prism)   The process of combining two or more prisms to obtain the equivalent prismatic effect expressed as a single prism.

concave An inward-curved surface.

conditioner, lens A specially formulated solution into which a plastic lens is immersed before being tinted. The purpose of lens conditioner is to prepare the lens for a fast and even uptake of dye.

conjugate foci See *foci, conjugate.*

contour plot See *plot, contour.*

convergence 1. An inward turning of the eyes, as when looking at a near object. 2. The action of light rays traveling toward a specific real image point.

convertible temple See *temple, convertible.*

convex An outward-curved surface.

coolant A liquid used to cool and lubricate the lens/grinding wheel interface during the grinding process.

coquille The thin nonpowered demonstration lens that comes in a spectacle frame to hold the shape of the frame as intended and to more realistically simulate the appearance of the frame for the prospective wearer. (Synonyms: *dummy lens, demo lens.*)

Corlon lens See *lens, Corlon.*

corrected curve lens See *lens, corrected curve.*

cosine For a right triangle, the ratio of the side adjacent the angle considered, to the hypotenuse.

$$\text{Cosine} = \frac{\text{Adjacent}}{\text{Hypotenuse}}$$

cosine-squared formula See *formula, cosine-squared.*

countersink curve See *curve, countersink.*

cover lens See *lens, cover.*

CR-39 A registered trademark of Pittsburgh Plate Glass Co. for an optical plastic known as Columbia Resin 39. It has been the standard material from which conventional plastic lenses are made.

crazed The cracked appearance of a lens with a damage or defective coating.

crest angle See *angle, crest.*

cribbing The process of reducing a semi-finished lens blank to a smaller size to speed the surfacing process or reduce the probability of difficulty.

cross curve See *curve, cross.*

cross, fitting A reference point 2 to 4 mm above the prism reference point on progressive-addition lenses. The fitting cross is positioned in front of the pupil.

cross, power A schematic representation on which the two major meridians of a lens or lens surface are depicted.

crown glass See *glass, crown.*

curl See *earpiece.*

Curvature The reciprocal of the radius of curvature of a curved surface, quantified in reciprocal meters (m^{-1}), and abbreviated by *R.*

curvature of field The lens aberration that causes the spherical power of the lens to be off in the periphery when compared with the center of the lens. For a flat object, this results in a curved image. (Synonym: *power error.*)

curve, back base The weaker back-surface curve of a minus cylinder-form lens. When the lens is a minus cylinder-form lens, the back base curve and the toric base curve are the same.

curve, base The surface curve of a lens that becomes the basis from which the other remaining curves are calculated.

curve, countersink For the manufacture of fused-glass semifinished bi- and trifocal lenses, the countersink curve is that curve that is ground into the main lens in the area where the segment is to be placed. The countersink curve matches the back curve of the bi- or trifocal segment. When the segment is placed on the countersink curve of the main lens, the two may then be fused together.

curve, cross The stronger curve of a toric lens surface.

curve, nominal base A 1.53-index-referenced number assigned to the base curve of a semifinished lens. For moderately powered crown-glass lenses the needed back surface tool curve may be found by subtracting the nominal base curve from the prescribed back vertex power.

curve, tool The 1.53-index-referenced surface power of a lap tool used in the fining and polishing of ophthalmic lenses.

curve, true base Synonym for true power.

cut, nasal The removal of an inferior, nasal portion of the lens shape to create a better frame fit.

cutting line See *line, cutting.*

cylinder A lens having a refractive power in one meridian only and used in the correction of astigmatism.

D

D An abbreviation for diopter of refractive power. See *diopter, lens.*

datum center See *center, datum.*

datum center distance See *distance, datum center.*

datum line See *line, datum.*

datum system See *system, datum.*

DBC Distance between centers.

DBL Distance between lenses.

DCD Datum center distance.

decentration 1. The displacement of the lens optical center or major reference point away from the boxing center of the frame's lens aperture. 2. The displacement of a lens optical center away from the wearer's line of sight for the purpose of creating a prismatic effect.

decentration, effective The distance from the axis of a decentered cylinder to the point from which decentration began.

demand, dioptric The inverse of the reading distance in meters, independent of actual bifocal addition power.

demo lens See *coquille.*

depth, mid-datum The depth of the lens measured through the datum center.

depth, reading The vertical position in the lens through which the wearer's line of sight passes when reading.

depth, sagittal (sag) The height or depth of a given segment of a circle.

depth, seg The longest vertical dimension of the lens segment before the lens has been edged.

deviation, angle of See *angle of deviation.*

diameter, effective Twice the longest radius of a frame's lens aperture as measured from the boxing center. Abbreviated ED.

difference, astigmatic The linear distance between the two line foci that occurs in oblique astigmatism. When expressed in diopters, this difference is called the *oblique astigmatic error.*

difference, frame In the boxing system, the difference between frame A and frame B dimensions, expressed in millimeters.

difference, pattern In the boxing system, the difference between pattern *A* and *B* dimensions, expressed in millimeters.

differential, wheel The difference in millimeters between the size of lens produced in roughing and finishing operations during edging

diopter, lens (D) Unit of lens refractive power, equal to the reciprocal of the lens focal length in meters.

diopter, prism (Δ) The unit of measurement that quantifies prism deviating power; one prism diopter (1Δ) is the power required to deviate a ray of light 1 cm from the position it would otherwise strike at a point 1 m away from the prism.

dioptric demand See *demand, dioptric.*

dispersion, mean The quantity ($n_F - n_C$)—the index of blue light minus the index of red light—that helps to define the chromatic nature of a lens material.

dispersive power See *power, dispersive.*

dissimilar segs See *segs, dissimilar.*

distance between centers (DBC) In a frame or finished pair of glasses, the distance between the boxing (geometrical) centers. (Synonym: *geometrical center distance.*)

distance between lenses (DBL) In the boxing system, the distance between the two boxed lenses as positioned in the frame. It is the shortest distance between a lens pair measured from the inside nasal eyewire grooves across the bridge area at the narrowest point (usually synonymous with *bridge size*).

distance reference point See *point, distance reference.*

distance, boxing center Synonym for distance between centers.

distance, datum center The distance between the datum centers in a frame or pair of glasses.

distance, frame center Synonym for distance between centers.

distance, geometric center The distance between the boxing (geometrical) centers of a frame.

distance, interpupillary (PD) The distance from the center of one pupil to the center of the other when either an infinitely distant object is being viewed (distance PD) or a near object is being viewed (near PD).

distance, near centration The distance between the geometrical centers of the near segments.

distance, vertex The distance from the back surface of the lens to the front of the eye.

distortion The lens aberration that causes the image to appear warped when compared with the object.

distortion, barrel The type of distortion normally caused by a plus lens that results in the image of a square object taking on a barrel-shaped appearance.

distortion, pattern The loss of correct edged lens shape resulting from use of a pattern that is too large or small in comparison with the lens size being edged.

distortion, pincushion The type of distortion normally caused by a minus lens that results in the image of a square object taking on a pincushion-shaped appearance.

divergence The action of light rays going out from a point source.

double gradient tint See *tint, double gradient.*

double-D lens See *lens, double-D.*

double-segment lens See *lens, double-segment.*

dress eyewear See *eyewear, dress.*

dress To reshape the cutting surface of a grinding wheel.

drop-ball test See *test, drop-ball.*

drop, blank seg The vertical distance from the blank geometric center to the top of the multifocal segment.

drop, seg 1. The vertical distance from the major reference point (MRP) to the top of the segment when the segment top is lower than the MRP. 2. The vertical distance from the horizontal midline to the top of the segment when the segment top is lower than the horizontal midline (laboratory usage). (Antonym: *seg raise.*)

DRP An abbreviation for distance reference point. See *point, distance reference.*

dummy lens See *coquille.*

E

ear That portion of the strap area on a rimless mounting that extends from the shoe, contacting the surface of the lens. (Synonym: *tongue*.)

earpiece That part of the temple that lies past the temple bend. (Synonym: *curl*.)

ED Effective diameter.

edge coating See *coating, edge*.

edge, rolled A lens edge configuration that reduces minus lens edge thickness by rounding out the back surface edge of the lens.

edger The piece of machinery used to physically grind the uncut lens blank to fit the shape of the frame.

edger, hand A grinding wheel made especially for changing a lens shape or smoothing a lens edge by hand.

edger, patterned A lens edger that uses patterns to produce the correct lens shape

edger, patternless An edger that uses an electronic tracing of a lens shape, rather than a physical pattern.

effective decentration See *decentration, effective*.

effective diameter See *diameter, effective*.

effective diameter angle See *angle, effective diameter*.

effective power See *power, effective*.

electrometallic wheel See *wheel, electrometallic*.

electroplated wheel See *wheel, electroplated*.

ellipse, Tscherning The elliptical-shaped graph that shows the best lens form(s) a lens can have for eliminating oblique astigmatism.

emmetrope A person without refractive error.

emmetropia The absence of refractive error.

endpiece angling pliers See *pliers, endpiece angling*.

endpiece One of the two outer areas of the frame front to the extreme left and right where the temples attach.

endpiece, American An older classification of metal endpiece that has a stop protruding from the single barrel on the temple, preventing the temple from opening out too far.

endpiece, butt-type An endpiece construction in which the front is straight and the temple butt is flat, and both meet at a 90-degree angle.

endpiece, English An older classification of metal endpiece that has a "stop" or "knuckle" that comes out around the hinge barrels and prevents the temples from opening out too widely.

endpiece, French An older classification of metal endpiece in which the temple is slotted between the two barrels and the stop is on the frame front as an extension of the single barrel.

endpiece, mitre-type An endpiece construction in which the frame front contact area and temple butt meet at a 45-degree angle.

endpiece, turn-back An endpiece design in which the frame front bends around and meets the temple end-to-end.

English endpiece See *endpiece, English*.

equation, Fresnel The formula for determining the amount of light that will be reflected from an uncoated lens surface, based on the index of refraction of the lens material.

Equithin A term used by the Varilux Corporation when referring to the use of yoked prism for thickness reduction on a pair of Varilux progressive-addition lenses. See also *prism, yoked*.

equivalent, spherical The sum of the spherical component and one half of the cylinder component of an ophthalmic lens prescription.

error, astigmatic Unwanted cylinder power found primarily in the inferior peripheral areas of a progressive addition lens.

error, oblique astigmatic The "astigmatic difference" that occurs in the aberration of oblique astigmatism as expressed in diopters.

error, power See *curvature of field*.

Executive bifocal See *bifocal, Executive*.

extractor, screw A device that resembles a screwdriver but has a barbed tip instead of a blade. The barbed tip digs into a damaged screw head or the remaining tip of a broken-off screw and is turned to remove the damaged or broken screw.

eyesize In the boxing system, the A dimension. (The horizontal dimension of the lens opening of a frame, which is bounded by two vertical lines tangent to the left and right sides of that lens opening.)

eyewear, dress Eyewear designed for everyday use.

eyewear, safety Eyewear designed to be worn in situations that could be potentially hazardous to the eyes and thus must meet higher standards of impact resistance than conventional eyewear.

eyewear, sports Eyewear designed to protect the eyes and/or enhance vision in specific sports situations. What is appropriate will vary dramatically, depending upon the sport.

eyewire The rim of the frame that goes around the lenses.

eyewire forming plier See *plier, eyewire forming*.

eyewire shaping plier Eyewire forming plier.

F

F Often used in equations to denote lens refractive power in diopters. Alternative symbol for F is D.

face form See *form, face*.

facet An edge configuration resembling the appearance of beveled glass that is sometimes used with high-minus lenses to reduce edge thickness and weight.

farsightedness   See *hyperopia*.

FDA   Food and Drug Administration.

Figure 8 liner   See *liner, figure 8*.

file, pillar   A general purpose file used in dispensing.

file, rat-tail   Used in dispensing on drilled lenses, to reduce lens thickness in an area to allow for proper lens strap grasp or to smooth the edges of the drilled lens hole.

file, ribbon   See *file, slotting*.

file, riffler   Spoon-shaped file used in dispensing, good for getting at small, hard-to-reach areas.

file, slotting   Used for reslotting screws or making a slot where none previously existed.

file, zyl   Used in dispensing to file plastic parts of a frame.

Filtron   A laser-absorbing lens series made by Gentex.

finger-piece pliers   See *pliers, finger-piece*.

fining   In surfacing, the process of bringing a generated lens surface to the smoothness needed so that it will be capable of being polished.

finished lens   See *lens, finished*.

finishing   The process in the production of spectacles that begins with a pair of uncut lenses of the correct refractive power and ends with a completed pair of spectacles.

first focal length   See *length, first focal*.

first principal focus   See *focus, first principal*.

fitting cross   See *cross, fitting*.

flash   Synonym for swarf.

flat surface touch test   See *test, flat surface touch*.

flat-top bifocal   See *bifocal, flat-top*.

focal point   See *point, focal*.

focal power   See *power, focal*.

foci, conjugate   Object and image points for a lens or lens system that correspond. Rays originating at one point will be focused at the other.

focimeter   Synonym for lensmeter.

focus, first principal   The point at which an object may be placed so that the lens will form its image at infinity. For positive lenses this is a real object position, for negative lenses, a virtual object position.

focus, second principal   That point at which parallel light entering a lens is brought to focus. For positive lenses the focal point is real, for negative, virtual.

fork, centering   A forklike device used to hold a lens in position for blocking or for placing a lens in an older-style edger at a specific orientation.

form, face   An expression of the extent to which the curve in the frame front varies from the classical four-point touch position.

form, minus cylinder   The form a prescription takes when the value of the cylinder is expressed as a negative number.

form, plus cylinder   The form a prescription takes when the value of the cylinder is expressed as a positive number.

former   British equivalent of *pattern*.

formula, accurate sag   The formula used to find sagittal depth, which states that

$$s = r - \sqrt{(r^2 - y^2)}$$

where *r* is the radius of curvature of the surface and *y* is the semidiameter of the chord.

formula, cosine-squared   A formula used to obtain the "power" of an oblique cylinder, usually in the 90-degree meridian.

formula, lensmaker's   A formula used to find the dioptric power of a surface or radius of curvature. The formula states that

$$D = \frac{(n' - n)}{r}$$

where *D* is the lens refractive power in diopters, n′ is the refractive index of the lens, and *n* is the refractive index of the media surrounding the lens.

formula, sine-squared   A formula used to obtain the "power" of an oblique cylinder, usually in the 180-degree meridian.

four-point touch   See *touch, four-point*.

frame center distance   See *distance, frame center*.

frame center distance   See *distance, geometrical center*.

frame difference   See *difference, frame*.

frame PD   Synonym for distance between centers or geometrical center distance.

frame tracer   See *tracer, frame*.

frame, combination   1. A frame having a metal chassis with plastic top rims and temples. 2. A frame having some major parts of plastic construction and some of metal.

frame, shell   An older expression referring to a plastic frame. Derived from when tortoise shell was used as a frame material.

Franklin bifocal   See *bifocal, Franklin*.

French endpiece   See *endpiece, French*.

Fresnel equation   See *equation, Fresnel*.

Fresnel lens   See *lens, Fresnel*.

Fresnel prism   See *prism, Fresnel*.

front vertex power   See *power, front vertex*.

front   That portion of the spectacles that contains the lenses.

front, wave   The outer border formed by rays diverging from their point of origin.

frontal angle   See *angle, frontal*.

front-to-bend (FTB)   Temple length expressed as the distance from the plane of the frame front to the bend of the temple.

FTB See *front-to-bend.*
full-field aspheric See *aspheric, full-field.*

G

g Symbol for the GOMAC system equivalent of the datum center distance.

gauge, Boley A gauge used to measure width of lenses or frame lens apertures.

gauge, circumference A device used to measure the distance around the outside of a previously edged lens or a coquille for the purpose of more accurately duplicating the size of an existing lens when edging a new lens.

GCD Geometrical center distance.

generating The process of rapidly cutting the desired surface curvature onto a semifinished lens blank.

geometrical center See *center, geometrical.*

geometric center distance See *distance, geometrical center.*

geometrically centered pattern See *pattern, geometrically centered.*

German silver See *nickel silver.*

glare control lenses See *lenses, glare control.*

glass, crown A commonly used glass lens material having an index of refraction of 1.523.

glazed lens See *lens, glazed.*

glazing 1. The insertion of lenses into a spectacle frame. 2. The clogging of empty spaces between the exposed abrasive particles of an abrasive wheel, resulting in reduced grinding ability.

GOMAC system See *system, GOMAC.*

GOMAC Groupement des Opticiens du Marche Commun. (A committee of Common Market opticians formed for the purpose of establishing European optical standards.)

gradient lens See *lens, gradient.*

gradient tint See *tint, gradient.*

grayness A lens surface defect caused by incomplete polishing.

grind, bicentric Synonym for slabing-off.

grinding allowance Synonym for wheel differential.

grinding, bicentric Grinding a portion of a lens so as to add a second optical center. Often used to create vertical prism in the lower portion of one lens for the purpose of alleviating vertical imbalance at near. (Synonym: *slabbing-off.*)

groover, lens The piece of equipment used to place a groove around the outer edge of a spectacle lens for the purpose of holding the lens in the frame with a nylon cord or thin metal rim.

guard arms See *arms, pad.*

H

half-eyes Frames made especially for those who need a reading correction but no correction for distance. They are constructed to sit lower on the nose than normal and have a vertical dimension that is only half the size of normal glasses.

hand edger See *edger, hand.*

hand stone *See stone, hand.*

HAZCOM Hazard Communication Standard (HCS). The Occupational Safety and Health Administration's *Hazard Communications Standard* requires all employers to provide their employees with information and training about any possible exposure to hazardous chemicals in the workplace. Information is to be in written form and should explain workplace policy on protection from hazards.

heat treating See *treating, heat.*

height, seg The vertically measured distance from the lowest point on the lens or lens opening to the level of the top of the segment.

Hide-a-Bevel Originally a trade name for an edge-grinding system that produces a shelf effect behind the bevel on thick-edged lenses. Now Hide-a-Bevel refers to this type of lens edge configuration in general.

high impact See *impact, high.*

high-index lens See *lens, high-index.*

high mass impact test See *test, high mass impact.*

high velocity impact test See *test, high velocity impact.*

hollow snipe-nosed pliers See *pliers, hollow snipe-nosed.*

horizontal alignment See *alignment, horizontal.*

horizontal midline See *midline, horizontal.*

hyperope A person with hyperopia.

hyperopia The refractive condition of the eye whereby light focuses behind the retina. Plus lenses are required to correct for hyperopia. (Synonyms: *hypermetropia* and *farsightedness.*)

I

Ilford mounting See *mounting, Balgrip.*

image jump See *jump, image.*

image, real An image formed by converging light and able to be focused on a screen.

image, virtual An image formed by tracing diverging rays leaving an optical system back to a point from which they appear to originate.

imbalance, vertical A differential vertical prismatic effect between the two eyes. At near this can be induced by right and left lenses of unequal powers when the wearer drops his or her eyes below the optical centers of the lenses.

impact, basic   The ANSI requirements for impact resistant safety eyewear that includes a minimum thickness requirement of 3.0 mm unless lenses are +3.00 D of power or higher in the highest plus meridian. In this case a 2.5 mm minimum edge thickness is permissible. Glass lenses are permissible. Lenses must be capable of withstanding the impact of a 1-inch steel ball dropped from 50 inches.

impact, high   The ANSI requirements for impact resistant safety eyewear that allows a minimum thickness of 2.0 mm when the lens material is capable of withstanding the impact of a $1/4$-inch steel ball traveling at 150 feet/second.

implant, intraocular lens   A plastic lens placed inside the eye as a replacement for the eye's natural crystalline lens. An intraocular lens implant is commonly used to replace a crystalline lens that has lost its clarity because of a developing cataract.

impregnated wheel   See *wheel, impregnated.*

index, absolute refractive   The ratio of the speed of light in a vacuum to the speed of light in another medium.

index, refractive   The ratio of the speed of light in a medium (such as air) to the speed of light in another medium (such as glass).

index, relative refractive   The ratio obtained by dividing the speed of light in a certain medium (usually air) by its speed in another medium.

index, UV   A measure of the amount of ultraviolet radiation present on a given day.

infrared   Invisible rays having wavelengths longer than those at the red end of the visible spectrum yet shorter than radio waves.

inset   The amount of lens decentration nasally from the boxing center of the frame's lens aperture. (Antonym: outset.)

inset, blank seg   The horizontal distance from the blank geometrical center to the center of the multifocal segment.

inset, geometrical   The lateral distance from the distance centration point to the geometrical center of the segment. (Synonym: *seg inset.*)

inset, net seg   The amount of additional seg inset (or outset) required to produce a desired amount of horizontal prismatic effect at near, added to the normal seg inset required by the near PD.

inset, seg   The lateral distance from the major reference point to the geometrical center of the segment.

inset, total   The amount the near segment must move from the boxing center to place it at the near PD (near centration distance).

intermediate   The area of a trifocal lens between the distance viewing portion and the near portion.

interpupillary distance   See *distance, interpupillary.*

intraocular lens implant   See *implant, intraocular lens.*

invisible bifocals   See *lens, blended bifocal.*

iseikonic lenses   See *lenses, iseikonic.*

isocylinder line   See *line, isocylinder.*

J

jig   Also called "third hand." A jig consists of adjustable clips mounted on a base. It is used to hold a frame in place while soldering.

jump, image   The sudden displacement of image as the bifocal line is crossed by the eye.

K

keyhole bridge   See *bridge, keyhole.*

knife-edge   A plus lens ground to an absolute minimum thickness such that the edge of the lens is so thin that it has a knifelike sharpness to it, that is, an edge thickness of zero.

L

ℓ   Symbol for the GOMAC system eyesize measure. It is equal to the boxed length of the lens (A dimension).

laminated lens   See *lens, laminated.*

lap   A tool having a curvature matching that of the curvature desired for a lens surface. The lens surface is rubbed across the face of the tool and, with the aid of pads, abrasives and polishes, the lens surface is brought to optical quality.

lateral chromatic aberration   See *aberration, lateral chromatic.*

law, Snell's   Concerning the passage of light from one medium to another, and stating that

$$n \sin i = n' \sin i'$$

where n and n' are the refractive indices of the two materials, i is the angle of incidence, and i' is the angle of refraction.

layout blocker   See *blocker, layout; marker/blocker.*

layout   The process of preparing a lens for blocking and edging.

LEAP   A 3M Company adhesive pad blocking system.

length, datum   The horizontal width of a lens or lens opening as measured along the datum line.

length, first focal   For a thin lens, the distance from the lens to the first principal focus.

length, overall temple   The length of a spectacle lens temple as measured from the center of the hinge barrel, around the temple bend, to the posterior end of the temple.

length, second focal For a thin lens, the distance from the lens to the second principal focus.

length-to-bend (LTB) Temple length measured from the center of the hinge barrel to the middle of the bend.

lens analyzer See *analyzer, lens.*

lens conditioner See *conditioner, lens.*

lens groover See *groover, lens.*

lens measure See *measure, lens.*

lens opening See *opening, lens.*

lens protractor See *protractor, lens.*

lens size See *size, lens.*

lens washer See *washer, lens.*

lens, aspheric lenticular A lenticular lens whose optically usable central portion has a front surface with a changing radius of curvature. The farther from the center of the lens, the longer the front surface radius of curvature becomes.

lens, best form See *lens, corrected curve.*

lens, blended bifocal Bifocal lenses with a segment area that is not visible to the observer. Blended bifocals are usually round-segment lenses that have the demarcation line between the distance portion and the bifocal portion smoothed away.

lens, blended myodisc A minus lens, lenticular in design, with the edges of the bowl blended so as to improve the cosmetic aspects of the lens.

lens, Corlon A glass lens that has been laminated on the back with a thin layer of polyurethane plastic. (Synonym: *C-Lite lens.*)

lens, corrected curve A lens whose surface curvatures have been carefully chosen with the intent of reducing those peripheral lens aberrations that are troublesome to the spectacle lens wearer. (Synonym: *best form lens.*)

lens, cover A thin lens that is temporarily glued to the surface of a semifinished blank to protect the surface of the lens and facilitate accurate grinding, as in the case of a slab-off grind on a glass lens.

lens, demo See *coquille.*

lens, double-D A multifocal lens with a flat-top bifocal-style segment in the lower portion of the lens and an inverted flat-top bifocal-style segment in the upper portion of the lens.

lens, double-segment A multifocal lens that has two segments, one in the lower and one in the upper portion of the lens.

lens, dummy See *coquille.*

lens, finished A spectacle lens that has been surfaced on both front and back to the needed power and thickness. A finished lens has not been edged for a spectacle frame but is still in uncut form.

lens, Fresnel A lens made from a thin flexible plastic material, having concentric rings of ever-increasing prismatic effect that duplicates the refractive effect of a powered spectacle lens.

lens, glare control Present usage of the term denotes a lens that absorbs wavelengths toward the blue end of the spectrum, reducing glare from scattered short, visible wavelength light.

lens, glazed 1. A prescription or nonprescription lens mounted in a frame. 2. The thin plastic demonstration lens that comes in a pair of spectacle frames. (Synonyms: *dummy lens, coquille.*)

lens, gradient A lens having a tinted upper portion that gradually lightens toward the lower portion of the lens.

lens, hand-flattened lenticular A negative lenticular lens with the lenticular produced on a hand edger and hand polished.

lens, high-index A lens with an index of refraction that is at the upper end of the range of available indices of refraction for lenses, yielding a lens that is thinner than other lenses of the same size and power.

lens, laminated An ophthalmic lens that is made up of more than one layer. Examples include polarized lenses, lenses that have a glass front and a polyurethane back surface, and plastic bifocal lenses made from front and back sections to bypass conventional surfacing procedures.

lens, lenticular A high-powered lens with the desired prescription power found only in the central portion. The outer carrier portion is ground so as to reduce edge thickness and weight in minus prescriptions and center thickness and weight in plus prescriptions.

lens, meniscus A lens having a convex front surface and a concave back surface.

lens, mineral Synonym for glass lens.

lens, minus cylinder form A lens ground such that it obtains its cylinder power from a difference in surface curvature between two back surface meridians.

lens, minus lenticular A high-minus lens that is lenticular in design, having a central area containing the prescribed refractive power and a peripheral carrier that is plus in power for maximum edge thinning.

lens, multidrop A high-plus, full-field aspheric lens in which the surface power drops rapidly as the edge of the lens is approached.

lens, multifocal A lens having a sector or sectors where the refractive power is different from the rest of the lens, such as bifocals or trifocals.

lens, myodisc 1. Traditional definition: a high-minus lens that is lenticular in design, having a central area containing the prescribed refractive power and a peripheral carrier that is plano in power. The front curve is either plano in power or very close to plano. 2. General usage: any high-minus lens that is lenticular in design.

lens, negative lenticular   A high-minus lens that has had the peripheral portion flattened for the purpose of reducing weight and edge thickness. (Synonym: *myodisc*.)

lens, Percival form   A lens design that concentrates on the elimination of power error instead of oblique astigmatism.

lens, photochromic   A lens that changes its transmission characteristics when exposed to light.

lens, plus cylinder form   A lens ground so that it obtains its cylinder power from a difference in surface curvature between two front surface meridians.

lens, point focal   A lens design that concentrates on the elimination of oblique astigmatism instead of power error.

lens, polarizing   A lens that blocks light polarized in one plane, such as light reflected from a smooth, non-diffusing surface.

lens, prism segment   A 10-mm deep ribbon-style segment containing a prismatic effect for near. The ribbon segment extends to the nasal edge of the lens blank.

lens, progressive-addition   A lens having optics that vary in power gradually from the distance to near zones.

lens, quadrafocal   A multifocal lens that has a flat-top trifocal segment in the lower portion of the lens and an inverted flat-top bifocal-type segment in the upper portion of the lens.

lens, reverse-slab   A slab-off lens that has base-down prism below the slab line, instead of base-up. Reverse-slab lenses are usually precast plastic.

lens, single-vision   A lens with the same sphere and/or cylinder power throughout the whole lens, as distinguished from a multifocal lens.

lens, spheric lenticular   A lenticular lens whose optically usable central portion has a front surface that does not vary in curvature but is entirely spherical.

lens, stock   A lens that is premade and does not have to be custom surfaced.

lens, uncut   A lens that has been surfaced on both sides but not yet edged for a frame.

lens, X-Chrom   A red contact lens used in an attempt to improve color vision for certain red-green color defectives.

lens, Younger seamless   Trade name for a blended bifocal made by Younger Optics.

lenses, iseikonic   A lens pair with their curvatures and thicknesses specially chosen in order to produce a difference in image magnification between the left and right eyes. Also known as size lenses.

lensmaker's formula   See *formula, lensmaker's*.

lensmeter   The instrument used for finding power and prism in spectacle lenses.

lensometer   A trade name for a type of lensmeter.

lenticular   A high-powered lens with the desired prescription power found only in the central portion. The outer carrier portion is ground so as to reduce edge thickness and weight in minus prescriptions and center thickness and weight in plus prescriptions.

lenticular lens   See *lens, lenticular* or *lenticular*.

lenticular, aspheric   A lenticular lens whose optically usable central portion has a front surface with a changing radius of curvature.

lenticular, hand-flattened   A negative lenticular lens with the lenticular portion produced on a hand edger and hand polished.

lenticular, negative   A high-minus lens that has had the peripheral portion flattened for the purpose of reducing weight and edge thickness. (Synonym: *myodisc*.)

lenticular, spheric   A lenticular lens whose optically usable central portion has a front surface that does not vary in curvature but is entirely spherical.

level, reading   A synonym for reading depth. See *depth, reading*.

library temple   See *temple, library*.

light box   See *box, light*.

line, 180-degree   A synonym for horizontal midline.

line, cutting   the 180-degree line marked on a lens after it has been properly positioned for cylinder axis orientation and decentration. It is used for reference in blocking and edging a lens.

line, datum   A line drawn parallel to and halfway between horizontal lines tangent to the lowest and highest edges of the lens. (Synonyms: *horizontal midline, 180-degree line*.)

line, isocylinder   One of the lines on the contour plot of a progressive addition lens denoting the location of unwanted cylinder of a given dioptric power.

line, mounting   1. The horizontal reference line that intersects the mechanical center of a lens pattern. 2. On metal or rimless spectacles the line that passes through the points at which the guard arms are attached, and that serves as a line of reference for horizontal alignment.

liner, figure-8   A liner that that fits into the top eyewire channel of some nylon cord frames.

longitudinal chromatic aberration   See *aberration, longitudinal chromatic*.

LTB   The length-to-bend measure of a frame temple.

M

major reference point   See *point, major reference*.

marginal astigmatism   See *astigmatism, oblique*.

marker   A centering device used to accurately position a lens and stamp it with horizontal and vertical reference lines for use in accurate lens blocking.

marker/blocker A device used to accurately position a lens and either stamp it with horizontal and vertical reference lines for use in accurate lens blocking, or block it directly while still in the device; that is, a centering device with stamping and blocking capability.

Material Safety and Data Sheet A single sheet of paper containing information about potentially hazardous chemicals found in the workplace. MSDS sheets should include physical and chemical characteristics, known acute and chronic health effects, exposure limits, precautionary measures, and emergency and first-aid procedures.

MBL Minimum between lenses

MBS Minimum blank size. See *size, minimum blank.*

mean dispersion See *dispersion, mean.*

measure, lens A small, pocket-watch–sized instrument for measuring the surface curve of a lens. Also called a *lens clock* or *lens gauge.*

meniscus lens See *lens, meniscus.*

meridian, axis The meridian of least power of a cylinder or spherocylinder lens; for a minus cylinder the least minus meridian, for a plus cylinder the least plus meridian.

meridian, major One of two meridians in a cylinder or spherocylinder lens. These meridians are 90 degrees apart and correspond to the maximum and minimum powers in the lens.

meridian, power The meridian of maximum power of a cylinder or spherocylinder lens; for a minus cylinder the most minus meridian, for a plus cylinder the most plus meridian.

metal bonded wheel See *wheel, metal bonded.*

metal saddle bridge See *bridge, metal saddle.*

mid-datum depth See *depth, mid-datum.*

midline, horizontal In the boxing system of lens measurement, the horizontal line halfway between the upper and lower horizontal lines bordering the lens shape. (Synonym: *180-degree reference line.*)

mini-bevel A lens edge configuration that has a bevel and an angled ledge.

minimum between lenses The datum system equivalent of the boxing system's distance between lenses (DBL).

minus add bifocal Bifocal, minus add.

minus cylinder form See *form, minus cylinder.*

minus cylinder form lens See *lens, minus cylinder form.*

minus lenticular lens See *lens, minus lenticular.*

mirror coating See *coating, mirror.*

Monel A whitish, pliable, nicely polishing metal frame material that is made from nickel, copper, and iron; it also contains traces of other elements.

monochromatic aberration See *aberration, monochromatic.*

monocular PD See *PD, monocular.*

mounting 1. The name for a spectacle lens frame when the lenses are held in place without the aid of an eyewire as with rimless or semi-rimless mountings. 2. The attaching of lenses to a rimless or semi-rimless spectacle frame.

mounting line See *line, mounting.*

mounting, Balgrip A mounting (frame) that secures the lens in place with clips attached to a bar of tensile steel that fits into a nasal and a temporal slot on each side of the lens.

mounting, Ilford Synonym for Balgrip mounting.

mounting, numont A lens mounting that holds the lenses in place only at their nasal edge. The lenses are attached at the bridge area and the temples are attached to a metal arm that extends along the posterior surface temporally. Thus each lens has only one point of attachment.

mounting, rimless A mounting that holds the lenses in place by some method other than eyewires or nylon cords. Usually the method of mounting is by screws through the lenses. (Synonym: *three-piece mounting.*)

mounting, semirimless Mountings similar to the rimless, except for a metal reinforcing arm, which follows the upper posterior surface of the lens and joins the centerpiece of the frame to the endpiece.

mounting, Wils-Edge A lens mounting (frame) that secures the lens in place by means of a grooved arm that grips the top of the lens.

MRP An abbreviation for major reference point. See *point, major reference.*

MSDS Abbreviation for Material Safety and Data Sheet.

multidrop lens See *lens, multidrop.*

multifocal A lens having a sector or sectors where the refractive power is different from the rest of the lens, such as bifocals or trifocals.

multifocals, segmented Multifocal lenses having a visible, clearly demarcated bi-or tri-focal area. Nonsegmented multifocals would be progressive addition lenses.

myodisc See *lens, myodisc.*

myope A person with myopia.

myopia The refractive condition of the eye whereby light focuses in front of the retina. Minus lenses are required to correct for myopia. (Synonym: *nearsightedness.*)

N

nasal The side of a lens or frame that is toward the nose (inner edge).

nasal add See *add, nasal.*

nasal cut See *cut, nasal.*

NBC   The abbreviation for nominal base curve.

near power   See *power, near.*

near reference point   See *point, near reference.*

near Rx   The net power resulting from the combination of the add power and the distance power.

nearsightedness   See *myopia.*

net seg inset   See *inset, net seg.*

neutralize   To determine the refractive power of a lens. Most often this is done with the aid of a lensmeter.

neutralizer   A solution used to reduce the color in or remove the color from a previously tinted lens.

nickel silver   A whitish-appearing metal frame material containing more than 50% copper, 25% nickel, and the rest zinc. (Synonym: *German silver.*)

nominal base curve   See *curve, nominal base.*

normal   A line perpendicular to a reflecting or refracting surface at the point of incidence.

NRP   An abbreviation for near reference point. See *point, near reference.*

number, set   The compensating number used with a pattern to arrive at a compensated eyesize setting for the edger.

Numont mounting   See *mounting, Numont.*

Numont pliers   See *pliers, Numont.*

nystagmus   A condition characterized by a constant, involuntary back-and-forth movement of the eye.

O

oblique astigmatic error   See *error, oblique astigmatic.*

oblique astigmatism   See *astigmatism, oblique.*

OC   Optical center.

Occupational Health and Safety Administration   The U.S. government agency responsible for setting workplace safety policy and ensuring worker safety.

OD   Latin, oculus dexter (right eye).

OLA   Abbreviation for the Optical Laboratories Association.

open temple spread   See *spread, open temple.*

opening, lens   The portion of the spectacle frame that accepts the spectacle lens. (Synonym: *lens aperture.*)

optical axis   See *axis, optical.*

optical center   See *center, optical.*

Optical Laboratories Association   A professional association of optical laboratories.

optically centered pattern   See *pattern, optically centered.*

Optyl   The trade name for an epoxy resin material used to make spectacle frames.

OS   Latin, oculus sinister (left eye).

OSHA   Occupational Health and Safety Administration.

outset   The amount of lens decentration temporally from the boxing center of the frame's lens aperture. (Antonym: *inset.*)

overall temple length   See *length, overall temple.*

P

p   Symbol for the GOMAC system distance between lenses. It is equal to the boxing DBL.

pad arms   See *arms, pad.*

pad-adjusting pliers   See *pliers, pad-adjusting.*

pads, build-up   Small nosepad-shaped pieces of plastic used to alter the fit of the bridge.

Panoptik   See *bifocal, Panoptik.*

pantoscopic angle or tilt   See *angle, pantoscopic.*

pantoscopic angling pliers   See *pliers, pantoscopic angling.*

parallax   The apparent change in position of an object as the result of a change in viewing angle.

paraxial rays   See *rays, paraxial.*

pattern difference   See *difference, pattern.*

pattern   A plastic or metal piece having the same shape as the lens aperture for a given frame. Used in lens edging as a guide for shaping the lens to fit the frame.

pattern, geometrically centered   A pattern with mechanical and geometrical centers on the same horizontal plane.

pattern, optically centered   A pattern with its mechanical center above boxing center.

patterned edger   See *edger, patterned.*

patternless edger   See *edger, patternless.*

PD   An abbreviation for interpupillary distance (see *distance, interpupillary*).

PD, binocular   The measured distance from the center of one pupil to the center of the other pupil without regard to how each eye may vary in its distance from the center of the bridge of the frame.

PD, distance   The wearer's interpupillary distance specified for a situation equivalent to when the wearer is viewing a distant object.

PD, frame   Synonym for geometrical center distance or distance between centers.

PD, monocular   Interpupillary distance specified for each eye individually. The center of the frame bridge is the reference point from which measurements are specified.

PD, monocular   The distance from the center of the frame bridge to the center of the wearer's pupil measured for each eye separately.

PD, near   The interpupillary distance as specified for a near viewing situation.

Percival form lens   See *lens, Percival form.*

peripheral rays   See *rays, peripheral.*

phoria The direction of the line of sight of one eye with reference to that of the partner eye when fusion is interrupted, as when one eye is covered.

photochromic lens See *lens, photochromic.*

photometer An instrument for measuring brightness. When used with lenses, the percent transmission of the lens is measured in a given spectral area or areas.

pillar file See *file, pillar.*

pincushion distortion See *distortion, pincushion.*

planes, variant A form of vertical misalignment of a spectacle frame in which the lens planes are out of coplanar alignment (one lens is further forward than the other).

plano (pl) A lens or lens surface having zero refracting power.

pliers, bridge-narrowing Used to narrow the bridge of a plastic frame.

pliers, bridge-widening Used to widen the bridge of a plastic frame.

pliers, chipping Pliers used to chip or break away the outer portions of an uncut or semifinished glass lens to either reduce its size or bring it into the rough shape needed to approximate the finished shape.

pliers, endpiece angling Pliers used in the adjustment of rimless mountings.

pliers, eyewire-forming Pliers with horizontally curved jaws used to shape or form the upper and lower eyewires of a metal frame to match the meniscus curve of the edged lens.

pliers, fingerpiece Pliers used for adjustment of the temple-fold angle of plastic frames. Fingerpiece pliers have parallel jaws and were originally designed for adjusting fingerpiece mountings. Also called *Fits-U pliers.*

pliers, hollow snipe-nosed Thin-nosed pliers with a hollowed-out central jaw area.

pliers, Numont Holding pliers specially designed for use with Numont mountings. Numont pliers serve the same purpose for Numont mountings as endpiece angling pliers do for standard rimless mountings.

pliers, pad-adjusting These pliers have one cupped jaw to conform to the face-portion of an adjustable nosepad; the other jaw is shaped to allow the back of the pad to be held securely while being angled.

pliers, snipe-nosed Pliers that taper to a small tip on both jaws, allowing use in tight places. Often used in the adjustment of pad arms.

pliers, square-round Used to adjust pad arms, these pliers have a small round section on one jaw and a squared off section on the other.

pliers, strapping Pliers having two flat jaws. One jaw extends beyond the other and then overlaps it. Used to adjust straps of a rimless or semirimless mounting.

plot, contour A line diagram used to plot the areas of unwanted cylinder, attainable visual acuity, or vertical imbalance over the viewing areas of a progressive addition lens.

plus cylinder form See *form, plus cylinder.*

plus-cylinder-form lens See *lens, plus cylinder form.*

point One tenth of a millimeter of lens thickness.

point focal lens See *lens, point focal.*

point, distance centration The British equivalent of the major reference point.

point, distance reference (DRP) That point on a lens where, according to the manufacturer, the distance power is to be measured. Distance power consists of sphere, cylinder and axis. DRP may not correspond to the prism reference point (PRP), as with progressive addition lenses.

point, focal A point to or from which light rays converge or diverge.

point, major reference (MRP) The point on a lens where the prism equals that called for by the prescription.

point, near reference (NRP) That point on the lens where, according to the manufacturer, the power of the near addition is to be measured.

point, prism reference (PRP) The point on a lens where prism power is to be verified. Also referred to as the *major reference point.*

polariscope See *colmascope.*

polarizing lens See *lens, polarizing.*

polyamide A strong, nylon-based frame material that allows a frame to be made thinner and lighter than it would ordinarily be if made from cellulose acetate frame material.

polycarbonate A 1.586-index lens material known for its strength.

power cross See *cross, power.*

power meridian See *meridian, power.*

power, actual Synonym for true power.

power, back vertex The reciprocal of the distance in air from the rear surface of the lens to the second principal focus, which serves as a specific measure of the power of a lens.

power, chromatic See *aberration, lateral chromatic.*

power, compensated Back vertex power that has been converted to a 1.53-index frame of reference. Used for the purpose of finding a 1.53-index-referenced tool curve for a lens with a different index of refraction.

power, dispersive The following quantity

$$\frac{n_F - n_C}{n_D - 1}$$

used for quantifying chromatic aberration of a given material. Dispersive power is abbreviated as the Greek letter omega, or ω.

power, effective 1. The vergence power of a lens at a

designated position other than that occupied by the lens itself. 2. That power lens required for a new position that will replace the original reference lens and yet maintain the same focal point.

power, focal   A measure of the ability of a lens or lens surface to change the vergence of entering light rays.

power, front vertex   The reciprocal of the distance in air from the front surface of a lens to the first principal focus.

power, near   The sum of the distance power and the near add. (Synonym: *near Rx.*)

power, nominal   An estimate of total lens power, calculated as the sum of front and back surface powers. (Not to be confused with nominal base curve.)

power, refractive   The dioptric value that accurately describes the ability of a lens or lens surface to converge or diverge light. For a lens surface in air the refractive power is expressed as

$$F = \frac{n-1}{r}$$

where n is the refractive index of the lens material and r is the radius of the surface expressed in meters.

power, true   The 1.53-index-referenced curvature of the base curve of a lens. True power is found by using a lens clock or sagometer (sag gauge) that is 1.53-index referenced.

precoat   A spray or brush-on liquid that when applied to a lens, protects the surface during processing, and/or makes the adhesion of a block to the lens possible.

Prentice's Rule   See *Rule, Prentice's.*

Prep, Lens   A trade name for lens conditioner.

prism   That part of an optical lens or system that deviates the path of light.

prism axis   See *axis, prism.*

prism diopter   See *diopter, prism.*

prism reference point   See *point, prism reference.*

prism, Fresnel   A prism made from thin flexible material and consisting of small rows of equal-powered prisms resulting in the same optical effect as that of a conventional ophthalmic prism.

prism, Rx   Prism in an ophthalmic lens prescription that has been called for by the prescribing doctor.

prism, yoked   Vertical prism of equal value ground on both right and left lenses of a progressive or Franklin-style lens for the purpose of reducing lens thickness.

progressive-addition lens   See *lens, progressive-addition.*

propionate   The common name for the frame material cellulose aceto-propionate. Propionate has many of the same characteristics as cellulose acetate and is better suited for injection molding.

protractor, lens   A millimeter grid on a 360-degree protractor used in the lens centration process for both surfacing and finishing.

PRP   An abbreviation for prism reference point. See *point, prism reference.*

Q

quadrafocal   See *lens, quadrafocal.*

R

radial astigmatism   See *astigmatism, oblique.*

raise, seg   1. The vertical distance from the major reference point to the top of the seg when the seg top is higher than the MRP. 2. The vertical distance from the horizontal mid-line of the edged lens to the top of the seg when the seg top is higher than the horizontal midline (laboratory usage). (Antonym: seg drop.)

rat-tail file   See *file, rat-tail.*

rays, paraxial   Those rays of light that pass through the central area of the lens.

rays, peripheral   Those rays of light that enter the lens nearer the edge than the center.

R-compensated segs   See *segs, R-compensated.*

reading center   See *center, reading.*

reading depth   See *depth, reading.*

reading level   See *level, reading.*

real image   See *image, real.*

Rede-Rite bifocal   See *bifocal, minus add.*

reduced thickness   See *thickness, reduced.*

reference point, distance   See *point, distance reference.*

reference point, near   See *point, near reference.*

reference point, prism   See *point, prism reference.*

reflex color   See *color, reflex.*

refraction   1. The bending of light by a lens or optical system. 2. The process of determining the needed power of a prescription lens for an individual.

refractive index   See *index, refractive.*

refractive power   See *power, refractive.*

relative refractive index   See *index, relative refractive.*

resolving (of prism)   The process of expressing a single prism as two prisms whose base directions are perpendicular to each other but whose combined effect equals that of the original prism.

retroscopic angle or tilt   See *angle, retroscopic.*

reverse-slab lens   See *lens, reverse-slab.*

ribbon bifocal   See *bifocal, ribbon.*

ribbon file   See *file, slotting.*

riding-bow temple   See *temple, riding-bow.*

riffler file   See *file, riffler.*

rim   See *eyewire.*

rimless   Having to do with frames (mountings) that hold lenses in place by some method other than eyewires. Most rimless mountings have two points of attachment per lens.

rimless mounting See *mounting, rimless.*

Rimway mounting See *mounting, semirimless.*

rolled edge See *edge, rolled.*

rolling A pulling of the eyewire such that it covers less of the front of the lens bevel than back or vice versa.

round-seg bifocal See *bifocal, round-seg.*

Rule, Prentice's A rule that states that the decentration of a lens in centimeters times the power of the lens is equal to the prismatic effect:

$$\Delta = cF$$

rule, three-quarter The three-quarter rule states that for every diopter of dioptric demand, the optical center of each reading lens, or the geometrical center of each bifocal addition, should be inset 0.75 (three-quarters) mm.

Rx prism See *prism, Rx.*

S

saddle bridge See *bridge, saddle.*

safety bevel See *bevel, safety.*

safety eyewear See *eyewear, safety.*

sag A synonym or abbreviation for sagittal depth. See also *depth, sagittal.*

sagittal depth See *depth, sagittal.*

scratch A furrowed-out line that has jagged edges.

screw extractor See *extractor, screw.*

second focal length See *length, second focal.*

second principal focus See *focus, second principal.*

seg See *segment.*

seg clock See *clock, seg.*

seg depth See *depth, seg.*

seg drop See *drop, seg.*

seg height See *height, seg.*

seg inset See *inset, seg.*

seg optical center See *center, seg optical.*

seg width See *width, seg.*

segment (seg) An area of a spectacle lens with power differing from that of the main portion.

segment, prism See *lens, prism segment.*

segmented multifocals See *multifocals, segmented.*

segs, dissimilar A method of correcting vertical imbalance at near that uses different bifocal segment styles for the right and left eyes.

segs, R-compensated A method for correcting vertical imbalance at near that uses ribbon-style bifocal segments that have been modified so that the segment optical center for one lens is high in one segment and low in the other.

semidiameter Diameter divided by 2. In ophthalmic optics, semidiameter refers to half of the chord for the arc of a given surface and is used in calculating the sagittal depth of the surface.

semifinished blank See *blank, semifinished.*

semifinished lap tool See *tool, semifinished lap.*

semirimless mountings See *mountings, semirimless.*

semisaddle bridge See *bridge, semisaddle.*

set number See *number, set.*

shell frame See *frame, shell.*

shield On a plastic frame, the metal piece to which rivets are attached to hold the hinge in place.

shields, side Protective shields attached to the spectacle frame at the outer, temporal areas to protect the eyes from hazards approaching from the side.

shoe That part of the strap area of a mounting that contacts the edge of the lens, bracing it. Also called *shoulder* or *collar.*

shop, back Synonym for surfacing laboratory.

shop, front Synonym for finishing laboratory.

shoulder See *shoe.*

side shields See *shields, side.*

sine For a right triangle, the ratio of the side opposite the angle considered, to the hypotenuse:

$$Sine = \frac{Opposite}{Hypotenuse}$$

sine-squared formula See *formula, sine-squared.*

single-vision lens See *lens, single-vision.*

size lenses See *lenses, iseikonic.*

size, lens In the boxing system, the A dimension of a lens or lens opening.

size, minimum blank The smallest lens blank that can be used for a given prescription lens and frame combination.

sizer A frame chassis or frame front used exclusively for checking edged lens size accuracy.

skewed bridge See *bridge, skewed.*

skull temple See *temple, skull.*

slab-off Grinding a portion of a lens so as to add a second optical center. Often used to create vertical prism in the lower portion of one lens for the purpose of alleviating vertical imbalance at near.

sleek A furrowed-out line on a lens, which resembles a scratch but whose edges are smooth instead of jagged.

slotting file See *file, slotting.*

smoothing, edge The process of bringing the bevel surfaces of an edged lens to a finer, smoother finish.

Snell's law See *law, Snell's.*

snipe-nosed pliers See *pliers, snipe-nosed.*

solid tint See *tint, solid.*

spectrophotometer A device used to measure the transmission of each wavelength of light across the spectrum.

sphere (sph) A lens having a single refractive power in all meridians.

spheric lenticular   See *lenticular, spheric.*

spherical aberration   See *aberration, spherical.*

spherical equivalent   See *equivalent, spherical.*

spherocylinder   The combination of sphere and cylinder powers into a single lens.

splay angle   See *angle, splay.*

sports eyewear   See *eyewear, sports.*

spotting   The placing of spots on a lens with a lensmeter in such a manner that the lens will be oriented correctly for axis and positioned for major reference point and horizontal meridian locations.

spread, open temple   That angle an open temple forms in relationship to the front of the frame (also called let-back).

square-round pliers   See *pliers, square-round.*

SRC   An abbreviation for scratch resistant coating.

standard alignment   See *alignment, standard.*

stars   Microchips at the lens surface/lens bevel interface.

stock lens   See *lens, stock.*

stock, lens   1. An inventory of lenses. 2. The material from which a semifinished blank is made, as in the amount of stock removal required to bring the blank to its needed thickness.

stone   1. An abrasive grinding wheel. 2. To sharpen the cutting ability of a grinding wheel by honing it with an abrasive stick.

stone, hand   Synonym for hand edger.

strabismus   The condition whereby one eye is pointed in a different direction than the other eye.

straight-back temple   See *temple, straight-back.*

strap   Mechanism for holding drilled lenses in a rimless or semirimless mounting.

strapping pliers   See *pliers, strapping.*

stria   A streak seen in a lens caused by a difference in the refractive index in the material. The streak causes a distortion in the object viewed and is not a physical streak like a mark on or in the lens. (The plural of stria is striae.)

surfacing   The process of creating the prescribed refractive power, prism, and major reference point location on a lens by generating the required curves and bringing the surface to a polished state.

swarf   Fibrouslike lens material resulting from the grinding process for certain types of lens material, such as polycarbonate.

system, boxing   A system of lens measurement based on the enclosure of a lens by horizontal and vertical tangents to form a box or rectangle.

system, datum   A system of lens measurement that defines the lens or eyesize as being the width of the lens along the datum line and the bridge size as the width of the bridge at the level of the datum line.

system, GOMAC   A European Economic Community standard incorporating portions of both the boxing and datum systems.

T

tables, sag   A set of tables used for finding sagittal depth when surface power and lens diameter are known.

tables, surfacing   Tables supplied by a lens manufacturer for the purpose of helping the surfacing laboratory accurately determine the tool curves and lens thicknesses needed to grind lenses to the specified back vertex power. Surfacing tables are now largely replaced by computer software programs.

tangent   For a right triangle, the ratio of the side opposite the angle considered to the side adjacent:

$$\text{Tangent} = \frac{\text{Opposite}}{\text{Adjacent}}$$

tap   Consists of a chuck on a handle in which threaders of varying size may be placed. It is used to restore threading that has been damaged.

tempering, chemical   The process of increasing the impact resistance of glass lenses by immersing them in a bath of molten salt. (Synonyms: *chemtempering, chem hardening.*)

temple   The part of a pair of spectacles that attaches to the frame front and hooks over the ears to hold spectacles in place.

temple, cable   Cable temples are of metal construction with the curl, or postear portion, constructed from a flexible coiled cable. The postear portion follows the crotch of the ear where the ear and the head meet and extends to the level of the earlobe. (Synonym: *Relaxo.*)

temple, comfort cable   See *temple, cable.*

temple, convertible   Temples that are straight through their entire length but are designed to be bent down to take on the form of a skull temple.

temple, library   The type of spectacle frame temple that begins with average width at the temple butt and increases in width toward the posterior end of the temple. Library temples are practically straight and hold the glasses on primarily by pressure against the side of the head. (Synonym: *straight-back temple.*)

temple, riding-bow   Plastic temples with thin, round postear portions that curve around the ear, following the crotch of the ear where the ear and the head meet and extend to the level of the earlobe. They often are used in children's and safety frames and are the plastic version of the metal comfort cable temple.

temple, skull   The type of spectacle frame temple that

bends down behind the ear and follows the contour of the skull, resting evenly against it.

temple-fold angle   See *angle, temple fold.*

temporal   The area of a lens or frame that is toward the temples (outer edge).

test, drop-ball   A test to determine impact resistance of ophthalmic lenses whereby either a $^5/_8$- or 1-inch steel ball is dropped onto the front surface of the lens from a height of 50 inches.

test, flat surface touch   A test for temple parallelism in which the spectacles are positioned upside-down on a flat surface with temples open.

test, high mass impact   A pointed, conical-tipped projectile weighing 17.6 ounces is dropped from 51.2 inches through a tube and onto the eyeglasses. The lens must not break, nor come out of the frame. (*Note:* A proposed change to this test modifies the distance from 51.2 to 50 inches.)

test, high velocity impact   This test simulates a high-velocity, low-mass object. In the high velocity impact test a series of $^1/_4$-inch steel balls traveling at 150 feet per second are directed at 20 different parts of the frame with lenses in place. A new frame is used for each impact. Neither the frame for the lens can break. Nor can the lens come out of the frame.

thickness, reduced   The thickness of a medium divided by its refractive index.

three-quarter rule   See *rule, three-quarter.*

tint, double gradient   A lens tint that has two colors, one at the top and a second at the bottom. The color at the top is darkest at the top and fades out towards the middle of the lens. The color at the bottom is most intense at the bottom and lighten toward the middle.

tint, gradient   The variation in light transmission of a lens from a low transmission (dark) to high transmission (light) from one area of the lens to another. Usually the lens is dark at the top and lightens at the bottom.

tint, solid   A tint that has the same color and light transmission over the entire lens.

tint, triple gradient   A lens with three colors. The color at the top is darkest at the top and fades out toward the middle of the lens. The color at the bottom is most intense at the bottom and lightens toward the middle. The third color is in the middle of the lens.

tongue   See *ear.*

tool, lap   A tool used for fining and polishing lens surfaces. The tool used must have a surface identical in curvature to that of the lens for which it is to be used; that is, if the lens surface is convex, the tool must be concave.

toric   A surface having separate curves at right angles to one another.

toric base curve   See *curve, toric base.*

toric transposition   See *transposition, toric.*

total inset   See *inset, total.*

touch, four-point   A check for vertical alignment carried out by placing a straight edge so that its edge goes across the inside of the entire front of the spectacles below the nosepad area.

tracer, frame   An instrument used to physically trace the inside groove of a frame's lens opening or the outside edge of a lens for the purpose of creating a digitized shape. That shape is then transmitted to a patternless edger so that the shape can be duplicated when the lens is edged.

Transitions   A trade name for a brand of plastic photochromic lenses.

transmission   The percent of light passing on through a lens and out the back surface, compared to the amount of light incident upon the first surface.

transposition, toric   The process of transposing a prescription from the form in which it is written to another form, such as from a plus to a minus cylinder form.

treating, heat   The process of hardening a glass lens by first heating it in a kiln, then quickly cooling by blowing forced air against both front and back surfaces. (Synonyms: *air hardening, heat hardening, heat tempering.*)

trifocals   Lenses having three areas of viewing, each with its own focal power. Usually the upper portion is for distance viewing, the lower for near, and the middle or intermediate portion for distance in between.

triple gradient tint   See *tint, triple gradient.*

Trivex   The brand name for a PPG Industries plastic lens material known for its high impact resistance and ability to be processed in a manner similar to that of other plastic lenses.

true   1. To bring a pair of glasses into a position of correct alignment. 2. To reshape the cutting surface of a worn grinding wheel so that it cuts at the angles and in the manner originally intended. 3. In surfacing, when using a hand pan, a step following roughing and smoothing, using a somewhat finer grade of abrasive in order to bring the lens to an exact curve.

true base curve   See *curve, true base.*

true power   See *power, true.*

trueing   See *true.*

Tscherning ellipse   See *ellipse, Tscherning.*

turn-back endpiece   See *endpiece, turn-back.*

U

ultraviolet   Rays having a wavelength somewhat shorter than those at the violet end of the visible spectrum.

uncut   A lens that has been surfaced on both sides but not yet edged for a frame.

upcurve bifocal   See *bifocal, minus add.*

UV index   See *index, UV.*

V

value, Abbé   The most commonly used number for identifying the amount of chromatic aberration for a given lens material. The higher the Abbé value, the less chromatic aberration present in the lens. Abbé value is the reciprocal of ω (dispersive power) and is the symbolized by the Greek letter nu, or ν. In other words:

$$\frac{1}{\omega} = \nu$$

(Synonyms: *nu value, constringence.*)

variant planes   See *planes, variant.*

V-bevel   See *bevel, V.*

vertex distance   See *distance, vertex.*

vertex power allowance   See *allowance, vertex power.*

vertical alignment   See *alignment, vertical.*

vertical angle   See *angle, vertical.*

vertical imbalance   See *imbalance, vertical.*

Vertometer   Trade name for a type of lensmeter.

virtual image   See *image, virtual.*

W

W bridge   See *bridge, metal saddle.*

washer, lens   Also called *lens liner,* a plastic material that is inserted between a loose lens and the eyewire.

wave   A defect in lens surface curvature causing a localized irregular variation in lens power.

wave front   See *front, wave.*

wheel differential   See *differential, wheel.*

wheel, electrometallic   Synonym for electroplated wheel.

wheel, electroplated   An abrasive wheel made by electrolytically depositing metal on the wheel in such a manner as to encompass diamond particles. This type of wheel is often used to grind plastic lenses

wheel, finishing   The wheel used in edging to bring the lens edge to its final configuration.

wheel, hogging   Synonym for roughing wheel.

wheel, impregnated   Synonym for a metal-bonded wheel.

wheel, metal-bonded   Abrasive wheels made by mixing diamond material with powdered metal that is heated in a mold until fusion of the metal occurs.

wheel, roughing   An edger wheel that rapidly cuts a lens to near its finished size.

width, seg   The size of a bi- or trifocal segment measured horizontally across its widest section.

Wils-Edge mounting   See *mounting, Wils-Edge.*

X

X-Chrom lens   See *lens, X-Chrom.*

X-ing   A vertical misalignment evidenced by a twisting of the frame front such that the planes of the lenses are out of coincidence with each other.

Y

yoked prism   See *prism, yoked.*

Younger blended myodisc   See *lens, blended myodisc.*

Younger seamless   See *lens, Younger seamless.*

Z

Z80.1   The identification number for the American National Standard for Ophthalmics–Prescription Ophthalmic Lenses–Recommendations.

Z87   The identification number for the American National Standard Practice for Occupational and Educational Eye and Face Protection, denoting safety lenses and frames.

zero inset method   See *method, zero inset.*

zone, blended   The blurred area between distance and near areas on an "invisible" bifocal. (Not to be confused with the progressive zone of a progressive-add lens.)

zone, progressive   That portion of a progressive-addition lens between the distance and near portions where lens power is gradually increasing.

zyl file   See *file, zyl.*

zyl   An abbreviation for the frame material zylonite. Often used to refer to plastic frames in general.

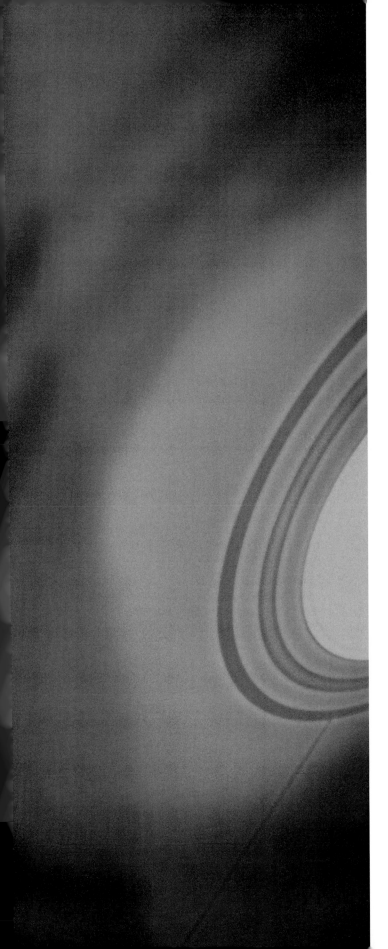

Centration Skills Series

This series of exercises is designed to develop proficiency in the layout of ophthalmic prescription lenses. The exercises may be carried out on real lenses and an actual centration device. However, these may not be readily available with home study.

In this case use the Centration Skills Figures CSS-1 and CSS-2 on p. 438 to make a mock centration device. To do this, photocopy Figure CSS-1 onto regular paper. This is a simulation of the background grid in a centration device. Photocopy Figure CSS-2 onto a sheet of clear transparency material. This is the same material as is used when making transparencies for an overhead projector.

If finished uncut lenses are available, use these lenses to do the exercises. If not, photocopy the lenses shown in Figure CSS-3 on pp. 439–440 onto transparency material and cut them out to serve as mock lenses.

Mock bifocal or trifocal lenses can be used for either the left or right eye by simply turning the "lens" over.

Each series of problems builds upon the previous set. When an instructor is available to check the accuracy of each student's work, the exercises may be used in a more formalized learning situation. Otherwise, students may check their own work by referring to the Centration Skills Series Answer Key immediately following these series of exercises.

A nonpermanent, water-soluble felt-tip marker such as is used for overhead projectors should be used to mark the real or mock lenses. Marks can be washed away or wiped off with a damp cloth and the lenses remarked.

The student should note that problems may contain more information than is needed to solve the problem.

This is done intentionally to reflect everyday practice situations, just as all prescription information is not needed to carry out certain specific tasks.

All figures associated with the Centration Skills Series have been placed at the end of the text, after the answer key for the last series of exercises. The student is encouraged to photocopy them for use during skills exercises. The legends for all of the figures associated with the Centration Skills Series appear on p. 444.

SERIES 1

Single Vision Lenses

Choose the single vision lens from the kit and place three dots on the lens, as would be applied ordinarily with a lensmeter. The center dot should appear at the center of the lens, and the other two dots should be approximately 15 mm to either side of the center dot.

1. (a) Place an *R* above the three dots on the back surface of your single vision lens to make it a right lens. With the lens front side up, decenter it 3 mm inward. Because *inward* is toward the nose, you must visualize whether the nose will be to the right or to the left of the lens (Figure CSS-4, p. 441). Which way did you move the lens to decenter it?

Reference: Pages 78, Figure 4-2, and 79, Box 4-1.

   (b) Now mark the lens with a cross to indicate the correct position for blocking (Figure CSS-5, p. 441). (This cross indicates what will become the geometrical or boxing center of the lens once it has been edged.) Is the cross you drew to the right or to the left of the center lensmeter spot?

Reference: Page 80.

2. Calculate the decentration required; place an *L* on the lens, and hand mark this left lens with a cross for blocking. Place the lens convex (front) side up.

   Frame A = 50
   DBL = 18
   Wearer's PD = 64 mm

   How much decentration per lens did you calculate? Was your marked cross to the right or to the left of your center lensmeter spot?

Reference: Pages 76 and 82.

3. Mark the lens with an *R*, calculate the decentration required, and hand mark the lens for blocking when the wearer has a PD of 67, the frame *A* dimension = 53, and the DBL = 17.

For each of the following, calculate decentration, place the lenses convex side up and mark the lenses to indicate the location of the center of the block. With the lens still convex side up, is the marked cross to the right or left of your center lensmeter spot?

4. Right lens

   A = 52 mm
   DBL = 16 mm
   Wearer's PD = 65 mm

5. Left lens

   A = 49 mm
   DBL = 17 mm
   Wearer's PD = 62 mm

6. Left lens

   A = 48 mm
   DBL = 20 mm
   Wearer's PD = 68 mm

7. Right lens

   A = 53 mm
   DBL = 19 mm
   Wearer's PD = 63 mm

8. Left lens

   A = 57 mm
   DBL = 18 mm
   Wearer's PD = 69 mm

9. Left lens

   A = 53 mm
   DBL = 17 mm
   Wearer's PD = 63 mm

10. Right lens

   A = 54 mm
   DBL = 16 mm
   Wearer's PD = 72 mm

SERIES 2

Single Vision Lenses

CENTRATION FOR MONOCULAR PDS AND PRACTITIONER-SPECIFIED MAJOR REFERENCE POINT HEIGHT

Reference: Page 96.

When interpupillary distances (PDs) are given monocularly, they must be calculated separately for right and left lenses. For each of the exercises in this section, perform the following steps:

- Dot the single vision lens with the three parallel lensmeter dots using your water-soluble overhead transparency pen.
- Calculate the correct decentration.
- Lay out the lens for the calculated decentration.
- Mark the lens with a cross to show where the center of the block will be.

1. A = 48 mm
   B = 45 mm
   DBL = 15 mm
   Monocular PDs: R = 26.5 mm; L = 28.5 mm
2. A = 56 mm
   B = 49 mm
   DBL = 18 mm
   Monocular PDs: R = 30 mm; L = 29 mm
3. A = 57 mm
   B = 49 mm
   DBL = 16 mm
   Monocular PDs: R = 29.5 mm; L = 31.5 mm
4. A = 54 mm
   B = 48 mm
   DBL = 17 mm
   Monocular PDs: R = 32 mm; L = 34 mm
5. A = 55 mm
   B = 47 mm
   DBL = 16 mm
   Monocular PDs: R = 31.5 mm; L = 32.5 mm
6. A = 60 mm
   B = 47 mm
   DBL = 14 mm
   Monocular PDs: R = 34 mm; L = 31 mm
7. A = 54 mm
   B = 51.5 mm
   DBL = 14 mm
   Monocular PDs: R = 31.5 mm; L = 28.5 mm

Reference: Pages 78 through 81.

In most cases, the major reference point (MRP) of a lens is placed along the horizontal midline so that the MRP falls halfway between the highest and lowest points on the edged lens. This corresponds to the horizontal reference line in the centration device. If the MRP is specified vertically, it is given in terms of its vertical distance from the lowest portion of the inside groove of the lower eyewire. For layout, the vertical decentration above or below the horizontal midline must be known. This is calculated as follows:

$$\text{Vertical decentration} = \text{MRP height} - \frac{B}{2}$$

For each of the exercises in this section, perform the following steps:

- Dot the single vision lens with the three parallel lensmeter dots.
- Calculate the correct horizontal decentration per lens.
- Calculate the correct vertical decentration per lens.
- Lay out the lens for the calculated horizontal and vertical decentration.
- Mark the lens with a cross to show the location of the lens block using your water-soluble transparency marker.

8. A = 54 mm
   B = 50 mm
   DBL = 14 mm
   PD = 61 mm
   MRP height = 27 mm
9. A = 56 mm
   B = 54 mm
   DBL = 17 mm
   PD = 64 mm
   MRP height = 30 mm
10. A = 54 mm
    B = 50 mm
    DBL = 14 mm
    PD = 57 mm
    MRP height = 26 mm

For the following exercises, calculate the horizontal decentration per lens for the monocularly specified PDs and also vertical decentration. Mark the lens with a cross to show the location of the lens block using a water-soluble transparency marker.

11. A = 50 mm
    B = 45 mm
    DBL = 22 mm
    Monocular PDs: R = 32 mm; L = 33 mm
    MRP height = 26 mm
12. A = 54 mm
    B = 51.5 mm
    DBL = 15 mm
    Monocular PDs: R = 27.5 mm; L = 30.5 mm
    MRP height = 27 mm
13. A = 50 mm
    B = 41.5 mm
    DBL = 17 mm
    Monocular PDs: R = 30.5 mm; L = 27.5 mm
    MRP height = 22 mm

SERIES 3

Single Vision Lenses

LENSES WITH PRESCRIBED PRISM

Reference: Pages 20 through 23.

Lenses with prescribed prism are decentered for prism during the spotting process using the lensmeter. This places the three dots off the optical center of the single vision lens. Yet once the lenses have been spotted, the centration process is identical to the centration process for single vision lenses without prism.

HORIZONTAL PRISM

For the following exercises, place the three lensmeter dots 5 mm to the *right of center, as viewed from the front.* Calculate the correct horizontal decentration and mark the lenses with a cross to show where the center of the block will be located. In addition, tell what the prism base direction would be, assuming the lenses are spheres.

Example

A right lens of minus power, spotted as described, will result in prism base
_____ .

A = 46 mm
DBL = 20 mm
PD = 60 mm

The lens will look like Figure CSS-6, *A,* (on p. 442) when spotted 5 mm to the right of center and viewed from the front. The prism base direction may be thought through by looking at a cross-section of the lens as shown in Figure CSS-6, *B* (on p. 442). As seen in Figure CSS-6, *B,* the prism base direction is base in.

Horizontal (distance) decentration is as follows:

$$\text{Decentration per lens} = \frac{A + DBL - PD}{2}$$
$$= \frac{46 + 20 - 60}{2}$$
$$= \frac{6}{2}$$
$$= 3 \text{ mm}$$

In lens layout, the MRP is moved 3 mm to the right. So the center lensmeter dot (where the MRP is) is 3 mm to the right of the marked cross, as in Figure CSS-6, *C* (on p. 442).

1. A right lens of minus power spotted as described will result in prism base _____ .

   A = 53 mm
   DBL = 14 mm
   PD = 60 mm

2. A right lens of plus power spotted as described will result in prism base _____ .

   A = 45 mm
   DBL = 17 mm
   PD = 41 mm

3. A left lens of minus power spotted as described will result in prism base _____ .

   A = 45 mm
   DBL = 21 mm
   PD = 63 mm

4. A left lens of plus power spotted as described will result in prism base _____ .

   A = 55 mm
   DBL = 14 mm
   PD = 61 mm

VERTICAL PRISM

For the following exercises, place the three lensmeter dots 5 mm above the center of the lens. This will result in vertical prism. Calculate the correct horizontal decentration and mark the lenses with a cross to show where the center of the block will be located. In addition, tell what the prism base direction will be, assuming the lenses are spheres.

5. A right lens of minus power spotted as described will result in prism base _____ .

   A = 56 mm
   DBL = 18 mm
   PD = 66 mm

6. A left lens of minus power spotted as described will result in prism base _____ .

   A = 44 mm
   DBL = 15 mm
   PD = 55 mm

7. A left lens of plus power spotted as described will result in prism base _____ .

   A = 52 mm
   DBL = 18 mm
   PD = 64 mm

8. A right lens of plus power spotted as described will result in prism base _____ .

   A = 55 mm
   DBL = 14 mm
   PD = 58 mm

HORIZONTAL AND VERTICAL PRISM

For the following exercises, place three lensmeter dots 5 mm to the left and 5 mm below the geometrical center of the single vision lens, as viewed from the front of the lens. Calculate the correct horizontal decentration and mark the lenses with a cross to show where the center of the block will be located. In addition, tell what the prism base direction will be, assuming the lenses are spheres.

9. A right lens of minus power spotted as described will result in prism base _____ and _____ .

A = 53 mm
DBL = 14 mm
PD = 60 mm

10. A right lens of plus power spotted as described will result in prism base
_____ and _____ .

A = 53 mm
DBL = 14 mm
PD = 62 mm

11. A left lens of minus power spotted as described will result in prism base
_____ and _____ .

A = 51 mm
DBL = 16 mm
PD = 64 mm

12. A left lens of plus power spotted as described will result in prism base
_____ and _____ .

A = 52 mm
DBL = 18 mm
PD = 60 mm

UNDERSTANDING PRISM

For each of the following exercises, look at the lens power, then decide the approximate position the three lensmeter dots would have after being spotted in a lensmeter. Place the dots in this location using your water-soluble overhead transparency marking pen. Calculate the correct horizontal decentration and mark the lenses with a cross to show where the center of the block will be located.

13. R: + 5.00 D   1Δ base-up prism

A = 54 mm
DBL = 18 mm
PD = 64 mm

14. R: -5.00 D   1Δ base-up prism

A = 56 mm
DBL = 18 mm
PD = 58 mm

15. R: + 5.00 D   2Δ base-out prism

A = 50 mm
DBL = 17 mm
PD = 55 mm

16. R: - 5.00 D   2Δ base-out prism

A = 56 mm
DBL = 16 mm
PD = 60 mm

17. R: - 5.00 D   2Δ base-in prism

A = 51 mm
DBL = 17 mm
PD = 61 mm

SERIES 4

Progressive Addition Lenses: Using the Fitting Cross

Reference: Pages 99 through 102.

Although progressive addition lenses have a near portion that is invisible to the casual observer, they should not be confused with invisible bifocals.

Invisible or *blended bifocals* are round-style segment lenses with the demarcation line smoothed over to be indistinct.

Progressive addition lenses differ from blended bifocals in that they increase in power gradually, beginning at the major reference point of the lens and gaining power the farther downward into the near area the wearer looks.

LAYOUT USING THE FITTING CROSS

Lay out the following progressive add lenses for edging using the fitting cross system. Carry out the proper layout procedures and mark the lens with a cross to show the location of the block.

1. A = 53 mm
   B = 50 mm
   DBL = 16 mm
   Monocular PDs: R = 30 mm; L = 29 mm
   Fitting cross heights: R = 27 mm; L = 27 mm
2. A = 48 mm
   B = 41 mm
   DBL = 20 mm
   Monocular PDs: R = 31 mm; L = 32 mm
   Fitting cross heights: R = 23 mm; L = 24 mm
3. A = 52 mm
   B = 49 mm
   DBL = 16 mm
   Monocular PDs: R = 32 mm; L: = 32 mm
   Fitting cross heights: R = 28 mm; L = 28 mm
4. A = 50 mm
   B = 48 mm
   DBL = 14 mm
   Monocular PDs: R = 31 mm; L: = 29 mm
   Fitting cross heights: R = 25 mm; L = 26 mm
5. A = 53 mm
   B = 49 mm
   DBL = 14 mm
   Monocular PDs: R = 32 mm; L: = 31 mm
   Fitting cross heights: R = 29 mm; L = 29 mm
6. A = 54 mm
   B = 49 mm
   DBL = 17 mm
   Monocular PDs: R = 31 mm; L: = 31 mm
   Fitting cross heights: R = 28 mm; L = 29 mm
7. A = 56 mm
   B = 44 mm

DBL = 18 mm
Monocular PDs: R = 32.5 mm; L = 33.5 mm
Fitting cross heights: R = 25 mm; L = 26 mm

8. A = 51 mm
B = 42 mm
DBL = 17 mm
Monocular PDs: R = 29 mm; L = 31 mm
Fitting cross heights: R = 25 mm; L = 26mm

9. A = 50 mm
B = 45 m
DBL = 15 mm
Monocular PDs: R = 28 mm; L = 29 mm
Fitting cross heights: R = 24 mm; L = 24 mm

SERIES 5

Progressive Addition Lenses: Using Hidden 'Circles'

Reference: Pages 102 through 105.

Laying out progressive lenses is possible using the hidden marks on a progressive lens instead of the fitting cross. Hidden circles are permanent marks on the lens and are not subject to error. Fitting crosses are removable marks placed on the lens using the hidden "circles" as reference.

For the exercises in this section, use the hidden circles to lay out the lens instead of the fitting cross and perform the following steps:

- Determine monocular distance decentration.
- Calculate hidden circle raise (or drop) based on the fitting cross height. (For these exercises, assume that the fitting cross is 4 mm above the level of the PRP and hidden "circles.")
- Lay the lens out for edging.
- Mark the lens with a cross to indicate the location of the block.

  1. A = 48 mm
     B = 38 mm
     DBL = 20 mm
     Monocular PDs: R = 32 mm; L = 32 mm
     Fitting cross heights: R = 24 mm; L = 24 mm
  2. A = 44 mm
     B = 32 mm
     DBL = 20 mm
     Monocular PDs: R = 30.5 mm; L = 31.0 mm
     Fitting cross heights: R = 19 mm; L = 19 mm
  3. A = 49 mm
     B = 34 mm
     DBL = 21 mm
     Monocular PDs: R = 31.5 mm; L = 30.5 mm
     Fitting cross heights: R = 20 mm; L = 21 mm
  4. A = 47 mm
     B = 36 mm
     DBL = 19 mm
     Monocular PDs: R = 32.0 mm; L = 31.5 mm
     Fitting cross heights: R = 24 mm; L = 23 mm
  5. A = 40 mm
     B = 30 mm
     DBL = 24 mm
     Monocular PDs: R = 30.0 mm; L = 31.0 mm
     Fitting cross heights: R = 19.5 mm; L = 20.0 mm
  6. A = 50 mm
     B = 38 mm
     DBL = 18 mm
     Monocular PDs: R = 33.0 mm; L = 32.5 mm
     Fitting cross heights: R = 23.5 mm; L = 25.0 mm
  7. A = 49 mm
     B = 39 mm
     DBL = 20 mm
     Monocular PDs: R = 34.0 mm; L = 32.5 mm
     Fitting cross heights: R = 26 mm; L = 27 mm

8. A = 47 mm
   B = 38 mm
   DBL = 19 mm
   Monocular PDs: R = 31.5 mm; L = 32.5 mm
   Fitting cross heights: R = 23.5 mm; L = 24.5 mm
9. A = 44 mm
   B = 37 mm
   DBL = 20 mm
   Monocular PDs: R = 32.5 mm; L = 31.0 mm
   Fitting cross heights: R = 21.5 mm; L = 22.0 mm
10. A = 46 mm
    B = 39 mm
    DBL = 19 mm
    Monocular PDs: R = 31.0 mm; L = 30.0 mm
    Fitting cross heights: R = 26.5 mm; L = 25.5 mm

SERIES 6

Flat-Top Bifocals

TOTAL INSET AND DROP CONSIDERED INDEPENDENTLY

Reference: Pages 112 through 114.

For the following problems, lay out a flat-top bifocal lens for the correct bifocal height. (For these exercises, do not be concerned about total inset.) Be concerned only with the vertical position of the segment line.

1. Frame B = 42 mm
   Segment height = 18 mm
2. Frame B = 42 mm
   Segment height = 21 mm
3. Frame A = 48 mm
   B = 38 mm
   Segment height = 17 mm
4. Frame A = 50 mm
   B = 43
   Segment drop = −4 mm
   (What is the segment height?)
5. Frame A = 52 mm
   B = 42 mm
   DBL = 18 mm
   Segment raise = +1 mm
   (What is the segment height?)
6. Frame A = 54 mm
   B = 41 mm
   DBL = 17 mm
   Segment height = 17 mm

For the following prescriptions, assume that the segment top moves −3 mm vertically for the segment drop. Position the lens for marking such that both the drop and the total inset are correct. (The lens does not need to be "spotted" ahead of time for this exercise.) The lens should be positioned front side up. Mark the lens with your water-soluble marker for blocking.

7. Right lens

   A = 48 mm
   DBL = 20 mm
   Near PD = 60 mm

8. Right lens

   A = 51 mm
   DBL = 17 mm
   Near PD = 60 mm

9. Left lens

   A = 50 mm
   DBL = 18 mm
   Near PD = 58 mm

10. Right lens

   A = 55 mm
   DBL = 18 mm
   Wearer's PD = 66/62

11. Left lens
   Lens power is +1.00 −0.75 × 180

   A = 53 mm
   DBL = 17 mm
   Wearer's PD = 64/60

12. Right lens

   A = 52 mm
   DBL = 17 mm
   ED = 57 mm
   Wearer's PD = 62/59

SERIES 7

Flat-Top Bifocals

TOTAL INSET AND DROP CONSIDERED SIMULTANEOUSLY

Reference: Pages 117 and 118.

For each of the following exercises, position the flat-top bifocal lens on the centration device for the amount of total inset and segment drop given. Assume the lens to be front side up and mark the lens for edging using your water-soluble overhead transparency marking pen.

1. Total inset = 4 mm
   Segment drop = –4 mm
2. Total inset = 5.5 mm
   Segment drop = –3 mm
3. Total inset = 7 mm
   Segment drop = –2 mm
4. Total inset = 2.5 mm
   Segment drop = –5 mm
5. Total inset = 4.5 mm
   Segment raise = +1 mm
6. Total inset = 3 mm
   Segment drop = –3.5 mm
7. Total inset = 5 mm
   Segment drop = –6 mm

For each of the following problems, lay out a flat-top bifocal lens for both the correct bifocal height and total inset. The lens should be positioned front side up for this exercise and does not need to be "spotted" ahead of time. Mark the lens with a cross with your water-soluble marking pen to indicate where the center of the block will be.

8. Right lens

   A = 53 mm
   B = 44 mm
   DBL = 18 mm
   Wearer's PD = 65/61
   Segment height = 18 mm

9. Right lens

   A = 49 mm
   B = 38 mm
   DBL = 18 mm
   Wearer's PD = 65/62
   Segment height = 18 mm

10. Left lens

   A = 51 mm
   B = 42 mm
   DBL = 17 mm
   Wearer's PD = 61/58
   Segment height = 19 mm

11. Left lens

     A = 54 mm
     B = 44 mm
     DBL = 16 mm
     Wearer's PD = 63/59
     Segment height = 18 mm

12. Right lens
    Lens power is $+8.00 -1.00 \times 17$

     A = 50 mm
     B = 41 mm
     DBL = 20 mm
     Wearer's PD = 66/61
     Segment height = 20 mm

13. Left lens
    Lens power is $-7.75 -0.50 \times 95$

     A = 48 mm
     B = 43 mm
     DBL = 19 mm
     Wearer's PD = 64/61
     Segment height = 17 mm

14. Right lens
    Lens power is $+1.00 -3.00 \times 18$

     A = 52 mm
     B = 42 mm
     DBL = 19 mm
     Wearer's PD = 61/57
     Segment height = 23 mm

SERIES 8

Curve-Top Bifocals

Reference: Pages 125 and 126.

Curve-top segments are positioned in a manner similar to that of flat-top bifocals. The highest part of the curve is placed at the millimeter line coinciding with the required drop. The outer segment corners must be on, or equidistant from, the same horizontal line to ensure straightness upon completion.

   Carry out the centration process with curve-top lenses, marking the lens with the front-side-up. (Do not forget to mark whether the lens is the right or left.)

1. Right lens

   A = 48 mm
   B = 45 mm
   DBL = 14 mm
   PD = 53/50
   Segment height = 18 mm

2. Right lens

   A = 52 mm
   B = 45 mm
   DBL = 22 mm
   PD = 64/62
   Segment height = 20 mm

3. Left lens

   A = 58 mm
   B = 47 mm
   DBL = 17 mm
   PD = 68/64
   Segment height = 18 mm

4. Right lens

   A = 54 mm
   B = 44 mm
   DBL = 16 mm
   PD = 67/63
   Segment height = 22 mm

5. Left lens

   A = 57 mm
   B = 53 mm
   DBL = 16 mm
   PD = 65/62
   Segment height = 23 mm

6. Left lens

   A = 54 mm
   B = 47 mm
   DBL = 16 mm
   PD = 61/58
   Segment height = 22 mm

7. Right lens

   A = 55 mm
   B = 48 mm
   DBL = 16 mm
   PD = 67/63
   Segment height = 25 mm

8. Left lens

   A = 46 mm
   B = 39 mm
   DBL = 22 mm
   PD = 64/61
   Segment height = 18 mm

9. Left lens

   A = 52 mm
   B = 47 mm
   DBL = 19 mm
   PD = 65/61
   Segment height = 19 mm

10. Right lens

    A = 52 mm
    B = 44 mm
    DBL = 19 mm
    PD = 62/59
    Segment height = 19 mm

11. Left lens

    A = 58 mm
    B = 48 mm
    DBL = 20 mm
    PD = 67/65
    Segment height = 22 mm

12. Right lens

    A = 46 mm
    B = 39 mm
    DBL = 20 mm
    PD = 65/62
    Segment height = 18 mm

SERIES 9

Trifocal Lenses

Reference: Page 125.

Trifocal lenses are centered in exactly the same manner as their corresponding bifocal styles. Always remember that the upper of the two segment lines is used for a segment height reference point.

Using a flat-top trifocal positioned front side up, lay out and mark the lens for each of the following.

1. Left lens

    A = 46 mm
    B = 37 mm
    DBL = 22 mm
    PD = 67/65
    Segment height = 20 mm

2. Right lens

    A = 50 mm
    B = 42 mm
    DBL = 19 mm
    PD = 52/49
    Segment height = 20 mm

3. Right lens

    A = 52 mm
    B = 42 mm
    DBL = 20 mm
    PD = 60/57
    Segment height = 17 mm

4. Right lens

    A = 54 mm
    B = 51.5 mm
    DBL = 16 mm
    PD = 67/64
    Segment height = 21 mm

5. Right lens

    A = 54 mm
    B = 46 mm
    DBL = 17 mm
    PD = 67/64
    Segment height = 24 mm

6. Left lens

    A = 54 mm
    B = 46 mm
    DBL = 24 mm
    PD = 69/66
    Segment height = 20 mm

7. Right lens

   A = 56 mm
   B = 52 mm
   DBL = 16 mm
   PD = 65/63
   Segment height = 22 mm

8. Right lens

   A = 48 mm
   B = 41 mm
   DBL = 19 mm
   PD = 58/56
   Segment height = 24 mm

9. Left lens

   A = 58 mm
   B = 50 mm
   DBL = 19 mm
   PD = 64/61
   Segment height = 21 mm

10. Left lens

   A = 57 mm
   B = 53 mm
   DBL = 16 mm
   PD = 65/63
   Segment height = 25 mm

SERIES 10

Flat-Top Bifocals

RELATING MAJOR REFERENCE POINT AND SEGMENT POSITIONS

Reference: Pages 117 through 121.

For each of the following exercises, perform the following steps:

- Find the total inset.
- Find the segment drop or raise.
- Lay out the lens front side up for blocking.
- Dot the location of the MRP as it should appear on the lens.
- Mark the lens with a cross to show where the center of the block should be. When drawing the cross, skip over the MRP dot so as not to hide it from view.

Example
Right lens

> A = 48 mm
> B = 38 mm
> DBL = 20 mm
> PD = 62/59
> Segment height = 16 mm

The following exercises describe how the different parts of the problem are solved.

A. *Total inset*

$$= \frac{[A + DBL] - \text{Near PD}}{2}$$

$$= \frac{[48 + 20] - 59}{2}$$

$$= \frac{68 - 59}{2}$$

$$= \frac{9}{2}$$

$$= 4.5$$

B. *Segment drop or raise*

$$= \text{Segment height} - \frac{B}{2}$$

$$= 16 - \frac{38}{2}$$

$$= 16 - 19$$

$$= -3 \text{ mm drop}$$

C. *Layout for the lens is shown in Figure CSS-7 on p. 443.*

D. *Location of the MRP is at the distance decentration.*

$$= \frac{[A + DBL] - \text{Distance PD}}{2}$$

$$= \frac{[48 + 20] - 62}{2}$$

$$= \frac{68 - 62}{2}$$

$$= \frac{6}{2}$$

$$= 3 \text{ mm}$$

The center lensmeter dot (MRP) is 3 to the right of the background grid center. Its location also may be figured backward from the location of the segment, as segment inset:

$$\text{Segment inset} = \frac{\text{Distance PD} - \text{Near PD}}{2}$$

$$= \frac{62 - 59}{2}$$

$$= \frac{3}{2}$$

$$= 1.5 \text{ mm}$$

So the center lensmeter dot is 1.5 mm to the left of the segment center (Figure CSS-8, p. 443).

E. *When the lens is marked with a cross to indicate the location of the center of the block, it will appear as shown in Figure CSS-9 on p. 443.*

1. Right lens

   A = 52 mm
   B = 38 mm
   DBL = 22 mm
   Wearer's PD = 66/62
   Segment height = 18 mm

2. Left lens
   Lens power is −0.75 −0.25 × 65

   A = 56 mm
   B = 50 mm
   DBL = 19 mm
   Wearer's PD = 67/63
   Segment height = 22 mm

3. Right lens
   Lens power is +1.25 −0.50 × 110

   A = 48 mm
   B = 42 mm
   DBL = 24 mm
   Wearer's PD = 64/61
   Segment height = 21 mm

4. Right lens

   A = 52 mm
   B = 44 mm
   DBL = 19 mm
   Wearer's PD = 61/59
   Segment height = 18 mm

5. Left lens

   A = 53 mm
   B = 51 mm
   DBL = 15 mm
   Wearer's PD = 62/59
   Segment height = 20 mm

6. Right lens

   A = 51 mm
   B = 48 mm
   DBL = 14 mm
   Wearer's PD = 54/52
   Segment height = 20 mm

7. Right lens
   Lens power is plano with 2Δ base-out prism

   A = 50 mm
   B = 40 mm
   DBL = 24 mm
   Wearer's PD = 71/68
   Segment height = 19 mm

SERIES 11

Round Bifocal Segment Lenses

Reference: Pages 126 through 131.

With round-segment lenses, first spot the lens to determine MRP location and, when applicable, the correct axis orientation. These exercises simulate centration of spheres. Therefore only the center dot of the three lensmeter spots is critical.

For this exercise, take the 22-mm round-segment bifocal lens and turn it so the segment is at the bottom of the lens and exactly in the middle. Measure up from the top of the segment an amount equal to the segment drop and place a dot on the lens with your water-soluble overhead transparency marker pen.* Now lay out the lenses according to the specifications given.

You may want to do some of the exercises using the blended bifocal and Ultex A bifocal lens (38 mm round-segment).

For blended bifocals, total segment inset may be done using either the outer edges of the segment or the center of the segment for reference.

1. Left lens

   A = 55 mm
   B = 46 mm
   DBL = 15 mm
   PD = 64/61
   Segment height = 19 mm

2. Left lens

   A = 54 mm
   B = 50 mm
   DBL = 14 mm
   PD = 63/59
   Segment height = 24 mm

3. Right lens

   A = 52 mm
   B = 44 mm
   DBL = 18 mm
   PD = 66/63
   Segment height = 22 mm

4. Left lens

   A = 51 mm
   B = 49 mm
   DBL = 16 mm
   PD = 59/56
   Segment height = 18 mm

---

*This technique will allow you to determine a correct drop and MRP location after the lens is turned during layout only because the differences between near and far PDs are small. Otherwise, the drop would decrease. In practice, this is taken into account during surfacing.

5. Right lens

   A = 50 mm
   B = 43 mm
   DBL = 16 mm
   PD = 58/54
   Segment height = 21 mm

6. Right lens

   A = 51 mm
   B = 42 mm
   DBL = 17 mm
   PD = 63/60
   Segment height = 18 mm

7. Left lens

   A = 50 mm
   B = 43 mm
   DBL = 19 mm
   PD = 63/60
   Segment height = 18 mm

8. Right lens

   A = 51 mm
   B = 47 mm
   DBL = 18 mm
   PD = 62/59
   Segment height = 19 mm

9. Right lens

   A = 52 mm
   B = 46 mm
   DBL = 18 mm
   PD = 60/56
   Segment height = 23 mm

10. Left lens

    A = 56 mm
    B = 54 mm
    DBL = 17 mm
    PD = 65/61
    Segment height = 22 mm

11. Left lens

    A = 52 mm
    B = 48 mm
    DBL = 16 mm
    PD = 62/58
    Segment height = 21 mm

12. Left lens

    A = 54 mm
    B = 51.5 mm
    DBL = 16 mm
    PD = 59/57
    Segment height = 19 mm

SERIES 12

Franklin-Style Bifocals

Reference: Page 131.

Franklin-style lenses* can be surfaced with a variety of methods. Two methods are as follows:

1. Drop, but no segment inset

   With this method the lens is surfaced such that the optical center will be above the segment line by an amount equal to the segment drop. The optical center is directly above the geometrical center of the segment. It is the same as if a flat-top bifocal were ground with equal distance and near PDs.

2. Adherence to both drop and segment inset amounts

   In this method the optical center is ground above the segment geometrical center by an amount equal to the drop *and* is outset by an amount equal to the segment inset.† When ground in this manner, the optics of the Franklin-style lens duplicate those of a large segment flat-top bifocal.

   Regardless of how Franklin-style lenses are surfaced, the layout for edging process is the same.

   For purposes of these exercises, place three lensmeter dots on the lens such that the center dot is exactly above the center of the segment line by an amount equal to the calculated drop. The other two dots must parallel the segment line. (In practice, the MRP may not be always in the center of the lens.)

   1. Right lens

      A = 56 mm
      B = 46 mm
      DBL = 20 mm
      PD = 69/66
      Segment height = 21 mm

   2. Right lens

      A = 48 mm
      B = 39 mm
      DBL = 14 mm
      PD = 49/47
      Segment height = 23 mm

   3. Left lens

      A = 52 mm
      B = 50 mm
      DBL = 16 mm
      PD = 60/57
      Segment height = 22 mm

---

*Franklin-style lenses are known more commonly as *Executive bifocals*. Executive is AO Sola's (Petaluma, Calif.) trade name for the Franklin-style lens.
†Some Franklin-style lenses are produced in semifinished form with the near optics already inset by a given amount. These semifinished lenses are marked for right and left eyes like flat-top lenses are.

4. Right lens
   A = 50 mm
   B = 43 mm
   DBL = 19 mm
   PD = 64/62
   Segment height = 15 mm

5. Left lens

   A = 52 mm
   B = 44 mm
   DBL = 19 mm
   PD = 64/60
   Segment height = 21 mm

6. Left lens

   A = 52 mm
   B = 49 mm
   DBL = 17 mm
   PD = 62/59
   Segment height = 19 mm

7. Left lens

   A = 57 mm
   B = 48 mm
   DBL = 19 mm
   PD = 67/64
   Segment height = 19 mm

8. Right lens

   A = 50 mm
   B = 40 mm
   ED = 55 mm
   DBL = 20 mm
   PD = 66/64
   Segment height = 15 mm

9. Left lens

   A = 56 mm
   B = 48 mm
   ED = 64 mm
   DBL = 14 mm
   PD = 70/67
   Segment height = 21 mm

10. Left lens

    A = 52 mm
    B = 47 mm
    ED = 59 mm
    DBL = 16 mm
    PD = 60/57
    Segment height = 16 mm

11. Right lens

A = 54 mm
B = 51 mm
ED = 63 mm
DBL = 14 mm
PD = 68/65
Segment height = 17 mm

SERIES 13

Centration Using Irregular Patterns

Reference: Pages 57 through 61.

Some "homemade" patterns have the central hole (mechanical center) slightly off center. Unless compensation is made in the centration process, the major reference point also will be displaced away from its intended location in the edged lens.

WHEN THE PATTERN CENTER IS OFF VERTICALLY

Unless otherwise indicated, for the following problems, assume that the MRP should be placed on the horizontal midline. For each of the following exercises, perform these steps:

- "Spot" the lens MRP.
- Calculate distance decentration.
- Calculate vertical compensation (how far the MRP must be dropped or raised to have it come out right for the nonstandard pattern).
- Lay out the lens for the calculated horizontal decentration and vertical compensation.
- Mark the lens with a cross to indicate where the center of the block will be.

  1. The central pattern hole is 3 mm above the pattern boxing center.
     Right lens

     A = 56 mm
     B = 47 mm
     ED = 64 mm
     DBL = 16 mm
     PD = 62 mm

  2. The central pattern hole is 1 mm above the pattern boxing center.
     Left lens

     A = 48 mm
     B = 42 mm
     ED = 50 mm
     DBL = 20 mm
     PD = 64 mm

  3. The central pattern hole is 0.5 mm above the pattern boxing center.
     Left lens

     A = 55 mm
     B = 46.5 mm
     ED = 63.5 mm
     DBL = 16 mm
     PD = 62 mm

  4. The central pattern hole is 1 mm above the pattern boxing center.
     Right lens

     A = 53 mm
     B = 45 mm
     ED = 62 mm
     DBL = 14 mm
     PD = 60 mm (Requested MRP height is 25 mm.)

5. The central pattern hole is 0.5 mm above the pattern boxing center.
   Right lens

   A = 58 mm
   B = 47 mm
   ED = 61 mm
   DBL = 20 mm
   PD = 62 mm (Requested MRP height is 26 mm.)

WHEN THE PATTERN IS OFF HORIZONTALLY

When patterns are made in the finishing laboratory, they should be checked upon completion to ensure that the hole is exactly in the center. If it is not, it can nevertheless be used if compensation is made. For each of the prescriptions listed below, mark the lens for blocking. For each of the following exercises, perform these steps:

- Spot the lens with the three parallel lensmeter dots.
- Determine how much inset or outset is required to simply compensate for the pattern error.
- Calculate normal inset per lens (or total inset, in the case of bifocals) as is normally done.
- Compensate the normal inset from step 3 by the amount of compensation you found in step 2.
- Mark the lens with a cross to indicate where the center of the block will be.

6. The central pattern hole is displaced 1 mm nasally.
   Left lens

   A = 44 mm
   B = 23 mm
   ED = 42 mm
   DBL = 22 mm
   PD = 60 mm

7. The central pattern hole is displaced 0.5 mm nasally.
   Right lens

   A = 50 mm
   B = 40 mm
   ED = 55.5 mm
   DBL = 20 mm
   PD = 73 mm

8. The central pattern hole is displaced 0.5 mm nasally.
   Right lens

   A = 54 mm
   B = 48 mm
   ED = 60 mm
   DBL = 14 mm
   PD = 61/58 mm
   Segment height = 20 mm

WHEN THE PATTERN IS OFF BOTH HORIZONTALLY AND VERTICALLY

9. The central pattern hole is displaced 1 mm nasally and is 0.5 mm too low.
    Left lens

    A = 51 mm
    B = 49.4 mm
    ED = 65.4 mm
    DBL = 16 mm
    PD = 56 mm

10. The central pattern hole is displaced 0.5 mm temporally and is 1 mm too high.
    Left lens

    A = 52 mm
    B = 48 mm
    ED = 54 mm
    DBL = 20 mm
    PD = 58/55
    Segment height = 18 mm

11. The central pattern hole is displaced 1.0 mm nasally and is 0.5 mm too low.
    Right lens

    A = 52 mm
    B = 42 mm
    ED = 57.5 mm
    DBL = 18 mm
    PD = 63/59
    Segment height = 18 mm

KEY SERIES 1

Single Vision Lenses

1. (a) To the right.
   (b) Viewed from the front, the cross should be 3 mm to the left of the center spot.
2. 2 mm in. Viewed from the front, the marked cross should be 2 mm to the right of the center dot.
3. The decentration per lens is 1.5 mm. When viewed from the front, the center dot is to the right of the marked cross.
4. 1.5 mm in
   To the left
5. 2.0 mm in
   To the right
6. 0 mm
   They are at the same location.
7. 4.5 mm in
   To the left
8. 3 mm in
   To the right
9. 3.5 mm in
   To the right
10. 1 mm out
    To the right

KEY SERIES 2

Single Vision Lenses

CENTRATION FOR MONOCULAR PDS AND PRACTITIONER-SPECIFIED MAJOR REFERENCE POINT HEIGHT

Answer Format

- R lens horizontal decentration = **a**
  (When viewed from the front of the lens, the center lensmeter dot is **a** mm to the right of the marked cross.)
- L lens horizontal decentration = **b**
  (When viewed from the front of the lens, the center lensmeter dot is **b** mm to the left of the marked cross.)

1. a = 5 mm
   b = 3 mm
2. a = 7 mm
   b = 8 mm
3. a = 7 mm
   b = 5 mm
4. a = 3.5 mm
   b = 1.5 mm
5. a = 4 mm
   b = 3 mm
6. a = 3 mm
   b = 6 mm
7. a = 2.5 mm
   b = 5.5 mm

Answer Format

- R lens horizontal decentration = **a**
  R vertical decentration = **b**
  (When viewed from the front, the center lensmeter dot is **a** mm to the right of and **b** mm above the marked cross.)
- L lens horizontal decentration = **c**
  L vertical decentration = **d**
  (When viewed from the front, the center lensmeter dot is **c** mm to the left of and **d** mm above the marked cross.)

8. a = 3.5 mm
   b = +2 mm raise
   c = 3.5 mm
   d = +2 mm raise
9. a = 4.5 mm
   b = +3 mm raise
   c = 4.5 mm
   d = +3 mm raise
10. a = 5.5 mm
    b = +1 mm raise
    c = 5.5 mm
    d = +1 mm raise

11. a = 4 mm
    b = +3.5 mm raise
    c = 3 mm
    d = +3.5 mm raise
12. a = 7 mm
    b = +1.25 mm raise
    c = 4 mm
    d = +1.25 mm raise
13. a = +3 mm
    b = 1.25 mm raise
    c = +6 mm
    d = 1.25 mm raise

KEY SERIES 3

Single Vision Lenses

LENSES WITH PRESCRIBED PRISM

Answer Format

- Prism base direction is base = **a**.
- Horizontal decentration = **b**.
  (When viewed from the front of the lens, the center lensmeter dot is **b** mm to the **c** of the marked cross.)

1. a = in
   b = 3.5 mm
   c = right
2. a = out
   b = 10.5 mm
   c = right
3. a = out
   b = 1.5 mm
   c = left
4. a = in
   b = 4 mm
   c = left
5. a = up
   b = 4 mm
   c = right
6. a = up
   b = 2 mm
   c = left
7. a = down
   b = 3 mm
   c = left
8. a = down
   b = 5.5 mm
   c = right

Answer Format

- Prism base direction is base = **a**.
- Horizontal decentration = **b**.
  (When viewed from the front of the lens, the center lensmeter dot is **b** mm to the **c** of the marked cross.)

9. a = out and down
   b = 3.5 mm
   c = right
10. a = in and up
    b = 2.5 mm
    c = right
11. a = in and down
    b = 1.5 mm
    c = left
12. a = out and up
    b = 5 mm
    c = left

Answer Format

When viewed from the front, the middle lensmeter dot is approximately **a** mm (above, below, to the right of, or to the left of) **b** the geometrical center of the lens blank. This same lensmeter dot should also be **c** mm to the **d** of the marked cross, since horizontal decentration = **c** mm.

13. a = 2 mm
    b = below
    c = 4 mm
    d = right
14. a = 2 mm
    b = above
    c = 8 mm
    d = right
15. a = 4 mm
    b = to the right of
    c = 6 mm
    d = right
16. a = 4 mm
    b = to the left of
    c = 6 mm
    d = right
17. a = 4 mm
    b = to the right of
    c = 3.5
    d = right

KEY SERIES 4

Progressive Addition Lenses: Using the Fitting Cross

1. Horizontal decentration

   R = 4.5 mm
   L = 5.5 mm

   Fitting cross raise:

   R = +2 mm
   L = +2 mm

2. Horizontal decentration

   R = 3 mm
   L = 2 mm

   Fitting cross raise:

   R = +2.5 mm
   L = +3.5 mm

3. Horizontal decentration

   R = 2 mm
   L = 2 mm

   Fitting cross raise:

   R = +3.5 mm
   L = +3.5 mm

4. Horizontal decentration

   R = 1 mm
   L = 3 mm

   Fitting cross raise:

   R = +1 mm
   L = +2 mm

5. Horizontal decentration

   R = 1.5 mm
   L = 2.5 mm

   Fitting cross raise:

   R = +4.5 mm
   L = +4.5 mm

6. Horizontal decentration

   R = 4.5 mm
   L = 4.5 mm

   Fitting cross raise:

   R = +3.5 mm
   L = +4.5 mm

7. Horizontal decentration

    R = 4.5 mm
    L = 3.5 mm

    Fitting cross raise:

    R = +3 mm
    L = +4 mm

8. Horizontal decentration

    R = 5 mm
    L = 3 mm

    Fitting cross raise:

    R = +4 mm
    L = +5 mm

9. Horizontal decentration

    R = 4.5 mm
    L = 3.5 mm

    Fitting cross raise:

    R = +1.5 mm
    L = +1.5 mm

KEY SERIES 5

Progressive Addition Lenses: Using Hidden 'Circles'

1. Horizontal decentration

   R = 2 mm
   L = 2 mm

   Hidden circle raise or drop:

   R = +1 mm
   L = +1 mm

2. Horizontal decentration

   R = 1.5 mm
   L = 1.0 mm

   Hidden circle raise or drop:

   R = −1 mm
   L = −1 mm

3. Horizontal decentration

   R = 3.5 mm
   L = 4.5 mm

   Hidden circle raise or drop:

   R = −1 mm
   L = 0 mm

4. Horizontal decentration

   R = 1.0 mm
   L = 1.5 mm

   Hidden circle raise or drop:

   R = +2 mm
   L = +1 mm

5. Horizontal decentration

   R = 2 mm
   L = 1 mm

   Hidden circle raise or drop:

   R = +0.5 mm
   L = +1.0 mm

6. Horizontal decentration

   R = 1.0 mm
   L = 1.5 mm

   Hidden circle raise or drop:

   R = +0.5 mm
   L = +2.0 mm

7. Horizontal decentration

   R = 0.5 mm
   L = 2.0 mm

   Hidden circle raise or drop:

   R = +2.5 mm
   L = +3.5 mm

8. Horizontal decentration

   R = 1.5 mm
   L = 0.5 mm

   Hidden circle raise or drop:

   R = +0.5 mm
   L = +1.5 mm

9. Horizontal decentration

   R = 0.5 mm out
   L = 1.0 mm in

   Hidden circle raise or drop:

   R = −1.0 mm
   L = −0.5 mm

10. Horizontal decentration

    R = 1.5 mm
    L = 2.5 mm

    Hidden circle raise or drop:

    R = +3.0 mm
    L = +2.0 mm

KEY SERIES 6

Flat-Top Bifocals

TOTAL INSET AND DROP CONSIDERED INDEPENDENTLY

1. The segment line is 3 mm below the horizontal reference line.
2. The segment is exactly on the line.
3. The segment line is 2 mm below the horizontal reference line.
4. The segment line is 4 mm below the horizontal reference line. (Segment height is 17.5 mm.)
5. The segment line is 1 mm above the horizontal reference line. (Segment height is 22 mm.)
6. The segment line is 3.5 mm below the horizontal reference line.
7. The center of the bifocal segment line is 4 mm to the right of and 3 mm below the center of the marked cross.
8. The center of the bifocal segment line is 4 mm to the right of and 3 mm below the center of the marked cross.
9. The center of the bifocal segment line is 5 mm to the left of and 3 mm below the center of the marked cross.
10. The center of the bifocal segment line is 5.5 mm to the right of and 3 mm below the center of the marked cross.
11. The center of the bifocal segment line is 5 mm to the left of and 3 mm below the center of the marked cross.
12. The center of the bifocal segment line is 5 mm to the right of, and 3 mm below the center of, the marked cross.

KEY SERIES 7

Flat-Top Bifocals

TOTAL INSET AND DROP CONSIDERED SIMULTANEOUSLY

For problems 1 through 7, if the lens is marked as a right lens, the mark should be left-of-segment-center by an amount equal to the total insert and above the seg top by an amount equal to the segment drop. If the lens is marked as a left lens, the mark should be right-of-segment-center by an amount equal to the total insert and above the seg top by an amount equal to the segment drop.

8. The center of the bifocal segment line is 5 mm to the right of and 4 mm below the center of the marked cross.
9. The center of the bifocal segment line is 2.5 mm to the right of and 1 mm below the center of the marked cross.
10. The center of the bifocal segment line is 5 mm to the left of and 2 mm below the center of the marked cross.
11. The center of the bifocal segment line is 5.5 mm to the left of and 4 mm below the center of the marked cross.
12. The center of the bifocal segment line is 4.5 mm to the right of and 0.5 mm below the center of the marked cross.
13. The center of the bifocal segment line is 3 mm to the left of and 4.5 mm below the center of the marked cross.
14. The center of the bifocal segment line is 7 mm to the right of and 2 mm above the center of the marked cross.

KEY SERIES 8

Curve-Top Bifocals

1. Distance decentration = 4.5 mm
   Total inset = 6 mm
   Segment drop = −4.5 mm
2. Distance decentration = 5 mm
   Total inset = 6 mm
   Segment drop = −2.5 mm
3. Distance decentration = 3.5 mm
   Total inset = 5.5 mm
   Segment drop = −5.5 mm
4. Distance decentration = 1.5 mm
   Total inset = 3.5 mm
   Segment drop = 0 mm
5. Distance decentration = 4 mm
   Total inset = 5.5 mm
   Segment drop = −3.5 mm
6. Distance decentration = 4.5 mm
   Total inset = 6 mm
   Segment drop = −1.5 mm
7. Distance decentration = 2 mm
   Total inset = 4 mm
   Segment raise = +1 mm
8. Distance decentration = 2 mm
   Total inset = 3.5 mm
   Segment drop = −1.5 mm
9. Distance decentration = 3 mm
   Total inset = 5 mm
   Segment drop = −4.5 mm
10. Distance decentration = 4.5 mm
    Total inset = 6 mm
    Segment drop = −3 mm
11. Distance decentration = 5.5 mm
    Total inset = 6.5 mm
    Segment drop = −2 mm
12. Distance decentration = 0.5 mm
    Total inset = 2 mm
    Segment drop = −1.5 mm

KEY SERIES 9

Trifocal Lenses

1. Distance decentration = 0.5 mm
   Total inset = 1.5 mm
   Segment raise = +1.5 mm
2. Distance decentration = 8.5 mm
   Total inset = 10 mm
   Segment drop = −1 mm
3. Distance decentration = 6 mm
   Total inset = 7.5 mm
   Segment drop = −4 mm
4. Distance decentration = 1.5 mm
   Total inset = 3.0 mm
   Segment drop = −4.75 mm
5. Distance decentration = 2 mm
   Total inset = 3.5 mm
   Segment raise = +1 mm
6. Distance decentration = 4.5 mm
   Total inset = 6 mm
   Segment drop = −3 mm
7. Distance decentration = 3.5 mm
   Total inset = 4.5 mm
   Segment drop = −4 mm
8. Distance decentration = 4.5 mm
   Total inset = 5.5 mm
   Segment raise = +3.5 mm
9. Distance decentration = 6.5 mm
   Total inset = 8.0 mm
   Segment drop = −4 mm
10. Distance decentration = 4 mm
    Total inset = 5 mm
    Segment drop = −1.5 mm

KEY SERIES 10

Flat-Top Bifocals

RELATING MAJOR REFERENCE POINT AND SEGMENT POSITIONS

1. The center of the bifocal segment line is 6 mm to the right of and 1 mm below the center of the marked cross. The MRP is 4 mm to the right of the center of the marked cross.
2. The center of the bifocal segment line is 6 mm to the left of and 3 mm below the center of the marked cross. The MRP is 4 mm to the left of the center of the marked cross.
3. The center of the bifocal segment line is 5.5 mm to the right of and on the same level as the center of the marked cross. The MRP is 4 mm to the right of the center of the marked cross.
4. The center of the bifocal segment line is 6 mm to the right of and 4 mm below the center of the marked cross. The MRP is 5 mm to the right of the center of the marked cross.
5. The center of the bifocal segment line is 4.5 mm to the left of and 5.5 mm below the center of the marked cross. The MRP is 3 mm to the left of the center of the marked cross.
6. The center of the bifocal segment line is 6.5 mm to the right of and 4 mm below the center of the marked cross. The MRP is 5.5 mm to the right of the center of the marked cross.
7. The center of the bifocal segment line is 3 mm to the right of and 1 mm below the center of the marked cross. The MRP is 1.5 mm to the right of the center of the marked cross.

KEY SERIES 11

Round Bifocal Segment Lenses

1. Distance decentration = 3 mm
   Total inset = 4.5 mm
   Segment drop = −4 mm
2. Distance decentration = 2.5 mm
   Total inset = 4.5 mm
   Segment drop = −1 mm
3. Distance decentration = 2 mm
   Total inset = 3.5 mm
   Segment drop = 0 mm
4. Distance decentration = 4 mm
   Total inset = 5.5 mm
   Segment drop = −6.5 mm
5. Distance decentration = 4 mm
   Total inset = 6 mm
   Segment drop = −0.5 mm
6. Distance decentration = 2.5 mm
   Total inset = 4 mm
   Segment drop = −3 mm
7. Distance decentration = 3 mm
   Total inset = 4.5 mm
   Segment drop = −3.5 mm
8. Distance decentration = 3.5 mm
   Total inset = 5 mm
   Segment drop = −4.5 mm
9. Distance decentration = 5 mm
   Total inset = 7 mm
   Segment drop = 0 mm
10. Distance decentration = 4 mm
    Total inset = 6 mm
    Segment drop = −5 mm
11. Distance decentration = 3 mm
    Total inset = 5 mm
    Segment drop = −3 mm
12. Distance decentration = 5.5 mm
    Total inset = 6.5 mm
    Segment drop = −6.75 mm

KEY SERIES 12

Franklin-Style Bifocals

1. Distance decentration = 3.5 mm
   Segment drop = −2 mm
2. Distance decentration = 6.5 mm
   Segment raise = +3.5 mm
3. Distance decentration = 4 mm
   Segment drop = −3 mm
4. Distance decentration = 2.5 mm
   Segment drop = −6.5 mm
5. Distance decentration = 3.5 mm
   Segment drop = −1 mm
6. Distance decentration = 3.5 mm
   Segment drop = −5.5 mm
7. Distance decentration = 4.5 mm
   Segment drop = −5 mm
8. Distance decentration = 2 mm
   Segment drop = −5 mm
9. Distance decentration = 0 mm
   Segment drop = −3 mm
10. Distance decentration = 4 mm
    Segment drop = −7.5 mm
11. Distance decentration = 0 mm
    Segment drop = −8.5 mm

KEY SERIES 13

Centration Using Irregular Patterns

1. When viewed from the front of the lens, the center lensmeter dot is 3 mm below and 5 mm to the right of the marked cross.
2. When viewed from the front of the lens, the center lensmeter dot is 1 mm below and 2 mm to the left of the marked cross.
3. When viewed from the front of the lens, the center lensmeter dot is 0.5 mm below and 4.5 mm to the left of the marked cross.
4. When viewed from the front of the lens, the center lensmeter dot is 1.5 mm above and 3.5 mm to the right of the marked cross.
5. When viewed from the front of the lens, the center lensmeter dot is 2 mm above and 8 mm to the right of the marked cross.
6. When viewed from the front of the lens, the center lensmeter dot is 2 mm to the left of the marked cross.
7. When viewed from the front of the lens, the center lensmeter dot is 2 mm to the left of the marked cross.
8. When viewed from the front of the lens, the marked cross is 4.5 mm to the left of and 4 mm above the center of the bifocal segment line.
9. When viewed from the front of the lens, the center lensmeter dot is 0.5 mm above and 4.5 mm to the left of the marked cross.
10. When viewed from the front of the lens, the marked cross is 9 mm to the right of and 7 mm above the center of the bifocal segment line.
11. When viewed from the front of the lens, the marked cross is 4.5 mm to the left of and 2.5 mm above the center of the bifocal segment line.

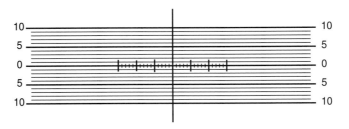

FIGURE **CSS-1**

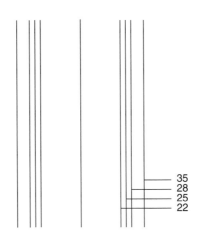

FIGURE **CSS-2**

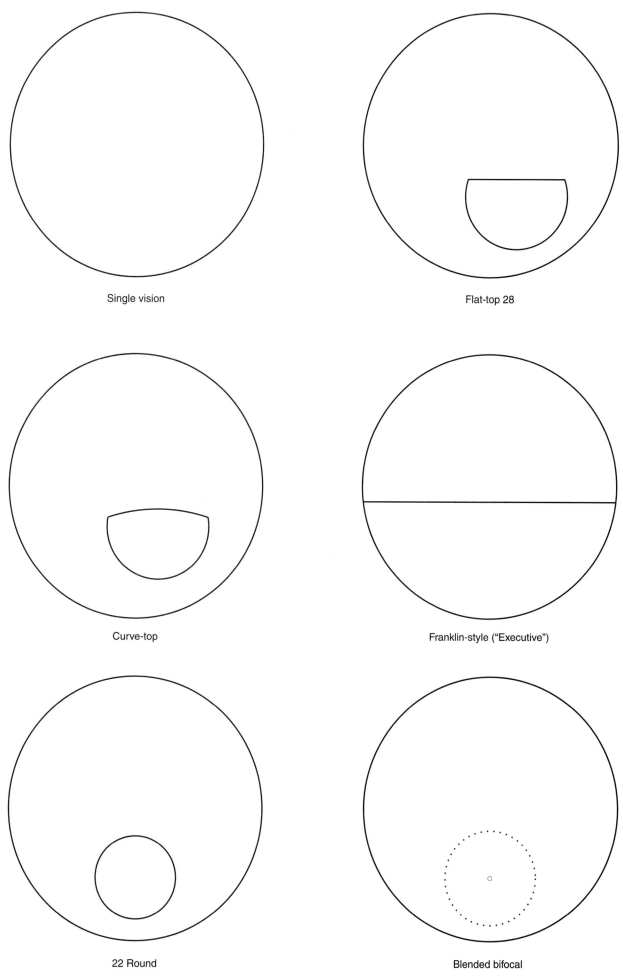

Single vision

Flat-top 28

Curve-top

Franklin-style ("Executive")

22 Round

Blended bifocal

FIGURE **CSS-3**

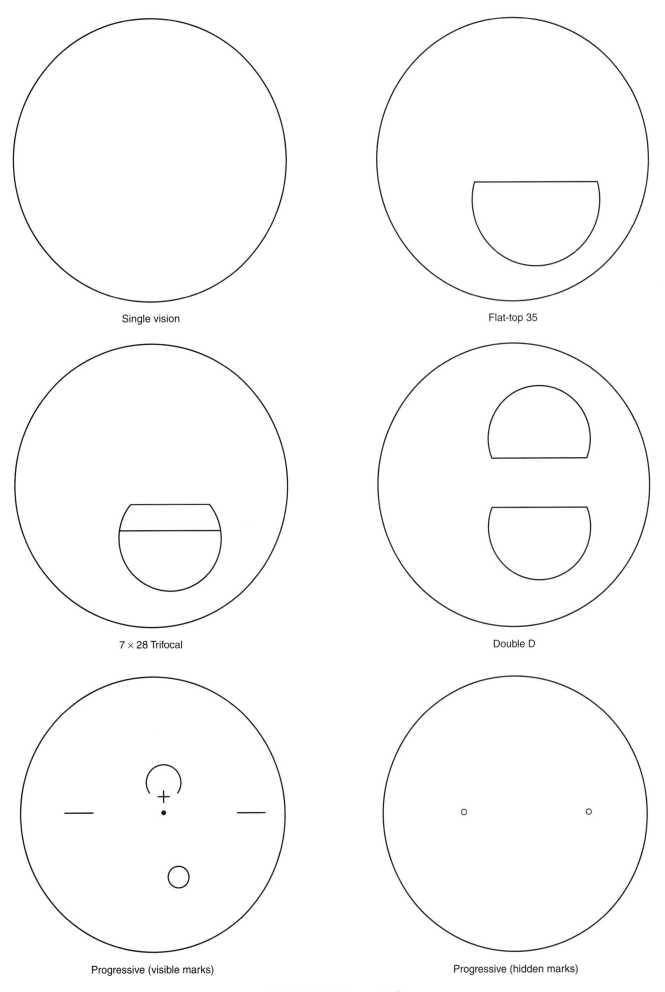

Single vision

Flat-top 35

7 × 28 Trifocal

Double D

Progressive (visible marks)

Progressive (hidden marks)

FIGURE **CSS-3, cont'd**

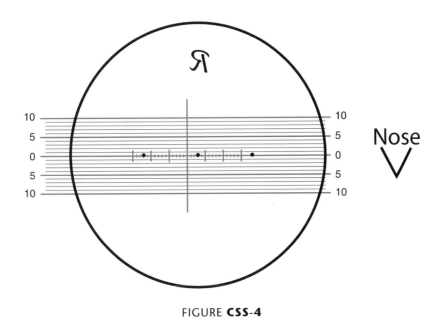

FIGURE **CSS-4**

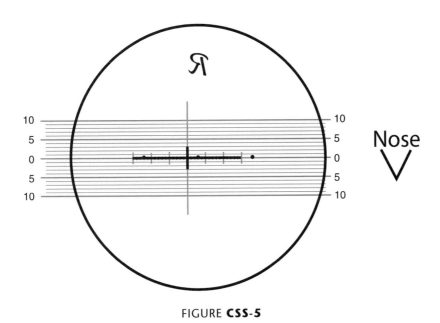

FIGURE **CSS-5**

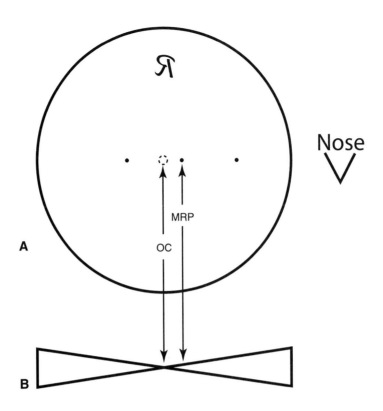

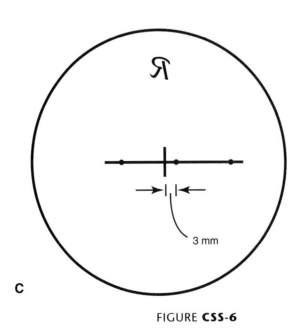

FIGURE **CSS-6**

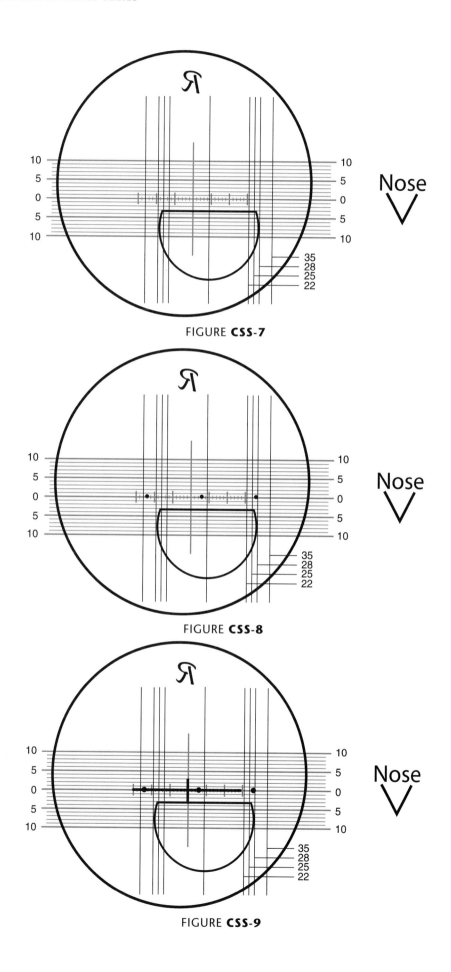

FIGURE **CSS-7**

FIGURE **CSS-8**

FIGURE **CSS-9**

FIGURE **CSS-1**   Photocopy this background grid on plain paper to use at home. To use for demonstration purposes with an overhead projector, copy the background grid onto a clear transparency.

FIGURE **CSS-2**   Photocopy these centering lines onto a clear transparency. Place it on top of the basic background grid to simulate a layout marker/blocker.

FIGURE **CSS-3**   Photocopy these lenses onto clear transparencies to simulate lenses. As shown, they are right lenses. Turn the transparency over to simulate a left lens.

FIGURE **CSS-4**   This right lens has been decentered 3 mm inward.

FIGURE **CSS-5**   This is how the lens in Figure CSS-4 would be marked with a cross to indicate the correct position for blocking.

FIGURE **CSS-6**   **A,** This right lens has been spotted to include prescribed prism. Notice that with prescribed prism, the optical center (OC) and major reference point (MRP) are not the same. The MRP is where the correct amount of prescribed prism is found. **B,** This lens is drawing schematically in cross-section as a minus lens. The eye will look through the MRP. The base of the prism is toward the nose—base in. **C,** In this example, decentration is 3 mm inward. The spotted MRP on this right lens is moved 3 mm to the right (inward).

FIGURE **CSS-7**   This flat-top 28 right lens has the proper centration for a total inset of 4.5 mm and a –3 mm drop.

FIGURE **CSS-8**   If the lens shown in Figure CSS-7 were properly surfaced and had been spotted, the center lensmeter spot should appear as shown 3 mm to the right of the center of the background grid or 1.5 mm to the left of the segment center. If this center lensmeter spot is not where it should be, the lens may not pass ANSI Z80.1 standards for prescription ophthalmic lenses.

FIGURE **CSS-9**   When the lens is marked to indicate the location of the center of the block, it appears as shown.

1.25D power
  change, 106f
  range, 108
1.66 HyperIndex lenses, 226
2-axis frame tracers. *See* Two-axis frame tracers
3-axis frame tracers. *See* Three-axis frame tracers
3M. *See* Blue Chip lens protector
7x28 trifocals, 440f
+8.00 D base curve lens, 264f
8.00 D bevel, 171
22 Round lenses, 439f
90-degree meridians, 120
180 line, 41
180-degree alignment, 263f
180-degree cutting line, horizontal orientation, 206f
180-degree line, 54, 129. *See also* Spotted 180-degree line
  0-degree side, angle, 41f
  block tilt, relationship, 313
  conformance, 312f
  correspondence. *See* Holes
  crossing, 20
  dots, placement, 79f
  drawing, 263f
  file marking. *See* Rimmed frame
  flat-top bifocals, reference, 222f
  marking, 29, 125f, 259f, 263
    lensmeter usage, 119f
  pattern tilt, 205
  setting, 127
  temporal hole, relationship, 265f
  tilt, 124-125
    relationship. *See* Segment top
180-degree meridian, lens orientation, 222f
180-degree midline, 31
180-degree mounting line, 222
180-degree reference dots, 115
180-degree reference line, 252, 311
  marking. *See* Horizontal 180-degree reference line
180-line orientation, 57

A
A dimension
  calculation, 316
  definition, 40
  measurement, 43f, 47f. *See also* Distance between
    lenses

A dimension *(Continued)*
  relationship. *See* Distance between centers
  usage. *See* Edger settings
Abrasive cone tool, usage, 255f
Abrasive particles, holding, 321f
Accidents, documentation, 337
Acetone replacer, 216
Adapter
  placement. *See* Frame tracers
  usage. *See* Mounting
Adhesion, breaking, 186f
Adhesive blocking pad. *See* Double-sided adhesive
    blocking pad
  usage, 170
Adhesive pad
  deblocker, 186f
  heat/humidity, exposure, 142
  holding area, relationship, 160f
  visual inspection, 145f
Adhesive pad blocking, 138, 140-146
  components, 140f
  high adds, usage, 143-146
  process, 143-146
  protective tape, usage, 146
  wide segments, usage, 143-146
Adhesive pad blocks, 311
  placement, 143f
  reedging, 168f
  usage, 261
Adhesive pad-blocked lenses, deblocking, 186-188
Adhesive padded block, 67
Adhesive-padded metal blocks, deblocking, 186-187
Adhesive-padded plastic blocks, deblocking, 187-188
Air chucking, 159
Air space, 84
Air Titanium frame design, type, 267f
Air Titanium Optician's Video, 263f
Aligned dots, placement, 17f
Alignment. *See* Bridge; Standard alignment; Temple;
    Vertical alignment
Allen screws, usage. *See* Translucent background grids
Alloy block, dropoff, 186f
Alloy finish blocking wastes, disposal, 340
Alloy-blocked lens, deblocking, 186f
American National Standards Institute (ANSI), 298
  OSHA, relationship, 298
  prescription standards, 121
  standards, 119. *See also* Safety frames
    exceeding, 203
  tolerances, 123

Page numbers followed by "f" indicate figures; page numbers followed by "t" indicate tables, page numbers followed by "b" indicate boxes.

American National Standards Institute (ANSI)
    (*Continued*)
    Z80.1 prescription lens standards, 293
    Z80.1-1999 standard, 92, 120-121, 202, 310
    Z87 standards, 302
    Z87.1, 298
        lens marking requirements, 299t
American Optical Company, 161, 162
ANSI. *See* American National Standards Institute
Antireflection (AR) coated lenses, 159, 201, 208
    back surface, protector disc application, 147f
    cleaning process, 228
    heating, 237
    light transmittance, 227
Antireflection (AR) coating, 3f, 6, 294-295
    crazing, 257
Antireflection (AR) spoilage, 170
Antireflection-coated (AR-coated) lenses, 170
    dyeing, 227-228. *See also* Pre-AR coated lenses
    edge polishing, 208
    hand edging, 202
AO Technica, 107t
    lens, design, 110f
Apex
    location, controlling. *See* Bevel
    placement. *See* Hand-beveled lenses
        automatic edger wheels, usage, 161
AR. *See* Antireflection
AR-coated. *See* Antireflection-coated
Aspheric form, usage, 171
Aspheric lenses, prism restrictions, 21
Aspheric lenticular lenses, OC blocking. *See* High plus
        aspheric lenticular lenses
Astigmatism, 5f
Atoric lenses, prism restrictions, 21
Autolensmeters
    spotting
        mechanism, 26f
        numerical readout, 23-27
        prescribed prism, inclusion, 23-27
        prescribed prism, noninclusion, 23
    usage, 225f. *See also* Spotting
Automated lensmeter usage, lens positioning. *See*
        Spotting
Automatic cycling, 152
Automatic edger wheels, usage. *See* Apex
Automatic edging, ceramic wheels (usage), 151-152
Automatic polishing machine, 208
Axis. *See* Cylinder axis; Oblique axis
    accuracy, checking. *See* Patterned edgers
    checking sequence. *See* Edgers
    errors, sources, 315t
    orientation, 28f
    position, lens rotation, 18

Axis (*Continued*)
    setting. *See* Lensmeter
    wheel, approach. *See* Major meridians

B
B dimension, 159
    calculation, 49
    definition, 40
    increase, 203. *See also* Frames
    reduction, 206
    subtraction, 81f
    usage, 132, 133
B frames, blocks (usage). *See* Narrow B frames
Back bevel surface, smoothing, 193f, 194
Back curves. *See* High-minus back curves
Back edge
    grooving, 283-284
    pin beveling, 200f. *See also* High-minus lens
Back mold, 5f
Back pin bevel, 199f
    application. *See* High-minus lens
Back surface, 283f
Back vertex power, verification. *See* Near power
Background grids, 438f
    readjustment. *See* Translucent background grids
Back-lighted crossed polaroids, usage. *See* Lenses
Back-to-back position. *See* Holding
Balgrip Lens Groovers, 258
Balgrip mountings, 248, 257
Bar coding, 182f
Base blocks, 141-142
Base curve
    change, 171
    determining, 3f
    dotted line, indication. *See* Front surface base curve
    drilling, 263f
    flatness, 251
    matching. *See* Lenses
    setting, 262
    steepness, 165f. *See also* High plus lens;
        Wrap-around frames
    usage, 164f
    variation, 165f
Base down prism
    addition, 101f
    usage, 101f
Base electric stand drills, 249
Base tints, 213
Base up prism, amounts, 100
Base-in prism, 89
Basic impact standard, 298
Basic-impact lenses, warning labels, 299-300
Basic-impact marking requirements, 298-299
Basic-impact requirements. *See* Safety eyewear

Basic-impact testing requirements, 298
Basic-impact thickness requirements, 298
Basing groove location, 284f
Batch testing
  contrast. *See* Individual testing
  performing, 294-295
Bath temperature, laboratory thermometer (usage), 216f
Bend-down end positions. *See* Temple
Bending pliers
  rotation, 244
  usage, 244f
Bevel
  alignment, 237f
    insertion, importance, 236f
  appearance, 181f
  configuration, ruining, 324
  cosmetic advantage. *See* Hidden bevel
  custom cut, 66f
  disengagement, 171
  drop off, 62
  edger, example. *See* Patterned bevel edger
  following. *See* Frame curvature; Front edge
  groove, 324f
  location, 181f
    changing, 324-325
  meniscus curvature, frame eyewire conformance, 239f
  occupation. *See* Edges
  placement, 152, 159-161, 165f
    judgment, 175f
    preprogrammed settings, 178f
  positioning, 164f
  rear surface, 325f
  shape, 65f
  sharpness, 196f
  snapping. *See* Lower nasal part
  style, 152
  surface
    edge smoothing. *See* Front bevel surface
    smoothing, 192f. *See also* Back bevel surface
  system. *See* Free-float bevel system; Guided bevel system
  tracking, 171f
  wheels, usage. *See* Hide-a-Bevel wheels; Mini-bevel wheels; V-bevel wheels
Bevel apex, 178f
  forward movement, 160-161, 325f
  location, controlling, 325t
  pin beveling, 198f
  placement, 324. *See also* Thick lenses; Thin lenses
  positioning, 194, 325
Beveled lenses, 6
Beveling. *See* Groove; Pin beveling
  process, 166
Biconcave lenses, testing exemption, 294

Bifocal lenses (bifocals). *See* Invisible bifocals; Stock finished bifocals
  definition, 2
  height, 45f, 58
  ledge, 145
  mass production. *See* Finished bifocals
  segment, 103. *See also* High bifocal segment; Tilted bifocal segments
  size. *See* Flat-top bifocals
  spotting. *See* Blended bifocals; Flat-top bifocals
Binocular distance PD
  indication, 90f
  usage. *See* Decentration per lens
Binocular PD, 51
  sufficiency, 106
Blade slipping, 256f
Blanks, 9f. *See also* Finished blanks; Semifinished blanks; Uncut lens blank; Uncut minus lens blank
  definition, 2
  proper size, ensuring, 83-92
  rotation. *See* Semifinished lens
  selection, 5, 9-11, 163f
  variety. *See* Patterns
Blanks, size, 9f. *See also* Minimum blank size
  addition. *See* Effective diameter
  adequacy, 87f, 88f
  determining, 3f
  effect. *See* Plus lenses
  minimum, 88f, 89f. *See also* Single vision minimum blank size chart
Blemished lenses, salvaging, 27-28
Blemished prism lenses, 27-28
Blemished sphere, 27
Blemished spherocylinder, 27
Blended bifocals, 129-131, 398, 439f. *See also* Factory-marked blended bifocal
  border, remarking, 130f
  centration
    dotted segment border, usage, 129
    process, 130f
    segment center, usage, 129-131
  spotting, 35b
  total segment inset, usage, 413
Blended round-segment lenses, 30
Blended zone, outermost borders, 130f
Blind holes/slots, 180
Blocked lenses
  drilling, 262-263
  edging, 175f
Blockers. *See* Centration; WECO blocker
  alignment, 312f
  checking, 312f
  grids, 181
  usage, 146-147, 173f. *See also* Marker/blocker

Blocking, 6, 138, 402. *See also* Adhesive pad blocking;
        Chipped portion; Lenses; Metal alloy
        blocking; Precast FreeBlock blocking; Pressure
        blocking
    definition, 6
    lens positioning, 174f
    preparation, 143
    process, 31f, 272f
    proficiency test questions, 147-148
    progressive addition lenses
        centering, hidden circles (usage), 105f
        positioning, 103-105
    suction, usage, 139
    system. *See* Gerber-Coburn Step Two blocking
        system
    types, 138
    usage. *See* Edging
Blocks. *See* Base blocks; Metal blocks; Plastic blocks
    advantages. *See* Plastic lenses
    attachment. *See* Finishing
    center, correspondence, 85f
    deblocking. *See* Adhesive-padded metal blocks;
        Adhesive-padded plastic blocks
    design, 152f
    dropoff. *See* Alloy block
    efficiency, 143f
    lens slippage, causes, 143b
    location, showing, 394, 396, 397
    matching. *See* Front lens curve
    placement. *See* Adhesive pad blocks; Centration
        device
    pressing, 144f, 174f
    removal. *See* Plastic blocks
    slippage, 314f
        prevention, 141-142
    usage, 140-141. *See also* Half-eye blocks; Half-eye
        lenses; Narrow B frames
Blue Chip lens protector (3M), 146
Bolt head, placement, 257f
Bonded roughing wheels, 161
Bonding
    material, 321f, 323
    type, 321-322
Boxing
    pattern size, 46
Boxing center, 40f, 41, 64f. *See also* Edged lenses
    definition, 80f
    determination, 63f
    equivalence. *See* Mechanical center
    measurement, 41f
    mechanical center, relationship, 59f
    nonequivalence. *See* Mechanical center
    position, 58
    rotational center, relationship, 81

Boxing system, 40f. *See also* Lenses
    definition, 39
    measurement, 76
    usage, 53f. *See also* Eyesize; Horizontal decentration;
        Vertical centration
Box-o-Graph, 167
    pattern measurement, 48f
    usage, 60
Bracing pliers, usage, 245
Bridge. *See* Skewed bridge
    alignment, 240-243
    horizontal/vertical preadjustments, 242
    size, 42, 173f
        measurements, 64
Brown lens, visible spectrum, 218f
Brown plastic lens, transmission curve, 219
Buffing compound, usage. *See* Rag wheel
Bulb filament, examination, 11f
Bushing, 257. *See also* Plastic bushing
Businesses
    Emergency Action Plan, usage, 336
    OSHA, impact. *See* Large businesses; Small
        businesses
By-hand lens tracing, laboratory requirements, 56-57

C
C dimension, 40f
    definition, 40
C size. *See* Lens shapes
Calibration, 309. *See also* Edgers; Power
    checking, 82
    checks, 309
    proficiency test questions, 317-319
Caliper
    line, 47f
    usage, 47f
Cast molding, 5f
Cement assembly lenses, testing exemption, 294
Center. *See* Boxing center; Enclosing box; Geometrical
        center
    finding, pattern makers (usage), 62
Center bevel placement. *See* Thick lenses
Center dot, 50
Center thickness, determining, 3f
Centering. *See* Centration device; Trifocal lenses
    pin
        locking. *See* Groover
        usage, 284f
    purpose, 75
    spring-connected coupling pins, positioning, 280f
Central hole placement, 60f, 418
Central lensmeter dot, raising/lowering, 84f
Central meridian, light color, 221
Centrally marked circles, 48f

Centration. *See* Curve-top segments; Decentration; Franklin-style lenses; Lens centration; Monocular PD; Practitioner-specified MRP height
  blockers, 311-313
  calculation, boxing system (usage). *See* Horizontal decentration; Vertical centration calculation
  chart, 104f
  compensation, 59f
  completion, 124f
  definition, 50
  importance, 21f
  instrument, usage, 80f. *See also* Lens centration
  irregular patterns, usage. *See* Centration skills series
  process, 31f, 50. *See* Curve-top lenses
  reference, 102f
  steps, protractor usage, 81b
  units
    ED circles, usage, 83
    superimposed patterns, usage, 83-86
  Centration device
  angled blocking, 313f
  block, placement, 85f
  concentric circles, usage, 86f
  example, 77
  horizontal reference line, 393-394
  lens centering, 144f
  lens-blocking mechanism, inclusion, 82
  movable vertical line, 131
  problem, 314f
  progressive addition lens positioning, 102
  shadow projection, usage, 88f
  usage. *See* Round-segment multifocals
Centration skills series (CSS), 389
  series 1 (single vision lenses), 391-392
    key, 421
  series 2 (single vision lenses), 393-394
    key, 422-423
  series 3 (single vision lenses), 395-397
    key, 424-425
  series 4 (progressive addition lenses), 398-399
    key, 426-427
  series 5 (progressive addition lenses), 400-401
    key, 428-429
  series 6 (flat-top bifocals), 402-403
    key, 430
  series 7 (flat-top bifocals), 404-405
    key, 431
  series 8 (curve-top bifocals), 406-407
    key, 432
  series 9 (trifocal lenses), 408-409
    key, 433
  series 10 (flat-top bifocals), 410-412
    key, 434

Centration skills series (CSS) *(Continued)*
  series 11 (round bifocal segment lenses), 413-414
    key, 435
  series 12 (Franklin-style bifocals), 415-417
    key, 436
  series 13 (centration, irregular pattern usage), 418-420
    key, 437
Ceramic block, usage, 285f
Ceramic hand-edging wheel, retruing, 191f
Ceramic wheel hand edgers, 190
  disadvantages, 191f
Ceramic wheels
  90-degree angle, usage, 285
  usage. *See* Automatic edging
Chamfering, 264, 269f. *See also* Drilled hole; Edges; Holes
Chase, George, 277, 296
Checklists. *See* Hazardous communication checklist; Insertion
  review, 337
Chemical Hazard Communication Standard (HAZCOM), 331-334
Chemical spills, 340
Chemical tempering, 303-305
  process, 304-305, 304f
  products, disposal, 340
  safety equipment, usage, 336
Chippage, 152f
  allowance, 88f
Chipped portion, marking/blocking, 27f
Chipping. *See* Holes; Patterned edging
  pliers, 150
  variety, 151f
  risk, reduction, 244f
Chips, removal, 205
Chuck pressure, reduction. *See* Edgers
Chucking, 145, 159f, 283. *See also* Air chucking; Electric chucking; Lenses; Manual chucking; Pneumatic chucking
  pressure, 145f-147f
  systems, 140f
Circles, 103. *See also* Centrally marked circles; Diameter
  location/dotting. *See* Engraved circles
Circular mires, crossing, 22f
Circumference. *See* Round pattern
  chart. *See* Lenses
    usage. *See* Edging
  gauge, usage, 56f, 169f. *See also* Edging
  knowledge, advantage, 168f
  tape, tightening, 169f
  usage. *See* Edger settings
Clamp-down holding system, 261

Clamping system, 263f
Clapper plate, position, 316
Cleaning products, disposal, 340
Clipped screw, rough ends, 257f
Clips
    appearance, 271f
    cleaning, 264
    lengths, 271f
    parallelism, 270f
    spring-tension effect, 267f
    usage, 263
    width, adjustment, 270f
Closure pliers. *See* Eyewires
    usage. *See* Lens size
Coating, 6
Colmascope
    crossed polarizing filter, 305f
    definition, 167, 200
    usage, 168f, 305
Color. *See* Solid tint
    accuracy
        checking, 217-218
        ensuring, 217-220
    balance, 218
    balancing
        recommendations. *See* Dyes
        table, 220t
    cross-contamination, prevention, 217
    matching, 218-219
        forced matching, 219
    usage. *See* Tints
Color coding lens holders, 217f
Color Primer, 216
Columbia Resin 39 (CR-39) (Pittsburgh Plate Glass
        Co.)
    1.498 index, 227
    lenses, 3f
    plastic, 249
    plastic lenses, 169, 226
        AR coating, 228
        light, transmittance, 227
    trademark, 169
    uncoated lenses, comparison, 295
Company policy. *See* Hazardous communication
        program
Computer lenses. *See* Specialty computer lenses
Computer-assisted drills, 249, 265-266
    advantages/disadvantages, 271f
Computer-assisted patternless edgers, 315
Concentration. *See* Diamond wheels
    factor, 321f
Cone tool
    absence, 255
    usage. *See* Abrasive cone tool; Holes; Notches

Cone-shaped tool, 264, 269f
Construction factors. *See* Diamond wheels
Containers, labels, 333
Contractor employers, 346
Convergence, definition, 76
Conversations, documentation, 337
Coolants. *See* Edgers
    change, 309, 317
    concentration, variation, 317
    disposal. *See* Edgers; Hand edgers
    flow, 176
        maintenance, 168
    presence, 164
    pump, disconnection, 323
Coquille, usage, 204. *See also* Shape tracing;
        Three-piece mountings
Cornea, limitation, 45f
Correctional modifications, 205-206
Corridor
    length, 98
    width. *See* Progressive corridor
CR-39. *See* Columbia Resin 39
Crackle-finish exteriors, 311
Crank handle, usage, 266f
Crazing. *See* Antireflection coating; Crown glass
    definition, 226
Crib lenses, 3f
Cross-contamination, prevention. *See* Color
Crossed polaroids, usage, 167
Crossed-line-target lensmeter, usage. *See* Single
        vision sphere spotting; Spherocylinder
        lenses
Crossing point. *See* Cylinder lines; Sphere lines
Crown glass, 168
    lenses
        crazing, 304f
        impact resistance, 305
C-size, definition, 56
CSS. *See* Centration skills series
Curing. *See* Lens-curing factor
    definition, 215
Curved cutting shears, usage, 55f
Curved upper segment border, lateral corners, 126f
Curved-rim frame, 179
Curved-top segment, 126f
Curve-top bifocals. *See* Centration skills series
Curve-top lenses, 439f
    centration process, 406
Curve-top segments, 406
    centration, 125-126
Cushion coatings, benefit, 296
Cutters, 151f, 320
    blades, 326
        usage, 166f, 278f

Cutters (Continued)
    matching, questions, 327-328
    proficiency test questions, 326-328
    wheels, 278
Cutting, 101f. See also Patterned edging
    center, 49
    nib, 277
    plane, 193f
    pliers, usage, 257f
    speed factors. See Hand edging
    spoon, 150f, 151f
        holding, position, 150f
    wheels, 150f
        cleanliness/coolness. See Groover
        usage. See Recessed metal rim
Cylinder axis, 25f, 30f, 34f. See also 121-degree cylinder
        axis; Prescribed cylinder axis; Required
        cylinder axis
    errors, 313f, 314f
    incorrectness, 63f
    position, approach, 91
    tolerance, 30
Cylinder component, 30f
Cylinder lenses, 28f
    decentration. See Plano cylinder lenses
Cylinder lines, 15f
    crossing point, 22f
    definition, 12
    focusing, 15f
    positioning, 20f
Cylinder power, 5f
    increase, 91
    variation, 98f
Cylinder values, 15f

D
Dab-on applicator, usage, 139
Datum line, definition, 41
Daylight-type bulbs, usage, 218
DBC. See Distance between centers
DBL. See Distance between lenses
Deblocker, mounting. See Layout
Deblocking, 3f, 6, 185. See also Adhesive pad; Adhesive
        pad-blocked lenses; Alloy-blocked lens; Metal
        alloy-blocked lenses; Suction-blocked lenses;
        Wax-blocked lenses
    definition, 6
    laboratory towel, usage, 187f
    methods, 188b
    occurrence, 186f
    proficiency test questions, 188-189
    reblocking, combination, 187f
Decals, usage, 35f, 104f
Decenter (finding), pattern makers (usage), 62

Decentered pattern
    option, 62
    usage, 63f
Decentering, 50, 64f, 87f. See also Minus lens
Decentration, 20f, 50, 51f. See also Left decentration;
        Plano cylinder lenses; Reading glasses; Right
        decentration; Total decentration; Vertical
        segment decentration
    amount, 88f, 311. See also Optical center
        addition, 89f
    calculation, 181
        boxing system, usage. See Horizontal
        decentration
    correction, 85f
    determination, monocular interpupillary distances
        (usage), 76
    direction, 79b, 80f
    inset, comparison, 115f
    occurrence, 51f
    requirement, 63f
Decentration per lens, 76
    binocular distance PD, usage, 52
Dehardening process, 202
Deionized water, usage, 213
Demarcation line, visibility, 2, 166f
Demo lenses, 158
    tracing, 66f
Dental pick, usage, 286f
Depressed-segment one-piece multifocals, testing
        exemption, 294
Diameter. See Effective diameter
    lens circle, 90f
Diamond wheels
    advantages, 191f
    concentration, 321
    dressing, 322-326
        sticks, 323f
    hand edgers, 190-192
    layer, depth, 321
    surfaces, construction factors, 320-322
    truing, 325
    usage, 164
Diamonds
    amount, reduction, 191f
    burr
        absence, 255
        usage, 254
    clogging, 161
    concentrations, 321t
    cutting surfaces, 325
    particles, 320
        exposure, 323f
        spacing, 162f
    powder, 321

Diamond-wheel edgers, capability, 278f
Difference measures, 115f
Direct plus cylinder power readings, 16
Displacement compensation. *See* Patterns
Distance between centers (DBC)
    definition, 43, 51
    determination, 51-52, 76
    A dimension, relationship, 44f
Distance between lenses (DBL), 42-43, 63f, 76. *See also*
        Frames
    measurement, 43f, 54. *See also* Grooved frame
Distance decentration, 105, 121, 129f. *See also* Left
        lens
    calculation, 418
    correction, 123f
    usage, 123, 126
Distance OC
    location, 31f
    vertical placement, 32f
Distance PD, 62f, 116
    alteration, 122b
    amount, 118
    favoring, 121-124
    maintenance, 122b
    near PD, relationship, 121-122
Distance portion, MRP (checking). *See* Flat-top
        multifocals
Distance power
    amount, 100f
    checking. *See* Major reference point
    completion, 5f
    verification. *See* Progressive addition lenses
        location, 99f
Distance prescription, 109f
Distance reference point (DRP), 98, 99f
    definition, 32, 98
    location, 33f, 104f
Distances, variations, 44f
Distilled water
    addition. *See* Dyes
    usage, 213
Documentation. *See* Accidents; Conversations; Injuries;
        Training
    maintenance, 336-337
Dots. *See* 180-degree reference dots; Center dot;
        Lensmeter dots
    circle, usage, 15f
    losing, 85f
    placement. *See* 180-degree line; Aligned dots;
        Spherocylinder lenses
    position, 129
    raising/lowering. *See* Central lensmeter dot
    reference usage, 105f
Dotted hidden circles, 105

Dotted lines
    appearance, 203f
    usage, 10f, 101f
Dotted MRP, usage, 131
Dotted segment border, usage. *See* Blended bifocals
Dotting. *See* Lenses
Double D lenses, 440f
Double gradients, 221f, 224
Double straps, distance, 273f
Double-bevel appearance, 205
Double-hole mountings, 260
Double-padded nylon jaw pliers, usage, 245
Double-segment lenses, 131-132
    centration, 132-133
    vertical lens area, sufficiency, 133f
Double-sided adhesive blocking pad, 82, 117
Double-sided adhesive pad, 140
Double-sided adhesive tape, usage, 260
Double-sided tape, usage, 140f. *See also* Drilling
Double-strap area, adjustments, 268-269
Double-strap mountings, usage, 266-273
Dress eyewear, requirements, 292-296
Dress ophthalmic lenses, minimum thickness, 293
Dressing. *See* Diamond wheels
    sticks. *See* Diamond wheels; Finishing wheels;
        Roughing wheels
        process, 323f
Drilled hole
    chamfering, 255f
    smoothing, rat-tail file (usage), 256
Drilled lens, attachment. *See* Mountings
Drilled mountings, 247
    bibliography, 273
    proficiency test questions, 274-275
Drill-guide, inclusion, 251
Drilling. *See* Free hand drilling; Lens drilling; Nasal
        hole; Polycarbonate lenses; Temporal hole
    bit, pressing, 269f
    chart, usage, 251f, 262, 267f
    effect. *See* Impact resistance
    guides. *See* Frames
        double-sided tape, usage, 261f
        usage, 262f
    sequence, template, 261f
    setup. *See* Nasal side
    system, 263f
Drill-mounting, quality, 265
Drillrite Automatic Lens Drill, 262
Drills. *See* Computer-assisted drills; In-edger drill
    bit
        lens, pressing, 266f
        pressing, 254f
    historical note. *See* Hand drills
    improvements. *See* Electric drills

Drills (Continued)
    movement, ability, 262
    small-millimeter gauge, inclusion, 253f
    stand, table construction, 263
    types. See Lenses
    usage. See Lens drilling
Driving, specialty lens (usage), 109f
Drop. See Segment drop
Drop ball test, 293-294
    timing, 294
Drop-ball tester, usage, 294f
Drop-ball testing. See Glass lenses
DRP. See Distance reference point
Drum tool, usage. See Polishing
Dry cut edgers, 164-167, 326
    emergency stops, 167
    problems, 338-339
    size accuracy, checking, 167
Dry edging. See Polycarbonate lenses
Dry-cut router-blade-type edger, usage, 277
Dummy lenses, 252-253
    usage, 204
Duty to Inform program, 296-297
Dyeing. See Antireflection-coated lenses; Hard-coated
       lenses; High-index lenses; Nylon cords; Plastic
       polarizing lenses; Simple gradient lens;
       Ultraviolet dyeing
    process
       lens coating, effects, 226-228
       lens material, effects, 226-228
Dyes, 213-215
    contamination, prevention, 214f
    disposal, 340
    distilled water, addition, 215f
    distribution. See Polycarbonate lenses
    life span, 215
    maintenance, 214-215
    manufacturer, color balancing recommendations,
       220t
    preparation, 213-214
    smells, laboratory reduction, 229

E
ED. See Effective diameter
Edge polishing, 206-208. See also Antireflection-coated
       lenses; Glass lenses; High-index plastic; Plastic
       lenses; Polycarbonate lenses
    edger, usage, 207
Edge smoothing, 192-194. See also Front bevel
    continuation, 199
    lens, proper holding, 193-194
    practicing, 197
    process, 193f, 199
    wheel, preparation, 192-193

Edge thickness. See Grooving; Rimless lenses
    dependence, 271f
    determining, 3f
    errors. See Plus lenses
    increase, 9
    lens, feeling, 172-175
    minimum, 285
    rolled edge, effect, 166f
    variation, 279f
Edged gradient lenses, 223
Edged lenses, 31f
    back-to-back holding, 313f
    boxing center, 51f, 81, 85f
    front-to-front, holding, 30f
    geometrical center, 85f
    line, drawing, 252f
    nasal half, 51f
    scratches, appearance, 28f
    thickness, measurement, 175f
Edger dials
    configuration, zero/plus-minus scale, 154-155
    marking, 154-155
       relationship. See Eyesize
    scales, combination, 155
Edger settings, accuracy
    adjustment
       circumference, usage, 316
       A dimension, usage, 316
       increasing, 155-157
Edger wheels, 320
    matching, questions, 327-328
    proficiency test questions, 326-328
    usage. See Apex placement
Edgers. See Dry cut edgers; WECO edger
    axis checking sequence, 313b
    calibration, 313-316
    chuck pressure, reduction, 170
    cleaning, 316-317
    coolants, 318
       disposal, 340
    cutting technique, 152
    frame tracer
       combination, 173f
       usage, 67
    frosted appearance, 197
    guided bevel system, usage, 171
    lens placement, 152f
    lubrication, 316-317
    manufacturer design, 139f
    pattern, placement, 62, 65f
    setting, 154f
    size, setting, 152-153
    sizing dial, 153
    stand-alone capabilities, 67

Edgers *(Continued)*
    tracers, placement, 69f
    types. *See* Hand edgers
    usage. *See* Dry-cut router-blade-type edger; Edge
        polishing; Grooving; Pattern making
Edges. *See* Thin edges
    bevel, occupation, 160f
    beveling, 255f
    chamfering, 255f
    configuration, destruction (avoidance), 192f
    gauge, 261
    groove, positioning, 279-284
    grooving. *See* Back edge; Front edge; Middle edge;
        Nylon cords
    locations, appearance. *See* High-plus lenses
    marking, 261f
    minimization. *See* Minus edges
    moderate thickness, 269-272
    padding, 187f
    temporal side appearance, 178f
    usage. *See* Polished edge; Rolled edges
    viewing screens, usage, 177-178
Edging, 3f, 6, 149, 159f. *See also* Blocked lenses; Glass
        lenses; Hand edging; Lenses; Patterned
        edging; Patternless edging; Plastic lenses;
        Pre-edging; Wrap-around frames
    blocking, usage, 83f
    center, 49
    ceramic wheels, usage. *See* Automatic edging
    circumference chart, 158t
    completion, 154f, 175f
    cycle, 315
    dimensions, 179f
    errors, catching. *See* Flat-top multifocals
    laboratory, 2
        personnel, checking, 296
    lenses, usage. *See* Wrap-around frames
    overall process, 161-167
    patternless systems, frame tracer (usage), 62-70
    process, 322f. *See also* Patterned edging
        layout, 415
        pliers, usage, 240f
    proficiency test questions, 182-184
    selection. *See* Polycarbonate lenses
    size
        accuracy (increasing), circumference
            gauge/chart (usage), 157-159
        compensation, usage. *See* Frames
        special situations, 170-171
        starting point, 195f
        stress. *See* Polycarbonate lenses
        variations. *See* Lenses
Effective diameter (ED), 41-42. *See also* Frames
    angle, 42

Effective diameter (ED) *(Continued)*
    blank size, addition, 89f
    circles, usage. *See* Centration
    definition, 41
    determination. *See* Lens shapes
    measurement, 41f, 42f
    showing, 83
    usage, 86f
Electric chucking, 159
Electric drills, improvements, 260-263
Electric stand drills, usage. *See* Lens drilling
Electrical hazards, 331
    awareness, 337-338
Electrometallic wheels, 322
Electronically controlled method, 162
Electroplated roughing wheels, 161
Electroplated wheels, cleaning, 325
Elongation, direction, 15f
Emergency Action Plan, usage. *See* Businesses
Emergency lights, example, 339f
Emergency telephone numbers, display, 336
Employee
    involvement. *See* Safety program
    participation, 331
    responsibilities, 344
    training, 333-334
Employee Right To Know laws, 330
Employee-identified problems, correction, 335
Employers. *See* Contractor employers
    responsibility, OSHA impact, 330-331
Enclosing box, center, 41f
Endpiece
    bending, 242-243
    gripping, 244f
    holding, 245f
    size, 245f
Engineering out the hazard. *See* Hazards
Engraved circles, location/dotting, 34f
Engraving, 3f, 6
Environmental concerns, 329, 339-341
    information, 341
    proficiency test questions, 342-343
    recommendations, 340-341
Environmental Protection Agency (EPA), 329, 330
EPA. *See* Environmental Protection Agency
Errors. *See* Human error; Optical center; Parallax;
        Pattern errors
    amount, 205
        parallax, effect, 34
    compensation. *See* Horizontal OC error; Major
        reference point
    sources, 314f. *See also* Axis
Essilor. *See* Interview; Varilux
Etchings, marking, 34

Executive bifocal, ledge, 171f
Executive lenses, 171, 201, 250, 439f
 positioning, 283
 rotation, 284
 testing, exemption, 294
Exit signs, display, 335
Explosion hazards, 331
Exposure limits, 333
Eyeglass correction. *See* Spherical eyeglass correction
Eyepiece
 focusing. *See* Lensmeter
 location, 12
Eyes
 decentration, 204
 suppression, 90
 tracing, 64
Eyesize, 44f. *See also* Frames
 adjustments. *See* Manual patterned edgers
 change, effect. *See* Lens shapes
 definition, 40
 edger dial marking, relationship, 154
 measurement, boxing system usage, 156f
 setting, 316
Eyesize/pattern size ratio, 54
Eyewear. *See* Safety eyewear; Sports eyewear
 categories, 292
 requirements. *See* Dress eyewear
Eyewires
 closure pliers, 239f
  usage, 240f
 conformance. *See* Bevel
 forming pliers, 239f
 groove, 90f
 horizontal/vertical preadjustments, 242
 inside groove, 394
 nasal edge, 236
 nasal sides, equidistance, 241
 screw, insertion/removal, 167f
 shape, change, 64
 touching. *See* Frames
 upper/lower rims, preshaping, 237f

F
Fabrication process, 19f
 overview, 1
 proficiency test questions, 7
Face form, 241
Face hand edger, spherical section, 201f
Facet, usage, 166
Faceted edge, usage. *See* Minus lens; Plus lenses
Face-type hand edger, 190
 effect, 191f
Factory-marked blended bifocal, 130f
Fault line, 296

FDA. *See* Food and Drug Administration
File marks. *See* Horizontal meridian
Fining, 3f
Finished bifocals. *See* Stock finished bifocals
 mass production, 2
Finished blanks, 3f
Finished lenses, 4f
 record keeping requirements. *See* Partially finished lenses
 sizes, 54
 terminology, 2-4
Finished PD, 57
Finished surfaces, 4f
Finishing
 cycle, 322
 laboratories, 1-2, 419
 lens block, attachment, 51f
 process, overview. *See* Lenses
Finishing wheels
 dressing, 324f. *See also* Metal-bonded finishing wheels
  sticks, 323f
 retruing, 326
  failure, 326f
 usage, 161-162
 wear, 325
Fire evacuation route, 336
Fire extinguishers, availability, 337
Fire hazards, 331
Fire prevention, 338
First aid kit, availability, 337, 338f
Fitting cross, 43-44, 98-99. *See also* Progressive addition lenses
 drop, 205
 height, 45f
  definition, 99f
  information, 173f
 importance, 99
 location, 102, 104f
 mismarking, 105f
 raise. *See* Progressive lenses
 system, usage. *See* Progressive lenses
 usage, 109, 398-399, 426-427. *See also* Layout
Fitting height. *See* Minimum fitting height
Five-layer AR-coated lenses, 295
Flat edges, usage. *See* Rimless style eyewear
Flat hand edger surface, disadvantage, 199f
Flat surface touch test, 242
 usage. *See* Parallelism testing
Flat-beveled lenses, 201f. *See also* Plastic flat-beveled lenses
Flat-front lenses, 179
Flat-top 28 lenses, 439f
Flat-top 35 lenses, 440f

Flat-top bifocals, 222, 237. *See also* Centration skills series
    bifocal segment size, 145f
    reference. *See* 180-degree line
    segment, 118, 125
    spotting, 30f
Flat-top lenses, layout, 32
Flat-top lines, 222
Flat-top multifocal centration
    device, usage, 118b
    instrument, usage, 117
    lens protractor, usage, 114-116; 116b
Flat-top multifocals, 4f, 114-117
    distance portion, MRP (checking), 118-121
    historical background, 114-116
    incorrect segment inset, 121-124
        checking, 121
    lens edging, errors (catching), 117-125
    mistakes, prevention, 124
    positioning, 127
    spotting, 31b
Flat-top trifocals
    positioning, 125
    usage, 408
Flat-top-segment multifocals, spotting, 29
Flat-top-style multifocals, 4f
Focimeter, 5
Focused target, 15f
Food and Drug Administration (FDA)
    compliance, 294
    laboratory labeling requirements, 297
    mandates, 293
    requirements, 297
    response, 296
Forced hot air, usage, 239
Forced matching. *See* Color
Forming pliers. *See* Eyewires
Four-point touch, 240-241
    checking, 241f
    conformance, 241f
Frame curvature
    bevel, following, 181f
    edger, following, 181f
    lens curve mismatch, 66f
Frame difference, 46f, 48f
    calculations, 48-49
    measurement, 46, 49
    stabililty, 49f
Frame tracers, 6, 39. *See also* Three-axis frame tracers;
        Two-axis frame tracers
    advantages/disadvantages, 64-67
    challenge questions, 74
    combination. *See* Edgers
    definition, 62
    disadvantage, 68

Frame tracers *(Continued)*
    layout blocker, integration, 70f
    lens/adapter, placement, 68f
    placement. *See* Remote-site dispensary
    proficiency test questions, 71-74
    third dimension, advantage, 179-180
    usage, 67-70. *See also* Edgers; Edging; Off-site
        location; Order entry
Frames. *See* Safety frames
    A + DBL, 240
    availability, 69f
    B dimension, 90f
        increasing, 204-205
    bridge, centering, 90f
    centering. *See* Pattern makers
    deformation, 177
    dimensions, 103
        ensuring, 70f
    distortion, 206f
    drilling guides, 260
    ED, 86
    edging, size compensation (usage), 157t
    eyesize, 86f
    eyewire
        conformance. *See* Bevel
        touching, 241f
    flexibility, 245f
    front, grasping, 244f
    groove
        alignment, 237f
        temporal edge, 236
    heating, 240b
    horizontal alignment, 240
    horizontal/vertical measurements, difference, 48f
    humping up, 206f
    lens blank size, effect, 104f
    lens opening, covering, 55f
    lenses, snapping, 157
    liners, inclusion. *See* Nylon cord frames
    materials
        requirements. *See* Patternless edging
        usage, 176f
    measurement system, 46f
    nasal rim, 203f
    old lens, usage, 253f
    PD, 51-52
        alignment/distance, 241f
    placement, 90f
    product introduction, 40f
    reshaping, 66f
    sample lens, usage, 253f
    setup. *See* Pattern making
    shape, 27
        three-dimensional tracing, 64-66

Frames *(Continued)*
    size, 28f
    thin metal rims, 277f
    usage. *See* Semirimless mountings
Frame's lens
    hand edging, 202-203
    reedging, 202-203
    shape, change, 203-205
    size, checking. *See* Metal frame lens size
Franklin-style bifocals. *See* Centration skills series
Franklin-style lenses, 171, 250, 439f
    centration, 132f
    hand edging, 201
    positioning, 283
    rotation, 284
    surfacing, 415
Franklin-style multifocals, 131
    centration, 131
Free hand drilling, 262f
Free-float bevel system, 162
Free-float method, usage, 324
Freehand scoring, 150
Fresnel Equation, 227
Front bevel
    edge smoothing, 199
    surface
        edge smoothing, 194
        smoothing, 193f
Front edge
    bevel, following, 180f
    grooving, 280-282
Front lens curve, block matching, 142f
Front surface base curve, dotted line (indication), 165f
Front vertex powers, usage. *See* Near add
Front-to-front holding, 207f
Front-to-front placement, 119

G
Gap, creation, 87f
GCD. *See* Geometrical center distance
General duty clause, 330
General-purpose-wear lens, 108f
Geometrical center, 40f, 41f. *See also* Edged lenses
    position, 84f
Geometrical center distance (GCD), 43, 82
Gerber-Coburn Step Two blocking system, 186
Glass. *See* Crown glass; High-index glass; Photochromic
    glass
Glass lenses, 3f
    cleaning, 208
    crazing. *See* Crown glass
    drop-ball testing, 294
    edge gloss, 207
    edge polishing, 206-207

Glass lenses *(Continued)*
    edging, 322f
    hardening, 303-305
    notes, 258-259
    pin bevel, 201f
    sandblasting, 299
    stress, exhibiting, 167
Glass pin bevels, size, 201f
Glasses, defining. *See* Safety glasses
Glaze, definition, 169
Glazed frame, 301
Glazed wheels, 322
Glazing, definition, 322
Good faith effort, 340
Gradient arm
    setting, 221
    usage, 222f
Gradient lenses. *See* Edged gradient lenses
Gradient lines
    achievement. *See* Level gradient line
    horizontality, 222f
    straightness, 223f
Gradients. *See* Double gradients; Reverse gradient;
        Triple gradients
    creation. *See* Smooth gradient
    lens, dyeing. *See* Simple gradient lens
    tints, 220-224; 221f
Graph paper, usage, 60f
Grinding
    allowance, checking, 315
    angles, comparison. *See* Hand edging
Grit. *See* Wheels
    size, 320-321
        factor, 321f
    types/purposes. *See* Hand-edger wheels
Groove. *See* Bevel; Eyewire groove
    centering, 286f
    cleaning, ultrasonic cleaner (usage), 282f
    cutting, 280f
    depth, 155. *See also* Wheels
    location, 279f, 283. *See also* Basing groove location;
        Right-hand lens groove location
    measurements, 43f
    mountings, 276
        proficiency test questions, 290-291
    positioning. *See* Edges
    rims, tightening, 277f
    safety beveling, 284-285, 285f
    touchup, 284
    usability, 283f
Groove position
    basing, setting, 283f
    control lever, turning, 283f
    lens type, effect, 284t

Grooved Executive lenses, 283f
Grooved frame
    DBL, measurement, 43
    A dimension, measurement, 43
Grooved lens, mounting, 286-289
Grooved wheel
    design, 192f
    hidden bevel edge configuration, 202f
Groover. *See* Santinelli groover
    centering pin, locking, 280f
    chucks, placement, 281f
    cutting wheel
        cleanliness/coolness, 279f
        flush placement. *See* Wheels
    depth dial, 278
    settings, change, 281-282
    setup, 278-279
    switches, 280
    zero-adjuster knob, 278
Grooving. *See* Back edge; Front edge; Middle edge;
        Polycarbonate lenses; Recessed metal rim
    capability, 278f
    edge thickness, 277
    edger, usage, 286
    effect. *See* Impact resistance
    guide arms, lens positioning, 281f
    lens preparation, 278-279
    methods, 277-286
    process, commencement, 281f
    screen, 286f
Guide arms. *See* Spring-controlled guide arms
    lens positioning. *See* Grooving
    lifting, 284
Guide wheel, usage, 164f
Guided bevel systems, 162-164
    usage, 171. *See also* Edgers
        example, 165f
Guided scoring, 150

H
Hairline cracks, 258
Half-eye blocks, usage, 141f
Half-eye lenses, blocks (usage), 141
Half-mounted lens, 260
Half-padded nylon jaw pliers, 288
Half-padded pliers, usage, 244f. *See also* Nylon
        cords
Hand drills, historical note, 258-259
Hand edgers. *See* Ceramic wheel hand edgers;
        Diamond wheels
    coolant, disposal, 340
    surface, disadvantage. *See* Flat hand edger surface
    types, 190-192
    V-bevel grooves, usage, 191-192

Hand edging, 3f, 190, 202f. *See also* Antireflection-
        coated lenses; Frame's lens; Franklin-style
        lenses; Polycarbonate lenses
    commencement, 196f
    cutting speed factors, 197b
    grinding angles, comparison, 198f
    mistake, 196f
    parts, 192
    pressure, monitoring, 194-195
    proficiency test questions, 209-211
    rationale, 190
    results, improvement rules, 194-197
    rules, summarizing, 197
    steps, order, 199t
    usage, 206f
    wheel, listening, 195-197
Hand reduction. *See* Lens size
Hand tools, usage, 338
Hand wheel, even wetting, 193f
Hand-beveled lenses, apex placement, 160-161
Hand-edger wheels, 199
    flat surfaces, usage, 200f
    grits
        fineness, 194
        types/purposes, 192t
Hand-edging process, 194
Hand-marking. *See* Lenses
Hard lenses, 215
Hard-coated lenses, dyeing, 226
Hardened residue, 215f
Hardening, 3f, 6
Hazard Communication Program, 332
Hazard Communication Standard (HCS), 332,
        345-346
Hazardous chemicals. *See* Potentially hazardous
        chemicals
    list, 332-333, 345, 348
    posting/labeling requirements, 335-336
    presence, 334
Hazardous communication checklist, 334b
Hazardous communication program
    company policy, 345-347
    sample, 345-347
Hazardous waste, 331
Hazards
    awareness. *See* Electrical hazards; Slippery hazards;
        Wet hazards
    control, 331
    correcting, 334
    engineering out, 340-341
    OSHA impact, 331
    prevention, 331
    standards. *See* Chemical Hazard Communication
        Standard

Hazards *(Continued)*
  warning, 333
  written communication program, 332
HAZCOM. *See* Chemical Hazard Communication
    Standard
HCS. *See* Hazard Communication Standard
Health effects, 333
Health hazard data, 350
Health training/education, 331
Heat sensitivities, 226
Heat transfer fluids, disposal, 340
Heat treating, 6
Heat-tempered glass, 303
Heat-tempered lens, dehardening, 305
Heat-treated lens, maltese-cross pattern identification,
    305f
Heat-treating process, 303
Heat-treating unit, 202
Height. *See* Major reference point height; Segment
    height
Hex wrench, usage, 255, 257f
Hidden bevel, 321
  cosmetic advantage, 161f
  edge configuration. *See* Grooved wheel
  edge shapes, 192f
Hidden circles, 103. *See also* Dotted hidden circles
  location, 35f
  raise, calculation, 400
  usage, 400-401, 428-429. *See also* Progressive
    addition lens centration; Progressive addition
    lenses
Hidden marks, 34. *See also* Progressive addition lenses
Hidden-bevel lenses, 191-192
  lens size reduction, 201
Hide-A-Bevel, 161
Hide-A-Bevel wheels
  placement, advice, 163f
  usage, 162
High adds
  power, amount. *See* Plastic flat-top lenses
  usage. *See* Adhesive pad blocking
High base metal blocks, 141f
High bifocal segment, 32f
High impact standard, 298
High mass impact test, 301
High minus lenses, 279f. *See also* Thick-edged high
    minus lenses
High near addition lens, creation, 123f
High plus aspheric lenticular lenses, OC blocking, 62
High plus lens
  base curve steepness, 142f
  plus direction, 284f
High-impact marking requirements, 301
High-impact requirements. *See* Safety eyewear

High-impact testing requirements, 300-301
High-impact thickness requirements, 300
High-index glass, 168-169
High-index lenses, 168-169
  dyeing, 226-227
High-index materials, 250
High-index minus lenses, thin centers, 277
High-index plastic, 169, 227, 250
  lenses, 3f
    edge polishing, 208
High-minus back curves, 199f
High-minus lens, 179f, 251
  back edge, pin beveling, 201f
  back pin bevel, application, 200f
  curvature, amount, 180f
  rear surface, pin beveling, 199
High-plus lenses, 179f
  edge locations, appearance, 164f
High-velocity impact test
  firing, 301
  survival, 300
Hinges, angling, 243f
Holding
  area, relationship. *See* Adhesive pad
  back-to-back position, 252, 313
  device, 18
  mechanism, 17f
  pliers, usage, 244f, 245f
  proper technique. *See* Edge smoothing
  system, 261
Holes. *See* Patterns
  180-degree line, correspondence, 47f
  back side, chipping, 254f
  chamfering/smoothing, 254-255
  chipping, 255f
  cone tools, usage, 259f
  diameters. *See* Variable-hole diameters
  drilling, 254f, 269f
    height, 261f
  location
    marking. *See* Temporal hole
    specifications, transfer ability, 262
  placement. *See* Central hole placement
Homemade patterns, 54, 418
Horizontal 180-degree reference line, marking, 252f
Horizontal alignment, MRP usage, 132f
Horizontal bar. *See* Pattern makers
Horizontal compensation, 60
Horizontal decentration, 82, 395
  calculation, 394, 396, 397
    boxing system, usage, 50-52, 75-76
  questions, 93
Horizontal eye, increase, 48f
Horizontal lens size, 40

Horizontal meridian
file marks, 224f
usage, 124f
Horizontal midline, 41, 113, 118
definition, 41
vertical decentration, 394
Horizontal misalignment. *See* Pattern centers
Horizontal MRP, location, 50f
Horizontal OC error, compensation, 91f
Horizontal pattern dimension, 61b
Horizontal prism, 395-397
calculation. *See* Progressive addition lenses
Horizontal protractor line, usage, 78
Horizontal reference
line, 82, 126. *See also* Centration device
equidistance, 126f
marks. *See* Non-water-soluble horizontal reference
marks
segment center usage, 116f
Horizontally displaced pattern centers, compensation,
59
Housekeeping program, 338
Hoya Desktop, 107t
Human error, 314f
Humphrey autolensmeter, upright design, 21
Humphrey Lens Analyzer, 23f, 24f, 219f
layout screen, 24f
usage. *See* Lenses
Humping. *See* Nasal humping
HyperIndex lenses. *See* 1.66 HyperIndex lenses

I
Identifying lens, 300
Immediate distances, progressive addition lenses
(usage), 105-110
Impact requirements. *See* Safety eyewear
Impact resistance, 292
drilling, effect, 296
grooving, effect, 296
lens coatings, effect, 295-296
lens processing, effect, 295-296
proficiency test questions, 306-308
reedging, effect, 296
surface scratches, effect, 296
test requirements, 293
testing, 3f
Impact-resistant lens material, 297
Impact-resistant quality, increase, 296
Impregnated wheels, 322
Incident light
amount, 227
reflection amount, 227
Incorrect segment inset, checking. *See* Flat-top
multifocals

Index mark, adjustment, 310
Individual testing, batch testing (contrast), 294-295
Industrial abrasives, 321
In-edger drill, 249, 266
Injuries, 338f
documentation, 337
Inking
amount. *See* Lensmeter
mechanism, 17f
Inserted lens, orientation, 238f
Insertion, 3f, 235. *See also* Metal frames; Plastic frames
checklist, 236-237
definition, 6
importance. *See* Bevel
plastic frame material differences, 238t
process, conclusion, 237f
proficiency test questions, 246
Inset. *See* Segment inset; Total inset
comparison. *See* Decentration
Instrument grid, origin, 82
Insurance. *See* Liability insurance
inclusion, 337
Intermediate viewing, 4f
straight-ahead position, 106
Intermediate/near progressive lenses
advantages, 105-106
full range, usage, 110
layout, 106-109
ordering, 106
variations, 107t
Intermediate/near specialty progressives
comparison. *See* Standard progressive
Internal lens stress, visibility, 167
Internal stress
control, 303f
creation, 202
Interpupillary distance (PD), 51f, 87f. *See also*
Binocular distance PD; Binocular PD;
Finished PD; Monocular PD; Near PD
accuracy, 92
ensuring, 122f
definition, 43
favoring. *See* Distance PD; Near PD
incorrect distance, 89-92
combination. *See* Oblique cylinder distances
information, 173f
measurements, 182
pushing, 89-92, 95
setting, 63f
standards, 92
usage, 63f. *See also* 69/60 PD; Decentration per lens
Interview (Essilor), 107t
Inverted prism lens, usage, 18f
Invisible bifocals, 398

Irregular patterns, usage. *See* Centration skills series
Iseikonic lenses, testing exemption, 294

J
Jaw pliers. *See* Half-padded nylon jaw pliers

K
Kiln, usage, 303

L
Labeling requirements. *See* Hazardous chemicals
Labels, usage, 346
Laboratory
    labeling requirements. *See* Food and Drug
        Administration
    space, saving, 70f
    thermometer, usage. *See* Bath temperature
    waste management, problems, 339-340
LAB-Tech DM-3 Drilling System, 262
Laminate lenses, testing exemption, 294
Laminated layer, notches (usage), 29f
Laminated lenses, 170
Large businesses, OSHA impact, 331
Large-jawed plier, usage, 186
Larger-than-standard patterns, 153
Latex gloves, usage, 336
Layout. *See* Edging; Intermediate/near progressive
        lenses
    blocker
        deblocker, mounting, 187f
        integration. *See* Frame tracers
    definition, 6
    fitting cross, usage, 398-399
    lens protractor, usage, 77f
    mode, 24f
        mires, usage, 26f
    verification, 34f
Ledge corners, 201
Left decentration, 78f
Left lens
    back view, 115f
    distance decentration, 118f
    segment
        drop, usage, 118f
        inset, usage, 118f
    total inset, 118f
Lens centration, 6
    centration instrument, usage, 82
    historical background, 76-78
    instruments, 81-82
    lens protractor, usage, 77-78
    mechanics, 75
Lens drilling, 251-257
    charts, usage, 251-252

Lens drilling *(Continued)*
    electric stand drills, usage, 253-255
    guides/templates, 251-252
    option, 180
Lens materials
    effects. *See* Dyeing
    removal, 194
    requirements. *See* Patternless edging
Lens Prep, 216
Lens protractor, 77
    degree scales, 77
    lens, positioning, 79f
    usage. *See* Flat-top multifocals; Layout; Lens
        centration
Lens shapes, 39
    C size, 40f
    challenge questions, 74
    change. *See* Frame's lens
    covering, 42f
    determination, 6
    ED, determination, 42f
    eyesize change, effect, 46-49
    proficiency test questions, 71-74
    tilting, 63f
    viewing screen, usage, 177, 177f
Lens size, 9, 287. *See also* Horizontal lens size; Vertical
        lenses
    accuracy, checking. *See* Dry cut edgers
        closure pliers, usage, 167f
    checking. *See* Metal frames
    edging, 168f
    hand reduction, 199-202
    information, 173f
    limitation, 20f
    reduction, 192f. *See also* Hidden-bevel lenses
        hand, bracing, 202f
Lens spotting, 5-6, 8. *See also* Polarizing lenses;
        Round-segment lenses
    challenge questions, 37-38
    prism
        inclusion, 20-21
        noninclusion, 16-18
    process, 124f
    proficiency test questions, 35-38
Lens-curing factor, 215-216
Lenses. *See* Antireflection-coated lenses; Laminated
        lenses; Plastic lenses; Polycarbonate lenses;
        Slotted lenses
    analyzer, 5
    back-to-back placement, 314f
    bevel. *See* Bevel
    blank. *See* Blanks
        size, effect. *See* Frames
    blocking. *See* Blocking

Lenses (*Continued*)

center thickness. *See* Minus lens center thickness

checking, back-lighted crossed polaroids (usage), 168f

chucking, 159

classification. *See* Trivex

cleaning, 208-209. *See also* Glass; Plastic lenses; Polycarbonate lenses

cleanup, 6

coating, effects. *See* Dyeing; Impact resistance

color. *See* Color

conditioner, 216

curvature
    amount, 65f, 66f
    mismatch. *See* Frame curvature

deblocking. *See* Adhesive pad-blocked lenses; Metal alloy-blocked lenses; Suction-blocked lenses; Wax-blocked lenses

defect, 12f

degree scale, 77

designation, 18f

different materials, edging variations, 167-170

dispensation. *See* Non-impact-resistant lenses

distance. *See* Distance between lenses

dotting, 80f

drilling. *See* Blocked lenses

drills, types, 249

dyeing. *See* Antireflection-coated lenses; Hard-coated lenses; High-index lenses; Plastic polarizing lenses; Polycarbonate lenses; Pre-AR coated lenses

edges. *See* Edges

edging. *See* Edging

feeling. *See* Edge thickness

finishing process, overview, 4-6

flaws, visual inspection, 10-11

front base curve, matching, 142f

front curve, 165f

generator, control, 67

grasping, 151f

guide, application, 261f

hand-marking, 80f, 312f

hardening. *See* Glass lenses
    determination, 305

holders, 222f. *See also* Color coding lens holders
    cleaning, 229
    usage, 217f

holding. *See* Holding

impact resistance. *See* Impact resistance

insertion. *See* Insertion; Metal frames; Plastic frames

insufficient size, 88-89

layout. *See* Layout

marking, 251-257. *See also* Visible lens marking
    requirements. *See* American National Standards Institute

Lenses (*Continued*)

measurement
    boxing system, 39-44
    Humphrey Lens Analyzer, usage, 225f

measuring instrument, 14f

minus cylinder form, reading, 12-16

mounting. *See* Mounting

notching, 257-260
    milling bit, usage, 258

off-center optical center, inclusion. *See* Stock lenses

opening, covering. *See* Frames

optical center, 18-19

optics, effect. *See* Peripheral lens optics

orientation, 29f, 125f. *See also* 180-degree meridian; Inserted lens; Prism
    improvement, 252f

pair, salvaging, 207f

patterns. *See* Patterns

pin beveling, 198-199

placement, 19f, 77, 78f

plus cylinder form, reading, 16

positioning. *See* Lens protractor; Prismatic lens; Segment

preparation. *See* Grooving; Tinting

prescription, 108f
    prism inclusion, 18-20
    verification. *See* Multifocal lenses

prism restrictions. *See* Aspheric lenses; Atoric lenses

processing
    effect. *See* Impact resistance
    sequence, 3f

protector discs, application. *See* Antireflection coated lenses

reedging. *See* Frames

refractive characteristics, 13f

removal, 245f, 287

replacement, problems. *See* One-lens replacement

retightening. *See* Loose lens

rotating pliers, 205

rotation. *See* Rotation

ruining, 27f

salvaging. *See* Blemished lenses; Off-axis lens

scratches, 28f
    appearance. *See* Edged lens

selection, 9-10

sizing, 287

slippage, causes. *See* Blocks

spoilage, reduction, 256f

standard alignment. *See* Standard alignment

surface, standard cross mark placement, 116f

table
    placement, 268f
    repositioning, 267f

terminology. *See* Finished lens; Semifinished lens

Lenses *(Continued)*
  testing. *See* Testing
  thickness. *See* Thickness
    incompatibility. *See* Straps
  tinting. *See* Tinting
  top, marking, 224
  tracing. *See* Tracing
  type, effect. *See* Groove
  usage. *See* Shape tracing
  verification, 6, 100
  waviness, 13f
Lenses only order, 57f, 157
Lensmeter
  accuracy, increasing, 83
  aperture, 15f, 100f
  axis setting, 124f
  care, 310-311
  exterior, cleaning, 311
  eyepiece
    focusing, 11-12
    setting, 13f
  inking, amount, 311
  optics, cleanliness, 310-311
  prism, accuracy, 310
  screen, representation, 24f
  spotting mechanism. *See* Autolensmeters; Manual
    lensmeter
  target, 20, 23
  usage, 11-16, 146-147, 395. *See also* Single vision
    sphere spotting; Spherocylinder lenses
  zero reading, 310f
Lensmeter dots, 395-397
  guide, 223f
  placement, 415
  position, 411
  raising/lowering. *See* Central lensmeter dot
  reference, usage, 252f
Lensmeter-measured imbalance, eliminates, 206
Lensometer, 5
Lenticular cataract lenses, testing exemption, 294
Lenticular lenses, 63f
  OC blocking. *See* High plus aspheric lenticular
    lenses
Level gradient line, achievement, 221-223
Liability insurance, 337
Light boxes
  definition, 220f
  usage, 218
Light scattering, 12f
Limbus, definition, 45f
Liners, inclusion. *See* Nylon cord frames
Lines, overlapping, 252f
Liquid resin, pouring, 5f
Liquid wastes, removal, 339

Lithium ions, usage, 303
Lock-glue
  adherence, 270f
  application, 270f, 271f
Locking mechanism, loosening, 264, 269f
Loose lens, retightening, 289
Low base metal blocks, 141f
Low minus lenses, 279-280
Lower nasal part, bevel (snapping), 237f
Low-minus-powered lenses, thinning, 101f
Low-plus-powered lenses, 280
Low-powered lens. *See* Thin-edged low-powered lens
Lubrication, 309

M
Machine hazards, 331
Magnetic stirrers, usage, 214
Maintenance, 309
  proficiency test questions, 317-319
  schedules, 309
Major meridians, 11f, 19
  axis wheel, approach, 15
  difference, 16
Major reference point (MRP), 21f, 41f, 43-44
  centering, 51f
  checking. *See* Flat-top multifocals
  definition, 19
  disappearance. *See* Multifocal lenses
  distance power, checking, 33f
  dot, positioning, 129f
  importance, 99f
  locating, dotting, 410
  lowering, 61
  marking, 27
  misplacement, 129f
  movement, 395
  placement, 119b, 393, 434, 442f
    errors, compensation, 122b
    problem, 119f
  position, 410-412
    checking, 122f
    correction, 122f
  positioning, 46f, 58
  relationship. *See* Optical center
  segment positions, relationship, 115f
  setting, 127
  spotting, 418
  usage, 101f. *See also* Dotted MRP; Horizontal
    alignment; Prism
  vertical position, 43, 84f
  vertical positioning, 90f
  vertical specification, 394
Major reference point (MRP) height, 29, 44, 81f
  centration. *See* Practitioner-specified MRP height

Major reference point (MRP) height (Continued)
    conversion, 79
    difference, 92
    specification, 113
Major reference point (MRP) location, 29, 49f, 85f.
        See also Horizontal MRP
    accuracy, checking. See Spotted MRP
    checking, 121
    determination, 413
    indication, 21
Maltese-cross pattern, identification. See Heat-treated
        lens
Management
    leadership, 331
        request. See Material Safety Data Sheet
    support. See Safety program
Manual chucking, 159
Manual lensmeter, spotting mechanism, 26f
Manual patterned edgers, eyesize adjustments, 316
Manufacturer, defining, 295
Marker/blocker, usage, 77
Marking. See Chipped portion; Etching; Lenses; Nasal
        hole; Safety frames
    alignment, 55
    coquilles, usage. See Three-piece mountings
    frames, usage. See Semirimless mountings
    methods. See Safety lenses
    pen, usage, 259
    pins, 311
    requirements. See American National Standards
        Institute; Basic-impact marking requirements;
        High-impact marking requirements
Marks. See Off-axis marks
    overlapping. See Reference
Masks, usage, 336
Matching. See Color; Uncuts
Material Safety Data Sheet (MSDS), 332-333, 345
    index, 348
    location, 346
    management request, 333
    sample, 349-350
Matte black background, 12f
MBS. See Minimum blank size
Mean fracture load, 295
Measuring mode, 24f
Mechanical center, 64f
    boxing center
        equivalence, 50
        nonequivalence, 52
    positioning. See Pattern
    usage, 58
Mechanically controlled method, 162
Meridians. See Major meridians
    light color. See Central meridian

Meridians (Continued)
    uniform power, 27
    usage, 15f
Metal alloy blocking, 138, 139
Metal alloy-blocked lenses, deblocking, 185-186
Metal blocks, 140. See also High base metal blocks; Low
        base metal blocks; Regular base metal blocks
    color-coded types, 141f
    selection criteria, 142f
    shape, molding, 140f
Metal frames
    indication, 176f
    lens insertion, 239
    lens size, checking, 199-200
    standard alignment, 243-246
Metal rims. See Frames
    grooving. See Recessed metal rim
Metal temple spread, 243-245
Metal-bonded finishing wheels, 322f
    dressing, 324
    performance, 324
Metal-bonded roughing wheels, 322
    dressing, 323-324
    performance, 323
Metal-bonded wheel (polishing usage), 322f
Micro-cracking, 226
Middle edge, grooving, 279-280
Milling bit
    ability, 263-264
    usage. See Lenses; Notching
Mini-bevel wheels, usage, 162
    examples, 164f
Minimum blank size (MBS), 41f, 86-88
    equation, 9
    questions, 94
Minimum fitting height, 98
Minus cylinder form, 12
    reading. See Lenses
Minus edges, minimization, 250
Minus lens
    blank. See Uncut minus lens blank
    center thickness, 9
    decentering, 91f
    faceted edge, usage, 166f
Minus lenticular lenses, testing exemption, 294
Mires
    crossing. See Circular mires
    usage. See Layout
Molten salt, 304f
Monocular distance decentration, determination, 400
Monocular PD, 76, 99
    centration, 393-394, 422-423
    request, 107
    usage, 101. See also Decentration

Mounting. *See* Balgrip mountings; Double-hole
       mountings; Drilled mountings; Groove;
       Grooved lens; Notched mountings; Rimless
       mountings; Slotted mountings
   adapter, usage, 67f
   definition, 6
   drilled lens, attachment, 255-257
   flaws, detection, 257
   line. *See* 180-degree mounting line
   marking
      coquilles, usage. *See* Three-piece mountings
      frames, usage. *See* Semirimless mountings
   system, 253
   table, usage, 268f
   usage. *See* Double-strap mountings
Movable line, 88f
   indication. *See* Single vision lenses
   presetting, 85f
Movable vertical line. *See* Single vision lenses
   usage, 82
MRP. *See* Major reference point
MSDS. *See* Material Safety Data Sheet
Multifocal lenses (multifocals), 5f, 98. *See also*
       Flat-top-style multifocals; Franklin-style
       multifocals; Segmented multifocal lenses
   categories, 97-98
   difficulties. *See* Noncentered pattern
   heights, 46f
   order, 114
   preparation, 2
   prescription verification, 29-32
   segment portion, major reference point
      disappearance, 31-32
   spotting, 29-32. *See also* Flat-top multifocals
   method. *See* Flat-top-segment multifocals;
      Round-segment-multifocals
   usage, 18f
Multifocal prescription, pattern usage, 62f
Myodisc lenses, testing exemption, 294

N
Narrow B frames, blocks (usage), 141
Nasal add, 203, 204
   achievement, 204f
Nasal corner, placement, 289f
Nasal cut, 203-204
   achievement. *See* Symmetrical nasal cut
Nasal direction, 289f
Nasal edge. *See* Eyewires
   relationship. *See* Nasal hole
Nasal flare, 204
Nasal half. *See* Edged lenses
Nasal hole
   horizontal zero point, 266f

Nasal hole *(Continued)*
   marking/drilling, 260f. *See also* Semirimless
      mountings
   nasal edge, relationship, 265f
Nasal humping, 238f
Nasal lens straps, bending, 268
Nasal rim. *See* Frames
Nasal side
   drilling setup, 265f
   matching, 65f
Nasal slots, positioning, 263
Nasalward segment rotation, 31f
Near add (determination), front vertex powers
      (usage), 100f
Near PD, 62f, 76
   accuracy, 121
   alteration, 122b, 124
   favoring, 121-124
   maintenance, 122b
   relationship. *See* Distance PD
Near portion, placement, 102f
Near power
   amount, 100f
   back vertex power verification, 100f
Near reference point (NRP), 33f, 98
   definition, 34, 98
   location, 104f
Near segment, centering, 122f
Near working distances, progressive addition lenses
      (usage), 105-110
Neoprene gasket, usage, 293-294
Neutralizer, 333
   disposal, 340
   process, 219
   sensitivities, 226
   usage. *See* Tints
No Smoking signs, display, 335
Non prismatic single vision lenses, 18f
Noncellular acetate, 237-239
Noncentered pattern, usage, 58-62
   consequences, 57-62
   multifocal lenses, difficulties, 58
Nonelectric hand-held drills, 249
Non-impact-resistant lenses, dispensation, 293
Non-premarked progressive lenses, 34-35
Nonproportionality, 48
Non-routine tasks, 346
Nonslip mat, usage, 339f
Non-water-soluble horizontal reference marks, 32,
      34
Non-water-soluble marks, usage, 102
Non-water-soluble progressive lens markings,
      34
Normal-thickness lenses, 267

Nosepads, 246
Notched mountings, 247
    bibliography, 273
    proficiency test questions, 274-275
Notches
    beveling, 259f
    cone tools, usage, 259f
    cutting, preparation, 266f
    usage. *See* Laminated layer
Notching. *See* Lenses
    accuracy, 266f
    milling bit, usage, 258f
NRP. *See* Near reference point
Nylon cord frames, 57, 66, 248
    liners, inclusion, 289-290
    types, 287f
    usage, 277f
Nylon cords, 276
    clipping, 287
    cutting, 287f
    dyeing, 228
    mounting, edge grooving, 3f
    pressing, half-padded pliers (usage), 288f
    proficiency test questions, 290-291
    removal, 286f
    replacement, 288f
    sizing, 288f
    stretching, 288
    tension, checking, 288-289, 290f
    threading, 287f, 289f
Nylon supras, 248

O
Oblique axis, 22f
Oblique cylinder distances, incorrect interpupillary
        distances (combination), 91-92
OC. *See* Optical center
Occupational progressives, 106
Occupational Safety and Health Administration
        (OSHA), 298, 329, 330
    complaints, 335
    Form 200, 337
    Form 300A, 344
    Hazard Communication Standard, 345
    impact. *See* Employers; Hazards; Large businesses;
        Small businesses
    inspections, 331
    poster, display, 335
    relationship. *See* American National Standards
        Institute
    requirements, 331, 334, 336
        agencies, relationship, 330
    standards, 330
    website, 341

Occupational Safety and Health (OSH) Act, 330, 337
    responsibilities, 344
Off-axis lens, salvaging, 205
    steps, 206f
Off-axis marks, 314f
Off-axis pattern, 54
Off-center optical center, inclusion. *See* Stock lenses
Off-center target, compensation difficulty, 311f
Off-site location, frame tracer usage, 70f
OLA. *See* Optical Laboratories Association
Old lens
    tracing, 66f
    usage. *See* Frames; Shape tracing
One-lens replacement, problem, 58
Open temple spread, 242
Ophthalmic lenses, minimum thickness. *See* Dress
        ophthalmic lenses
Optical center (OC). *See* Lenses; Sphere lenses
    accuracy amount, requirement, 92
    blocking. *See* High plus aspheric lenticular lenses
    centering, 15f
    decentration, amount, 86
    displacement, 21f
    error, compensation. *See* Horizontal OC error
    location, 29, 31f, 442f. *See also* Distance OC
    MRP, relationship, 98, 127
    not in line of sight, 19-20
    placement, errors, 91f
    positioning, 25f
    vertical placement. *See* Distance OC
Optical clarity, variation, 98f
Optical endpoint, 27f
Optical Laboratories Association (OLA), 249, 276-277
    program, 297
    Tech Topics, 296
Optical laboratory, 1-2
Optics, cleanliness. *See* Lensmeter
Order entry, 3f, 177
    area, frame tracer (usage), 67
OSH Act. *See* Occupational Safety and Health Act
OSHA. *See* Occupational Safety and Health
        Administration
Overplussed straight-ahead gaze, 109f
Over-thinning, 101f

P
Paired spherocylinder lens, custom surfacing, 2
Pantoscopic angle, 242
    change, 245f
Parallax
    definition, 77
    effect. *See* Errors
    error, 77
    prevention, 205

Parallelism testing, flat surface touch test (usage), 242f
Partially finished lenses, record keeping requirements, 295
Pattern centers
    compensation. *See* Horizontally displaced pattern centers; Vertically displaced pattern centers
      displacement compensation, 61b
        amount, determination, 61b
      horizontal misalignment, 419
      horizontal/vertical misalignment, 420
      vertical misalignment, 418-419
Pattern errors
    checking, 59-60
    direction/amount, determination, 60-62
    vertical compensation, 81
Pattern makers, 39
    frame centering, 53f
    horizontal bar, 54f
    models, 53
    usage. *See* Center; Decenter
Pattern making, 52-57
    edgers, usage, 57
    frame setup, 53-54
    lens tracing, usage, 54-57
    matching, 55-56
Pattern size, 46
    calculation, 84
    check, grid (usage), 60f
    standard (36.5 mm), 153
    usage, 155f
Patterned bevel edger, example, 165f
Patterned edgers, 39
    axis accuracy, checking, 313-315
    definition, 6
    eyesize adjustments. *See* Manual patterned edgers
    options, 180
Patterned edging, 149-171
    cutting/chipping, 150-151
    historical background, 149
    process, 152-167
Patternless edgers, 39. *See also* Computer-assisted patternless edgers
    definition, 6
    electronic link. *See* Tracers
    features, 286
    laboratory interface, 181-182
    options, 180
    patterns, usage, 172
      capability, 69f
    questions, 176f
    usage, 171-172
    viewing screens, 177-180; 177f, 178f
Patternless edging, 149, 171-182
    electronic shape, 172

Patternless edging *(Continued)*
    frame materials, requirements, 176-177
    lens materials, requirements, 176-177
    possibilities, 172-182
    systems, 155
      input, 173f
      technology, 165f
Patterns, 39. *See also* Homemade patterns; Larger-than-standard patterns; Lenses
    blanks
      mounting, 57
      variety, 55f
    challenge questions, 74
    creation, 419
    cutter, usage, 56f
    cutting, 55f
    difference, 46
    dimension. *See* Horizontal pattern dimension; Vertical pattern dimension
    distortion (prevention), larger patterns (usage), 153
    holes, 48f
    measurements, 44-50. *See also* Box-o-Graph
      system, 46f
    mechanical center, 49-50
      positioning, 50-52
      relationship. *See* Boxing center
    placement. *See* Edgers
    proficiency test questions, 71-74
    rotational center, 81
    roughness, smoothing, 56
    shadow system, 84
    stock, maintenance, 40f
    system, function, 47-48
    terminology, 44-50
    usage, 49f, 54-55. *See also* Multifocal prescription; Patternless edgers; Shape tracing consequences. *See* Noncentered pattern
    vertically displaced mechanical centers, usage, 59f
PD. *See* Interpupillary distance
Peripheral lens optics, effect, 171
Personal protective equipment, 336
Photochromic glass, 168
Photochromic lenses
    temperature, importance, 304
    tempering, 303
Photochromic process, 305
Photochromic salt bath, 304f
Photometer, usage, 217, 218f
Pin beveling, 192, 197-199. *See also* Back edge; Bevel apex; High-minus lens; Lenses; Rimless lenses
    breakage prevention, 197
    cosmetic considerations, 197

Pin beveling *(Continued)*
    reasons, 197-198
    wearer safety, 197-198
Pins
    bevel. *See* Glass lenses; Plastic lenses
    movement. *See* Spring-coupled pins
    usage. *See* Centering
Pittsburgh Plate Glass Co. *See* Columbia Resin 39
Plano cylinder lenses, decentration, 19
Plastic. *See* High-index plastic
    removal, 269f
Plastic blocks, 140-141
    removal, 188f
Plastic bushing, 255
Plastic flat-beveled lenses, 201f
Plastic flat-top lenses
    high add power, amount, 146f
    segment amount, 146f
Plastic frames
    lens insertion, 235-236; 236b
    materials, differences. *See* Insertion
    shape, retaining, 64
    standard alignment, 239-243
    stretching, 167
Plastic lenses, 169. *See also* Columbia Resin 39
    blocks, advantages, 141f
    cleaning, 209
    edges
        luster, ensuring, 208f
        polishing, 207-208
    edging, 166f, 322f
    marking, 299
    pin bevel, 201f
    regular bevel, 201f
    sandblasting, 299
    twist, 186f
    warping, 167, 200
Plastic polarizing lenses, dyeing, 228
Plastic sludge, removal, 316-317
Plastic strap, usage, 290f
Plus cylinder form, 12
    reading. *See* Lenses
Plus cylinder power readings. *See* Direct plus cylinder
        power readings
Plus edges, thickness (amount), 250
Plus lenses
    blank size effect, 9-10
    edge thickness errors, 250-251
    faceted edge, usage, 166f
Plus-minus scale, 154. *See also* Edger dials
    zero setting, 155f
Plus-minus-powered lenses, thinning, 101f
Pneumatic chucking, 159
Polariscope, usage, 305

Polarizing lenses
    spotting, 28-29, 29f
    testing exemption, 294
Polaroids, usage. *See* Crossed polaroids; Lenses
Polished edges, usage, 166
Polishing, 3f. *See also* Glass; Plastic lenses
    drum tool, usage, 208
    machine. *See* Automatic polishing machine
    rag wheel, usage, 207-208
Polycarbonate lens edging, 166f
    process, completion, 170
    stress, 170
    wheels, usage, 162
Polycarbonate lenses, 3f, 169-170
    classification, 277
    cleaning, 209
    drilling, 258
    dye distribution, 226
    edge polishing, 208
    edging process, 170
    grooving, 285
    hand edging, 201-202
    stress, 170
    thin centers, 277
    tinting, 226
        suggestions, 227b
    wet/dry edging, selection, 170
Polycarbonate material, curled threads, 202f
Posting requirements. *See* Hazardous chemicals
Potassium nitrate, usage, 303
Potentially hazardous chemicals, 332b
Power. *See* Cylinder power
    calibration, 310
    change, 106f
    cross, imagining/sketching, 124f
    increase, 398
    range. *See* 1.25D power
    reading. *See* Direct plus cylinder power readings
        progressive zone changing power, impact, 100f
    tools, usage, 338
    variation, 11
    verification, 34f. *See also* Spheres; Spherocylinders
        crossed-line-target lensmeter, usage. *See*
            Spherocylinder lenses
    wheel, turning, 13
Practitioner-specified MRP height, centration, 393-394,
        422-423
Pre-AR coated lenses, dyeing, 228
Precast FreeBlock blocking, 138, 139-140
Pre-edging, 161
Prefinished bifocals, spherocylinder lenses
        (matching), 2
Premarked line, scoring, 150f
Premarked progressives, verification, 32-34

Prentice's Rule, 19-20
  usage, 120. *See also* Prism
Prescribed cylinder axis, 5f
Prescribed prism, 98-100, 127, 395, 424-425
  horizontal/vertical components, inclusion, 21
  inclusion. *See* Autolensmeters
  noninclusion. *See* Autolensmeters
Prescription (Rx), 23
  accuracy, 310
    ethical factors, 92
  fabrication, 41f
  lens, manufacture/mounting, 66f
Pressure blocking, 138-139
Primer coatings, benefit, 296
Prism. *See* Base-in prism; Yoked base down prism
  accuracy. *See* Lensmeter
  amount. *See* Base up prism
    calculation, 91
    lens orientation, 26f
  calculation. *See* Progressive addition lenses
  compensation devices, instrument checking, 311f
  correction. *See* Unwanted vertical prism
  figuring, Prentice's rule (usage), 124f
  horizontal/vertical components. *See* Prescribed
    prism
  inclusion/noninclusion. *See* Lens spotting
  induction, 19
  lenses. *See* Blemished prism lenses
    usage. *See* Inverted prism lens
  restrictions. *See* Aspheric lenses; Atoric lenses
  segment multifocals, testing exemption, 294
  standards. *See* Unwanted prism
  thinning, 34
  understanding, 397
  usage. *See* Base down prism
  verification, MRP usage, 99f
Prism reference point (PRP), 33f, 98
  change, 98f
  definition, 19, 34, 98, 99f
  lens verification, 101f
  location, 104f
  usage, 102f
Prismatic effect, 22f, 120f
  change, 123
  creation, 20f
  verification, 101f
Prismatic lens, positioning, 22f
Program evaluation, 331
Progressive addition lens centration, 97
  conventional steps, 102b
  hidden circles
    steps, 103b
    usage, 102-105
  proficiency test questions, 110-111

Progressive addition lenses, 4, 32-35. *See also* Centration
    skills series; Occupational progressives;
    Specialty progressive addition lenses
  conventional centration, 99-102
  description, 98-105
  distance power, verification, 100f
  fitting cross, 45f
    vertical position, 44
  hidden marks, 440f
  horizontal prism, calculation, 101
  impact. *See* Upper distance portion
  marked 180-degree reference marks, 237
  mistake, 310
  positioning. *See* Blocking; Centration
    hidden circles, usage, 103
  power, 33f
  reference points, 33f, 98-99
  usage. *See* Immediate distances; Near working
    distances
  verification. *See* Premarked progressives
  vertical position, calculation, 102
  vertical prism, 100-101
  visible marks, 440f
Progressive corridor, 33f
  width, 98f
Progressive lenses. *See* Non-premarked progressive
    lenses
  fitting cross raise, 49f
  fitting cross system, usage, 102f
  markings. *See* Non-water-soluble progressive lens
    markings
Progressive zone, 33f, 101f
  changing power, impact. *See* Power
Protective tape, usage. *See* Adhesive pad blocking
Protractor. *See* Lenses
  line. *See* Vertical protractor line
    usage. *See* Horizontal protractor line
  usage. *See* Centration
PRP. *See* Prism reference point
Pupil
  center, 45f
  location, 51f
  vertical plane, 50f

Q
Quality
  control, 12f
  sacrificing, 27f

R
Radius, doubling, 42f
Rag wheel
  buffing compound, usage, 208f
  usage. *See* Polishing

Rainbow effect, 168f
Raised center type, 52
Raised multifocal lenses, testing exemption, 294
Rat-tail files, 255
    tapering, 256f
    usage, 273. *See also* Drilled hole
Reactivity data, 350
Reader replacements, 106
Reading glasses, decentration, 76
Rear bevel, pressure application, 199
Reblocking, 187f
    combination. *See* Deblocking
Recessed metal rim, grooving, 285-286
    cutting wheels, usage, 285-286
Reedging. *See* Frame's lens
    effect. *See* Impact resistance
Referee test, 293
Reference
    height, 45f
    line. *See* Horizontal reference; Vertical reference
    marks, overlapping, 313f
    points. *See* Distance reference point; Major
        reference point; Near reference point; Prism
        reference point; Progressive addition lenses
    scale, 77
Reflective screen, usage, 262
Refraction, index, 227
Refractive power, limitation, 20f
Regular base metal blocks, 141f
Remote-site dispensary, tracer placement, 67-70
Replacement lens, 58
Required cylinder axis, 125f
Reshaping, hand (bracing), 202f
Respotting, 207f
Restringing, procedure, 286-289
Reverse gradient, 224
Riffler file, usage, 257
Right decentration, 78f
Right lens, removal, 207f
Right round-segment lens, total decentration, 128f
Right-hand lens groove location, 156f
Rimless frames, 57, 66, 248
Rimless lenses
    edge thickness, 250-251
Rimless lenses, pin beveling, 199
Rimless mountings, 248f, 249f, 273f
    defined, 247-249
    description, 255, 257
    parts, 248-249
    types, 247-248
Rimless pattern, marking, 161
Rimless style eyewear, flat edges (usage), 161
Rimless three-piece mounting, 248f
Rimless use, materials comparison, 249

Rimmed frame, 180-degree line (file marking), 224f
Rims
    preshaping. *See* Eyewires
    tightening. *See* Groove
Rodenstock Office, 107t
    intermediate/near design specialty progressive lens,
        comparison. *See* Standard progressive
Rolled edge
    effect. *See* Edge thickness
    usage, 166
Rotated lens, 240
Rotation, 17f, 28f. *See also* Semifinished lens;
        Spherocylinder lenses
    checking, 237
    direction, 196f
        indication, 195f
    speed, 194-195, 198
    usage, 194f
Rotational center, 49. *See also* Patterns
    relationship. *See* Boxing center
Rough file surface, 257f
Roughing wheels. *See* Bonded roughing wheels;
        Electroplated roughing wheels
    dressing. *See* Metal-bonded roughing wheels
        sticks, 323f
    retruing, 325-326
    usage, 161
Roughness, smoothness. *See* Patterns
Round bifocal segment lenses. *See* Centration skills series
Round lenses. *See* 22 Round lenses
Round pattern, circumference, 316
Round-segment centration, process, 130f
Round-segment lenses, 126-129, 413. *See also* Blended
        round-segment lenses; Spherically powered
        round-segment lenses; Spherocylindrically
        powered round-segment lenses
    centration
        centration instrument, usage, 127-129
        device, usage, 128
    spotting, 35b
    total decentration. *See* Right round-segment lens
Round-segment multifocals
    centration device, usage, 128b
    spotting, 29-31
        alternative method, 32
Round-style segment lenses, 398
Rubber mask
    lens placement, 300
    sandblasting, 300
    stenciling, 300
Ruler
    positioning, 156f
    usage, 80f. *See also* T-seg style ruler
Ruler-wide markings, advantages, 156f

S

Safety bevel, 269f
  amount, 201f
Safety beveling, 192, 278. *See also* Groove
Safety concerns, 329
  information, 341
  proficiency test questions, 342-343
Safety equipment. *See* Chemical tempering
Safety eyewear, 292, 298
  basic-impact requirements, 298-300
  high-impact requirements, 300-301
  impact requirements, 298
  regulation, 298
Safety frames, 301-303
  ANSI standards, 301
  marking requirements, 302b
  Z87-2 marking, 302
  Z87-type, appropriateness, 305
Safety glasses, 336
  defining, 302
  sports eyewear, contrast, 305f
Safety lenses
  identifying marking, 300
  marking methods, 299
  requirements, 301t
Safety program
  effectiveness, 334-339
  employee involvement, 335
  enforcement plan, 335
  implementation/oversight, 334-335
  management support, 334-335
Safety program, development, 331
Safety signs, display, 335, 336f
Safety training/education, 331
Salt bath, usage, 239
Salt replacement, 304
Sand particles, scratching, 300
Sandblasting. *See* Glass lenses; Plastic lenses
Santinelli groover, 284f
Sclera, limitation. *See* White sclera
Scored lenses, breakage, 151f
Scored line, creation, 150f
Scoring. *See* Freehand scoring; Guided scoring
Scratched lenses, unacceptability, 10
Scratches. *See* Lenses
  appearance. *See* Edged lenses
  location, 28f
Scratching, prevention, 17f, 30f
Scratch-resistant coatings, 146, 295
Scratch-resistant-coated lenses, 295
Screw
  mechanism, usage, 262
  placement, 257f
  smoothing, 257f

Screwdrivers, plastic sleeve (inclusion), 256f
Segment. *See* Curved-top segment; High bifocal
      segment
  amount. *See* Plastic flat-top lenses
  border, lateral corners. *See* Curved upper segment
      border
  bordering lines, lens positioning, 128f
  center, usage, 130f. *See also* Blended bifocals;
      Horizontal reference
  centering. *See* Near segment
  centration. *See* Curve-top segments
  decentration. *See* Vertical segment decentration
  height, lowering, 61
  information, 173f
  line, cracking/indenting/chipping, 145f
  movement, 129f
  outlining, 130f
    distortion, circular area, 130f
  positions, 410-412, 434
    relationship. *See* Major reference point
  raise, 49f, 112-113
    calculation, 410
    segment height, conversion, 113
  rotation. *See* Nasalward segment rotation
  size. *See* Flat-top bifocals
Segment drop, 30f, 49f, 112-113
  amount, 117, 404, 415
  calculation, 59f, 410, 413
  position, calculation, 129f
  requirement, 130
  segment height, conversion, 113
  usage, 113f. *See also* Left lens
Segment height, 43-44, 49f, 112
  achievement, 59f
  allowance, 130f
  amount, 62f
  judgment, 125
  usage, 113f
Segment inset, 30f, 114. *See also* Total segment
      inset
  amount, 415
  checking. *See* Flat-top multifocals
  confusion, 115f
  increase/decrease, 101f
  usage. *See* Left lens
Segment top, 32f
  180-degree line tilt, relationship, 125f
  movement, 402
  usage. *See* Vertical alignment; Vertical reference
  vertical position, 113f
Segmented multifocal lenses, 2, 97, 112-114
  centration, 112
    proficiency test questions, 133-137
Self-diagnostics, calibrations, 180-181

Self-inspections, scope, 338b

Semifinished blanks, 3f, 216

Semifinished lenses, 4f
    blank, rotation, 101f
    definition, 2
    terminology, 2-4

Semirimless mountings, 248f, 260f. *See also* Spring
        tension semirimless mounting
    marking, frame usage, 259-260
    nasal hole, drilling/mounting, 260f

Set numbers, 153
    absolute value, addition, 84

Shadow projection, usage. *See* Centration device

Shape determination. *See* Lenses

Shape tracing, 57f
    coquille, usage, 66-67
    old lens, usage, 66-67
    pattern, usage, 66-67

Shapes, superimposition, 252f

Shoe
    contact, 269
    usage, 248

Shoulder, usage, 248

Side shields, 302-303
    removability, 302f

Sighting eye, positioning, 251f

Silhouette, usage, 260

Simple gradient lens, dyeing, 221

Simple gradient tint, 220-221

Single vision lenses, 2, 50f, 439f, 440f. *See also*
        Centration skills series; Non prismatic single
        vision lenses
    centration, 75
        challenge questions, 95-96
        general questions, 95-96
        proficiency test questions, 93-96
    movable line, indication, 84f
    movable vertical line, 82
    spotting, 20-21

Single vision minimum blank size chart, 90f

Single vision sphere spotting, crossed-line-target
       lensmeter (usage), 18b

Single-use bottles, usage, 214f

Skewed bridge, 240

Slab-off lenses, testing exemption, 294

Slippery hazards, awareness, 337

Slot centers
    vertical/horizontal lines, intersection, 268f

Slot centers, dotting, 267f

Slotted lenses, 263-266

Slotted mountings, 247
    bibliography, 273
    proficiency test questions, 274-275

Small businesses, OSHA impact, 331

Small-millimeter gauge
    inclusion. *See* Drills
    positioning/locking, 254f

Smart Drill, The, 261, 265f, 266f

Smooth gradient, creation, 223-224

Smooth-finish exteriors, 311

Smoothing. *See* Back bevel surface; Bevel; Holes
    necessity, 54
    tasks, performing, 192

Sodium ions, usage, 303

Sodium nitrate, usage, 303

Softening point, 303f

Sola Access, 107t

Sola Access intermediate/near specialty progressive,
       comparison. *See* Standard progressive

Solid tint, color/transmission, 221f

Solids, 220

Space bar, usage, 263

Specialty computer lenses, 110

Specialty progressive addition lenses, 105-110

Special-V bevel, 162

Spectrophotometer, usage, 217

Speed, control, 196f

Sphere lenses, OC, 28

Sphere lines
    crossing point, 22f
    definition, 12
    focusing, 15f
    positioning, 20f

Sphere/cylinder target intersection, 20

Spheres. *See* Blemished sphere
    power, 15f
        verification, 16
    spotting, 16

Spherical eyeglass correction, 13f

Spherical lens, examination, 13

Spherically powered round-segment lenses, 35b

Spherocylinder lenses
    custom surfacing. *See* Paired spherocylinder lens
    dots, placement, 30f
    examination, 13-16
    illuminated target, center, 22f
    matching. *See* Prefinished bifocals
    power (verification), crossed-line-target lensmeter
        (usage), 16b
    rotation, 101f
    spotting, crossed-line-target lensmeter (usage),
        18b
    verification, 16-18

Spherocylinders. *See* Blemished spherocylinder
    power
        requirements, 23
        verification, 16-18
    spotting, 16-18

Spherocylindrically powered round-segment lenses, 35b
Spills, cleanup, 340
Spoon-shaped riffler file, usage, 257f
Sports eyewear, 292, 305
    contrast. *See* Safety lenses
    sample, 305f
Spotted 180-degree line, 124, 124f
Spotted MRP, 115, 117, 121
    location accuracy, checking, 123f
Spotted point, 119
Spotting. *See* Lens spotting; Major reference point;
        Multifocal lenses; Respotting; Single vision
        lenses; Spheres; Spherocylinders
    autolensmeters, usage, 21-27
    automated lensmeter usage, lens positioning, 25f
    crossed-line-target lensmeter, usage. *See* Single
        vision sphere spotting; Spherocylinder lenses
    definition, 5
    mechanism. *See* Autolensmeters
    process, 395
Spring tension semirimless mounting, 257
Spring water, problems, 213
Spring-connected coupling pins, positioning. *See*
        Centering
Spring-controlled guide arms, 280
Spring-coupled pins, movement, 282f
Stainless-steel stirring rod, rinsing, 214f
Stand drill, 253
Stand table, movement, 266f
Standard alignment, 3f, 6, 235. *See also* Metal frames;
        Plastic frames
    definition, 6
proficiency test questions, 246
Standard cross mark, placement. *See* Lenses
Standard progressive
    intermediate/near specialty progressive,
        comparison, 106f
    Rodenstock Office intermediate/near design
        specialty progressive lens, comparison, 109f
    Sola Access intermediate/near specialty progressive,
        comparison, 108f
Standard V-bevel wheels, 162
Static load form testing, 295
Stationary vertical line, 121
Stock finished bifocals, 2
Stock lenses
    contrast. *See* Surfaced lenses
    off-center optical center, inclusion, 28
Stock removal, definition, 194
Stock single vision lenses, 2, 4f
Straight-ahead gaze, 109f. *See also* Overplussed
        straight-ahead gaze
Straight-ahead viewing, 109f

Strain points, 168f
Strapping pliers, usage, 270, 273f
Straps
    angling, 272f
    area
        adjustments. *See* Double-strap area
        close-up, 249f
    distance. *See* Double straps
    lens thickness, incompatibility, 272-273
    misrotation, 272f
    mountings, usage. *See* Double-strap mountings
    positioning, 272f
Stylus, definition, 64
Suction
    blocking, 138
    cup, adapter attachment, 139f
    usage. *See* Blocking
Suction-blocked lenses, deblocking, 185
Surfaced lenses, stock lenses (contrast), 216
Surfaces. *See* Finished surfaces
    cracking, 249
    curvature, 5f
    deficiencies, 11
    generation, 3f
    irregularities, 11f
    scratches
        effect. *See* Impact resistance
        prevention, 280
Surfacing, 3f
    process, 77f
Surfacing laboratories, 1-2, 32f, 99f
    data, transferring, 67
    functions, 3
    software programs, usage, 119
Symmetrical nasal cut, achievement, 203f

T
Tap water, problems, 213
Taps, usage, 272f
Target center, reference, 22f
Target clarity, degradation, 13f
Tattooing, 299
Technica. *See* AO Technica
Temple
    bend-down end positions, 245
    ends, alignment, 243
    opening, 272f
    parallelism, 242-243, 245-246
    re-angling, 245f
    spread, 242, 244f. *See also* Metal temple spread;
        Open temple spread
        decrease, 244f
        reduction, 244f
Temple-fold angle, 243, 246

Temporal edge. *See* Frames
Temporal hole
    drilling, 260f
    location, marking, 260f
    relationship. *See* 180-degree line
Temporal lens straps, bending, 268
Temporal movement, 289f
Temporal slots, positioning, 263
Testing, 292. *See also* Impact resistance
    proficiency test questions, 306-308
    requirements. *See* Basic-impact testing
            requirements; High-impact testing
            requirements
Thick lenses, center bevel placement, 160f
Thick-edged high minus lenses, 279f
Thick-edged plus lenses, edging, 163f
Thickness
    amount. *See* Plus edges
    determining. *See* Center thickness
    errors. *See* Plus lenses
    incompatibility. *See* Straps
    increase, 101f
    measurement. *See* Edged lenses
    requirements, 41f. *See also* Basic-impact thickness
            requirements; High-impact thickness
            requirements
    variation, 273f
Thin centers. *See* High-index minus lenses;
            Polycarbonate lenses
Thin edges, 250-251
Thin lenses, bevel apex placement, 160f
Thin metal rims. *See* Frames
Thin-edged low-powered lens, 279f
Thinning. *See* Low-minus-powered lenses; Over-
            thinning; Plus-minus-powered lenses
Three-axis frame tracers, 66
Three-dimensional tracing. *See* Frames
Three-piece mountings. *See* Rimless three-piece
            mounting
    marking, coquilles (usage), 252-253
Tilted 180-degree line. *See* 180-degree line
Tilted bifocal segments, 313f
Tilting ability, 261-262
Tint unit, 212-213
    availability, 213f
    dial, marking, 216f
    powering down, 228-229
Tinted lenses, transmission, 218f
Tinting, 3f, 6, 212, 216-217. *See also* Polycarbonate
            lenses; Uncuts
    bibliography, 234
    fluids, disposal, 340
    lens preparation, 216
    process, explanation, 212-216

Tinting *(Continued)*
    proficiency test questions, 231-234
    suggestions. *See* Polycarbonate lenses
    temperatures, 215
    troubleshooting, 229t-231t
Tints. *See* Base tints; Gradients; Simple gradient tint
    color, usage, 217f
    removal, neutralizer (usage), 219
    styles, 220-225
    tanks
        cleaning, 229
        variety, 213f
    temperature, 229
Top bar, connection, 248f
Total decentration, 52
Total drop
    independent consideration, 402-403, 430
    simultaneous consideration, 404-405, 431
Total inset, 114. *See also* Left lens
    confusion, 115f
    determination, 410
    independent consideration, 402-403, 430
    simultaneous consideration, 404-405, 431
Total segment inset, 114, 128
    usage. *See* Blended bifocals
Toxic substances, 331
Tracers
    patternless edger, electronic link, 172f
    placement. *See* Edgers; Remote-site dispensary
Tracing. *See* Demo lens; Eyes; Frame shape; Old lens;
            Shape tracing
    dimensions, 179f
    laboratory requirements. *See* By-hand lens tracing
    lens, right/left distinction, 67f
    process, 54f
    usage. *See* Pattern making
Training, 346
    documentation, 336-337
    sessions, 346
Translucent background grids, readjustment (Allen
            screws, usage), 312f
Translucent white plastic, back-lighting, 220f
Transmission. *See* Solid tint; Tinted lenses; Ultraviolet
            light; Visible light
    accuracy, ensuring, 217-220
    areas, 218f
    curve, 219f. *See also* Brown plastic lens
    measuring, 217
    reading, 225f
Tray up order, 3f
Trifocal lenses (trifocals), 4f. *See also* 7x28 trifocals;
            Centration skills series
    centering, 408
    definition, 2

Trifocal lenses (trifocals) *(Continued)*
  positioning. *See* Flat-top trifocals
  selection, 105
Triple gradients, 221f; 224-225
Trivex, 249, 250
  lenses
    classification, 277
    materials, 258
Truing, definition, 6
T-seg device, usage, 155
T-seg style ruler, usage, 156f
Two-axis frame tracers, 66

U
Ultrasonic cleaner, usage, 280. *See also* Groove
Ultraviolet (UV) dyeing, 225-226
Ultraviolet (UV) light
  effect, 217
  transmission, 218f
Ultraviolet (UV) liquid, disposal, 340
Ultraviolet (UV) radiation, 225
Ultraviolet (UV) region, inclusion, 219f
Unblemished lens, 12f
Uncut lens blank, 10f
Uncut minus lens blank, 10f
Uncut-finished stage, testing, 294
Uncuts, 2, 4f
  drawing, 252f
  tinting/matching, 219-220
Unwanted prism, standards, 92
Unwanted vertical prism, correction, 205-206
Upper distance portion, progressive addition lenses
    (impact), 98f

V
Variable-hole diameters, 262
Variant alignment, 241
Variant planes, 241-242
Varilux (Essilor), 104f
V-bevel blade, 277
V-bevel grooves
  apex, 326f
  usage. *See* Hand edgers
V-bevel wheels. *See* Standard V-bevel wheels
  usage, 162
V-bevels, 321
Ventilation, need, 338-339
Vertical alignment, 240-241
  segment top, usage, 132f
Vertical centration
  calculation, boxing system (usage), 78-83
  ensuring, 90f
Vertical compensation, 60. *See also* Pattern errors
  calculation, 418

Vertical decentration. *See* Horizontal midline
  questions, 93-94
Vertical lens
  area, sufficiency. *See* Double-segment lenses
  size, 40-41
Vertical line. *See* Single vision lenses; Stationary vertical
    line
  centering, 438f
Vertical misalignment. *See* Pattern centers
Vertical pattern dimension, 61b
Vertical placement, specification, 79-81
Vertical position. *See* Major reference point; Segment
    top
  calculation. *See* Progressive addition lenses
Vertical prism, 207f, 396-397. *See also* Progressive
    addition lenses
  amount, 91
  correction. *See* Unwanted vertical prism
  evaluation, 120f
  usage, 206
Vertical protractor line, 116
Vertical reference
  line, 88f
    movement, 82
  segment top, usage, 116f
Vertical segment decentration, 59
Vertically displaced mechanical centers, usage. *See*
    Patterns
Vertically displaced pattern centers, compensation,
    58-59
Vertometer, 5
V-grooved wheel, 191
Viewing screens. *See* Patternless edgers
  usage. *See* Edges; Lens shapes
Visible lens marking, 34
Visible light, transmission, 218f
Visible spectrum, inclusion, 219f
Vision, area (increase), 106f
Vision lenses. *See* Non prismatic single vision lenses;
    Stock single vision lenses
Vision Safety Notice, 297

W
Warning, forms, 346
Warpage, 209
Waste
  disposal, ease (rules), 339-340
  generator, 330
  management, problems. *See* Laboratory
  removal. *See* Liquid wastes
Waviness. *See* Lenses
  checking, 13f
Wax-blocked lenses, deblocking, 186
Wearer safety issues, 249, 276-277

WECO blocker, 266, 272f
WECO edger, 272f
Wet edging. *See* Polycarbonate lenses
Wet hazards, awareness, 337
Wet sponge, usage, 279
Wet surfaces, danger, 339f
Wheel differential
   adjustment, 316
   checking, 315
      sequence, 315b
   measuring, 315
Wheels. *See* Bonded roughing wheels; Edger wheels;
      Electroplated roughing wheels; Glazed wheels
   cleaning. *See* Electroplated wheels
   concentration. *See* Diamond wheels
   dome, groover cutting wheel (flush placement),
      279f
   dressing, 323-325. *See also* Diamond wheels; Metal-
      bonded finishing wheels; Metal-bonded
      roughing wheels
   grits, 192
      types/purposes. *See* Hand-edger wheel grits
   groove depth, 161
   preparation. *See* Edge smoothing
   retruing. *See* Ceramic hand-edging wheel; Roughing
      wheels
   rounded corner, usage, 200f
   sounds, 197
   surface, lens removal (frequency), 196f
   truing. *See* Diamond wheels
   types, 322f
      specification factors, 321f
   upward pull, advantage, 194f
   usage. *See* Finishing; Hide-a-Bevel wheels; Mini-bevel
      wheels; Polycarbonate lens edging; Roughing
      wheels; V-bevel wheels
   wear, automatic recalibration, 155

White sclera, limitation, 45f
Wide segments, usage. *See* Adhesive pad blocking
Workplace
   analysis, 331
   cleanup, 335
   hazards, 331
Work-related illness/injury, 336
Wraparound, 241
Wrap-around effect, 171
Wrap-around frames
   base curve, steepness, 171
   lenses, edging, 170-171

X
X coordinate, 179f
X-ing, 241, 243
   identification, 241f

Y
Y coordinate, 179f
Yoked base down prism, 100

Z
Z coordinate, 179f
Z80 standards, questions, 94-95
Z80.1-1999 standard. *See* American National Standards
      Institute
Z87.1 lens marking requirements. *See* American
      National Standards Institute
Z87.1-1989 standards, 302b
Z-axis dimension, 65
Zeiss RD, 107t
Zero scale. *See* Edger dials
Zero-adjuster knob. *See* Groover